ESSENTIAL ATLAS OF

Infectious Diseases

FOR PRIMARY CARE

ESSENTIAL ATLAS OF
Infectious Diseases
FOR PRIMARY CARE

Gerald L. Mandell, MD, Editor-in-Chief
Professor of Medicine
Owen R. Cheatham Professor of the Sciences
Chief, Division of Infectious Diseases
University of Virginia Health Sciences Center
Charlottesville, Virginia, USA

CONTRIBUTING EDITORS

Thomas P. Bleck, MD
Professor of Neurology and Neurological Surgery
Director, Nerancy Neurosocience Intensive Care Unit
Division of Critical Care, Department of Neurology
University of Virginia Health Sciences Center
Charlottesville, Virginia

Itzhak Brook, MD
Professor, Department of Pediatrics
Georgetown University School of Medicine
Washington, DC
Senior Investigator, Naval Medical Research Institute
Bethesda, Maryland

Robert Fekety, MD
Professor Emeritus of Internal Medicine
University of Michigan Medical School
Ann Arbor, Michigan

Bennett Lorber, MD
Thomas M. Durant Professor of Medicine
Chief, Section of Infectious Diseases
Temple University Health Sciences Center
Philadelphia, Pennsylvania

Donna Mildvan, MD
Professor of Medicine
Albert Einstein College of Medicine
Bronx, New York
Chief, Division of Infectious Diseases
Beth Israel Medical Center
New York, New York

Michael F. Rein, MD
Professor of Internal Medicine
Division of Infectious Diseases
University of Virginia Health Sciences Center
Charlottesville, Virginia

Michael S. Simberkoff, MD
Associate Professor of Medicine
New York University School of Medicine
Chief, Infectious Diseases Section
New York Veterans Affairs Medical Center
New York, New York

Jack D. Sobel, MD
Professor of Medicine
Wayne State University School of Medicine
Chief, Division of Infectious Diseases
Detroit Medical Center
Detroit, Michigan

Dennis L. Stevens, MD, PhD
Professor of Medicine
University of Washington
Seattle, Washington
Chief, Infectious Diseases Section
Veterans Affairs Medical Center
Boise, Idaho

With 174 contributors

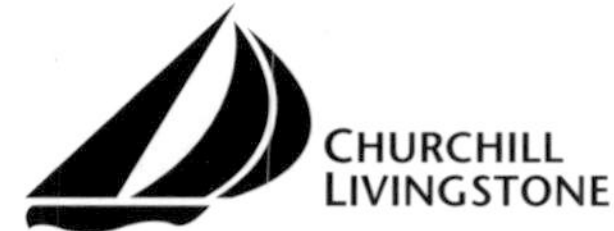

DEVELOPED BY CURRENT MEDICINE, INC.
PHILADELPHIA

CURRENT MEDICINE
400 MARKET STREET, SUITE 700
PHILADELPHIA, PA 19106

Library of Congress Cataloging-in-Publication Data

Essential atlas of infectious diseases for primary care/editor-in-chief, Gerald L. Mandell; chapter editors, Thomas P. Bleck . . . [et al.].
p. cm.
Includes bibliographical references and index.
ISBN 0-443-07961-7 (hardcover)
1. Communicable diseases—Atlases. 2. Primary care (Medicine)—Atlases. I. Mandell, Gerald L. II. Bleck, Thomas P., 1951– .
[DNLM: 1. Communicable Diseases—atlases. 2. Primary Health Care—atlases.
WC 17 E78 1997]
RC113.2.E84 1997
616.9—dc21
DNLM/DLC
for Library of Congress 96-45957
CIP

Managing Editor: ....**Lori J. Bainbridge**
Editor: ....**Elena Coler**
Art Director: ....**Paul Fennessy**
Cover Design: ....**Patrick Ward**
Interior Design: ....**Patrick Whelan**
Layout: ....**Patrick Ward and Lisa Weischedel**
Illustration Director: ....**Ann Saydlowski**
Illustrator:...**Beth Starkey**
Production: ....**Lori Holland**
Indexer: ....**Ann Cassar**

Printed in Hong Kong by Paramount Printing Group Limited.

10 9 8 7 6 5 4 3 2

Preface

The diagnosis and management of patients with infectious diseases is based in large part on visual clues. Skin and mucous membrane lesions, eye findings, imaging studies, gram stains, culture plates, insect vectors, preparations of blood, urine, pus, cerebrospinal fluid, and biopsy specimens are studied to establish the proper diagnosis and choose the most effective therapy. The Atlas is a modern, complete collection of those images. Superb color reproduction and state-of-the-art computer imaging facilities have enabled the publisher to produce a beautiful and instructive volume. All physicians and health care workers involved in primary care will find this atlas with available slides to be an effective educational tool.

A panel of distinguished editors with a wealth of experience in various aspects of infectious disease have put together a uniquely valuable volume. They have selected images and figures that will be most useful for physicians in the "front lines" of medical care.

Gerald L. Mandell, MD
Charlottesville, Virginia

Contributors

Rodolfo M. Abalos, MD
Leonard Wood Memorial Leprosy Research Center
Cebu, Philippines

Sebastian R. Alston, MD
Assistant Professor of Pathology (Neuropathology)
Department of Pathology
University of Virginia Health Sciences Center
Charlottesville, Virginia

Donald Armstrong, MD
Professor of Medicine
Cornell University Medical College
Chief, Infectious Diseases Service
Department of Medicine
Memorial Sloan-Kettering Cancer Center
New York, New York

Neil Barg, MD
Associate Professor of Medicine
University of Michigan Medical School
Assistant Chief of Infectious Diseases
Department of Veterans Affairs Medical Center
Ann Arbor, Michigan

Stephen G. Baum, MD
Professor of Medicine
The Albert Einstein College of Medicine
Chairman, Department of Medicine
Beth Israel Medical Center
New York, New York

Joseph R. Berger, MD, FACP
Professor and Chairman
Department of Neurology
Professor, Department of Internal Medicine
University of Kentucky College of Medicine
Lexington, Kentucky

Michel G. Bergeron, MD, FRCP(C)
Professor and Chairman
Department of Microbiology
Laval University Faculty of Medicine
Centre Hospitalier de l'Université Laval
Québec City, Québec
Canada

Robert F. Betts, MD
Professor of Medicine
Director, Educational Programs
University of Rochester School of Medicine and Dentistry
Strong Memorial Hospital
Rochester, New York

Roger C. Bone, MD
Professor of Medicine
Office of the Dean
Rush Presbyterian-St. Luke's Medical Center
Chicago, Illinois

Jose M. Bonnin, MD
Neuropathologist
Methodist Hospital of Indiana
Indianapolis, Indiana

Edward J. Bottone, PhD
Professor of Medicine, Microbiology, and Pathology
Mount Sinai School of Medicine
Director of Consultative Microbiology
Division of Infectious Diseases
The Mount Sinai Hospital
New York, New York

David G. Brock, MD
Neurointensivist
Pennsylvania Hospital and Wills Eye Hospital
Philadelphia, Pennsylvania

Richard E. Bryant, MD
Director, Infectious Diseases Section
Oregon Health Sciences University
Portland, Oregon

Helen Buckley, PhD
Professor, Microbiology and Immunology
Temple University School of Medicine
Director, Clinical Mycology Laboratory
Temple University Hospital
Philadelphia, Pennsylvania

Jason Calhoun, MD
Chairman
Department of Orthopedic Surgery & Rehabilitation
University of Texas Medical Branch
Galveston, Texas

Roland V. Cellona, MD, DPH
Leonard Wood Memorial Leprosy Research Center
Cebu, Philippines

Mary Ann Chiasson, DrPH
Assistant Commissioner
Bureau of Disease Intervention Research
The New York City Department of Health
New York, New York

Michael J. Chiu, MD
Assistant Professor
Department of Internal Medicine
University of Texas Southwestern
Dallas, Texas

Bruce H. Clements, MD
Chief, Clinical Branch
Gillis W. Long Hansen's Disease Center
Carville, Louisiana

Clay J. Cockerell, MD
Associate Professor
Departments of Dermatology and Pathology
University of Texas Southwestern Medical Center
Dallas, Texas

David A. Cooper, MD, DSc
Professor of Medicine
University of New South Wales
Director, National Centre in HIV Epidemiology and Clinical Research
St. Vincent's Hospital
Sydney, Australia

Lawrence Corey, MD
Professor of Laboratory Medicine and Medicine
University of Washington School of Medicine
Fred Hutchinson Cancer Research Center
Seattle, Washington

Sidney E. Croul, MD
Assistant Professor of Pathology
Allegheny University of the Health Sciences
MCP-Hahnemann School of Medicine
Philadelphia, Pennsylvania

Adnan S. Dajani, MD
Professor of Pediatrics
Wayne State University School of Medicine
Director, Infectious Diseases
Children's Hospital of Michigan
Detroit, Michigan

Scott F. Davies, MD
Professor of Medicine
University of Minnesota
Director, Division of Pulmonary and Critical Care Medicine
Hennepin County Medical Center
Minneapolis, Minnesota

Janet L. Davis, MD
Associate Professor
Department of Ophthalmology
University of Miami School of Medicine
Bascom Palmer Eye Institute
Miami, Florida

Claude Delage, MD, FRCP(C)
Professor of Pathology
Laval University Faculty of Medicine
L'Hôtel-Dieu de Québec Hospital
Québec City, Québec
Canada

Thomas A. Deutsch, MD
Professor and Chairman
Department of Ophthalmology
Rush Medical College of Rush University
Chicago, Illinois

Gregory J. Dore, MBBS, BSc
Lecturer in Epidemiology/Clinical Assistant
National Centre in HIV Epidemiology and Clinical Research
University of New South Wales
Clinical Assistant
HIV Unit
St. Vincent's Hospital
Sydney, Australia

D. Peter Drotman, MD, MPH
Clinical Assistant Professor
Department of Preventive and Family Medicine
Emory University School of Medicine
Acting Associate Director for Epidemiologic Science
National Center for Infectious Diseases
Centers for Disease Control and Prevention
Attending Physician
Infectious Diseases Section
Department of Medicine
Veterans Affairs Medical Center
Atlanta, Georgia

J. Stephen Dumler, MD
Associate Professor of Pathology
The Johns Hopkins University School of Medicine
Director, Division of Medical Microbiology
Department of Pathology
The Johns Hopkins Medical Institutions
Baltimore, Maryland

W. Christopher Ehmann, MD
Associate Professor
Department of Medicine
Division of Hematology/Oncology
The Pennsylvania State University College of Medicine
Hershey, Pennsylvania

James N. Endicott, MD
Professor of Surgery
Division of Otolaryngology
University of South Florida
Tampa, Florida

Janine Evans, MD
Assistant Professor of Internal Medicine
Yale University School of Medicine
New Haven, Connecticut

Thomas G. Evans, MD
Associate Professor of Internal Medicine
Division of Infectious Diseases
University of Rochester School of Medicine
Rochester, New York

E. Dale Everett, MD
Division Director, Infectious Diseases
University of Missouri Health Science Center
Columbia, Missouri

M. Elaine Eyster, MD
Distinguished Professor
Department of Medicine
Division of Hematology/Oncology
The Pennsylvania State University College of Medicine
Hershey, Pennsylvania

Tranquilino T. Fajardo, MD, DPH
Leonard Wood Memorial Leprosy Research Center
Cebu, Philippines

Ann R. Falsey, MD
Assistant Professor of Medicine
University of Rochester School of Medicine and Dentistry
Rochester General Hospital
Rochester, New York

Judith Feinberg, MD
Associate Professor of Clinical Medicine
University of Cincinnati College of Medicine
Cincinnati, Ohio

Patricia Ferrieri, MD
Professor of Laboratory Medicine & Pathology and Pediatrics
University of Minnesota Medical School
Director, Clinical Microbiology Laboratory
University of Minnesota Hospital
Minneapolis, Minnesota

Theodore W. Fetter, MD
Assistant Professor of Surgery (Otolaryngology)
Uniformed Services University of the Health Sciences
Bethesda, Maryland
Clinical Assistant Professor of Otolaryngology
Georgetown University Medical School
Washington, DC
Attending Physician
Fairfax Hospital
Falls Church, Virginia

Sydney M. Finegold, MD
Professor, Departments of Medicine & Microbiology and Immunology
University of California at Los Angeles School of Medicine
Staff Physician, Infectious Disease Section
Veterans Affairs Medical Center West Los Angeles
Los Angeles, California

Margaret A. Fischl, MD
Professor of Medicine
Director, Comprehensive AIDS Program
University of Miami School of Medicine
Miami, Florida

Jay A. Fishman, MD
Assistant Professor of Medicine
Harvard Medical School
Associate Chief and Clinical Director
Infectious Disease for Transplantation
Massachusetts General Hospital
Boston, Massachusetts

Nicholas J. Fiumara, MD, MPH
Clinical Professor of Dermatology
Tufts University School of Medicine
Clinical Professor Emeritus
Boston University School of Medicine
Boston, Massachusetts

Julie S. Francis, MD
Assistant Professor of Pediatrics, Dermatology
Director of Cutaneous Laser Surgery
University of Washington School of Medicine
Seattle, Washington

Alvin E. Friedman-Kien, MD
Professor of Dermatology and Microbiology
New York University Medical Center
New York, New York

John Froude, MB, BS, MRCP
Clinical Professor
Department of Medicine
New York University
Bellevue Hospital Medical Center
New York, New York

Harry A. Gallis, MD
Clinical Professor of Medicine
Department of Internal Medicine
University of North Carolina School of Medicine
Chapel Hill, North Carolina
Vice President, Regional Medical Education
Carolinas Healthcare System
Charlotte, North Carolina

Robert A. Gatenby, MD
Professor of Radiology
Diagnostic Imaging
Temple University School of Medicine
Section Chief, Abdominal Imaging
Department of Diagnostic Imaging
Temple University Hospital
Philadelphia, Pennsylvania

Robert Gelber, MD
Medical Director, San Francisco Regional Hansen's Disease Program
Clinical Professor, University of California-San Francisco
San Francisco, California

Robert M. Genta, MD
Professor of Pathology, Medicine, Microbiology, and Immunology
Baylor College of Medicine
Pathologist, Department of Pathology
Veterans Affairs Medical Center
Houston, Texas

Marlin E. Gher, Jr, DDS, MEd
Diplomate, American Board of Periodontics
Diplomate, American Board of Oral Medicine
Private Practice
Chula Vista, California

Bruce C. Gilliland, MD
Associate Dean for Clinical Affairs
University of Washington School of Medicine
Seattle, Washington

Janet R. Gilsdorf, MD
Professor of Pediatrics and Communicable Diseases
University of Michigan Medical School
Director, Pediatric Infectious Diseases
University of Michigan Hospital
Ann Arbor, Michigan

Dominique Giroux, MD, FRCP
Lecturer
Department of Radiology
Laval University Faculty of Medicine
L'Hôtel-Dieu de Québec Hospital
Québec City, Québec
Canada

Jonathan D. Glass, MD
Assistant Professor of Neurology
Department of Neurology
Emory University
Atlanta, Georgia

Christopher D. Gocke, MD
Assistant Professor of Pathology
The Pennsylvania State University College of Medicine
Hershey, Pennsylvania

Ellie J. C. Goldstein, MD
Clinical Professor of Medicine, UCLA School of Medicine
Director, R. M. Alden Research Lab
Santa Monica, California

Barney Graham, MD, PhD
Professor of Medicine
Assistant Professor of Microbiology and Immunology
Vanderbilt University School of Medicine
Nashville, Tennessee

David Y. Graham, MD
Professor of Medicine and Molecular Virology
Chief, Gastroenterology
Baylor College of Medicine
Chief, Digestive Disease Section
Veterans Affairs Medical Center
Houston, Texas

Deborah Greenspan, BDS, DSc, ScD(hc)
Clinical Professor of Oral Medicine
Department of Stomatology
Clinical Director, Oral AIDS Center
School of Dentistry
University of California San Francisco
San Francisco, California

John S. Greenspan, BSc, BDS, PhD, FRCPath, ScD (hc)
Professor of Oral Biology and Oral Pathology
Chair, Department of Stomatology
Director, Oral AIDS Center
School of Dentistry
Professor of Pathology
Director, AIDS Clinical Research Center
University of California San Francisco
San Francisco, California

Clark Gregg, MD
Associate Professor of Medicine
University of Texas Southwestern
Chief of Infectious Diseases
Department of Veterans Affairs Medical Center, Dallas
Dallas, Texas

David Gregory, MD
Associate Professor of Medicine
Vanderbilt University School of Medicine
Associate Chief of Staff for Ambulatory Care
Department of Veterans Affairs Medical Center
Nashville, Tennessee

Kenneth M. Grundfast, MD, FACS, FAAP
Vice-Chairman, Department of Otolaryngology
Director of Ear and Hearing Disorders Clinic
Children's National Medical Center
Washington, DC

Carl Grunfeld, MD, PhD
Professor of Medicine
Metabolism and Infectious Diseases Sections
University of California San Francisco
Medical Service
Department of Veterans Affairs Medical Center
San Francisco, California

Richard L. Guerrant, MD
Thomas H. Hunter Professor of International Medicine
University of Virginia
Chief, Division of Geographic and International Medicine
University of Virginia Hospital
Charlottesville, Virginia

Ricardo S. Guinto, MD, MPH[†]
Leonard Wood Memorial Leprosy Center
Cebu, Philippines

Laura T. Gutman, MD
Associate Professor
Departments of Pediatrics and Pharmacology
Duke University Medical Center
Durham, North Carolina

Caroline B. Hall, MD
Professor of Pediatrics and Medicine in Infectious Diseases
University of Rochester School of Medicine and Dentistry
Strong Memorial Hospital
Rochester, New York

Daniel F. Hanley, MD
Professor of Neurology
Johns Hopkins University School of Medicine
Director of Neurosciences Critical Care Unit
Johns Hopkins Hospital
Baltimore, Maryland

James J. Herdegen, MD
Assistant Professor
Pulmonary and Critical Care Medicine
Rush Presbyterian-St. Luke's Medical Center
Chicago, Illinois

Sharon L. Hillier, PhD
Associate Professor of Obstetrics, Gynecology, and Reproductive Sciences
University of Pittsburgh School of Medicine
Director, Reproductive Infectious Disease Research
Magee-Womens Research Institute
Pittsburgh, Pennsylvania

Jan Hirschmann, MD
Professor of Medicine, University of Washington School of Medicine
Assistant Chief of Medicine, Seattle Veterans Affairs
Seattle, Washington

Karen R. Houpt, MD
Assistant Professor
Department of Dermatology
University of Texas Southwestern Medical Center
Dallas, Texas

Jaishree Jagirdar, MD
Associate Professor of Pathology
New York University Medical Center
Chief of Surgical Pathology
Bellevue Hospital
New York, New York

Peter Jensen, MD
Clinical Professor of Medicine
University of California San Francisco
Chief, Infectious Diseases Section
Department of Veterans Affairs Medical Center
San Francisco, California

Richard T. Johnson, MD
Chairman, Department of Neurology
Johns Hopkins University School of Medicine
Baltimore, Maryland

Robert B. Jones, MD, PhD
Professor of Medicine, Microbiology, and Immunology
Vice Chairman, Clinical Affairs
Department of Medicine
Indiana Universtiy School of Medicine
Indianapolis, Indiana

Elaine C. Jong, MD
Clinical Professor of Medicine, Department of Medicine
University of Washington School of Medicine
Director, Hall Health Primary Care Center
Seattle, Washington

Carol A. Kauffman, MD
Professor of Internal Medicine
University of Michigan Medical School
Chief, Infectious Diseases Section
Veterans Affairs Medical Center
Ann Arbor, Michigan

Elaine T. Kaye, MD
Clinical Instructor
Department of Dermatology
Harvard Medical School
Assistant in Medicine
Division of Dermatology
Children's Hospital Medical Center
Boston, Massachusetts

Harold A. Kessler, MD, FACP
Professor of Medicine and Immunology/Microbiology
Associate Director, Section of Infectious Disease
Rush Presbyterian-St. Luke's Medical Center
Chicago, Illinois

Edward D. Kim, MD
Assistant Professor
Scott Department of Urology
Baylor College of Medicine
Houston, Texas

John N. Krieger, MD
Professor of Urology
University of Washington School of Medicine
Seattle, Washington

Susan E. Krown, MD
Professor of Medicine
Cornell University Medical College
Member and Attending Physician
Memorial Sloan-Kettering Cancer Center
New York, New York

Rajendra Kumar, MD
Professor of Radiology
Director, Musculoskeletal Division
University of Texas Medical Branch
Galveston, Texas

Sandra A. Larsen, PhD
Chief, Treponemal Pathogenesis and Immunology Branch
Division of Sexually Transmitted Diseases Laboratory Research
Centers for Disease Control and Prevention
Atlanta, Georgia

[†]*Deceased*

Rande H. Lazar, MD, FICS
Director, Pediatric Otolaryngology Fellowship Training
LeBonheur Children's Medical Center
Memphis, Tennessee

Howard L. Leaf, MD
Assistant Professor of Clinical Medicine
New York University School of Medicine
Infectious Diseases Section
New York Veterans Affairs Medical Center
New York, New York

Philip E. LeBoit, MD
Associate Professor of Clinical Pathology and Dermatology
Director of Dermatopathology Service
University of California, San Francisco
San Francisco, California

Jon T. Mader, MD
Professor
Division of Infectious Diseases, Internal Medicine
University of Texas Medical Branch
Chief, Hyperbaric Medicine
Marine Biomedical Institute
Galveston, Texas

Stephen E. Malawista, MD
Professor of Medicine
Section of Rheumatology
Department of Internal Medicine
Yale University School of Medicine
New Haven, Connecticut

Per-Anders Mårdh, MD, PhD
Professor of Clinical Bacteriology
University of Uppsala
Uppsala, Sweden

Andrew M. Margileth, MD, FAAP, FACP
Clinical Professor of Pediatrics
University of Virginia Health Sciences Center
Charlottesville, Virginia

Melanie J. Maslow, MD, FACP
Clinical Assistant Professor of Medicine
New York University School of Medicine
Assistant Chief, Infectious Diseases Section
New York Veterans Affairs Medical Center
New York, New York

Justin C. McArthur, MBBS
Assistant Professor of Neurology
Department of Neurology
Johns Hopkins University School of Medicine
Baltimore, Maryland

G. Diego Miralles, MD
Division of Infectious Disease and International Medicine
Duke University Medical Center
Durham, North Carolina

Birger Möller, MD
Department of Obstetrics and Gynecology
University of Odense
Odense, Norway

Susan Morgello, MD
Associate Professor of Pathology/Neurobiology
Neuro-AIDS Research Center
The Mount Sinai Medical Center
New York, New York

Daniel M. Musher, MD
Professor of Medicine
Professor of Microbiology and Immunology
Baylor College of Medicine
Chief, Infectious Disease Section
Veterans Affairs Medical Center
Houston, Texas

John Neff, MD
Associate Dean, Professor of Pediatrics
University of Washington School of Medicine
Medical Director, Children's Hospital and Medical Center
Seattle, Washington

J. Curtis Nickel, MD, FRCSC
Professor of Urology
Queen's University
Kingston General Hospital
Kingston, Ontario
Canada

Lindsay E. Nicolle, MD, FRCPC
H.E. Sellers Professor and Chair
Department of Internal Medicine
University of Manitoba Health Sciences Centre
St. Boniface General Hospital
Winnipeg, Manitoba
Canada

Moses Nussbaum, MD
Professor of Surgery
The Albert Einstein College of Medicine
Chairman, Department of Surgery
Beth Israel Medical Center
New York, New York

Paul Nyirjesy, MD
Assistant Professor
Departments of Obstetrics, Gynecology, & Reproductive Sciences and Medicine
Temple University School of Medicine
Philadelphia, Pennsylvania

Steven M. Opal, MD
Associate Professor of Medicine
Department of Internal Medicine
Brown University
Providence, Rhode Island
Staff Physician
Memorial Hospital of Rhode Island
Pawtucket, Rhode Island

Jorma Paavonen, MD
Associate Professor
Department of Obstetrics and Gynecology
University of Helsinki
Helsinki, Finland

Alan G. Palestine, MD
Clinical Associate Professor of Ophthalmology
Georgetown University
Washington, DC

Josephine Paredes, MD
Assistant Attending Physician
Memorial Sloan-Kettering Cancer Center
New York, New York

Richard D. Pearson, MD
Professor of Medicine and Pathology
University of Virginia School of Medicine
Attending Physician
University of Virginia Health Sciences Center
Charlottesville, Virginia

David H. Persing, MD, PhD
Associate Professor of Microbiology and Laboratory Medicine
Mayo Medical School
Director, Molecular Microbiology Laboratories
Director, Legionella and Lyme Serology Laboratories
Mayo Clinic
Rochester, Minnesota

C.J. Peters, MD
Chief, Special Pathogens Branch
Division of Viral and Rickettsial Diseases
Centers for Disease Control and Prevention
Atlanta, Georgia

Hans-Walter Pfister, MD
Department of Neurology
Klinikum Grosshadern
Ludwig-Maximilians-University of Munich
Munich, Germany

George Quintero, DDS
Former Professor of Periodontology
Naval Dental Hospital
Private Practice
Atlanta, Georgia

Lionel Rabin, MD, CM
Clinical Associate Professor
Division of Hepatic Pathology
Veterans Administration Special Reference Laboratory for Pathology
Department of Hepatic and Gastrointestinal Pathology
Armed Forces Institute of Pathology
Washington, DC

Justin D. Radolf, MD
Associate Professor
Internal Medicine and Microbiology
University of Texas Southwestern Medical Center
Dallas, Texas

David A. Ramsay, MB, ChB, DPhil, FRCP(C)
Neuropathologist
Departments of Pathology and Clinical Neurological Sciences
London Health Sciences Center
London, Ontario
Canada

Gregory J. Raugi, MD
Chief of Dermatology
Seattle Veterans Affairs
Seattle, Washington

Richard Reid, MD
Assistant Professor
Department of Obstetrics and Gynecology
Wayne State University School of Medicine
Director, Gynecologic Laser Services
Department of Obstetrics and Gynecology
Sinai Hospital
Detroit, Michigan

D.A. Relman, MD
Assistant Professor of Medicine and Microbiology & Immunology
Stanford University School of Medicine
Stanford, California
Staff Physician
Veterans Affairs Palo Alto Health Care System
Palo Alto, California

Herbert Y. Reynolds, MD
J. Lloyd Huck Professor of Medicine
Chairman, Department of Medicine
The Milton S. Hershey Medical Center
The Pennsylvania State University College of Medicine
Hershey, Pennsylvania

Richard B. Roberts, MD
Professor and Vice-Chairman, Department of Medicine
The New York Hospital-Cornell Medical Center
New York, New York

P.E. Rollin, MD
Chief, Pathogenesis and Immunology Section
Special Pathogens Branch
Division of Viral and Rickettsial Diseases
Centers for Disease Control and Prevention
Atlanta, Georgia

Allan Ronald, OC, MD, FRCP(C), FACP
Professor of Medicine and Medical Microbiology
Associate Dean of Research
University of Manitoba and St. Boniface General Hospital
Winnipeg, Manitoba
Canada

Karen L. Roos, MD
Associate Professor of Neurology
Indiana University School of Medicine
Indianapolis, Indiana

Mark J. Rosen, MD
Professor of Medicine
Albert Einstein College of Medicine
Chief, Division of Pulmonary and Critical Care Medicine
Beth Israel Medical Center
New York, New York

Robert H. Rubin, MD
Osborne Chair in Health Sciences and Technology
Harvard Medical School
Chief, Infectious Disease for Transplantation
Massachusetts General Hospital
Boston, Massachusetts

Michael S. Saag, MD
Associate Professor of Medicine
Director, AIDS Outpatient Clinic
Associate Director for Clinical Care and Therapeutics, AIDS Center
The University of Alabama at Birmingham
Birmingham, Alabama

Oren Sagher, MD
Assistant Professor of Neurosurgery
University of Michigan
Chief of Neurosurgery
Ann Arbor Veterans Administration Hospital
Ann Arbor, Michigan

Christopher J. Salmon, MD
Assistant Professor of Radiology
Director, Thoracic Imaging
Oregon Health Sciences University
Portland, Oregon

George A. Sarosi, MD
Chief, Medical Service and Professor of Medicine
Indiana University School of Medicine
Richard L. Roudebush VA Medical Center
Indianapolis, Indiana

Anthony J. Schaeffer, MD
Herman L. Kretschmer Professor and Chairman
Department of Urology
Northwestern University Medical School
Northwestern Medical Faculty Foundation, Inc.
Chicago, Illinois

W. Michael Scheld, MD
Professor of Medicine and Neurosurgery
Associate Chair for Residency Programs
Department of Medicine
University of Virginia School of Medicine
Attending Physician
University of Virginia Health Sciences Center
Charlottesville, Virginia

David M. Scollard, MD, PhD
Associate Professor of Pathology
Louisiana State University School of Medicine
New Orleans, Louisiana
Chief of Pathology
Gillis W. Long Hansen's Disease Center
Carville, Louisiana

Janet Seper, MD
Resident
Division of Otolaryngology
University of South Florida
Tampa, Florida

Robert D. Shaw, MD
Assistant Professor of Medicine
State University of New York at Stony Brook
Stony Brook, New York
Staff Physician, Gastroenterology
Northport Veterans Affairs Medical Center
Northport, New York

Thomas Shope, MD
Associate Professor of Pediatrics and Communicable Diseases
University of Michigan Medical School
Staff Physician
University of Michigan Hospitals
Ann Arbor, Michigan

Navjeet K. Sidhu-Malik, MD
Assistant Professor of Dermatology
University of Virginia Health Sciences Center
Charlottesville, Virginia

David Simmons, PhD
Professor, Department of Surgery
Department of Orthopedics and Rehabilitation
University of Texas Medical Branch
Galveston, Texas

David M. Simpson, MD
Associate Professor of Neurology
Director, Neuro-AIDS Research Center
Director, Clinical Neurophysiology Laboratories
The Mount Sinai Medical Center
New York, New York

Rosemary Soave, MD
Associate Professor of Medicine and Public Health
Cornell University Medical College
Associate Attending Physician
New York Hospital-Cornell Medical Center
New York, New York

David E. Soper, MD
Professor
Departments of Obstetrics & Gynecology and Medicine
Division of Infectious Diseases
Medical University of South Carolina
Charleston, South Carolina

Anastacio de Q. Sousa, MD
Associate Professor of Medicine
Universidade Federal de Ceara
Nucleo de Medicina Tropical
Fortaleza, Ceara
Brazil

Harris R. Stutman, MD
Associate Professor of Pediatrics
University of California, Irvine
Director, Pediatric Infectious Disease
Memorial Miller Children's Hospital
Long Beach, California

Richard L. Sweet, MD
Professor and Chair
Department of Obstetrics, Gynecology, and Reproductive Sciences
University of Pittsburgh School of Medicine/Magee-Womens Hospital
Pittsburgh, Pennsylvania

Michele Tagliati, MD
Clinical Instructor
Department of Neurology
Neuro-AIDS Research Center
The Mount Sinai Medical Center
New York, New York

Hedy Teppler, MD
Adjunct Assistant Professor of Medicine
Thomas Jefferson University
Philadelphia, Pennsylvania
Associate Director
Infectious Diseases
Clinical Research
Merck & Co., Inc.
Blue Bell, Pennsylvania

John J. Treanor, MD
Associate Professor of Medicine
University of Rochester School of Medicine and Dentistry
Strong Memorial Hospital
Rochester, New York

Debra A. Tristram, MD
Assistant Professor of Pediatrics
Department of Pediatrics
State University of New York at Buffalo
Director of Bacteriology
Division of Infectious Diseases
Children's Hospital of Buffalo
Buffalo, New York

Milan Trpis, PhD
Professor
Department of Molecular Microbiology and Immunology
The Johns Hopkins University School of Hygiene and Public Health
Baltimore, Maryland

Allan R. Tunkel, MD, PhD
Associate Professor of Medicine
Allegheny University of the Health Sciences
MCP-Hahneman School of Medicine
Philadelphia, Pennsylvania

Sten H. Vermund, MD, PhD
Professor and Chair
Department of Epidemiology
Director
Division of Geographic Medicine
Department of Medicine
University of Alabama at Birmingham
Birmingham, Alabama

Ellen R. Wald, MD
Professor of Pediatrics & Otolaryngology
University of Pittsburgh School of Medicine
Division Chief, Allergy, Immunology, and Infectious Diseases
Children's Hospital of Pittsburgh
Pittsburgh, Pennsylvania

Gerald P. Walsh, PhD
Leonard Wood Memorial Leprosy Research Center
Cebu, Philippines

Christine A. Wanke, MD
Assistant Professor of Medicine
Division of Infectious Diseases
Harvard Medical School
New England Deaconess Hospital
Boston, Massachusetts

Kent J. Weinhold, PhD
Department of Surgery
Duke University Medical Center
Durham, North Carolina

Mark H. Wener, MD
Associate Professor of Laboratory Medicine and Rheumatology
Head and Director of Division of Immunology
University of Washington School of Medicine
Seattle, Washington

Lars Weström, MD, PhD
Department of Obstetrics and Gynecology
Lund University
Lund, Sweden

Harold C. Wiesenfeld, MD, CM
Assistant Professor
Department of Obstetrics, Gynecology, and Reproductive Sciences
University of Pittsburgh School of Medicine/Magee-Womens Hospital
Co-Director
Sexually Transmitted Diseases Program
Allegheny County Health Department
Pittsburgh, Pennsylvania

Ayal Willner, MD
Department of Otolaryngology
Long Beach Medical Center
Long Beach, California

Eberhard Wilmes, MD
Department of ENT and Head and Neck Surgery
Klinikum Grosshadern
Ludwig-Maximilians-University of Munich
Munich, Germany

Barbara B. Wilson, MD
Associate Professor of Dermatology
University of Virginia Health Sciences Center
Charlottesville, Virginia

Samuel E. Wilson, MD
Professor and Chair
Department of Surgery
University of California at Irvine College of Medicine
Irvine, California

Edward S. Wong, MD
Associate Professor of Medicine
Medical College of Virginia
Chief, Infectious Diseases Section
McGuire Veterans Affairs Hospital
Richmond, Virginia

Thomas C. Wright, Jr, MD
Associate Professor of Pathology
Department of Obstetrics and Gynecologic Pathology
College of Physicians and Surgeons of Columbia University
New York, New York

Ram Yogev, MD
Professor of Pediatrics
Northwestern Universtiy Medical School
Director, Section of Pediatric and Maternal HIV Infection
The Children's Memorial Hospital
Chicago, Illinois

G. Bryan Young, MD, FRCP(C)
Professor
Department of Clinical Neurological Sciences
University of Western Ontario
London, Ontario
Canada

Herman Zaiman, MD
Editor, A Pictorial Presentation of Parasites
Valley City, North Dakota

S.R. Zaki, MD, PhD
Chief, Molecular Pathology and Ultrastructure Activity
Division of Viral and Rickettsial Diseases
Centers for Disease Control and Prevention
Atlanta, Georgia

Jonathan M. Zenilman, MD
Associate Professor
Division of Infectious Diseases
Johns Hopkins University School of Medicine
Baltimore, Maryland

Stephen H. Zinner, MD
Professor and Interim Chairman
Department of Medicine
Brown University School of Medicine
Director, Division of Infectious Diseases
Rhode Island Hospital and Roger Williams Medical Center
Providence, Rhode Island

CONTENTS

Chapter 1
AIDS
Donna Mildvan

Epidemiology, Natural History, and Prevention 1.2
Sten H. Vermund and D. Peter Drotman

Human Immunodeficiency Virus 1.4
Michael S. Saag

Host Response 1.9
Hedy Teppler, G. Diego Miralles, and Kent J. Weinhold

Classification and Spectrum 1.12
Gregory J. Dore and David A. Cooper

Cutaneous Manifestations 1.15
Alvin E. Friedman-Kien

Ophthalmic Manifestations 1.19
Janet L. Davis and Alan G. Palestine

Oral Cavity Manifestations 1.22
Deborah Greenspan and John S. Greenspan

Pulmonary Complications 1.24
Mark J. Rosen

Gastrointestinal Manifestations 1.25
Christine A. Wanke

Neurologic Manifestations 1.27
David M. Simpson, Susan Morgello, and Michele Tagliati

Metabolic Manifestations 1.30
Carl Grunfeld and Peter Jensen

Hematologic Manifestations 1.32
W. Christopher Ehmann, Christopher D. Gocke, and M. Elaine Eyster

Microbiology of Opportunistic Infections 1.35
Edward J. Bottone

Clinical Manifestations of Opportunistic Infections 1.37
Harold A. Kessler

Treatment and Prophylaxis of Opportunistic Infections 1.39
Judith Feinberg

AIDS-Associated Malignancies 1.42
Josephine Paredes and Susan E. Krown

Pediatric HIV Infection 1.44
Ram Yogev

HIV Infection in Women 1.47
Mary Ann Chiasson and Thomas C. Wright, Jr

Rationale and Strategies for Antiretroviral Therapy in HIV-1 Infection 1.50
Donna Mildvan

Antiviral Treatments 1.53
Margaret A. Fischl

Chapter 2
Skin, Soft Tissue, Bone and Joint Infections
Dennis L. Stevens

Introduction 2.2
Dennis L. Stevens

Staphylococcal Soft Tissue Infections 2.3
Jan Hirschmann

Streptococcal Infections of Skin and Soft Tissues 2.5
Dennis L. Stevens

Animal Bite Infections 2.7
Ellie J. C. Goldstein

Infections Associated With Animal Contact 2.9
E. Dale Everett

Fungal and Yeast Infections of the Skin, Appendages, and Subcutaneous Tissues 2.10
Gregory J. Raugi

Viral Infections of the Skin and Soft Tissues 2.13
Julie S. Francis and John Neff

Ectoparasitic Diseases of the Skin 2.15
Milan Trpis

Parasitic Diseases of the Skin and Soft Tissues 2.17
Herman Zaiman and Elaine C. Jong

Leprosy (Hansen's Disease) 2.19
Robert Gelber, Rodolfo M. Abalos, Roland V. Cellona, Tranquilino T. Fajardo, Gerald P. Walsh, and Ricardo S. Guinto

Spirochetal Infections of the Skin 2.22
Michael J. Chiu, Clay J. Cockerell, Karen R. Houpt, and Justin D. Radolf

Clostridial Infections 2.23
Dennis L. Stevens

Osteomyelitis 2.25
Jon T. Mader, Rajendra Kumar, David Simmons, and Jason Calhoun

Joint Infections and Rheumatic Manifestations of Infectious Diseases 2.28
Bruce C. Gilliland and Mark H. Wener

Chapter 3
Central Nervous System and Eye Infections
Thomas P. Bleck

Acute Bacterial Meningitides 3.2
Karen L. Roos and Jose M. Bonnin

Subacute and Chronic Meningitides 3.3
Allan R. Tunkel and Sidney E. Croul

Viral Encephalitis and Related Conditions 3.5
Daniel F. Hanley, Jonathan D. Glass, Justin C. McArthur, and Richard T. Johnson

Brain Abscesses 3.8
Brian Wispelwey

Parasitic Diseases of the Nervous System 3.10
Joseph R. Berger

Epidural Abscess and Subdural Empyema 3.12
David G. Brock

Venous Sinus Infections 3.14
Oren Sagher

Infections of the Skull and Bony Sinuses 3.16
Hans-Walter Pfister and Eberhard Wilmes

The Nervous System in Sepsis and Endocarditis 3.17
David A. Ramsay and G. Bryan Young

Ocular and Orbital Infections 3.19
Thomas A. Deutsch

Prion Diseases 3.21
Thomas P. Bleck and Sebastian R. Alston

Chapter 4

Upper Respiratory and Head and Neck Infections

Itzhak Brook

Eye and Orbit Infections 4.2
Ellen R. Wald

Otitis Media and Infections of the Inner Ear 4.4
Ayal Willner, Kenneth Grundfast, and Rande Lazar

Infections of the External Ear 4.6
Theodore W. Fetter

Sinusitis 4.8
Ellen R. Wald

Infectious Diseases of the Oral Cavity 4.10
Marlin E. Gher, Jr, and George Quintero

Pharyngotonsillitis 4.12
Harris R. Stutman

Epiglottitis, Croup, Laryngitis, and Tracheitis 4.14
Debra A. Tristram

Cervical Lymphadenopathy 4.17
Andrew M. Margileth

Parotitis and Thyroiditis 4.19
Stephen G. Baum and Moses Nussbaum

Deep Neck Infections and Postoperative Infections 4.20
James N. Endicott and Janet Seper

Chapter 5

Sexually Transmitted Diseases

Michel F. Rein

Gonorrhea 5.2
Jonathan M. Zenilman

Chlamydial Infections 5.3
Robert B. Jones

Bacterial Vaginosis 5.4
Sharon L. Hillier

Pelvic Inflammatory Disease 5.6
Per-Anders Mårdh, Birger Möller, Jorma Paavonen, and Lars Weström

Trichomoniasis 5.7
John N. Krieger and Michael F. Rein

Vulvovaginal Candidiasis 5.9
Jack D. Sobel

Syphilis:Epidemiology and Laboratory Testing 5.10
Sandra A. Larsen

Primary and Secondary Syphilis 5.11
Nicholas J. Fiumara

Late Syphilis 5.14
Michael F. Rein and Daniel M. Musher

Congenital Syphilis 5.15
Laura T. Gutman

Human Papillomavirus-Associated Diseases 5.17
Richard Reid

Ectoparasitic Infestations 5.18
Navjeet K. Sidhu-Malik and Michael F. Rein

Molluscum Contagiosum 5.19
Barbara B. Wilson

Herpes Simplex Virus Infections 5.20
Lawrence Corey

Chancroid 5.21
Allan Ronald

Chapter 6

Pleuropulmonary and Bronchial Infections

Michael S. Simberkoff

Gram-Positive Bacterial Infections of the Lungs 6.2
Richard B. Roberts

Gram-Negative Bacterial Infections of the Lungs 6.3
Melanie J. Maslow

Atypical Pneumonia Due to Higher Bacteria 6.6
Melanie J. Maslow and Jaishree Jagirdar

Tuberculosis and Other Mycobacterial Infections of the Lungs 6.7
Melanie J. Maslow

Fungal Infections 6.9
Scott F. Davies and George A. Sarosi

Anaerobic Lung Infections, Lung Abscesses, and Nosocomial Pneumonias 6.11
Howard L. Leaf

Viral Pneumonias 6.12
Robert F. Betts, Ann R. Falsey, Caroline B. Hall, and John J. Treanor

Protozoan and Helminthic Infections of the Lungs 6.15
John Froude

Pleural Effusion and Empyema 6.16
Christopher J. Salmon and Richard E. Bryant

Pneumonias in Cancer Patients 6.18
Donald Armstrong
Respiratory Infections in Transplant Recipients 6.21
Jay A. Fishman and Robert H. Rubin
Pulmonary Manifestations of Extrapulmonary Infection 6.23
James J. Herdegen and Roger C. Bone
Acute and Chronic Bronchitis and Bronchiolitis 6.24
Herbert Y. Reynolds and Michael S. Simberkoff

Chapter 7

Intra-abdominal Infections, Hepatitis, and Gastroenteritis

Bennett Lorber

Intra-abdominal Infections and Abscesses 7.2
Sydney M. Finegold and Samuel E. Wilson
Hepatitis 7.5
Lionel Rabin
Bacterial Enteritis 7.9
Richard L. Guerrant
Helicobacter pylori Infection 7.14
David Y. Graham and Robert M. Genta
Viral Enteritis 7.17
Robert D. Shaw
Parasitic Enteritis 7.19
Rosemary Soave
Fungal Enteritis 7.23
Helen Buckley
Diagnostic Imaging 7.25
Robert A. Gatenby

Chapter 8

External Manifestations of Systemic Infections

Robert Fekety

Viral Exanthems of Childhood 8.2
Janet R. Gilsdorf and Thomas Shope
Infective Endocarditis 8.6
W. Michael Scheld
Sepsis and Bacteremia 8.9
Steven M. Opal and Stephen H. Zinner
Streptococcal Infections 8.12
Adnan S. Dajani and Patricia Ferrieri
Staphylococcus aureus Infections 8.14
Neil Barg, Barney Graham, Clark Gregg, and David Gregory
Lyme Disease 8.16
Janine Evans and Stephen Malawista
Ehrlichiosis and Babesiosis 8.19
J. Stephen Dumler and David H. Persing
Bartonella Infections 8.22
David A. Relman and Philip E. LeBoit
Leprosy 8.25
Bruce H. Clements and David M. Scollard
Viral Hemorrhagic Fevers 8-27
C.J. Peters, S.R. Zaki, and P.E. Rollin
Systemic Fungal Infections 8.29
Carol A. Kauffman
Manifestations of Protozoal and Helminthic Diseases in Latin America 8.32
Anastacio de Q. Sousa, Thomas G. Evans, and Richard D. Pearson
Cutaneous Manifestations of Infection in the Immunocompromised Host 8.34
Donald Armstrong

Chapter 9

Urinary Tract Infections and Infections of the Female Pelvis

Jack D. Sobel

Cystitis 9.2
Edward S. Wong
Pyelonephritis 9.4
Michel G. Bergeron, Dominique Giroux, and Claude Delage
Complicated Urinary Tract Infections 9.6
Lindsay E. Nicolle
Infections of the Prostate 9.8
Edward D. Kim and Anthony J. Schaeffer
Candiduria 9.10
Harry A. Gallis and Jack D. Sobel
Catheter-Associated Urinary Tract Infections 9.12
J. Curtis Nickel
Infections of the Vulva 9.14
Elaine T. Kaye
Cervicitis and Endometritis 9.16
David E. Soper
Septic Abortion 9.18
Paul Nyirjesy
Tuboovarian Abscesses 9.20
Harold C. Wiesenfeld and Richard L. Sweet
Index I.1

Chapter 1

AIDS

Editor

Donna Mildvan

Contributors

Edward J. Bottone
Mary Ann Chiasson
David A. Cooper
Janet L. Davis
Gregory J. Dore
D. Peter Drotman
W. Christopher Ehmann
M. Elaine Eyster
Margaret A. Fischl
Christopher D. Gocke
Deborah Greenspan
John S. Greenspan
Carl Grunfeld
Judith Feinberg
Alvin E. Friedman-Kien
Peter Jensen
Harold A. Kessler
Susan E. Krown
G. Diego Miralles
Susan Morgello
Alan G. Palestine
Josephine Paredes
Mark J. Rosen
Michael S. Saag
David M. Simpson
Michele Tagliati
Hedy Teppler
Sten H. Vermund
Christine A. Wanke
Kent J. Weinhold
Thomas C. Wright, Jr
Ram Yogev

Epidemiology, Natural History, and Prevention

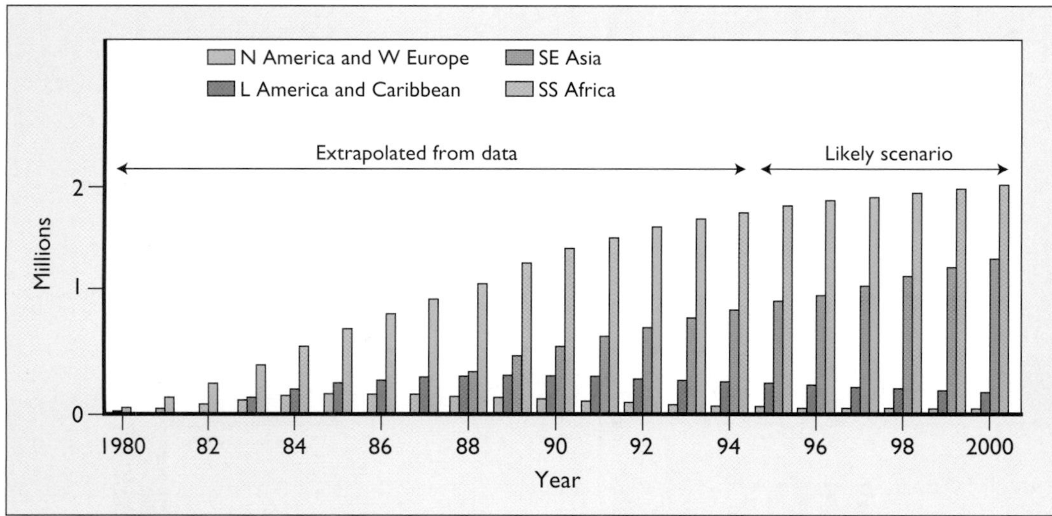

Figure 1-1 Annual HIV infection rates have been projected to the year 2000 by the World Health Organization based on conservative assumptions from HIV and AIDS reports and estimates. The epidemics in North America and Europe have stabilized, with the number of new infections and the number of deaths from AIDS coming into equilibrium. The epidemic in Latin America substantially exceeds that in North America. The epidemic in Asia began in the late 1980s but has been growing at least as rapidly as did the African epidemic 5 to 10 years earlier. New Asian cases may exceed 1 million/year by 2000. The African epidemic is of almost unimaginable magnitude; the projected decline in incident HIV cases in the late 1990s is largely a consequence of a saturation with HIV infection of at-risk persons, *ie*, the number of *new* HIV infections will be limited by a decreasing pool of susceptible persons [1]. (Dr. James Chin, personal communication, 1994.)

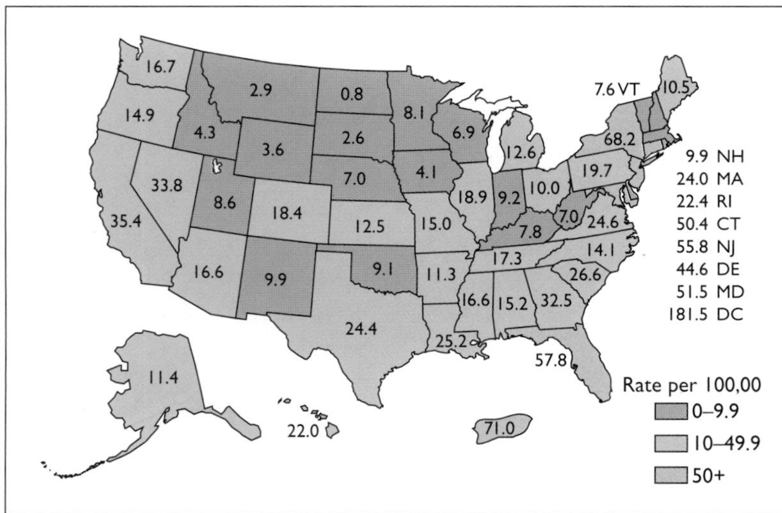

Figure 1-2 The states and territories in the United States with the highest annual AIDS rates in 1995. They included the District of Columbia, Puerto Rico, and New York, with over 68 cases/100,000 population reported. States with 33 to 58 cases/100,000 included Florida, New Jersey, Maryland, Connecticut, Delaware, California, and Nevada [2]. (*Courtesy of* Centers for Disease Control and Prevention.)

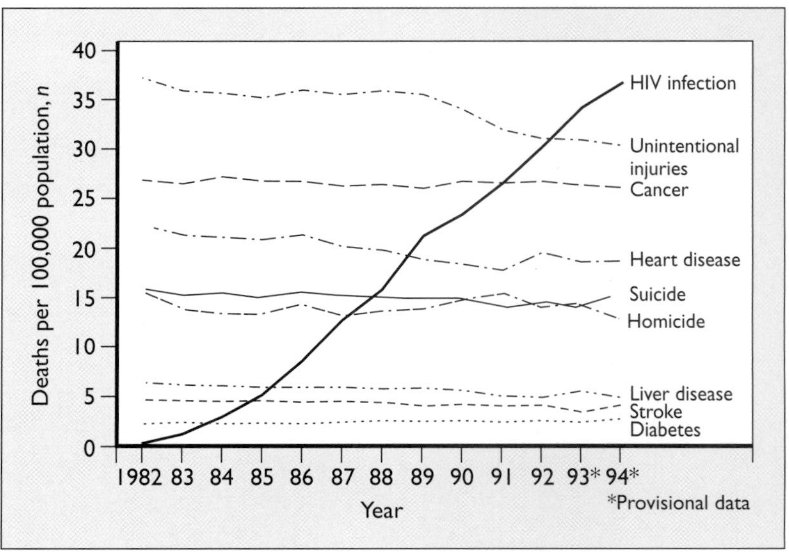

Figure 1-3 Since 1993 AIDS has been the leading cause of death among Americans aged 25 to 44 years [3,4].

1993 Revised classification system for HIV infection and expanded AIDS surveillance case definition for adults and adolescents ≥ 13 years of age*

	Clinical categories		
CD4⁺ T-cell categories	**(A) Asymptomatic, acute (primary) HIV, or PGL**	**(B) Symptomatic, not (A) or (C) conditions**	**(C) AIDS-indicator conditions**
(1) ≥ 500/µL	A1	B1	C1†
(2) 200–499/µL	A2	B2	C2†
(3) < 200/µL	A3†	B3†	C3†

*HIV-infected persons classified in A3, B3, or any C cell meet the 1993 AIDS surveillance case definition.
† AIDS-defining.
PGL—persistant generalized lymphadenopathy.

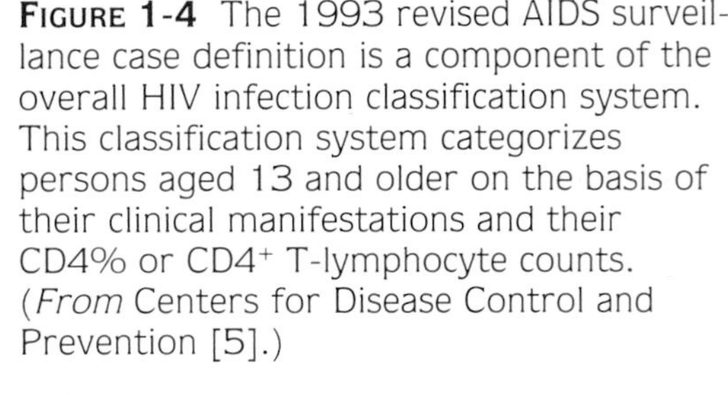

Figure 1-4 The 1993 revised AIDS surveillance case definition is a component of the overall HIV infection classification system. This classification system categorizes persons aged 13 and older on the basis of their clinical manifestations and their CD4% or CD4⁺ T-lymphocyte counts. (*From* Centers for Disease Control and Prevention [5].)

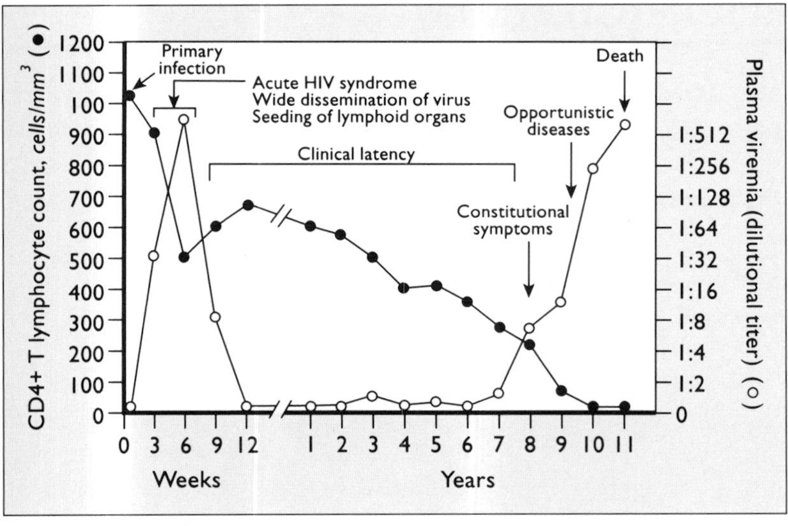

Figure 1-5 Typical course of HIV infection. Primary infection is a devastating immunologic event which typically results in the loss of 30% of circulating CD4⁺ T-cell volume (*solid circles*). As the host immune response is mounted, viremia (*open circles*) drops and some immunologic recovery is typical. However, many cells have been seeded by HIV, and typically, 60 CD4⁺ T cells/mm³ are lost per year. AIDS may typically manifest approximately a decade after infection, though there is wide variation. As the immune system deteriorates, more or less unbridled viral replication may ensue. (For recent review of viral load, *see* Saag *et al.* [6].) (*Adapted from* Pantaleo *et al.* [7].)

A. Interventions for HIV prevention: Sexual transmission

Reduce sexually transmitted diseases
Expand use of condoms
Improve barrier technologies for women
Treat HIV-infected persons with antiviral medication
Expand and improve behavioral interventions (risk reduction)

B. Interventions for HIV prevention: Perinatal transmission

Identify HIV-positive pregnant women and offer prenatal care and antiviral therapy
Provide noninvasive prenatal and intrapartum care to reduce blood exposures
Provide sexually transmitted disease diagnosis and treatment
Consider mild antiseptic wash of vagina and newborn if prolonged membrane rupture
Minimize time of delivery after membrane rupture
Do cesarean section, when indicated

Figure 1-6 HIV prevention strategies. It is widely accepted that more could be done with existing prevention modalities to control HIV. In addition, many important research projects can be performed to assess whether novel control strategies are efficacious. **A**, Regarding sexual transmission, it is not known to what extent different sexually transmitted disease control strategies might work to prevent HIV transmission. Although male condoms are important to prevent HIV, many female-controlled methods remain untested, such as available virucides, female condoms, or cervical caps and diaphragms. Treating HIV-infected persons with antiviral medications may reduce their infectiousness, but the duration or magnitude of any protective effect is not known. Finally, practical and effective behavioral interventions remain elusive. (For virucide and microbicide review, *see* Elias and Heise [8]; for sexually transmitted disease control for HIV prevention; *see* Grosskurth *et al.* [9].) **B**, Perinatal transmission. In the wake of 1994 results suggesting that zidovudine given antepartum, intrapartum, and to the newborn infant prevents 67% of perinatal HIV transmission, a number of challenges remain in efforts to block perinatal transmission. These efforts include the effective identification of HIV-infected women to offer state-of-the-art prenatal care, including antiviral therapy when indicated and intrapartum and postpartum care designed to avoid potentially infectious blood contaminations to the infant. Sexually transmitted diseases can be screened and treated in pregnancy. (*continued*)

C. Interventions for HIV prevention: Parenteral transmission
Medical exposure
Provide clean blood supply
Prevent nosocomial and iatrogenic spread
Universal precautions for health care workers
Consider antiretroviral chemoprophylaxis for health care worker exposures
Injection drug use
Expand drug prevention and treatment programs
Provide needle exchange programs, including "clean works" education
Minimize sexual transmission

Figure 1-6 (*continued*) Several studies suggest that prolonged rupture of membranes increases risk of perinatal transmission. Cesarean section might be protective for infants born to HIV-infected mothers, and studies should assess the costs and benefits to enable women and their health care providers to make informed decisions. (For perinatal transmission prevention, *see* Minkoff *et al.* [10]; Biggar *et al.* [11]; and Connor *et al.* [12].) **C**, Parenteral transmission can result from a contaminated blood supply where HIV testing is not readily available, such as in developing countries. Occupational or iatrogenic exposures must be minimized for health care workers by using universal precautions for all patients with unknown or HIV-seropositive status. Providing treatment to all drug users who wish to take advantage is a goal to which we should strive. Until treatment is available to all and for those who do not avail themselves of treatment opportunities, needle exchange and education to clean the needle injection equipment might be expected to slow the epidemic of HIV among injecting drug users. Many drug users are exposed through high-risk sexual activities. (For needle exchange discussion, *see* Kaplan [13].)

Human Immunodeficiency Virus

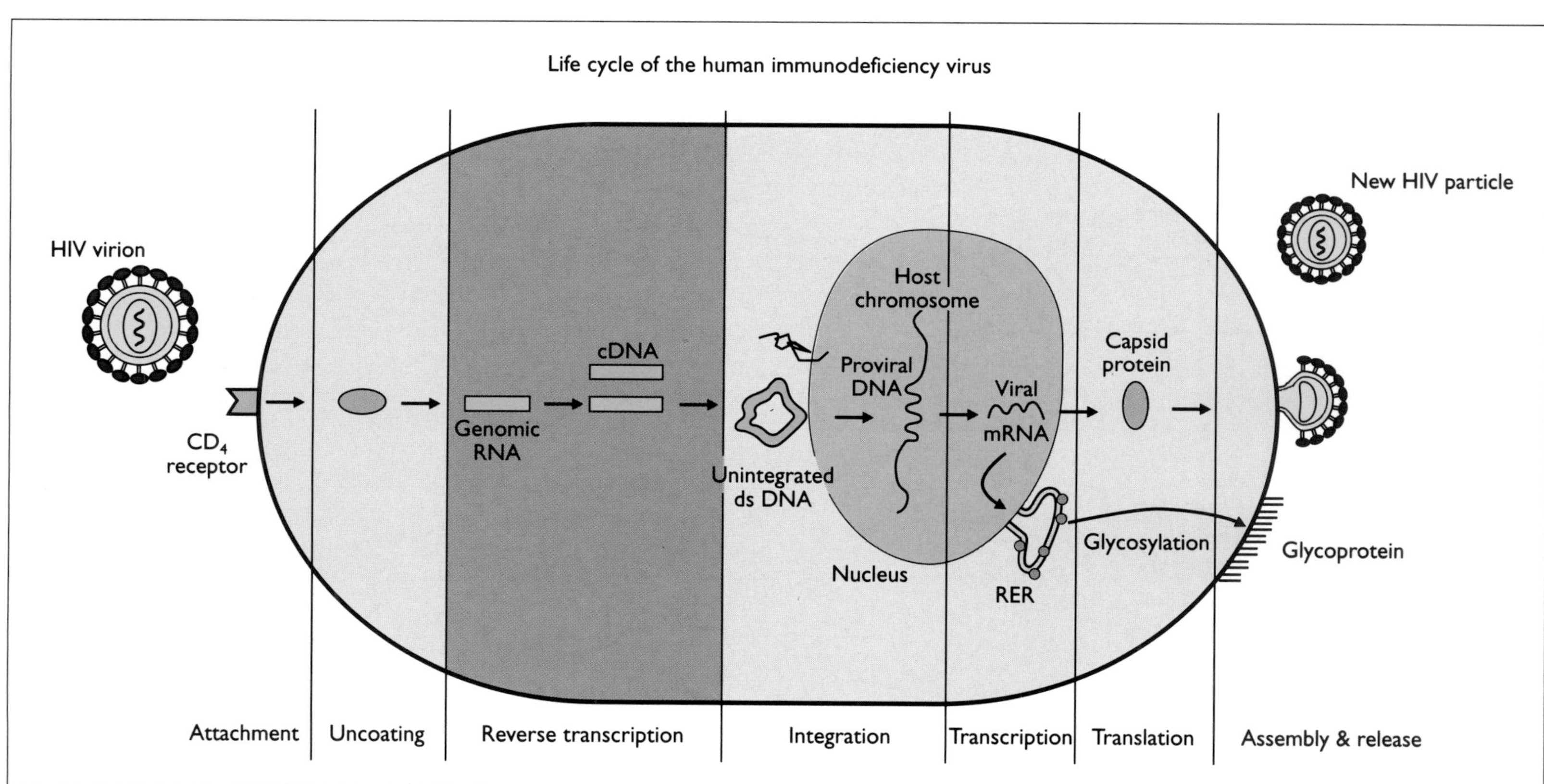

Figure 1-7 Lifecycle of HIV-1 (not drawn to scale). The HIV-1 virus binds to the CD4 receptor complex on the surface of $CD4^+$ cells. The virion then enters the cell, uncoats, and undergoes the process of reverse transcription (*magenta area*) in which viral RNA is transcribed into complementary DNA (cDNA). This is the portion of the lifecyle at which all currently available antiretroviral agents are designed to intercede. After reverse transcription, the DNA becomes double-stranded and migrates to the cell nucleus, where it is integrated into the host genomic DNA as a provirus. The virus can then be transcribed back into messenger RNA (mRNA) and genomic RNA, and the resultant proteins and genomic RNA are assembled near the surface of the cell and packaged into a new virion, which buds from the cell membrane [14].

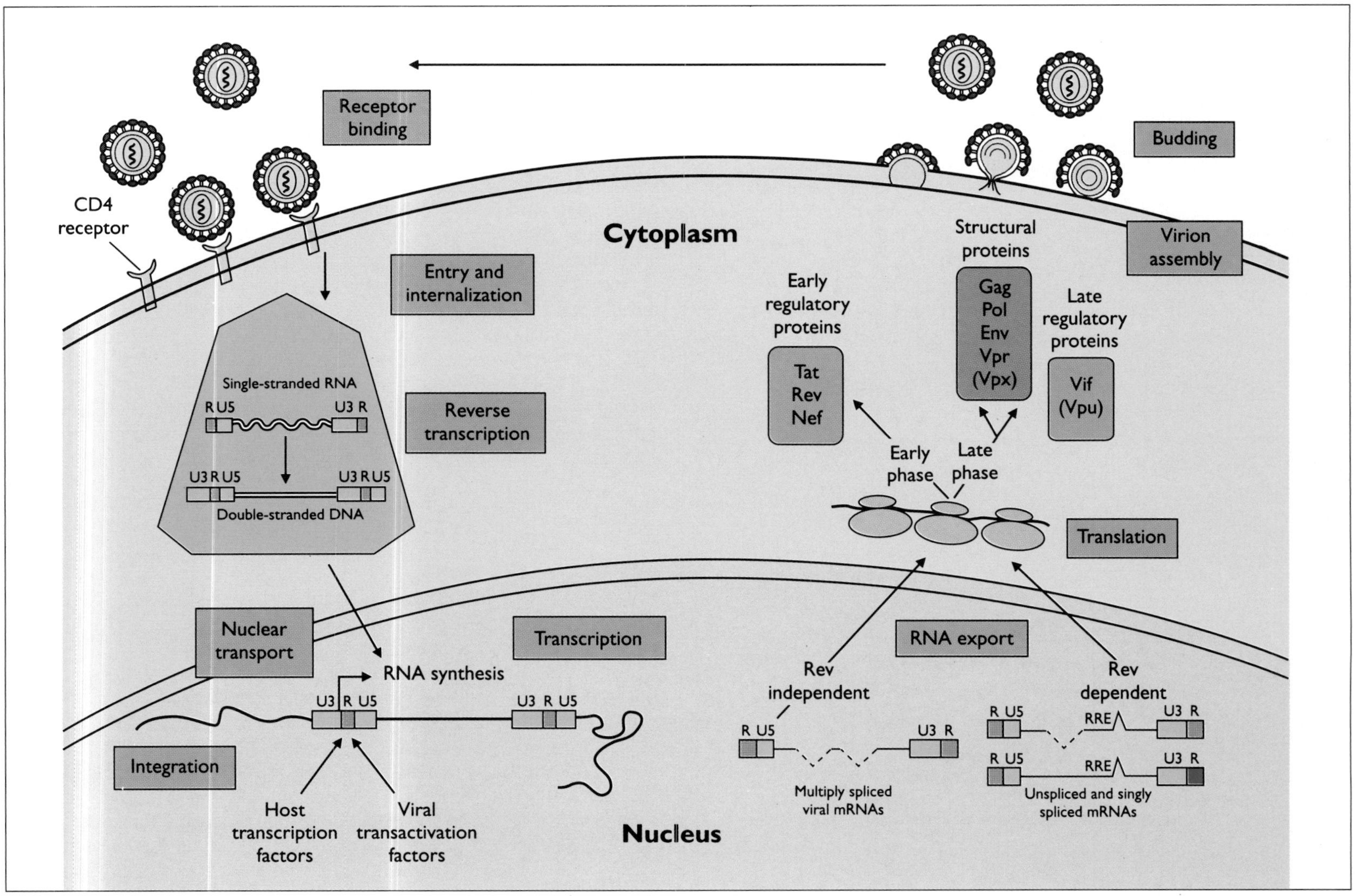

FIGURE 1-8 Viral replication. Once HIV enters a cell, undergoes reverse transcription, and is integrated into the nucleus (integration), several host transcriptional and viral activational factors stimulate viral replication (transcription). Regulatory proteins, such as Tat, Rev, and Nef, are generally produced early and, in the case of Tat, stimulate the virus to replicate. Rev-dependent messenger RNA (mRNA) usually results in unspliced or singly spliced RNA products via the "chaperone" effect of Rev, which escorts the unspliced message from the nucleus to the cytoplasm. Once in the cytoplasm, the long messages are translated into structural proteins, such as Gag, Pol, and Env, usually as a later event in the replication cycle (translation, late regulatory proteins). The production of these proteins is augmented by the help of late regulatory proteins such as Vif. Once the proteins and genomic RNA have been produced, they aggregate near the cell surface, where an immature virion buds on the cell membrane. After release of the immature virion from the cell, the activity of the protease gene results in development of a mature virion [15]. (RRE—Rev-responsive elements.) (*Adapted from* Hahn [16].)

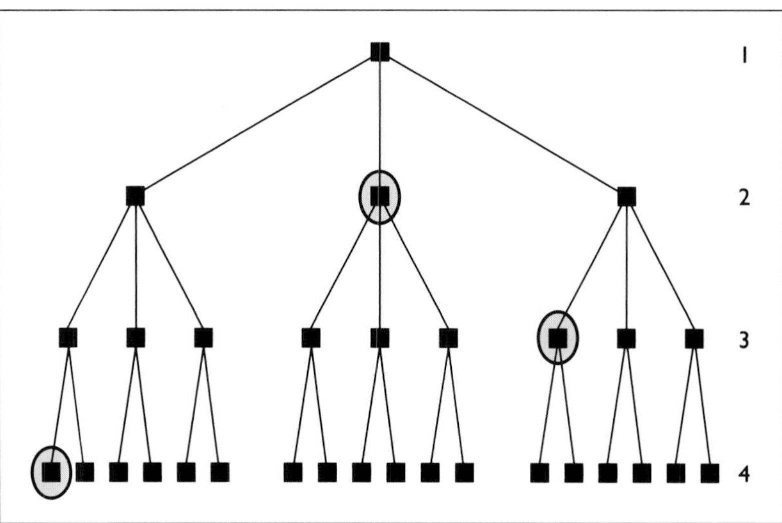

FIGURE 1-9 Genotype selection in HIV infection. Antigenic variation is a hallmark of HIV infection. It is believed that an individual is initially infected with a single genotype. However, this virus rapidly evolves over a period of weeks into a complex mixture of highly related, yet genetically distinct, viral variants. This figure represents the evolution of a family of viruses in an infected patient from a single genotype (*top of tree*) into the typical genetic quasi-species of HIV-1. At any given timepoint, a predominant genotype can be identified in either the plasma or peripheral blood mononuclear cells; however, other variants continue to exist simultaneously. Changes in selective pressure, due to either the immune response or the initiation of antiretroviral therapy, shift the population of viral variants such that another genotype becomes the most prevalent (represented by circled variants at a given timepoint) [17].

Methods for diagnosing HIV-1 infection

Method	Product measured
Culture in PBMCs	Infectious virus (as measured by reverse transcriptase activity or p24 antigen)
Antibody detection techniques	
ELISA	Anti-HIV antibody or p24 antigen
Western blot	Anti-HIV antibody
PCR	Proviral DNA Transcribed complementary DNA
Quantitative-competitive PCR	Viral RNA or DNA
Branched-chain DNA amplification	"Labeled" viral RNA

ELISA—enzyme-linked immunosorbent assay; PBMCs—peripheral blood mononuclear cells; PCR—polymerase chain reaction.

Figure 1-10 Methods for diagnosing HIV-1 infection. Many methods are available to detect HIV in patients. The most direct is to culture HIV via co-cultivation of patient peripheral blood mononuclear cells (PBMCs) with stimulated PBMCs from uninfected donors. Under the proper conditions, this *in vitro* culture system results in an explosive viral infection, leading to the production of millions of virions. The culture is read as positive by detecting either reverse transcriptase activity or p24 antigen in the virus culture supernatant. Due to the technical difficulty and expense of performing viral culture, other techniques have been developed to detect the presence of HIV infection. Many of these techniques rely on detection of the antibody response to HIV rather than detection of the virus itself. The two most commonly employed antibody tests are the enzyme-linked immunosorbent assay and the Western blot test, both of which are highly sensitive (> 99%) tests. Newer techniques for detecting HIV include polymerase chain reaction (PCR), quantitative-competitive–PCR, and branched DNA, but their roles in clinical staging and predicting progression of HIV disease remain undefined.

1. Antigen is bound to microtiter well

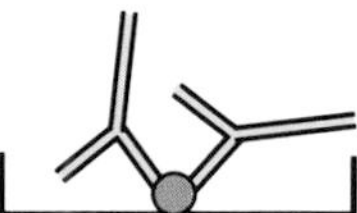

2. Antibody from serum added; wash

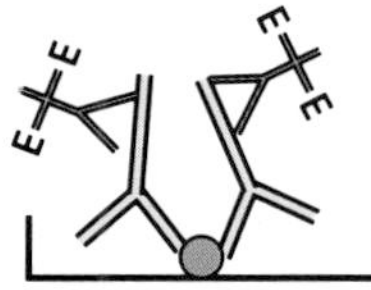

3. Antihuman immunoglobulin antibody conjugated with enzyme (E) added; wash

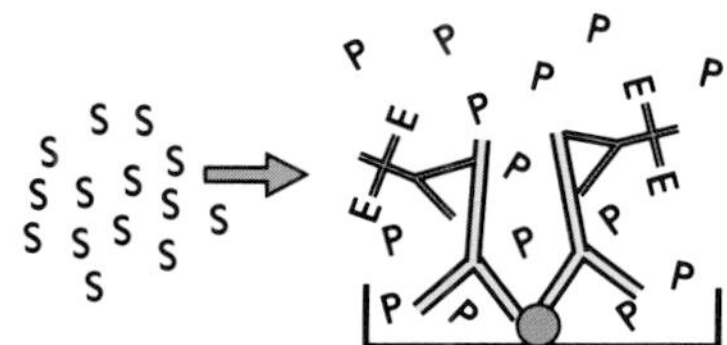

4. Add enzyme substrate (S); color formed (P)

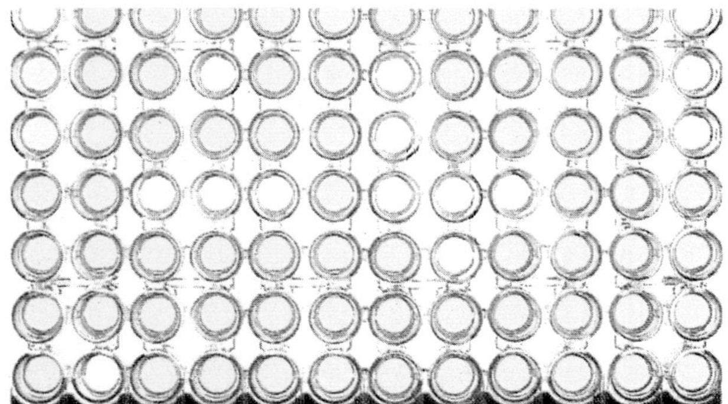

5. Color formed is proportional to amount of antibody in serum

Figure 1-11 Enzyme-linked immunosorbent assay (ELISA) antibody test. The ELISA test is based on the capture of anti-HIV-specific antibodies by viral antigens that are coated on a microwell (*1*). Once the antibody binds to the HIV antigens, a washing procedure is performed (*2*) followed by incubation with a goat antihuman immunoglobulin antibody that is conjugated with an enzyme (*3*). The goat antihuman antibody binds tightly and specifically to any human antibody that has bound to HIV antigen, and after a washing procedure, an enzyme substrate is added, which is cleaved by the enzyme to form a product that yields a color (*4*). The relative amount of color present in the well (*5*) is proportional to the amount of human anti-HIV antibody present in the patient's sera [18]. (*Adapted from* Brock and Madigan [19].)

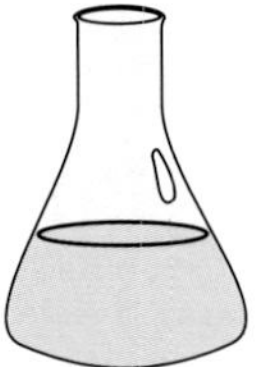

1. Tissue culture for HIV yields cellular lysate (proteins)

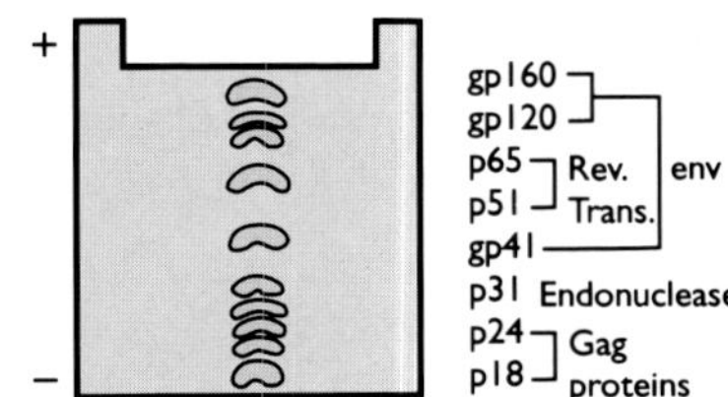

2. Mixture subjected to polyacrylamide gel electrophoresis; proteins separate by MW

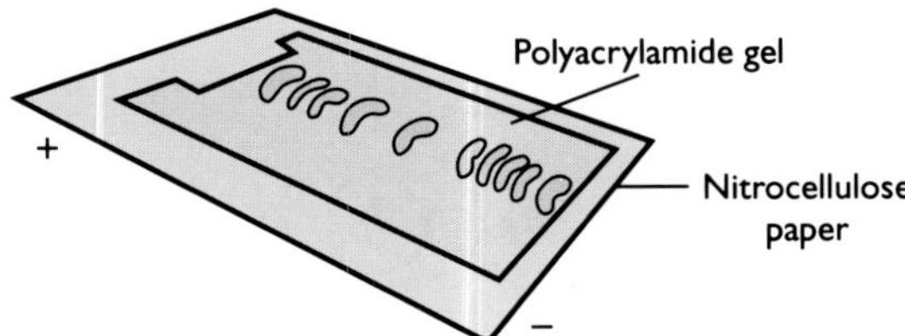

3. Transfer the separated proteins from the gel to nitrocellulose paper; cut into strips

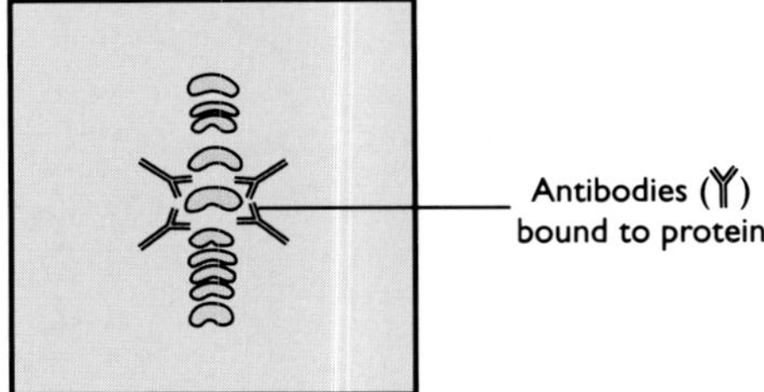

4. Nitrocellulose paper containing blotted proteins is incubated with patient sera; if antibody is present, it recognizes and binds to a specific protein

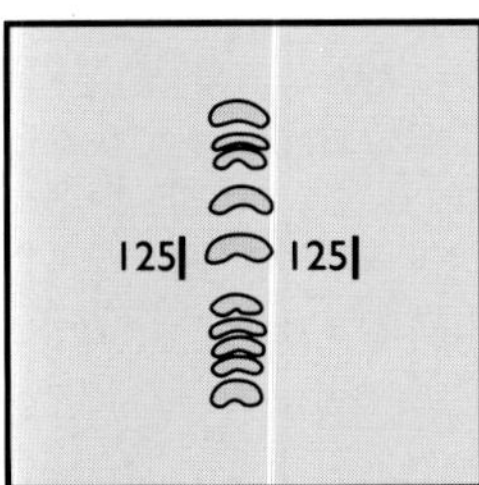

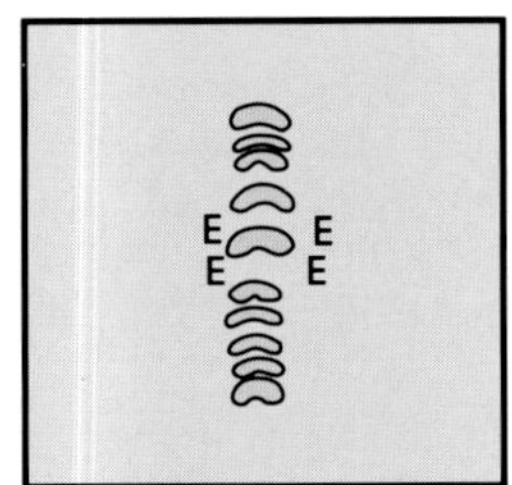

5. Add marker to bind to antigen–antibody complexes, either radiolabeled protein (*left*) or antibody-containing conjugated enzyme (*right*)

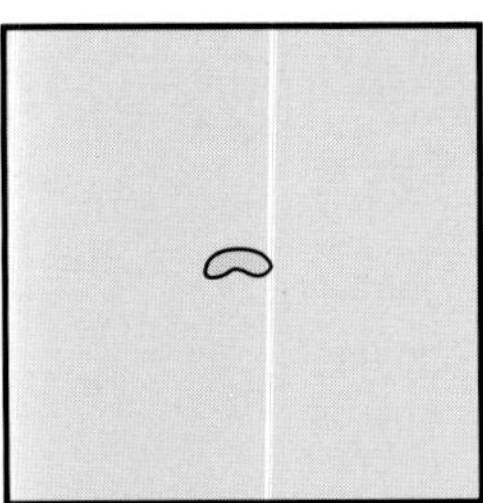

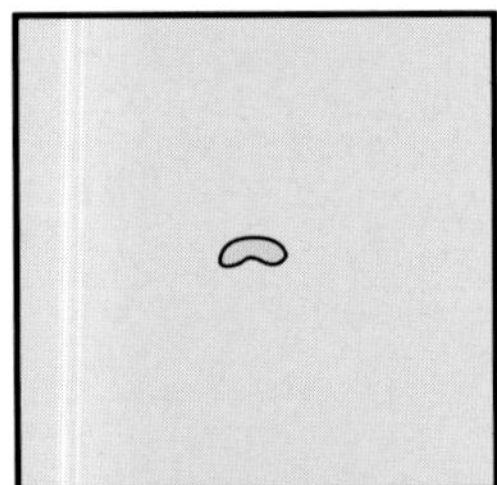

6. Develop blot by either exposing blot to x-ray film (*left*) or adding substrate of enzyme (*right*); dark spot appears where antibody bound to antigen on blot

Figure 1-12 Western blot. The Western blot antibody test works on the same principle as enzyme-linked immunosorbent assay (ELISA) *ie*, capturing antibody with HIV-specific antigens. In contrast with the ELISA, the antigens on the Western blot are separated on a polyacrylamide gel (*2*) and transferred to nitrocellulose paper (*3*). The nitrocellulose paper is cut into strips, which are incubated with the patient's sera (*4*). If antibody is present, it binds specifically at the point where the antigen migrated. This allows accurate determination of the specific antigen against which the antibody is targeted [18]. (MW—molecular weight.) (*Adapted from* Brock and Madigan [19].)

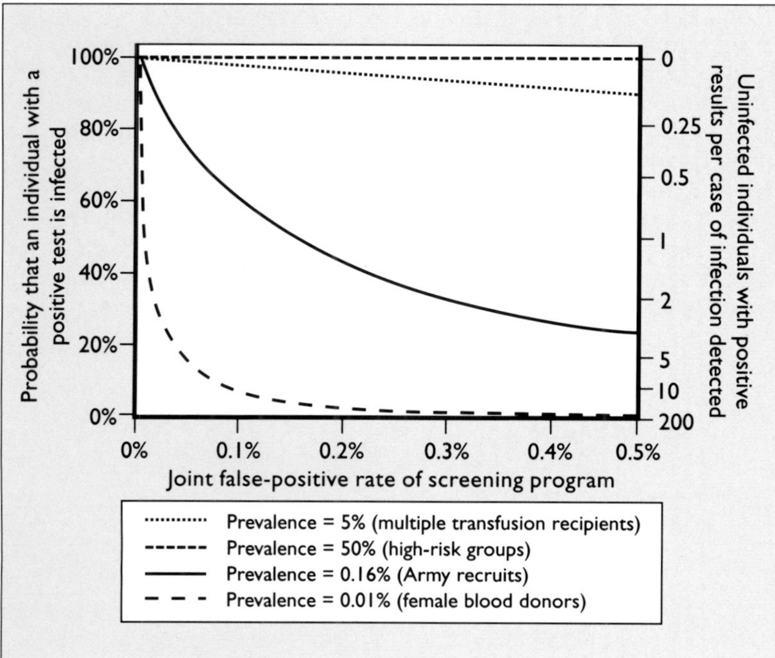

FIGURE 1-13 Positive predictive value of enzyme-linked immunosorbent assay (ELISA) and Western blot. Although the sensitivity and specificity of the ELISA and Western blot tests are high, the positive predictive value of the two tests, even when used in combination, depends on the population of patients being tested. If the prevalence of HIV infection is high (*eg*, intravenous drug users from the inner city), the probability that an individual with a positive test is truly infected remains at 100% even when the joint false-positive rate is 0.5%. Conversely, if the prevalence of HIV infection is very low (0.01%), such as with female blood donors, even a joint false-positive rate of 0.02% will lead to at least half of the individuals who test positive having a false-positive test. This concept is a critically important one to consider when making decisions about universal testing. (*Adapted from* Meyer and Paulker [20].)

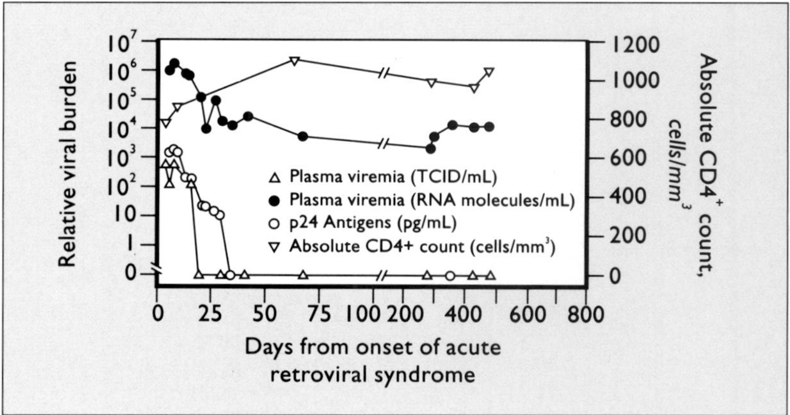

FIGURE 1-14 Viral replication profile. A representative patient from the time of acute seroconversion with serial CD4$^+$ count measurements, p24 antigen, culturable free virus in plasma, and plasma viremia measured via quantitative competitive polymerase chain reaction (QC-PCR). Coincident with the development of an effective immune response, the levels of p24 antigen and culturable free virus in plasma drop to undetectable levels within 20 to 30 days after seroconversion. In contrast, although the viral burden as measured by QC-PCR drops by over 100-fold, the levels do not approach the undetectable range and remain in the 1000 to 10,000 range over the course of the next year. These data indicate that viral replication is an ongoing process throughout the period of clinical latency and underscores the increased sensitivity of QC-PCR methods over standard p24 antigen or plasma culture assays. (TCID—tissue culture infective dose.) (*Courtesy of* J. Lifson, MD.)

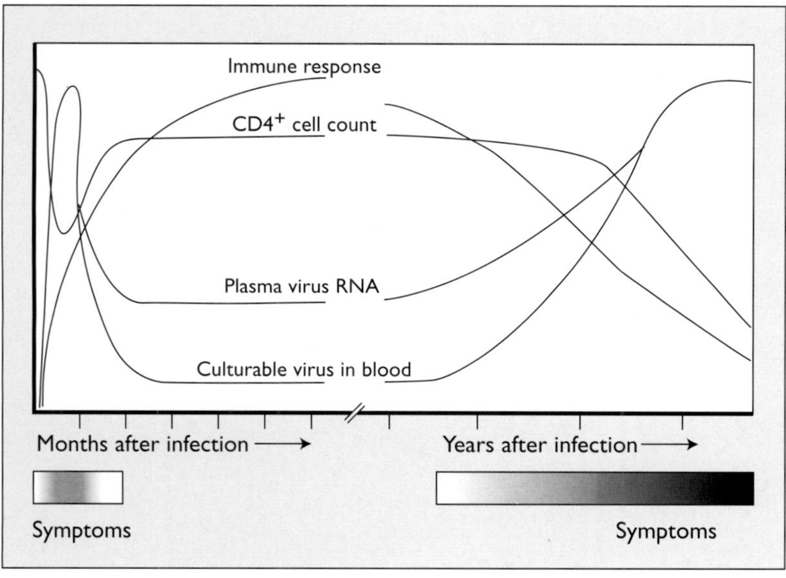

FIGURE 1-15 Hypothetical course of HIV infection in adults. High levels of plasma viremia as measured by either culturable free virus from plasma or plasma RNA titer decrease dramatically as the immune system response is established after acute seroconversion. Over time, as the CD4$^+$ cell count begins to decline, the level of viral burden begins to increase coincident with the development of symptomatic HIV disease. (*Adapted from* Saag *et al.* [21].)

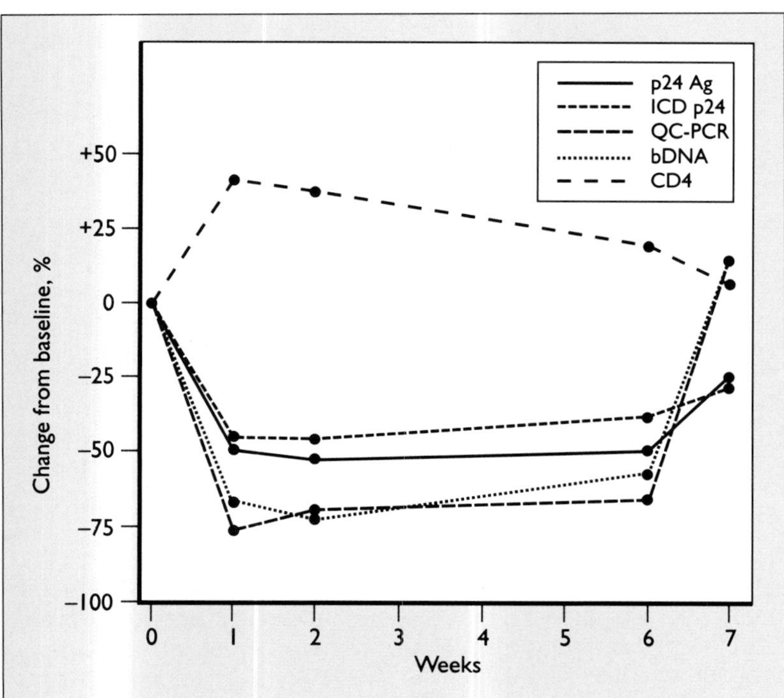

FIGURE 1-16 Virologic response to antiretroviral therapy. Nucleoside antiretroviral therapy has been shown to increase survival and delay disease progression. The application of surrogate markers, such as the CD4⁺ count, p24 antigen, and viral RNA markers of quantitative competitive polymerase chain reaction (QC-PCR) and branched-chain DNA (bDNA), are beginning to be used to determine the relative activity of antiretroviral drugs. This figure depicts the percent change from baseline over 6 weeks when zidovudine therapy is initiated. Therapy is stopped at week 6, and the patient receives no antiretroviral therapy between weeks 6 and 7. Note the dynamic decrease in viral burden as measured by QC-PCR and bDNA within 1 week of therapy and a sharp rebound after withholding drug for just 1 week. Also, note the strong concordance between the decrease in viral burden as measured by plasma RNA values and the reciprocal increase in $CD4^+$ cell counts. (ICD—immune complex dissociated.)

HOST RESPONSE

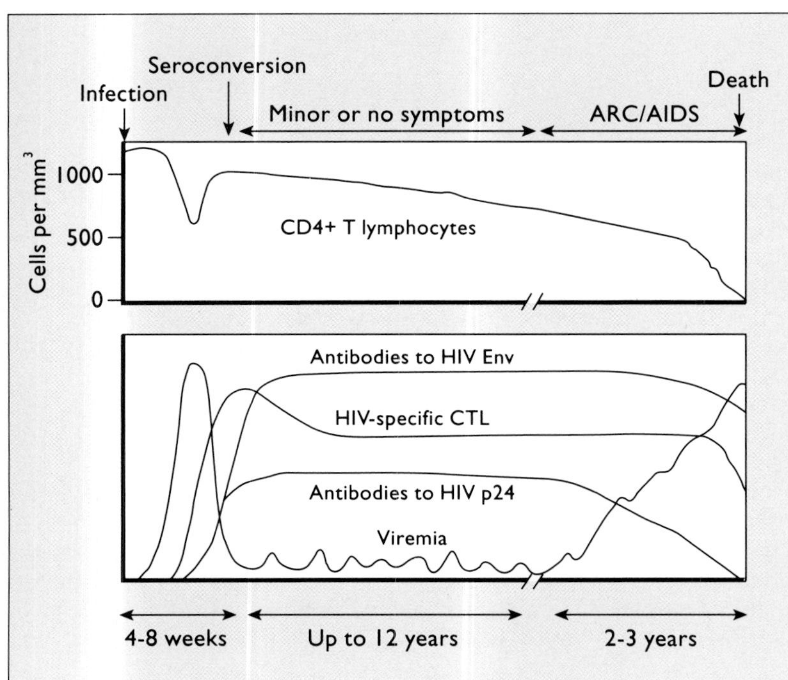

FIGURE 1-17 Natural history of HIV infection and the immune response. Acute HIV infection is associated with a steep but transient decrease in the number of circulating $CD4^+$ T cells, followed by a slower gradual loss over many years of latent disease. Initial viremia leads to seeding of virus throughout the body. With the development of immune responses to the virus, especially HIV-specific cytotoxic T cells (CTL), there is containment of the plasma viremia. HIV-specific antibodies are detectable only after the viremia has declined, suggesting that control of the viremia is due to the cytotoxic effector cells, rather than antibodies. Antibodies to HIV envelope are detectable within months after the acute infection and their levels remain elevated, whereas anti-p24 antibody levels decline in later stages of disease. The period of clinical latency may last 12 years or longer, during which few or no symptoms are present. Viremia during the clinical latency is at a low or undetectable level, although active viral replication persists within lymphoid tissue. Changes in the immune response and/or the virus itself lead to a resurgence of viral replication and viremia, progressive immune dysfunction, and the clinical signs and symptoms of HIV disease. (ARC—AIDS-related complex.) (*Adapted from* Weiss [22].)

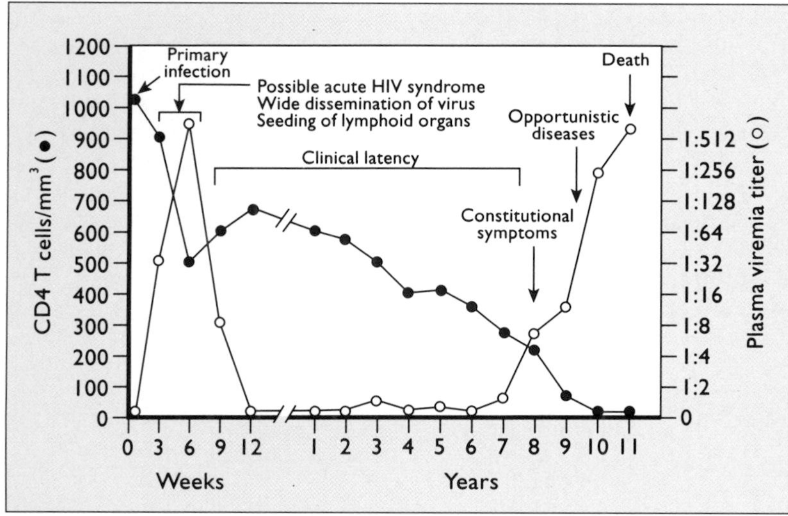

FIGURE 1-18 Typical clinical course of HIV infection. After initial infection with HIV, there is wide dissemination of virus and seeding of lymphoid tissues throughout the body, accompanied by a transient decline in CD4⁺ T-lymphocyte counts. This decline may be associated with the acute HIV illness. With the onset of the immune response, plasma viremia declines dramatically. During the period of clinical latency, there are few or no symptoms and low levels of virus detectable by quantitative culture. However, despite low levels of viremia, viral RNA may be detected at this and all stages of infection. Ultimately, viral replication escapes the control of the immune system. Increasing viremia is associated with decreasing CD4⁺ T-lymphocyte counts and progressive immune dysfunction. This leads to the constitutional symptoms of AIDS-related complex and later to the opportunistic diseases characteristic of AIDS. (*Adapted from* Pantaleo *et al.* [23].)

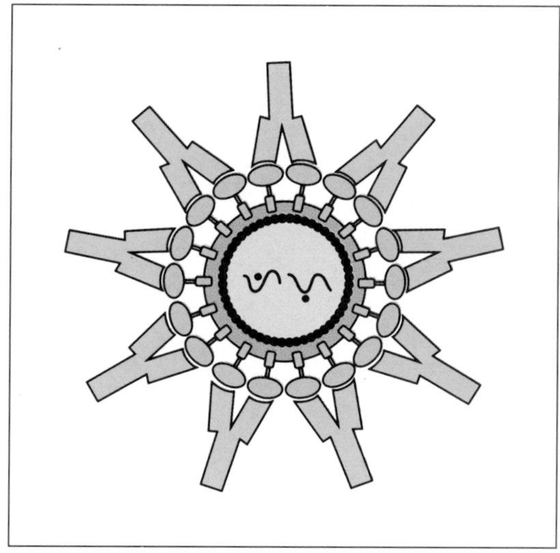

FIGURE 1-19 Neutralizing antibodies. Neutralizing antibodies are defined *in vitro* as antibodies that inhibit the infectivity of HIV by interacting with the viral envelope. Group-specific antibodies are capable of neutralizing many viral strains, whereas type-specific antibodies neutralize only a given strain. For vaccine development, it would be optimal to elicit group-specific neutralizing antibodies to confer protection against many strains of HIV.

Is effective clearance or containment of HIV infection possible?

Nonprogressors
Estimated at 5% of total HIV-infected population
Demonstrable infection but little detectable virus and no immunologic decline
Variety of explanations
Strong and effective virus-specific immunity
Attenuated virus

Clearance of HIV infection in perinatally infected infant
- Well-documented case of an infant with established perinatal infection who cleared infection by age 12 mos and has remained without demonstrable evidence of HIV infection at age 5 yrs

FIGURE 1-20 Is effective clearance or containment of HIV infection possible? There is evidence that HIV-1 infection is not uniformly progressive or fatal. Studies of long-term nonprogressors, who make up approximately 5% of the HIV-infected population, indicate that these individuals have lived with controlled HIV infection without any clinical or laboratory evidence of immunologic deterioration. Multiple factors may be responsible, including strong host immune responses and some attenuation of the pathogenicity of the infecting virus. There is at least one well-documented case of a perinatally infected infant who showed evidence of HIV infection on multiple occasions in the first months of life, yet by age 12 months was negative for all evidence of HIV infection by multiple laboratory parameters. The child remained free of laboratory and clinical evidence of HIV infection 5 years later. The reasons for this outcome are not elucidated but offer hope that a protective and perhaps curative immune response is possible in HIV infection [24–29].

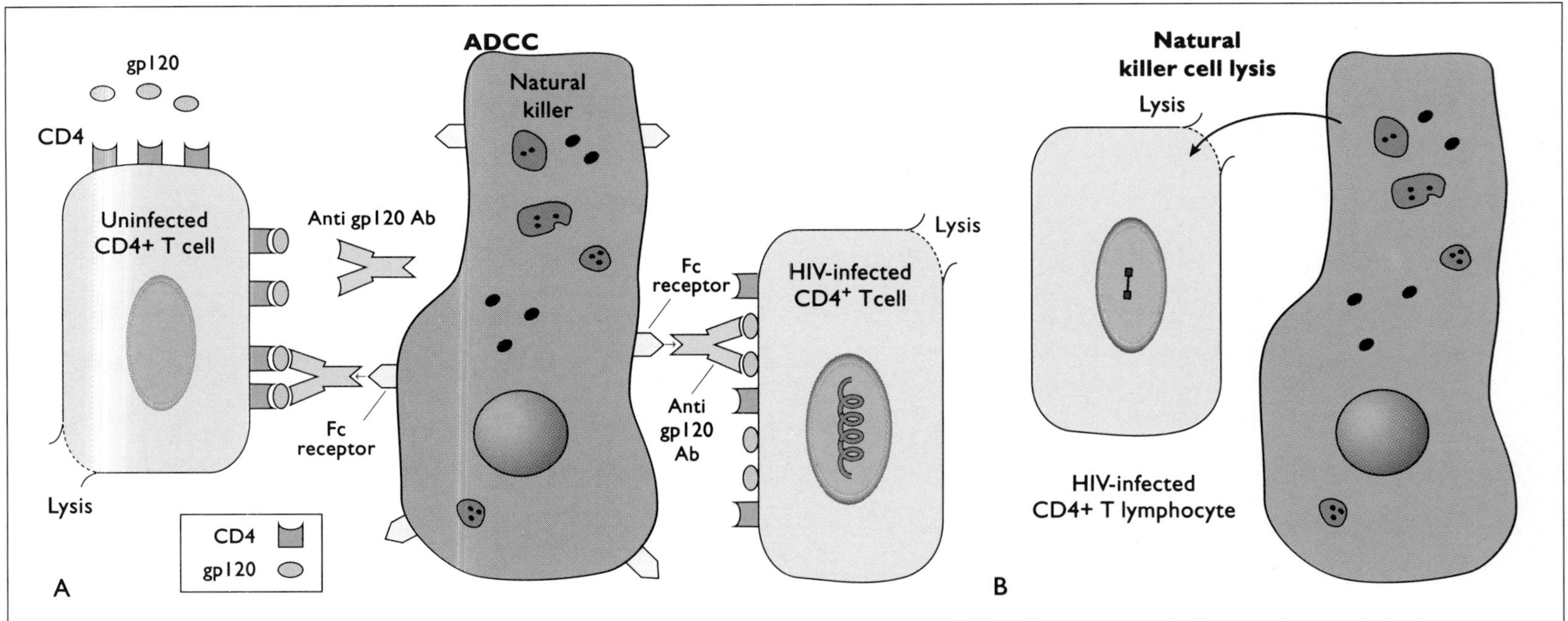

FIGURE 1-21 Natural killer cell responses. **A**, Antibody-dependent cellular cytotoxicity (ADCC) is a form of cellular immunity mediated by natural killer cells. HIV-specific antibodies can form complexes with whole virions or, as illustrated, with envelope components of HIV. These HIV components, such as gp120, may be expressed on the surface of an infected cell (*right cell*) or, in soluble form, may bind to the surface of an uninfected $CD4^+$ cell (*left cell*). Natural killer cells effect cell lysis when their surface Fc receptors bind to the constant Fc portion of these antibodies. Therefore, although the antibody responsible is HIV-specific, the effector cell is not. Because ADCC can kill both infected and innocent bystander uninfected cells, its effect may be protective or pathogenic. **B**, Natural killer cells also can kill HIV-infected cells in the absence of antibody.

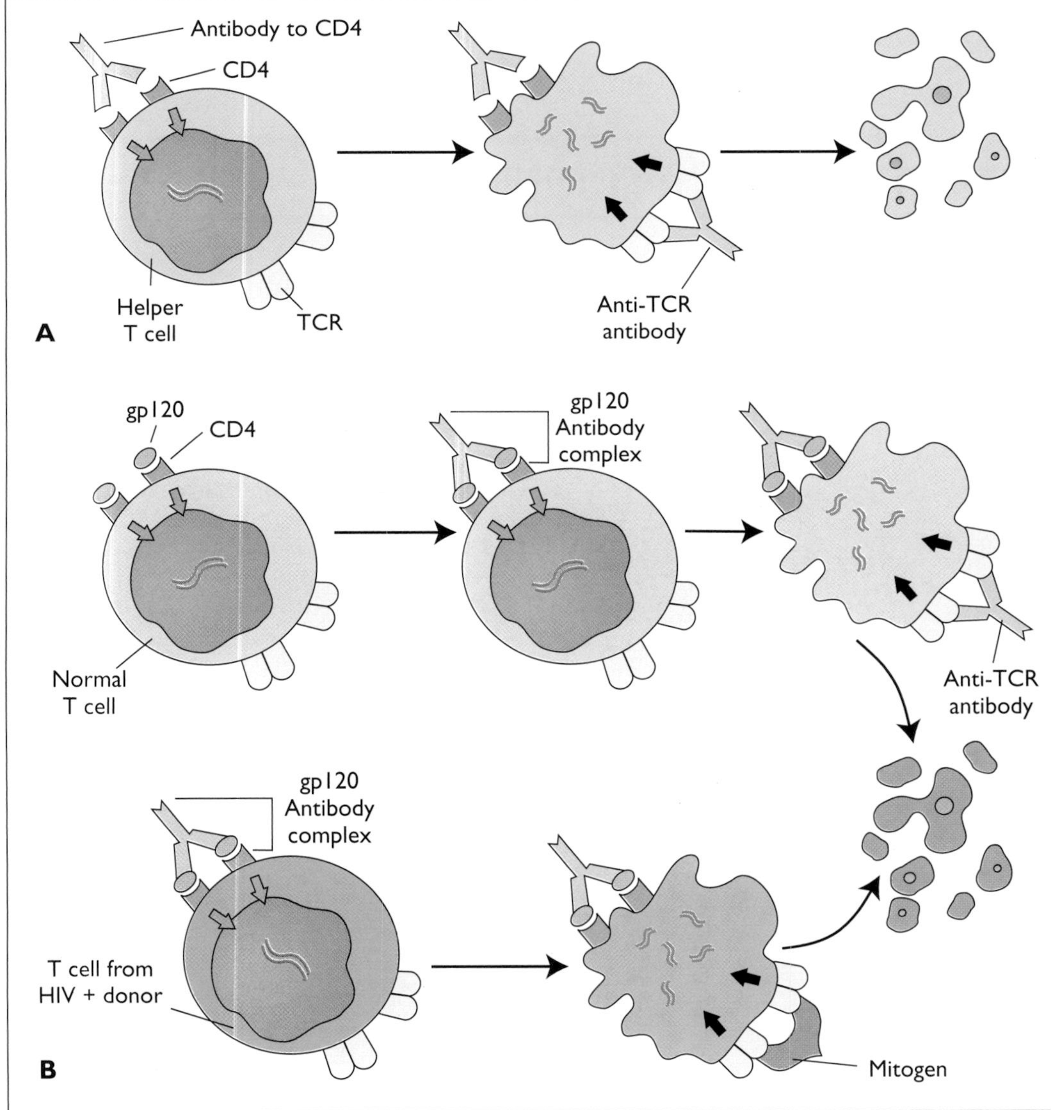

FIGURE 1-22 HIV-induced apoptosis. **A**, Apoptosis is a particular mechanism of cell death in which the cell actively fragments and is phagocytosed without associated inflammatory responses. The hallmarks of apoptosis are DNA fragmentation and formation of membrane blebs. During immunologic development, apoptosis allows the clonal deletion of autoreactive T cells in the thymus. Apoptosis also has been postulated as one of the mechanisms responsible for CD4 cell depletion in HIV infection. In normal CD4 cells, simultaneous activation of CD3 and CD4 receptors leads to T-cell proliferation. However, when CD4 activation precedes T-cell receptor (TCR) stimulation, the T cell undergoes cell death by apoptosis [30]. **B**, If T cells from uninfected individuals are crosslinked with gp120/anti-gp120 and then their TCR is stimulated by anti-TCR, mitogens, or superantigens, they also undergo apoptosis. The same findings have also been confirmed in peripheral blood mononuclear cells from HIV-infected individuals. These findings suggest that circulating CD4 cells from infected individuals are primed to die by apoptosis upon signals that would otherwise mediate proliferation. The role of this process in CD4 cell depletion *in vivo* remains unknown [31]. (*Adapted from* Cohen [32].)

Cytokine regulation of HIV expression and regulation

Cytokine	Target cells(s)	Effect
Bulk supernatant	T,M	↑
IL-1	T,M	↑
IL-2	T	↑
IL-3	M	↑
IL-4	T,M	↑↓
IL-6	M	↑
IL-10	M	↑↓
IL-13	M	↓
TNF-α, TNF-β	T,M	↑
TGF-β	T,M	↑↓
M-CSF	M	↑
GM-CSF	M	↑
IFN-α, IFN-β	T,M	↓
IFN-γ	M	↑↓

GM-CSFL—granulocyte-macrophage colony-stimulating factor; IFN—interferon; IL—interleukin; M—monocytes/macrophages; M-CSF—moncyte colony- stimulating factor; T—T lymphocyte; TGF—transforming growth factor; TNF—tumor necrosis factor.

Figure 1-23 Cytokine regulation of HIV expression. Many cytokines have been tested under a variety of *in vitro* conditions for their effect on HIV replication and expression. The most potent inducers of HIV replication are tumor necrosis factor -α, and -β, and interleukin (IL)-6. Potent inhibitors of HIV replication are interferon -α and -β. Several cytokines, such as IL-4 and transforming growth factor -β, have dual effects on HIV expression. Target cells, either T lymphocytes or monocytes/macrophages, are cell types in which the effect was observed [33]. (*Adapted from* Fauci [34].)

Rationale for immune-based therapies

Restore immune competence
Inhibit host-derived cofactors of viral replication
Inhibit host mechanisms that cause complications of HIV disease
Improve immunity for treatment/prevention of opportunistic complications

Figure 1-24 Rationale for immune-based therapies. Given the modest benefit afforded by currently available antiretroviral therapies and the increasing understanding of the immunopathologic aspects of HIV disease, interest is growing in therapeutic strategies that target the immune response. These therapies include the obvious aim of restoring overall immune function and of interrupting the host-derived mechanisms, which may contribute to viral pathogenesis, but also novel strategies to improve immunity for the treatment and prevention of opportunistic infections and neoplasms that characterize AIDS.

Classification and Spectrum

A. 1993 Revised classification system for HIV infection and expanded AIDS surveillance case definition for adults and adolescents ≥ 13 years of age*

	Clinical categories		
CD4+ T-cell categories	(A) Asymptomatic, acute (primary) HIV, or PGL	(B) Symptomatic, not (A) or (C) conditions	(C) AIDS-indicator conditions
(1) ≥ 500/μL	A1	B1	C1
(2) 200–499/μL	A2	B2	C2
(3) < 200/μL AIDS-indicator T-cell count	A3	B3	C3

*HIV-infected persons classified in A3, B3, or any C cell meet the 1993 AIDS surveillance case definition.
PGL—persistent generalized lymphadenopathy.

B. Category B conditions

Bacillary angiomatosis
Candidiasis, oropharyngeal (thrush)
Candidiasis, vulvovaginal
Cervical dysplasia
Cervical carcinoma *in situ*
Constitutional symptoms
Hairy leukoplakia, oral
Herpes zoster (shingles)
Idiopathic thrombocytopenic purpura
Listeriosis
Pelvic inflammatory disease
Peripheral neuropathy

Figure 1-25 1993 revised classification for HIV/AIDS. The CDC in 1993 revised the classification system for HIV infection to emphasize the clinical importance of the CD4+ T-lymphocyte count in the categorization of HIV-related clinical conditions. Consistent with the 1993 revised classification system, the CDC also expanded the AIDS surveillance case definition to include all HIV-infected persons who have < 200 CD4+ T lymphocytes/μL or a CD4+ T-lymphocyte percentage of total lymphocytes of < 14%. This expansion adds three clinical conditions—pulmonary tuberculosis, recurrent pneumonia, and invasive cervical cancer—and retains the 23 clinical conditions in the AIDS surveillance case definition published in 1987. **A**, The expanded AIDS surveillance case definition. Persons with AIDS-indicator conditions (category C) as well as those with CD4+ T-lymphocyte counts < 200/μL (categories A3 or B3) became reportable as AIDS cases in the United States and territories, effective 1 January 1993. **B**, Category B conditions are listed. Category C includes the clinical conditions listed in the AIDS surveillance case definition [35].

Clinical manifestations of primary HIV-1 infection

General	Dermatologic
Fever	Erythematous maculopapular rash
Pharyngitis	Diffuse urticaria
Lymphadenopathy	Desquamation
Arthralgia	Alopecia
Myalgia	Mucocutaneous ulceration
Lethargy/malaise	
Anorexia/weight loss	**Gastrointestinal**
Neuropathic	Oral/oropharyngeal candidiasis
Headache/retro-orbital pain	Nausea/vomiting
Meningoencephalitis	Diarrhea
Peripheral neuropathy	
Radiculopathy	
Brachial neuritis	
Guillain-Barré syndrome	
Cognitive/affective impairment	

FIGURE 1-26 Clinical manifestations of primary HIV-1 infection. The main clinical features of primary HIV-1 infection reflect both the lymphocytopathic and neurologic tropism of HIV-1. Patients typically present with an illness of acute onset characterized by fever, lethargy, malaise, myalgias, headaches, retro-orbital pain, photophobia, sore throat, lymphadenopathy, and maculopapular rash. Meningoencephalitis may also occur. The time from exposure to HIV-1 until the onset of the acute clinical illness is typically 2 to 4 weeks. The clinical illness lasts 1 to 4 weeks. This acute clinical illness associated with seroconversion for HIV-1 has been reported in 53% to 95% of cases [36,37].

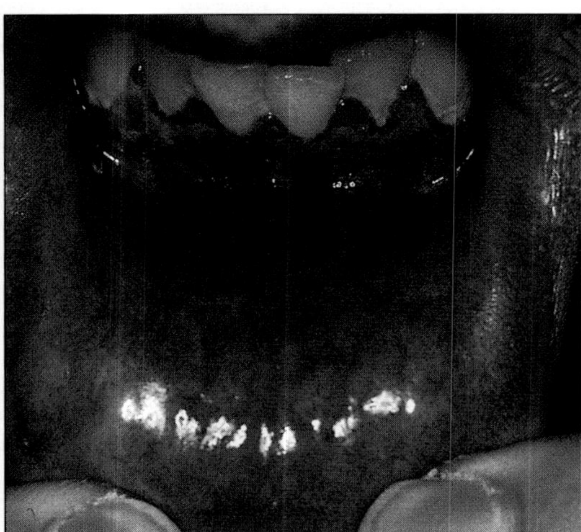

FIGURE 1-27 Mucocutaneous inflammation in primary HIV-1 infection. Mucocutaneous inflammation and ulceration are distinctive features of primary HIV-1 infection. Inflammation of the buccal mucosa and gingiva is common, and ulceration has been reported at these sites as well as the palate and esophagus. The ulcers are generally round or oval and sharply demarcated, with surrounding mucosa that appears normal [38–40].

Differential diagnoses of primary HIV-1 infection
Epstein-Barr virus mononucleosis
Cytomegalovirus mononucleosis
Toxoplasmosis
Rubella
Viral hepatitis
Secondary syphilis
Disseminated gonococcal infection
Primary herpes simplex virus infection
Other viral infection
Drug reaction

FIGURE 1-28 Differential diagnoses of primary HIV-1 infection. Although originally described as "mononucleosis-like" and still described as such in the Centers for Disease Control and Prevention classification system of HIV-1 disease, symptomatic primary HIV-1 infection is a distinct and recognizable clinical syndrome [41]. The skin rash associated with primary HIV-1 infection is a valuable differential diagnostic aid. Skin eruptions are rare in patients with Epstein-Barr virus infection (unless antibiotics have been given), toxoplasmosis, and cytomegalovirus infection and do not affect the palms and soles in patients with rubella. Mucocutaneous ulceration is a fairly distinctive finding because it is unusual in most of the other differential diagnoses.

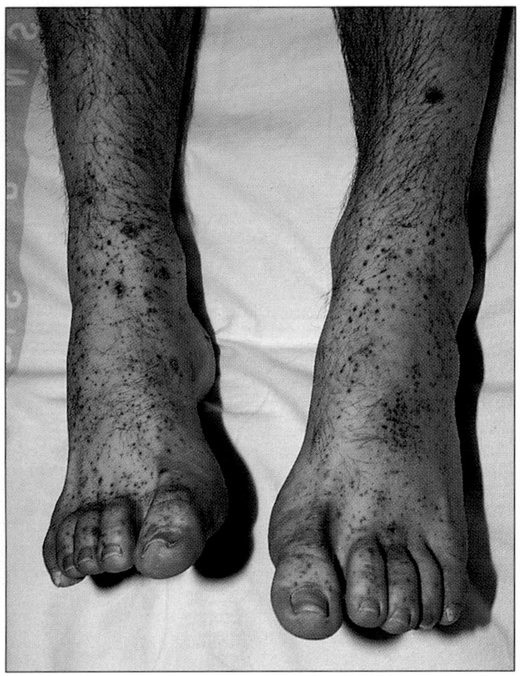

FIGURE 1-29 HIV vasculitis. This patient demonstrates cutaneous vasculitis, which occurred prior to the development of an AIDS-defining illness. A wide range of inflammatory vascular diseases have been described in patients infected with HIV at all stages of the illness. These have included necrotizing arteritis, polyarteritis nodosa, Henoch-Schönlein purpura, and drug-induced hypersensitivity vasculitis. The systemic vasculitis seen in HIV-infected patients most commonly involves the skin, peripheral nerves, skeletal muscles, and central nervous system [42].

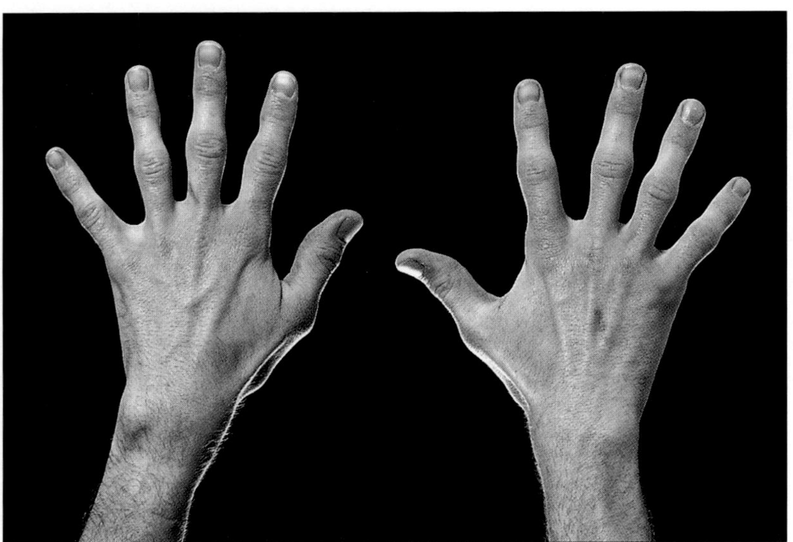

FIGURE 1-30 HIV polyarthritis. A symmetric polyarthritis involving the small joints of both hands developed prior to the onset of an AIDS-defining illness in this patient. In a prospective study, the musculoskeletal system was found to be involved in 70% of patients with HIV infection, with active arthritis developing in 24%. Although arthralgias are the most common manifestation, other associated disorders appear to be reactive arthritis, including Reiter's syndrome, psoriatic arthritis, Sjögren's syndrome, polymyositis, and necrotizing vasculitis. Oligoarthritis affecting the lower limbs appears to be the most common form of arthritis, but an inflammatory polyarthritis in HIV patients has been increasingly recognized in populations such as Africans in Zimbabwe, where rheumatologic disorders are uncommon [43–45].

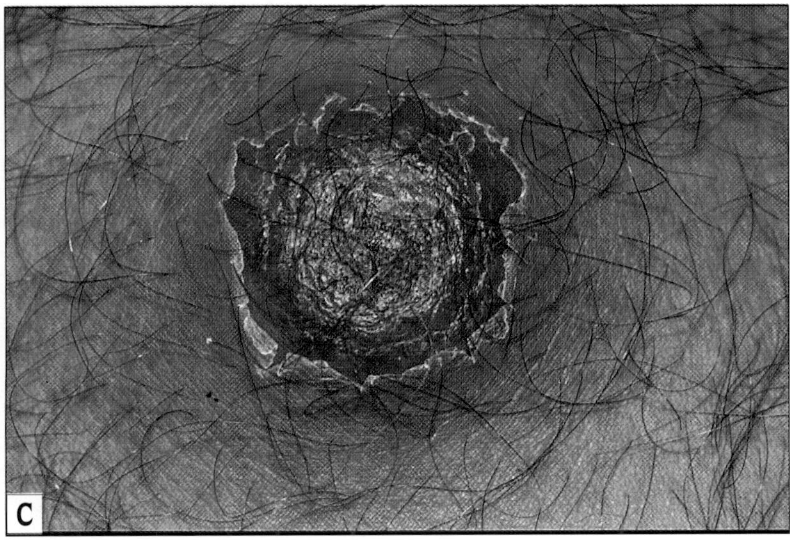

FIGURE 1-31 Unusual skin manifestations. Cryptococcosis, cytomegalovirus disease, and non-Hodgkin's lymphoma (shown here) are common AIDS illnesses that generally present when immune deficiency is severe (CD4+ T-lymphocyte count < 100/μL). Although unusual, all three conditions can manifest as skin lesions. Non-Hodgkin's lymphoma was diagnosed following biopsy of a large (4–5 cm diameter), partly necrotic lesion involving the lower limb.

Cutaneous Manifestations

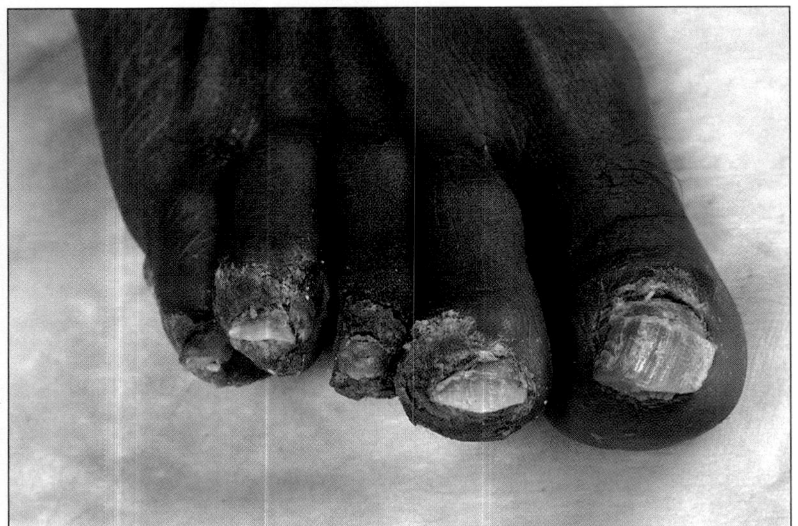

Figure 1-32 Onychomycosis. Tinea infections of the nails usually cause marked thickening and discoloration with opacification of several nails in these patients. Although topical antifungal preparations are not useful, systemic antifungal agents such as Lamisil, fluconazole, and itraconazole are effective treatment for fungal infections of the nails. In general, those patients who are prone to such fungal infections tend to have rather extensive involvement of their skin and nails, which is resistant to the conventional forms of treatment.

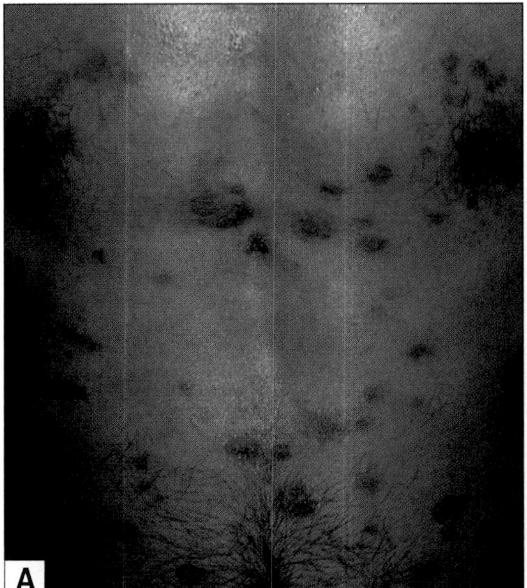

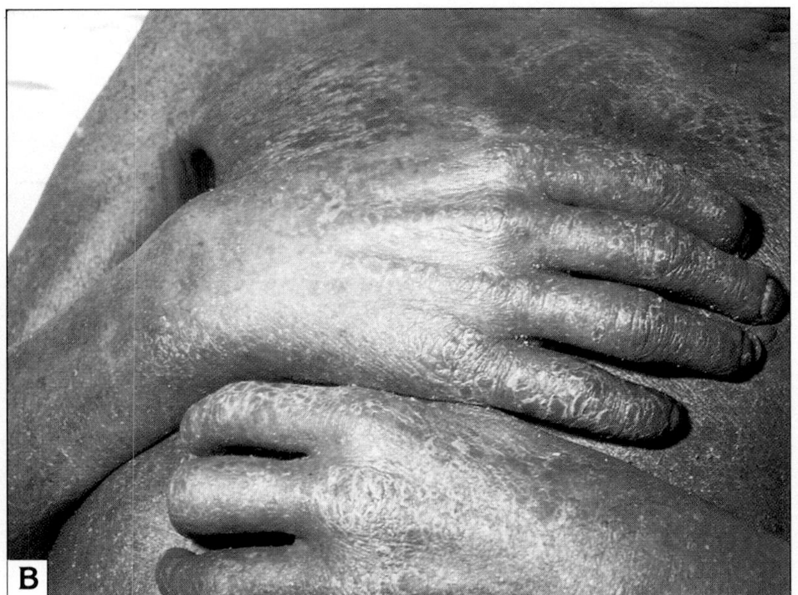

Figure 1-33 Psoriasis. Those AIDS patients who have a prior history of psoriasis often experience a worsening of the symptoms of this condition as their HIV disease progresses. Some HIV-infected patients who have never had psoriasis may suddenly develop this condition. **A**, Psoriasis in the HIV-infected host tends to be more severe, characterized by widely disseminated, thickened, salmon-colored plaques, with superimposed thick adherent and silvery scales located over the glabrous skin and scalp. **B**, Generalized, exfoliative psoriatic erythroderma may be seen in the HIV-infected host as well. "Psoriatic arthritis," usually involving the distal phalanges joints, may occur. The nails on the feet and hands are frequently "pitted" and thickened, and they take on a yellowish opaque color, which mimics onychomycosis. The vigorous use of topical tar preparations and high-potency topical steroid creams, as well as ultraviolet light or PUVA therapy, conventionally used for psoriasis, may only be partially effective in alleviating this condition in patients with HIV disease.

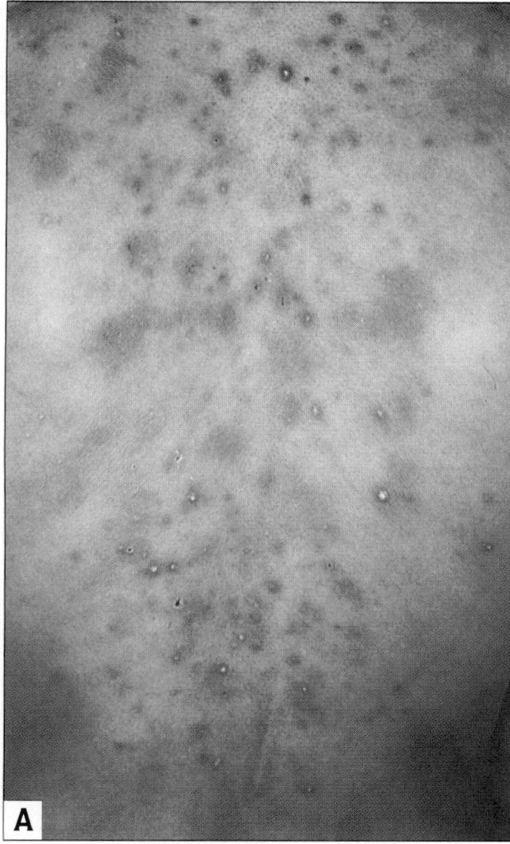

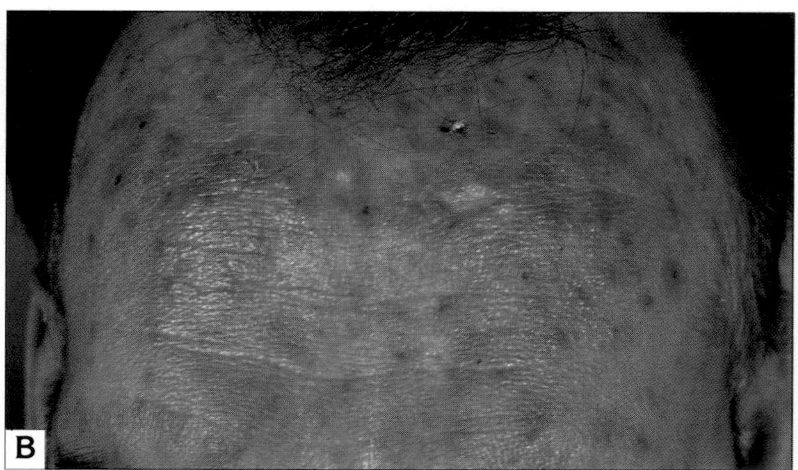

Figure 1-34 "Itchy red bump disease" (pruritic papular dermatoses of HIV disease) and eosinophilic pustular folliculitis. **A**, A common skin condition seen in HIV-infected persons is characterized by discrete "itchy red bumps," perifollicular papules that initially appear to be pustular or acneiform but rapidly become excoriated. This rash is most frequently seen on the chest, back, and face but may be widespread on other parts of the body. An unrelenting pruritus is usually associated with this eruption. It may appear at any time during the course of disease in the HIV-infected host. **B**, A particular variant of the "itchy red bump disease" associated with HIV infection is known as *eosinophilic pustular folliculitis*. Histologically, biopsy specimens of these lesions show a perifollicular inflammatory infiltrate, which frequently includes an abundance of eosinophils surrounding the hairbulb; however, eosinophils are often not present in these papules. Treatment includes the use of various topical steroid creams or lotions containing 0.25% menthol and 0.25% phenol, which may provide temporary relief for the severe itching that accompanies these conditions. Various antihistamines and hydroxyzine (10–50 mg given every 4–6 hours) may be helpful and can provide temporary relief. About 30% to 60% of patients with this condition respond to the antifungal drug itraconazole (Sporanox, 200 mg three times daily), although there is no evidence that any fungal organism is involved in this condition.

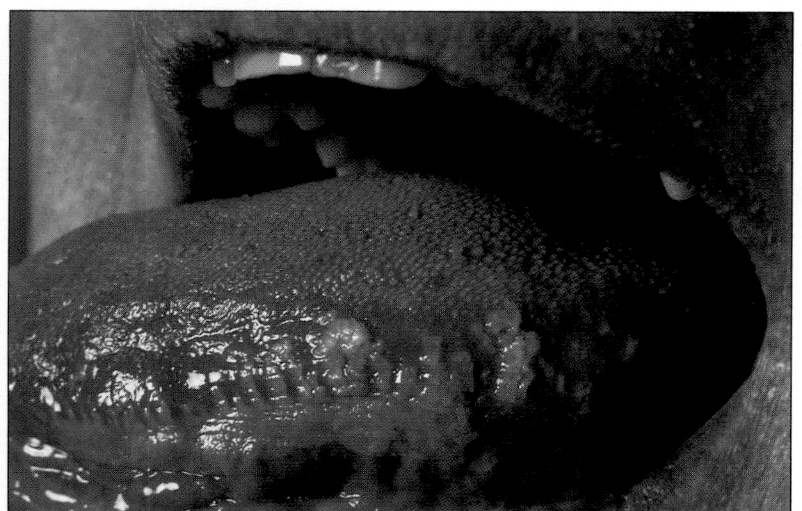

Figure 1-35 Oral hairy leukoplakia. The appearance of symptomatic verrucous white excrescences on the lateral margins of the tongue (hairy leukoplakia) is frequently seen in HIV-positive persons, often prior to the development of symptomatic HIV disease. These lesions are believed to be due to the Epstein-Barr virus, which is found to be present under electron microscopic examination. Occasionally, such lesions occur on the other mucosal surfaces of the mouth. The lesions clinically mimic "thrush" but are not readily scraped off as with oral candidiasis.

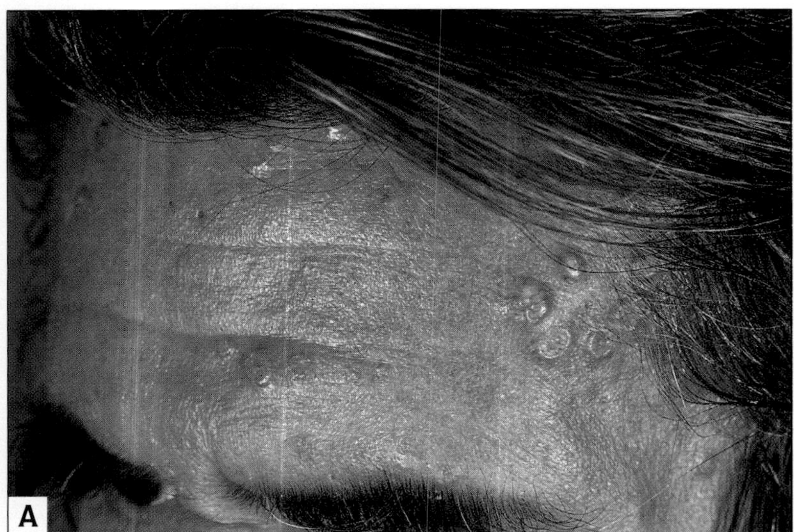

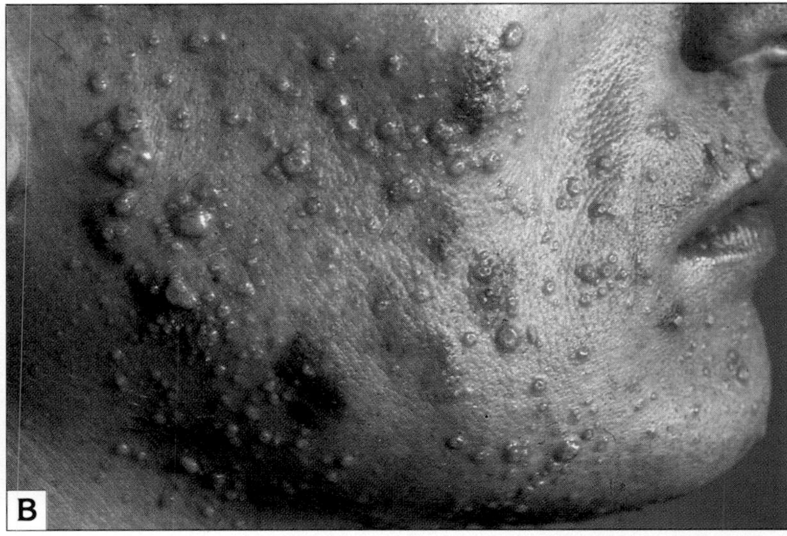

FIGURE 1-36 Molluscum contagiosum. Widespread papular skin lesions of molluscum contagiosum, which is due to the human poxvirus, are frequently seen in HIV-infected hosts, especially those with low $CD4^+$ lymphocyte counts. **A** and **B**, The asymptomatic, "waxy," skin-colored to pink papules of molluscum contagiosum (*panel 36A*), which can vary in size from 1 mm to > 1 cm, are often found widely scattered on the skin or form localized clusters, sometimes coalescing into "giant" molluscum lesions (*panel 36B*). In the center of each papule is a slightly depressed crusted "core," which when squeezed exudes a "cheesy" white matter. Local destructive surgical treatments including curettage and electrocauterization are usually effective, although immunocompromised patients tend to develop new lesions throughout the course of their illness. The skin lesions of disseminated systematic fungal infections such as cryptococcosis may mimic molluscum contagiosum in AIDS patients.

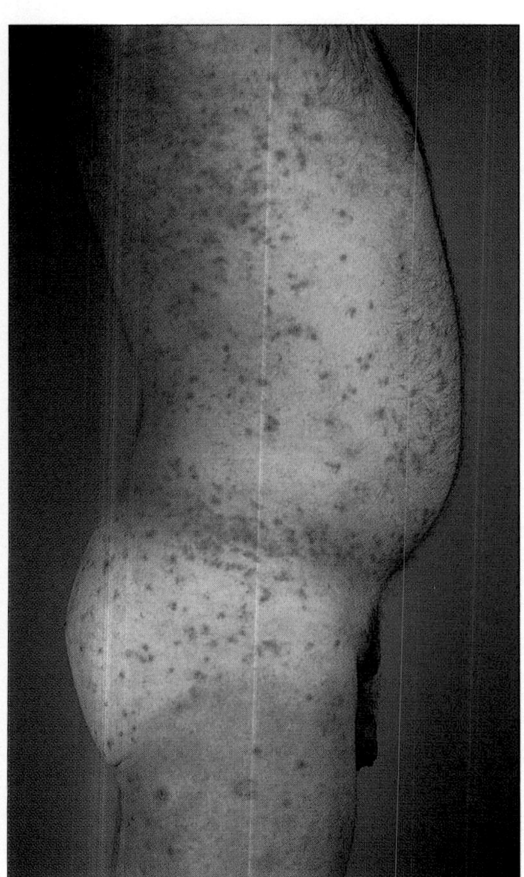

FIGURE 1-37 Scabies. Ectoparasitic infection of the skin with scabies tend to be more severe and widespread in patients who are immunocompromised. Widespread excoriated pruritic, tiny red papules develop that are usually more concentrated in the anogenital regions (especially the glans penis), wrist, axillae, waist, webs between the fingers, as well as the intertriginous folds. Microscopic examination of the scrapings or biopsy specimens from these papules reveal the presence of scabitic mites *Sarcoptes scabiei* and their eggs located within burrows in the epidermis. Repeated topical treatments with lindane (Kwell), crotamiton (Eurax), or permethrin (Elimite) will usually rid the host of infestation. The itchy red papules may persist for sometime despite adequate treatment, due to a localized delayed hypersensitivity reaction to the residual proteins from the killed parasites within the skin. In such cases, both the physician and patient often assume that the infestation has not been adequately treated. Such posttreatment reactions are effectively treated with an antihistamine and the topical application of topical steroid creams, until the symptoms subside.

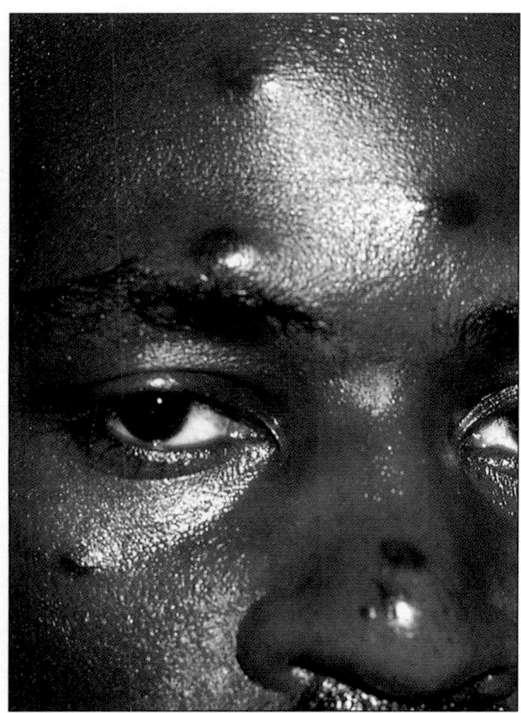

FIGURE 1-38 Bacillary epithelioid angiomatosis (BEA). BEA is an unusual infection characterized by multiple, tender, red vascular lesions of the skin and subcutaneous tissues caused by *Bartonella henselae*, a species of *Rickettsia* closely related to the organisms that cause "cat scratch" disease. This agent is sensitive to a variety of systemic antibiotics including erythromycin and tetracycline. The vascular proliferative lesions of BEA are most frequently seen in the skin but also occur subcutaneously and can involve the internal organs in patients with AIDS. These skin lesions may clinically resemble those of Kaposi's sarcoma, although histologically, BEA is similar to pyogenic granuloma rather than Kaposi's sarcoma. The causative organisms of BEA are readily detectable in specially stained tissue sections. The skin lesions of BEA can also mimic the skin eruption associated with verruca peruana due to infection with another bacteria, *Bartonella* sp. Because BEA can be fatal, early diagnosis and initiation of appropriate antibiotic treatment can be life-saving.

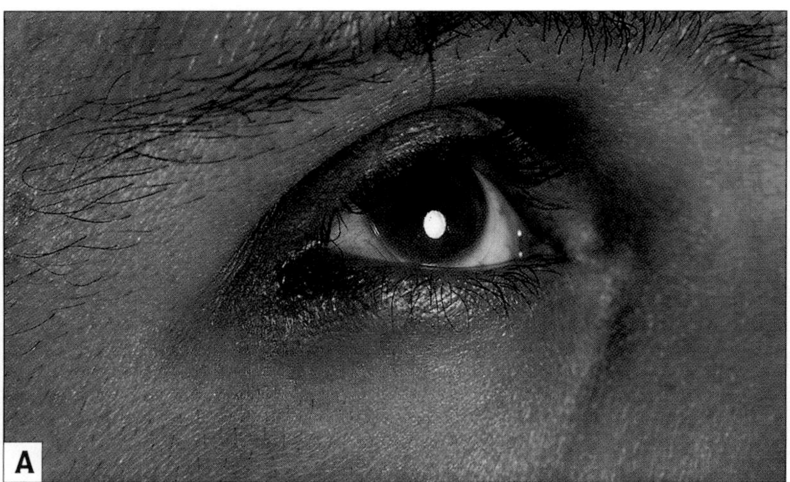

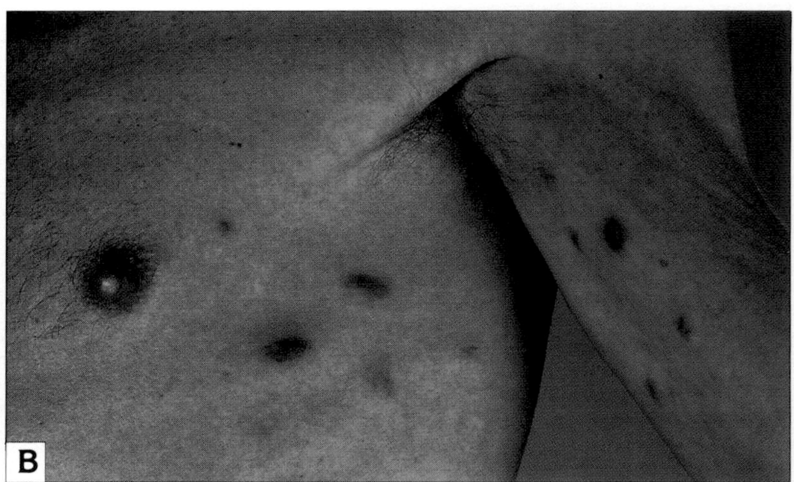

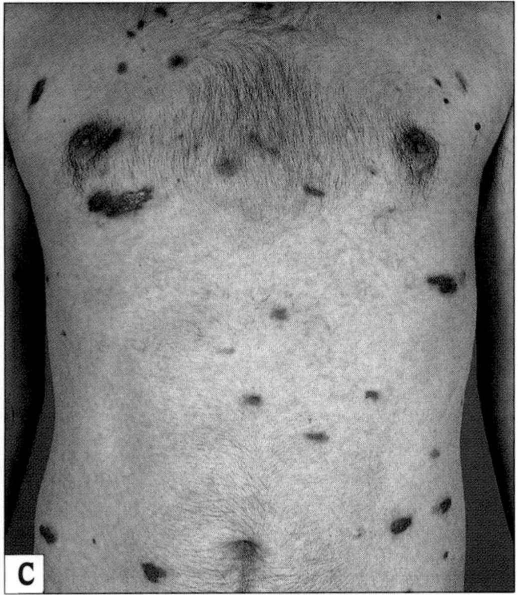

FIGURE 1-39 AIDS-related Kaposi's sarcoma. An aggressive and disseminated form of Kaposi's sarcoma is the most frequently reported neoplastic disorder associated with AIDS. Remarkably, 95% of all of the AIDS-related "epidemic" form of Kaposi's sarcoma occurring in North America, Europe, and Australia has been seen among homosexual or bisexual men, suggesting that in this population, Kaposi's sarcoma may be due to a sexually transmissible agent other than HIV. The Kaposi's sarcoma tumors are seen most often on the skin and mucosa as asymptomatic, pink to deep purple or dark brown, round to oval-shaped patches, which eventually become thickened plaques and nodular tumors. They appear as single lesions or in clusters, at the same or distant sites. **A**, A faint early patch-stage lesion, which resembles a bruise, can even occur in the lower eyelid area. **B** and **C**, Remarkably, in AIDS patients, the lesions almost always have a symmetric distribution over the skin along the lines of skin cleavage.

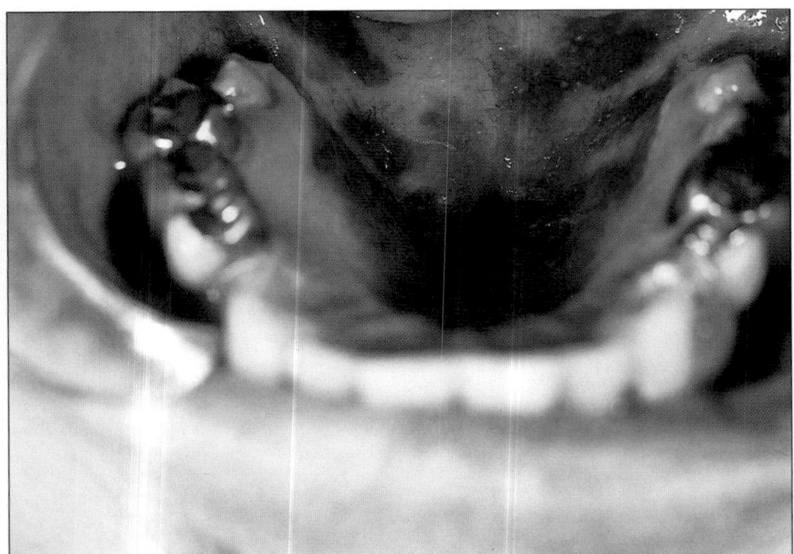

Figure 1-40 Oral Kaposi's sarcoma lesions are usually flat asymptomatic patches or plaques on the hard or soft palate. Nodular tumor lesions on the oral mucosa, including the pharynx, tongue, or gingival, can interfere with swallowing and speech. These lesions tend to ulcerate and bleed, become secondarily infected, and be very painful. Although usually asymptomatic, tumor lesions of the gastrointestinal tract may cause occasional bleeding.

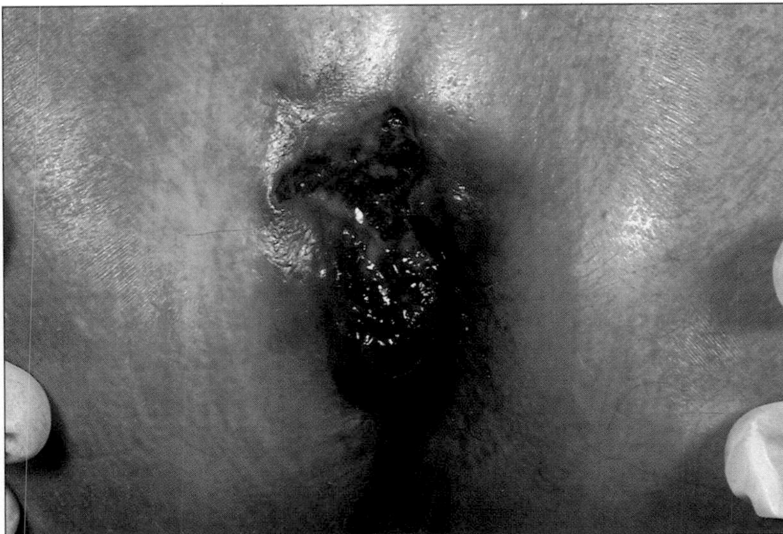

Figure 1-41 B-cell lymphoma of the skin. Patients with AIDS have an increased incidence of lymphomas, occurring in about 3% of the cases. On rare occasion, cutaneous lesions of lymphomas are seen; in this patient, a large nodular tumor suddenly developed, which proved to be a B-cell lymphoma of the skin, associated with a disseminated lymph node and eventually brain involvement.

Ophthalmic Manifestations

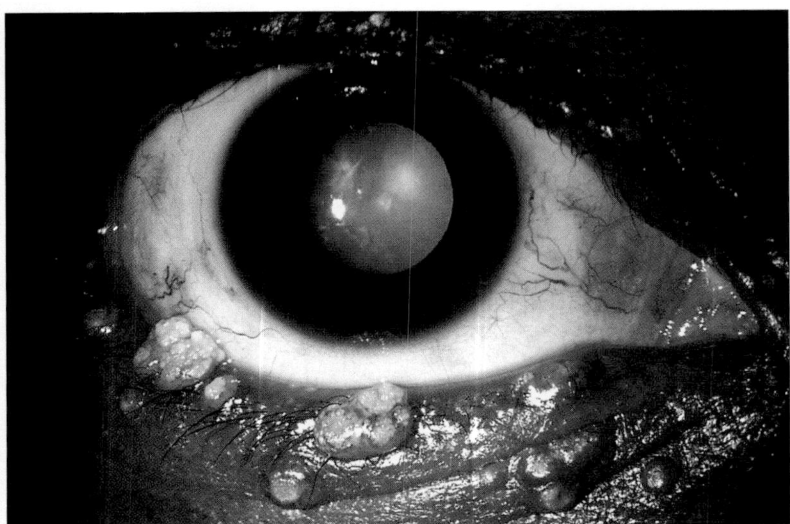

Figure 1-42 Molluscum contagiosum of the eyelid margin. Progressive infection of the eyelids and face with this large DNA pox virus is associated in HIV-infected patients with advanced stages of AIDS [46]. Secondary keratoconjunctivitis can occur; epibulbar nodules are rare. Curettage, local excision, and cryotherapy can be attempted for eyelid margin lesions but recurrence is likely [47]. Recurrence may occur because of subclinical infection of epidermis up to 1.0 cm lateral to clinically visible lesions.

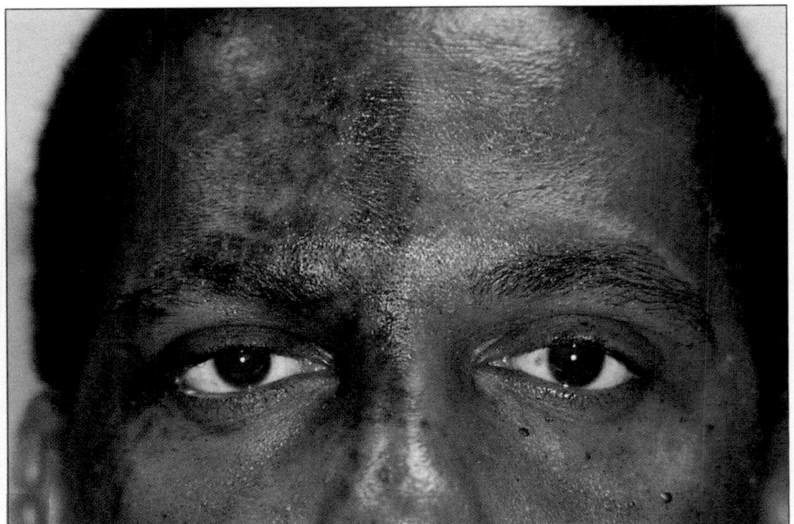

Figure 1-43 Herpes zoster ophthalmicus (HZO). A 38-year-old Haitian man was diagnosed with HIV infection after presenting with HZO. Intravenous acyclovir was begun 6 days after the vesicular eruption, and the skin lesions are shown healed 1 month after treatment. Punctate keratopathy and corneal anesthesia of the right eye developed, but elevated intraocular pressure was not documented. HZO in young adults may be a marker of early HIV infection or of AIDS [48]. Complications such as optic neuritis and retinitis may be more common in the HIV-infected population [49]. Treatment with intravenous acyclovir has been recommended for patients in whom HIV infection is suspected or confirmed. Two weeks after onset, while on acyclovir, the patient noted decreased vision in the right eye consistent with zoster-related retrobulbar optic neuritis [50]. The right optic nerve was cupped with pallor. The vision was counting fingers in a small temporal island. The left optic nerve was normal in appearance. Vision was 20/15.

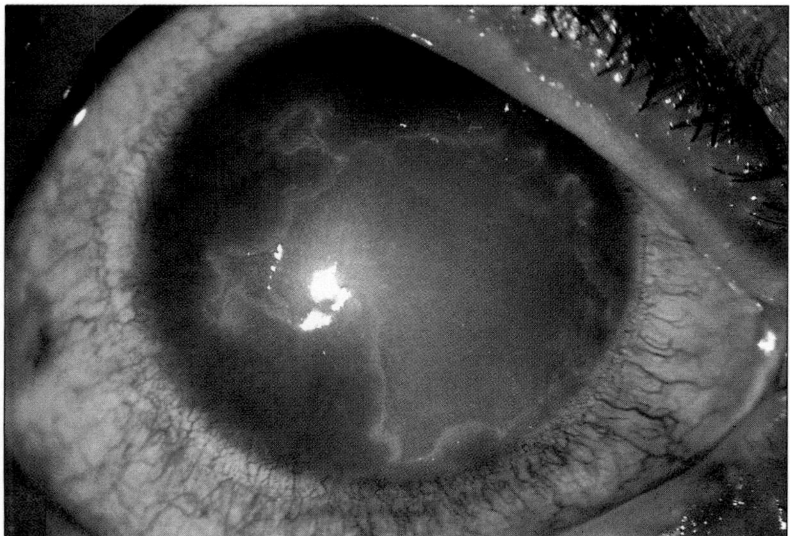

Figure 1-44 Herpes simplex keratitis. Nonhealing corneal ulcer of the right eye due to culture-positive herpes simplex I infection in a 15-year-old woman with AIDS dementia. Treatment with oral acyclovir, topical trifluridine, vidarabine, or idoxuridine for 2 months failed to sterilize the cornea. Interferon alfa-2A, 12 MU/mL, was given as a topical eye drop twice daily. Complete healing of the corneal ulcer after 3 weeks of treatment with interferon topical drops [51] was observed. Dendritic herpes simplex virus infection of the left cornea developed subsequently. Stromal scars and neovascularization from previous recurrences are seen. Frequent recurrences of dendritiform or geographic herpetic infections with prolonged healing times on topical antivirals may be typical for HIV infection [52].

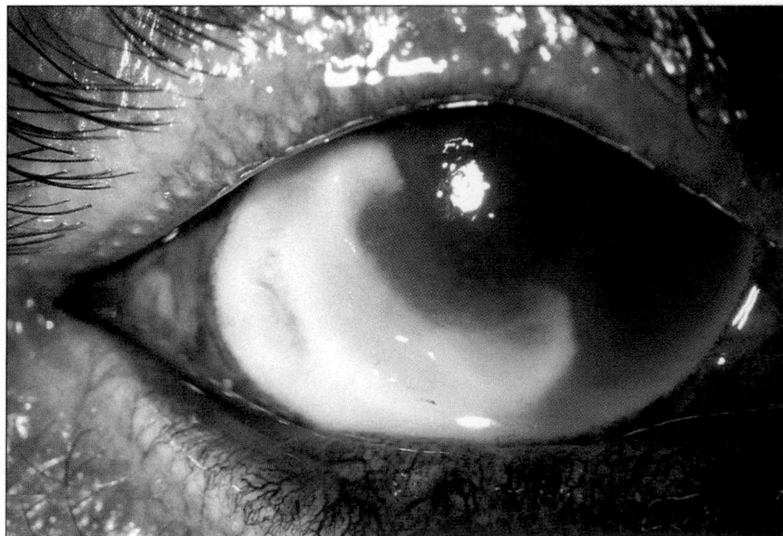

Figure 1-45 Pseudomonas sclerokeratitis. The patient presented with a 10-day history of pain and eyelid erythema and edema (not shown). The pseudomonas ulcer involved the peripheral cornea and extended into the sclera. Intensive topical and intravenous therapy with tobramycin and ceftazidime for 10 days as well as local cryotherapy failed to sterilize the eye. Progressive necrosis of the sclera with impending perforation occurred and enucleation was recommended [53].

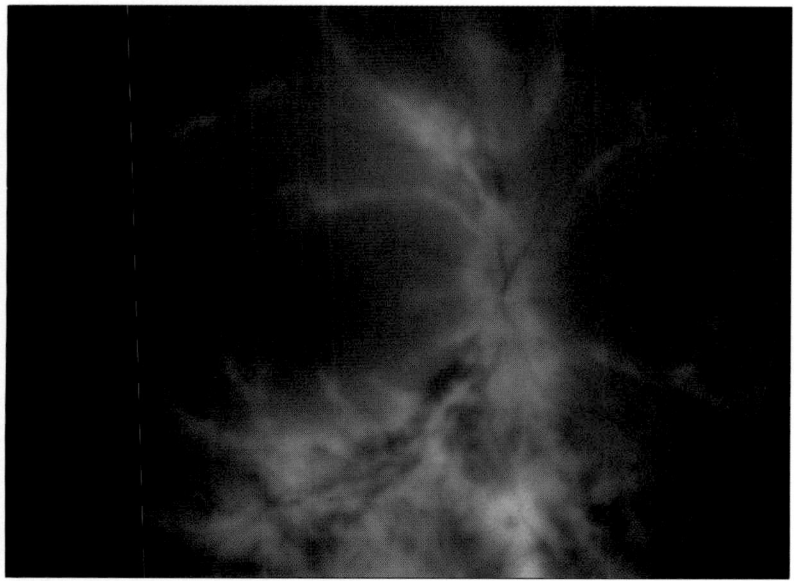

Figure 1-46 Fulminant, edematous cytomegalovirus retinitis complicated by a mild vitreous reaction and diffuse periphlebitis or "frosted branch angiitis" [54]. Two months later, the retinitis was in remission on ganciclovir, 5 mg/kg daily. The retinal vessels appeared normal. The median time to complete response to medication was 31 ± 10 days [55]. Recurrent retinitis with progression into new areas of retina was noted after 150 days of therapy. The median time to progression after treatment is started is 60 days [56]. Despite an increase in ganciclovir dose, the retinitis continued to progress and a new lesion appeared next to the optic nerve head. In addition, retinal detachment became present in the temporal half of the retina due to hole formation in the area of active retinitis. Retinal detachment occurs in about 25% of patients with cytomegalovirus retinitis [57].

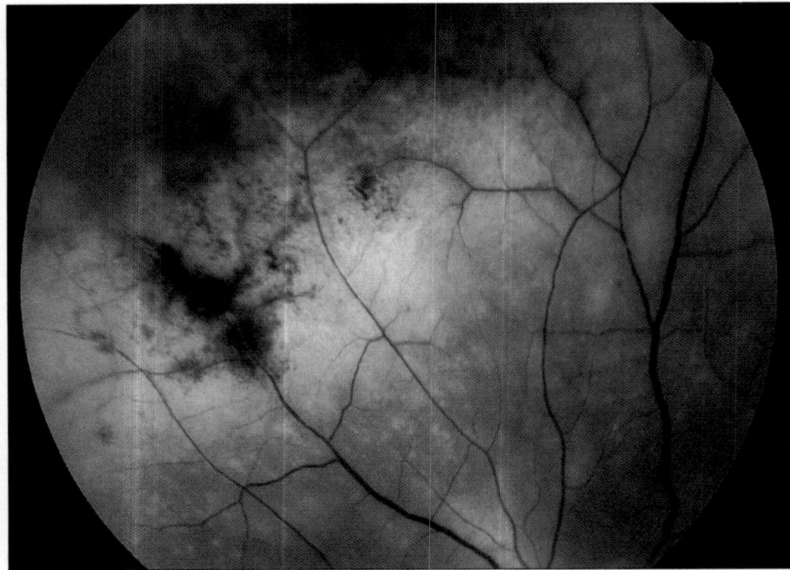

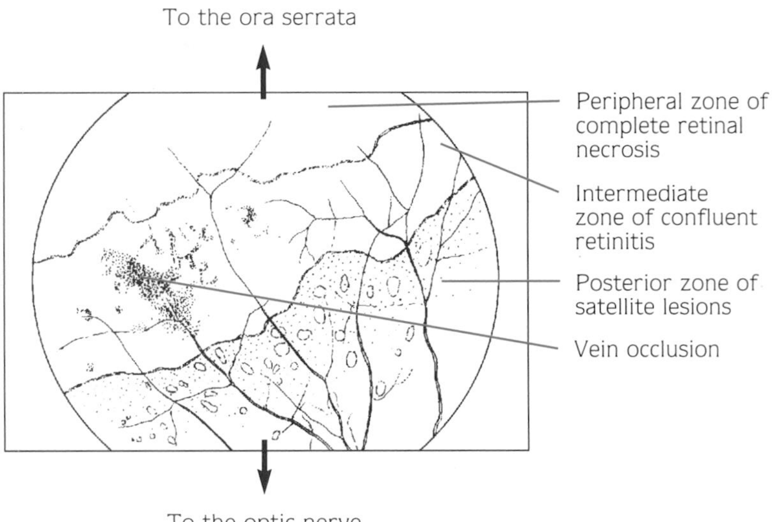

FIGURE 1-47 Confluent, peripheral, herpetic necrotizing retinitis in the left eye. Older, total necrosis of the retina is seen at the top of the frame, confluent retinal whitening with venous obstruction in the middle of the frame, and fresh, large, indistinct lesions of retinitis at the bottom of the frame. For orientation, the peripheral edge of the retina (ora serrata) is superior to the frame and the optic nerve is inferior to the frame. The photograph demonstrates the orderly progression of the retinitis from peripheral to posterior retina in approximately 60° wedge; all 360° of the retinal periphery were similarly involved in both eyes. Treatment consisted of combination therapy with intravenous foscarnet and ganciclovir and retinal detachment repair with silicone oil. The patient retains ambulatory vision in the left eye 9 months after onset. The right eye is blind.

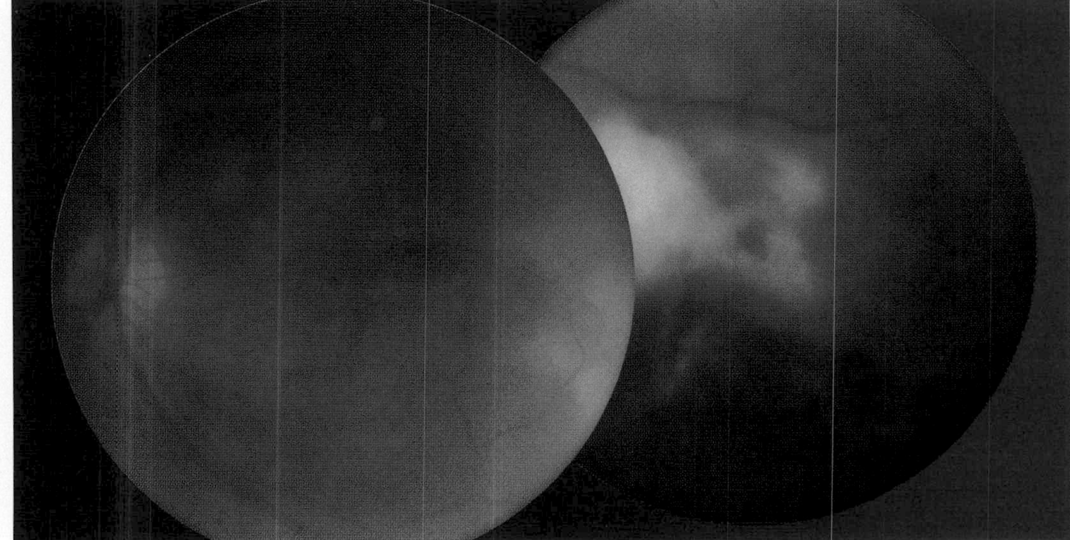

FIGURE 1-48 Toxoplasmic chorioretinitis. This episode is the second reactivation of toxoplasmic chorioretinitis in this 32-year-old man. The first episode was complicated by retinal detachment, which was successfully repaired with 20/25 vision. The chorioretinitis remained under good control on sulfadiazine 500 mg twice daily and pyrimethamine 25 mg daily for 4 years. Reactivation occurred suddenly with decrease in vision to 4/200 due to vitreous cellular inflammation and subretinal fluid exudation in the macula. The figure is hazy due to vitreous opacification. Dark gray pigmentation corresponds to the old, healed lesion. The yellow exudate is the active lesion. The marked vitreous opacification, large amount of subretinal exudation, full-thickness involvement of retina, and response to increased doses of sulfadiazine and pyrimethamine distinguish this lesion from the more common cytomegalovirus retinitis. Clindamycin or atovaquone are possible alternate treatments in patients who cannot tolerate sulfa medications [58–60].

Oral Cavity Manifestations

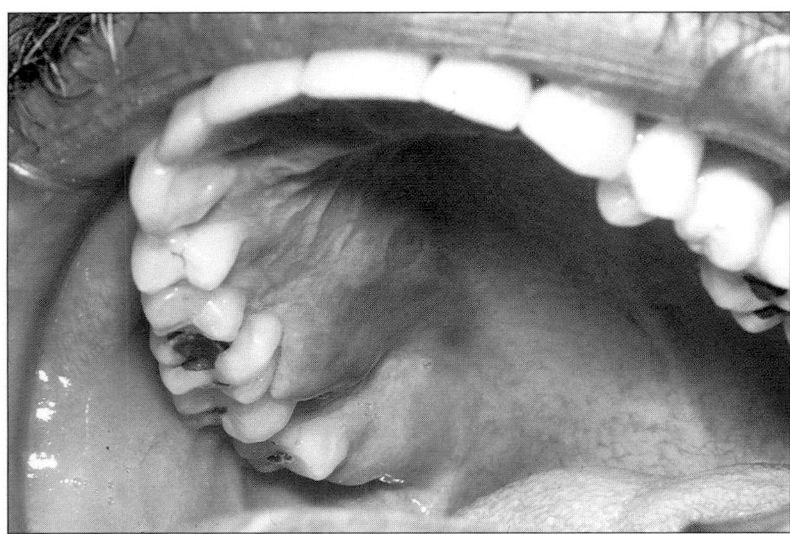

Figure 1-49 Kaposi's sarcoma of the palate. The oral mucosa is one of the commonest sites for Kaposi's sarcoma and is often the first or presenting location, with the palate being the most common intraoral site. A nodular purple lesion is seen in this patient, but larger lesions may ulcerate and can become secondarily infected. These lesions can be treated with intralesional chemotherapy, *eg*, vinblastine. Very extensive lesions may warrant radiation therapy [61,62].

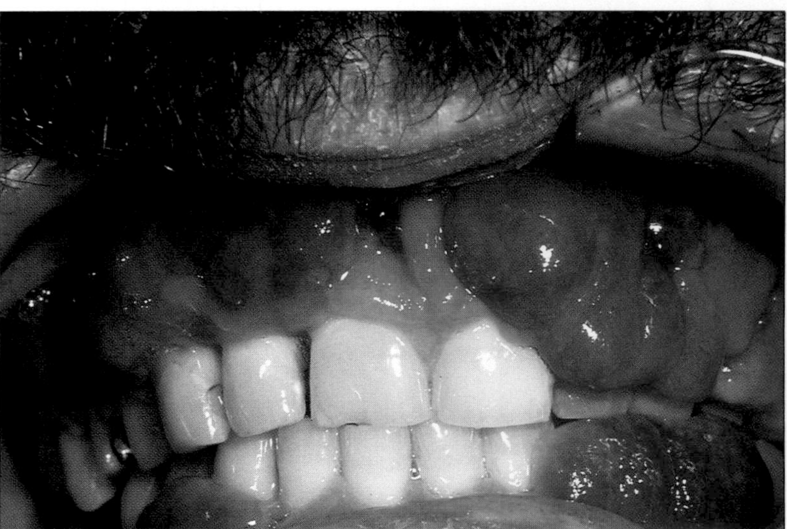

Figure 1-50 Kaposi's sarcoma of the maxillary and mandibular gingiva. Multiple and extensive nodular purple lesions are apparent on the gingiva in this patient. The gingiva is the second commonest intraoral site, and these lesions often become infected with dental plaque microorganisms, causing severe pain. Careful debridement, scaling, and curettage result in reduction of inflammation, making surgical excision or radiotherapy more effective.

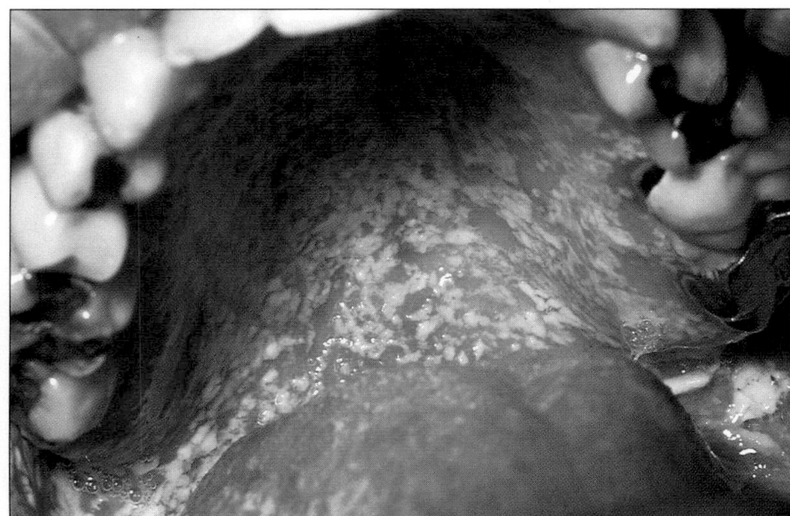

Figure 1-51 Pseudomembranous candidiasis of the palate. A creamy-white plaque consisting of fungal hyphae, desquamated epithelial cells, and polymorphonuclear cells can be easily removed, leaving a red surface. These lesions can appear at any location in the mouth and oropharynx. There may be symptoms of burning or changes in taste [63].

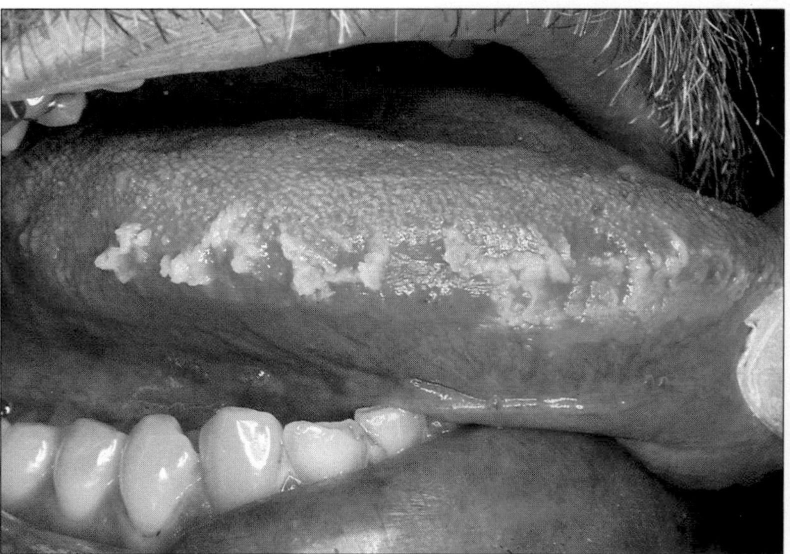

Figure 1-52 Hairy leukoplakia of the tongue. The lesion, consisting of corrugations on the lateral margin continuous with flat areas on the ventral surface, is seen most commonly on the lateral tongue. Originally described in HIV-positive individuals, in whom it is common, hairy leukoplakia has now been seen in a number of other immunodeficient groups, including transplant recipients and those on long-term steroid therapy. Like oral candidiasis, hairy leukoplakia is predictive of progression to AIDS in HIV-infected individuals [64–67].

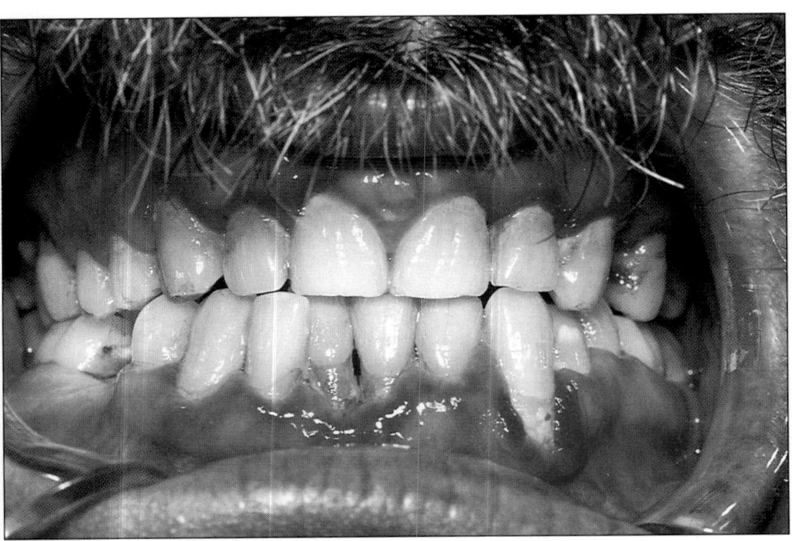

Figure 1-53 Necrotizing periodontitis ("HIV periodontitis"). This rapidly destructive inflammation, seen here on the anterior mandible, is associated with the same wide range of anaerobic bacteria as is found in conventional periodontal disease in immunocompetent individuals. The lesions respond to thorough local debridement (scaling and root planing) plus local antibacterial irrigation supplemented with systemic antibiotics [68,69].

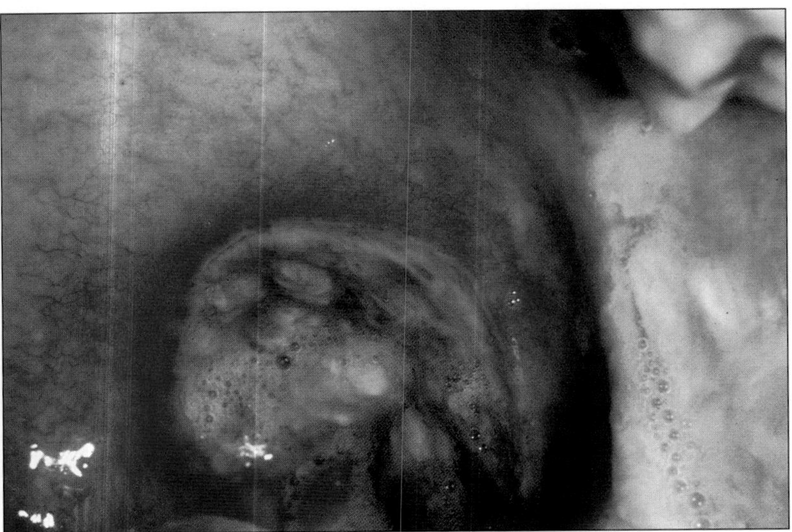

Figure 1-54 Severe major recurrent aphthous ulcers. Such lesions, as seen on the right soft palate in this patient, can be the cause of significant pain and difficulty with speech, mastication, and swallowing. Biopsy is usually indicated to rule out lymphoma and other chronic ulcerative lesions. A recent clinical study (ACTG 251) has confirmed the efficacy of thalidomide.

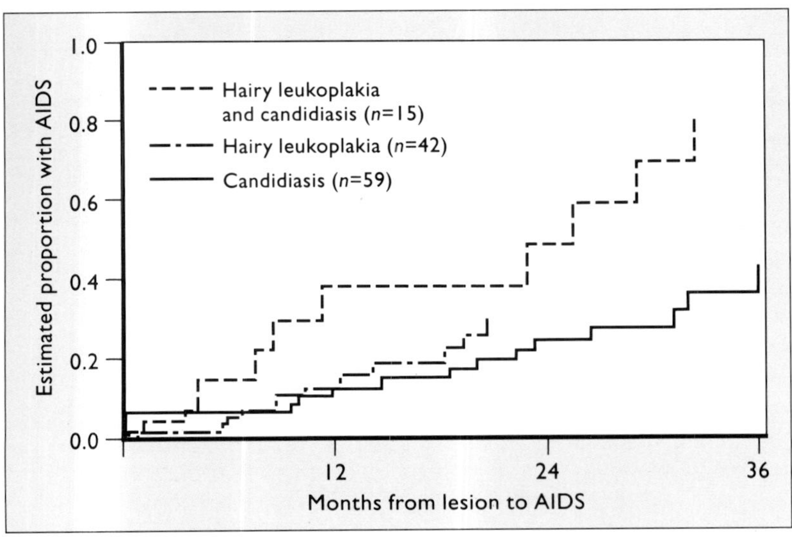

Figure 1-55 Progression to AIDS, according to the presence of oral manifestations. In three San Francisco cohorts, both oral candidiasis and hairy leukoplakia proved to be indicators of progression of HIV disease. After CD4 counts were adjusted for, men with hairy leukoplakia and candidiasis on baseline examinations had a significantly higher rate of progression to AIDS than men with normal oral findings. (*Adapted from* Katz *et al.* [67].)

PULMONARY COMPLICATIONS

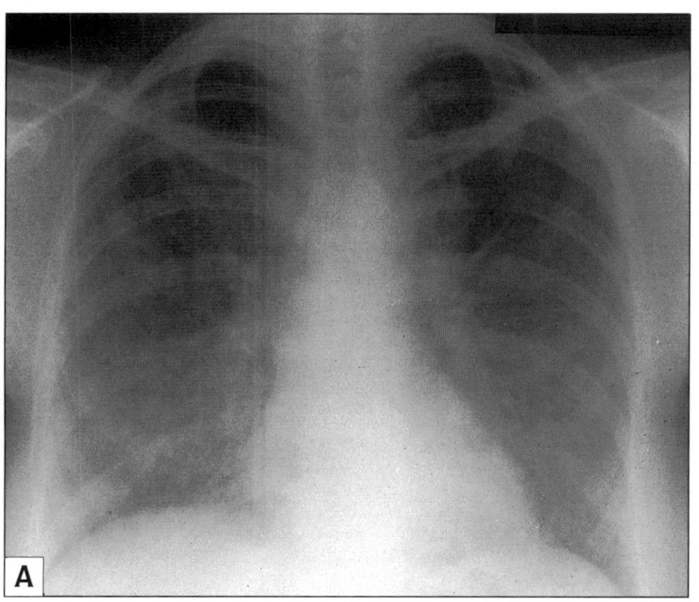

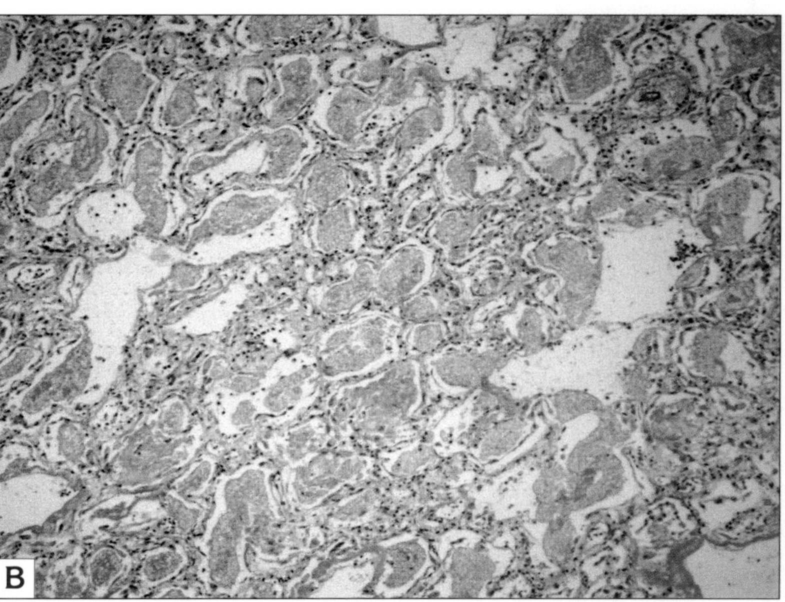

FIGURE 1-56 *Pneumocystis carinii* pneumonia. **A**, Chest radiograph showing typical changes of *P. carcinii* pneumonia. There are bilateral diffuse pulmonary infiltrates [70]. **B**, An open lung biopsy (hematoxylin-eosin stain) shows most alveoli are filled with foamy pink material, typical of *P. carinii* pneumonia. Profound ventilation-perfusion mismatching causes severe hypoxemia [71].

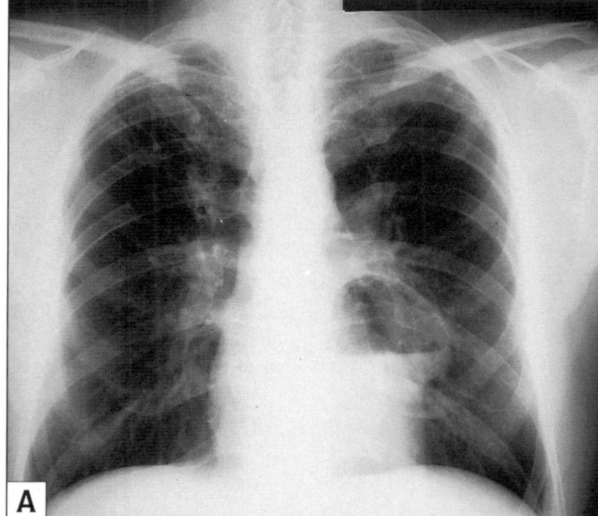

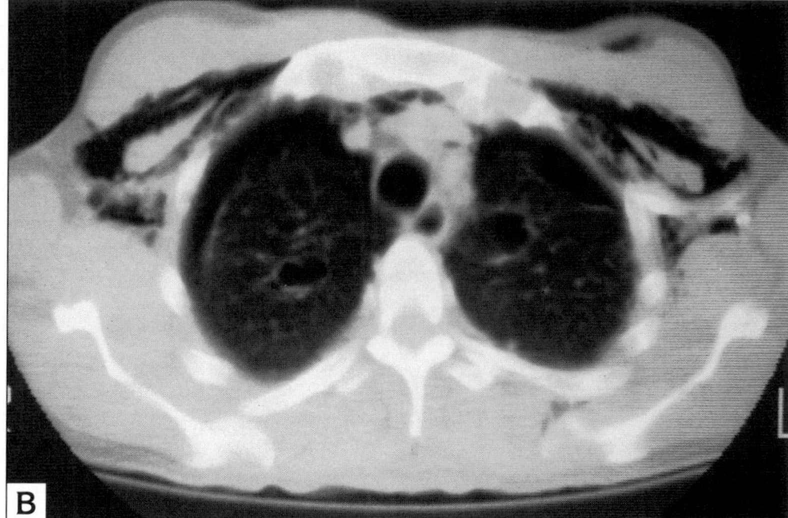

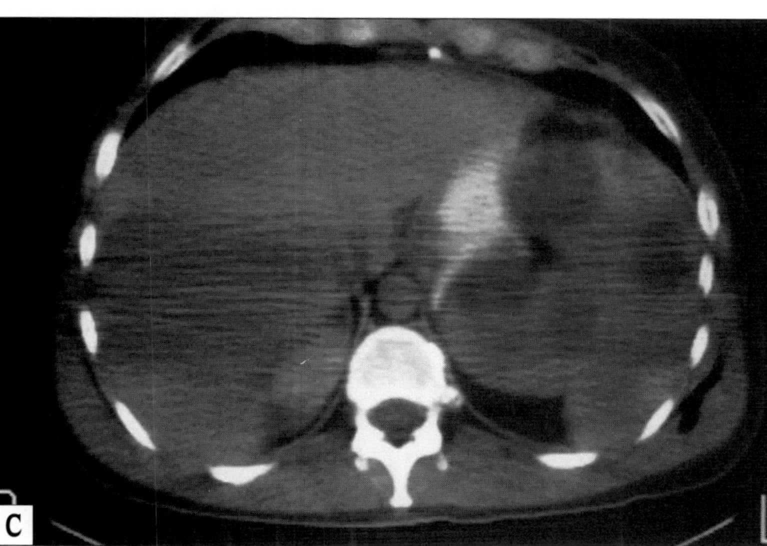

FIGURE 1-57 *Pneumocystis carinii* pneumonia in a patient receiving aerosolized pentamidine prophylaxis. **A**, Chest radiograph showing a large cystic space with an air-fluid level and bilateral upper lobe linear densities. Bronchoscopic washings confirmed the presence of *P. carinii* pneumonia. **B**, Computed tomography (CT) scan of the chest in the same patient shows cystic changes in both upper lung fields, small bilateral pneumothoraces, and subcutaneous emphysema. Upper lobe cystic changes and pneumothoraces are common complications of *P. carinii* pneumonia in patients taking aerosolized pentamidine prophylaxis [70]. **C**, CT scan of the abdomen in the same patient shows the presence of mass lesions in the spleen. These are presumed to be due to *P. carinii*, because they later resolved following anti-*Pneumocystis* treatment. Extrapulmonary *P. carinii* infection occurs more frequently in the setting of aerosolized pentamidine prophylaxis, presumably because the drug is distributed only to the lung.

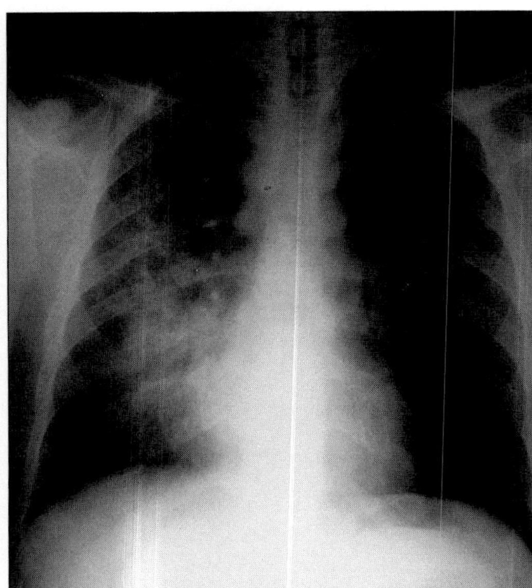

Figure 1-58 A chest radiograph in a patient with HIV infection and a low CD4 lymphocyte count (150×10^6/L) shows right lower lobe consolidation and paratracheal lymphadenopathy [72].

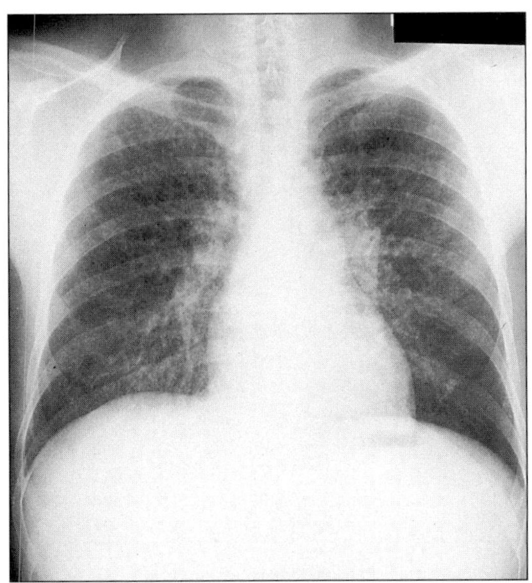

Figure 1-59 Miliary tuberculosis in a patient with HIV infection.

Gastrointestinal Manifestations

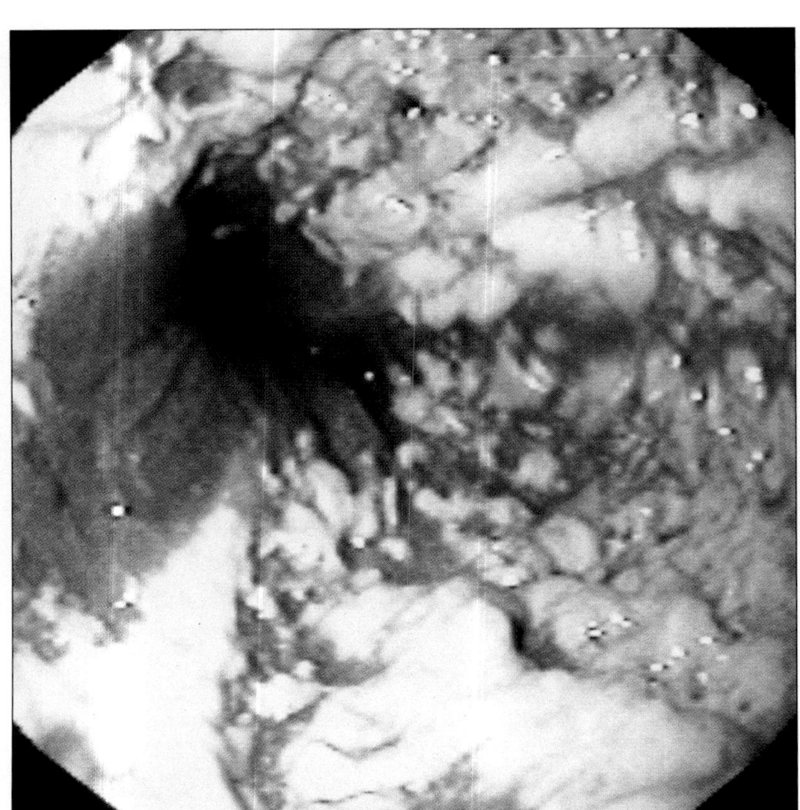

Figure 1-60 Candidal esophagitis. Manifestations of HIV infection extend throughout the gastrointestinal tract. Candidal infection of the oral cavity or thrush may be one of the first manifestations of immune compromise in an HIV-infected patient. Apthous ulcers of unclear etiology also occur. Some of these can be persistent, painful, and refractory to therapy, although some response to thalidomide has been seen. Esophagitis caused by *Candida albicans* is a frequent complication in AIDS patients and may develop as an extension of untreated oral thrush. The use of the effective oral prophylactic antifungal agent, fluconazole, has decreased the incidence of this opportunistic infection. Severe disease may also be treated by a short course of intravenous amphotericin B. The appearance of severe candidal esophagitis is distinctive as seen in this figure, but confirmation of the diagnosis depends on scrapings demonstrating the classic gram-positive candidal forms [73].

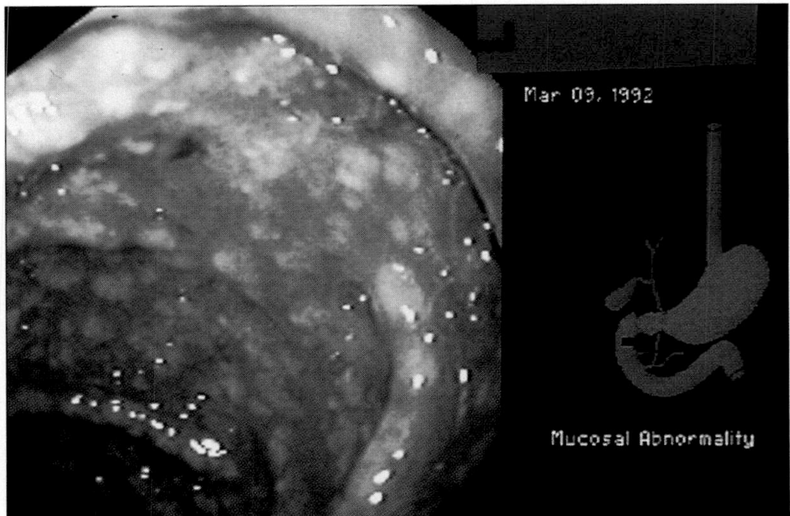

Figure 1-61 *Mycobacterium avium* complex may infiltrate the small bowel of AIDS patients with low CD4 counts. In addition to systemic symptoms such as fever, it may result in severe malabsorption with weight loss and diarrhea. Such malabsorption also complicates therapy, as the oral drugs routinely used to treat *M. avium* complex would be poorly absorbed in this situation. When biopsy and culture-proven infiltration of the small bowel occurs, therapy may need to include intravenous modalities as well, such as amikacin and one of the intravenous quinolones [74,75]. (*Courtesy of* D. Pleskow, MD.)

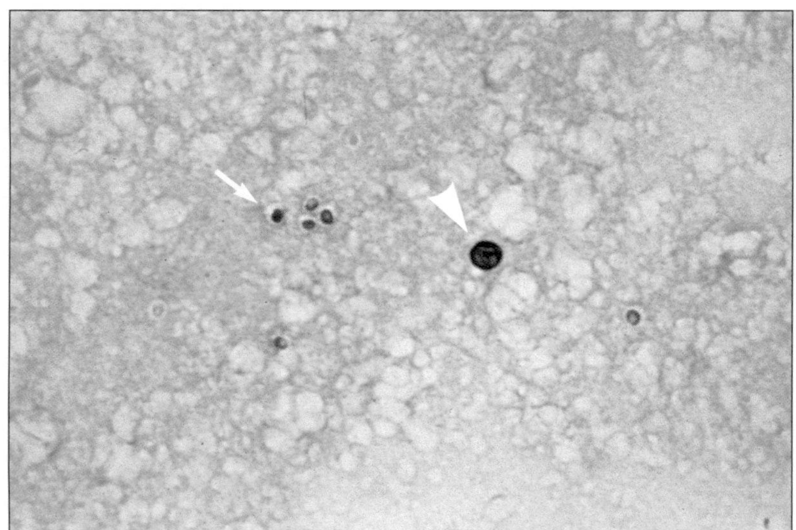

FIGURE 1-62 Cryptosporidial organisms. Cryptosporidial organisms (*arrow*) may be identified in stool by modified acid-fast stain or fluorescent antibody stains. *Cyclospora cayatenensis* (*arrowhead*) is a recently recognized parasite, which may also be detected by modified acid-fast stain. This organism has been described in travelers and in sporadic cases in noncompromised hosts, but is similar to cryptosporidium in the prolonged nature of the diarrheal illness in immunocompromised hosts. Other protozoan parasites, such as *Isospora belli*, *Giardia lamblia*, or the controversial *Blastocystis hominis*, may also be identified in stool by the modified acid-fast (*Isospora*) or trichrome stain [76,77]. (*Courtesy of* J. Fishman, MD.)

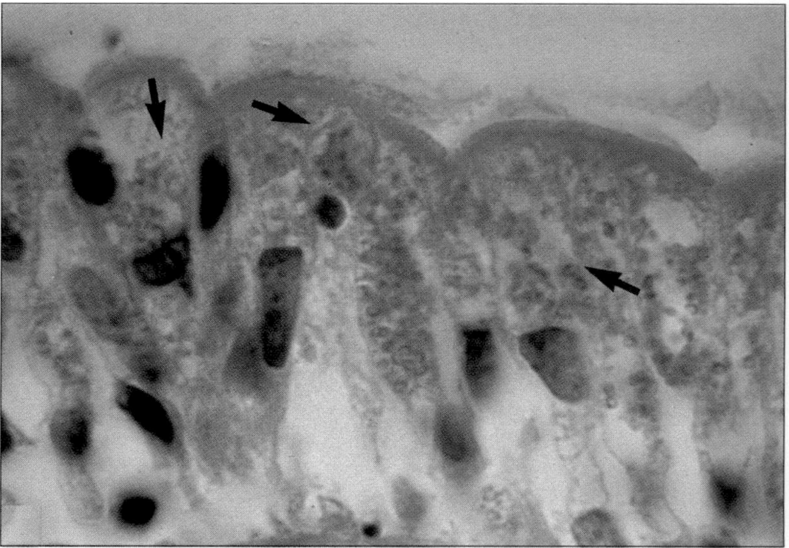

FIGURE 1-63 Microsporidiosis. Microsporidial species have been recently recognized as potentially associated with up to 40% to 50% of the persistent diarrhea seen in patients with advanced AIDS. Although several microsporidial species are able to infect humans, to date only two species are known to infect the intestine. These organisms primarily infect the small bowel. Microsporidial organisms may be missed on routine histopathologic examination, although to an experienced observer they are readily visible (as in this hematoxylin-eosin–stained biopsy section), where they may be expected to occur supranuclearly (*arrows*). Speciation of microsporidia cannot be done at a light microscopic level [78].

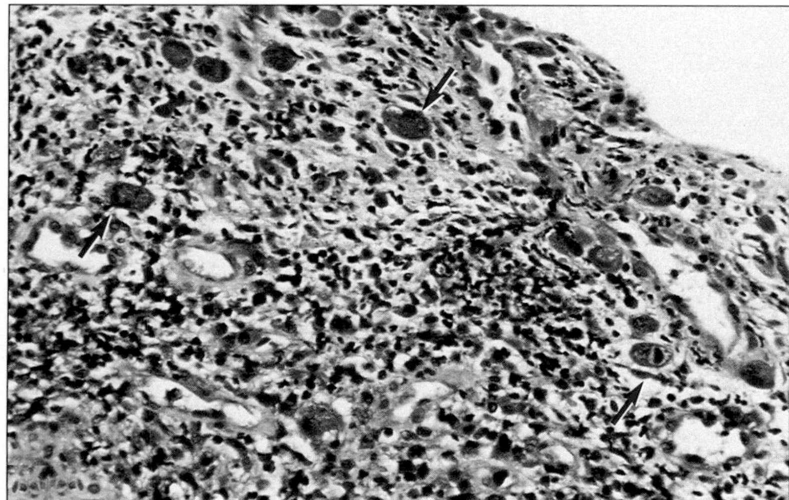

FIGURE 1-64 Colitis in AIDS patients may be caused by viral pathogens such as cytomegalovirus (CMV). CMV colitis is often, but not invariably, seen in patients who have other end-organ evidence of CMV disease. Diagnosis requires biopsy with identification of the typical inclusion bodies and inflammation. The true efficacy of therapy for CMV colitis with either ganciclovir or foscarnet remains unclear. CMV may produce a full spectrum of disease in the colon, from mild ulcerations to deeply inflamed ulcerations. Typical CMV inclusion bodies (*arrows*) with inflammation on a colonic biopsy as seen by electron microscopy. Diarrheal disease may be either fulminant and watery or scant and bloody. Diarrheal disease caused by CMV is often accompanied by fever. Other viral causes of colitis in this population, such as adenovirus, must also be diagnosed by biopsy and demonstration of organisms by electron microscopy [79,80].

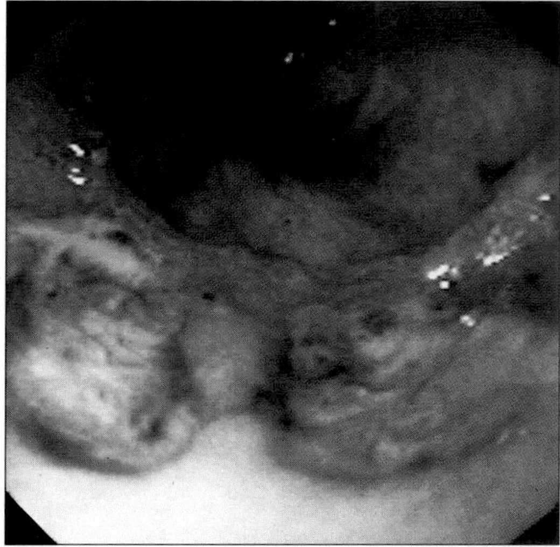

FIGURE 1-65 More distal colonic lesions or proctitis may be caused by a variety of organisms including herpes simplex virus, as seen on this endoscopic view. These patients may also have perianal disease (not shown) with severe pain as well as diarrhea. Patients who have been repeatedly exposed to acyclovir may develop refractory disease with resistant viral strains. Proctitis may also be caused by chlamydial organisms and spirochetes [81].

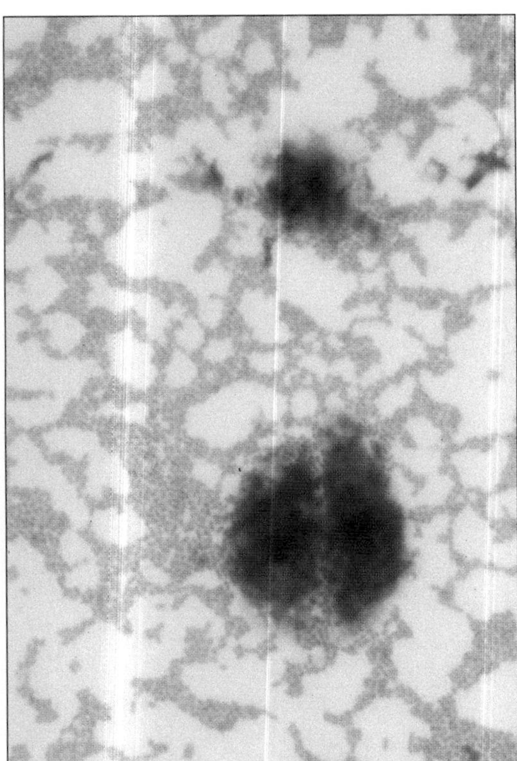

FIGURE 1-66 Potential gastrointestinal pathogens in HIV. Other bacterial pathogens have been postulated as potential causes of diarrheal disease in patients infected with HIV. These pathogens include the enteroaggregative *Escherichia coli*, which previously have been associated with persistent diarrheal disease and weight loss in children in the developing world and can be identified only by an adherence bioassay in research laboratories as shown in this figure [82,83]. Toxigenic *Bacteroides fragilis* is another potential bacterial pathogen in this patient population.

NEUROLOGIC MANIFESTATIONS

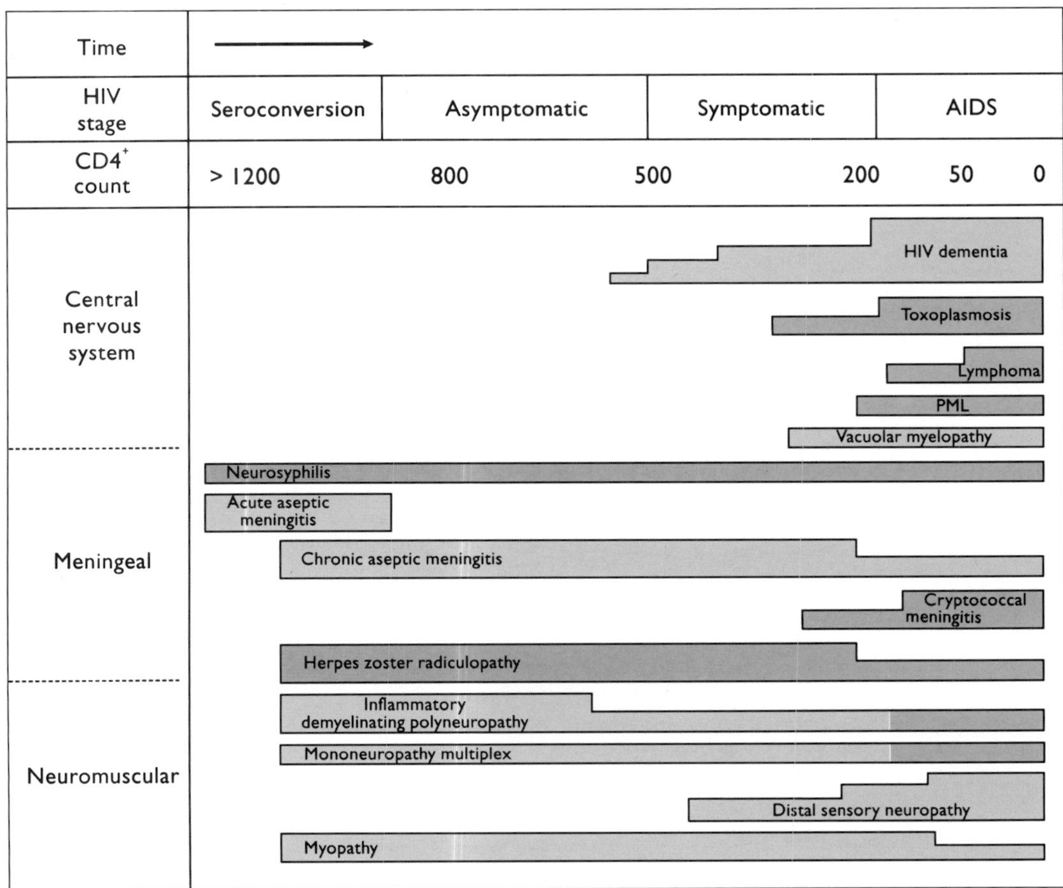

FIGURE 1-67 Time line of primary (*blue*) and secondary (*red*) neurologic complications of HIV infection. As patients progress from seroconversion to progressive HIV disease, a constellation of central and peripheral neurologic complications may occur, in isolation or together. The CD4 cell count is the best predictor of the likelihood of a specific disorder and thus provides guidance for empiric and prophylactic therapy. (*Adapted from* Johnson *et al.* [84].)

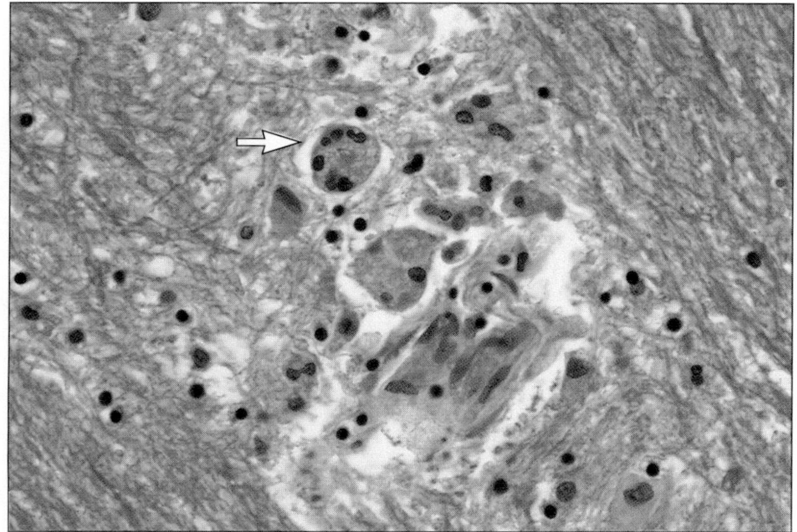

Figure 1-68 HIV encephalitis. Primary central nervous system infection with HIV is characterized by a microglial nodule encephalitis with multinucleated cells (*arrow*). (Hematoxylin-eosin stain.) Virus is located within these nodules, which are present in subcortical structures and are often accompanied by white matter pallor (not shown). The relationship between HIV encephalitis and dementia is unclear because many patients with dementia do not display this histopathology. The histopathologic substrate of dementia in this latter group is unclear [85].

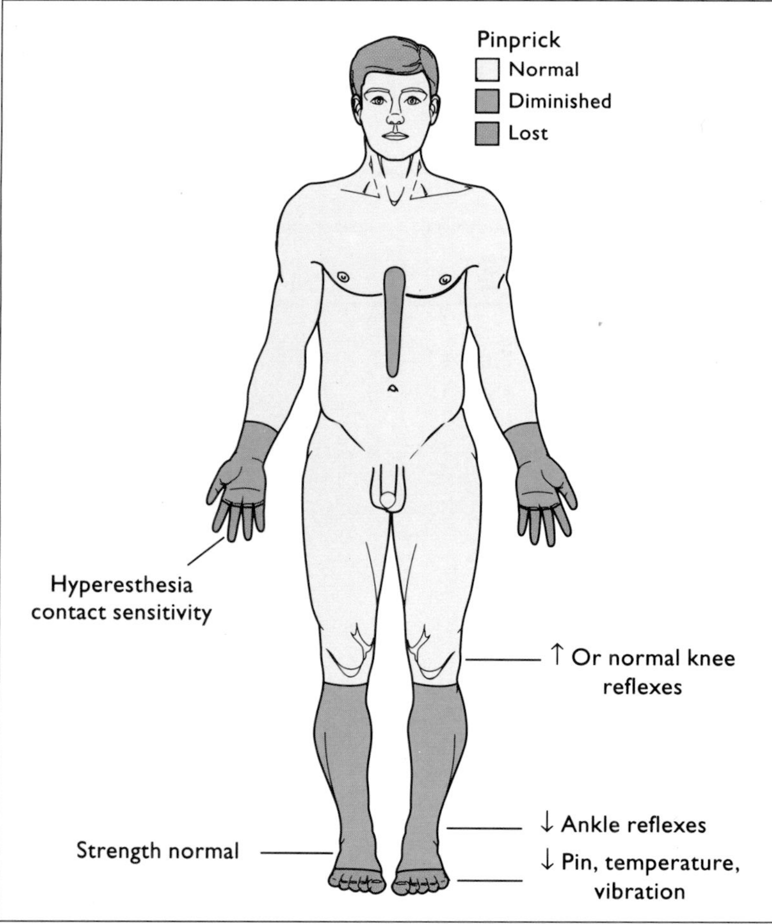

Figure 1-69 Typical "stocking-glove" pattern of sensory impairment in distal symmetrical polyneuropathy. This condition is a primary manifestation of HIV infection or may result from metabolic or nutritional abnormalities (*eg*, vitamin B12 deficiency). Neurotoxins such as vincristine, didanosine (ddI), zalcitabine (ddC), and stavudine (d4T) may initiate or exacerbate neuropathic symptoms, particularly in patients with preexisting HIV neuropathy. (*Adapted from* Schaumberg *et al.* [86].)

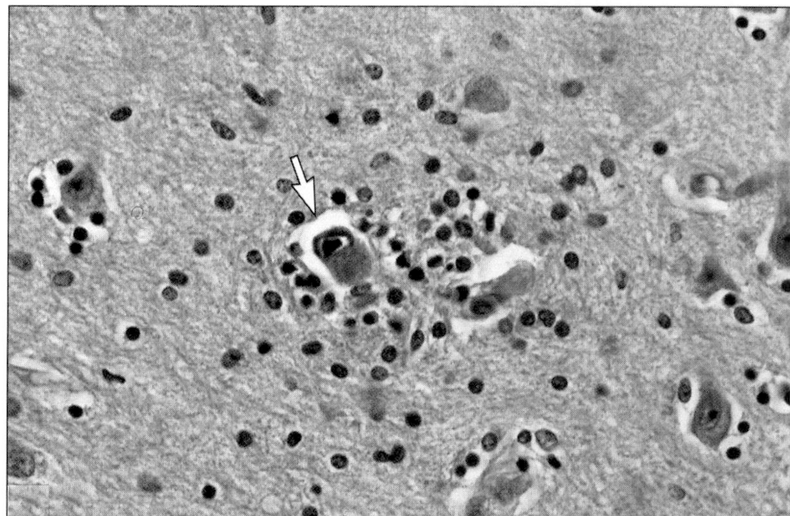

Figure 1-70 Cytomegalovirus (CMV) encephalitis. The clinical manifestations of central nervous system infection with CMV are diverse and include dementia, brainstem syndromes, and myelitis. Central nervous system involvement often occurs in the setting of systemic CMV infection. The most common finding in the brain is a microglial nodule encephalitis with rare CMV inclusions. The *arrow* indicates inclusion in the nodule seen. (Hematoxylin-eosin stain.) Most patients with CMV-related encephalitis are not detected antemortem.

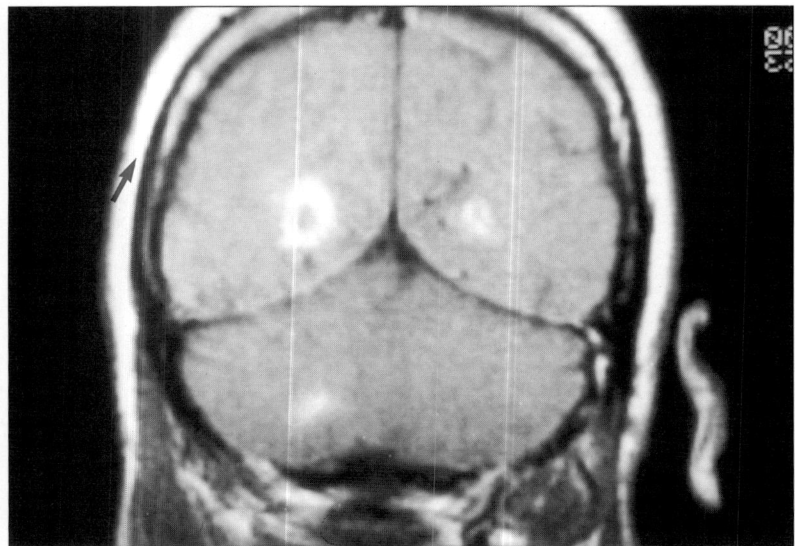

FIGURE 1-71 Cerebral toxoplasmosis. Coronal brain magnetic resonance imaging reveals multiple subtentorial and supratentorial contrast-enhancing toxoplasma lesions. Central nervous system toxoplasmosis is the most common brain mass lesion in AIDS and generally represent the reactivation of latent infection. Empirical therapy with sulfadiazine, pyrimethamine, or clindamycin generally results in rapid clinical and radiologic improvement [87].

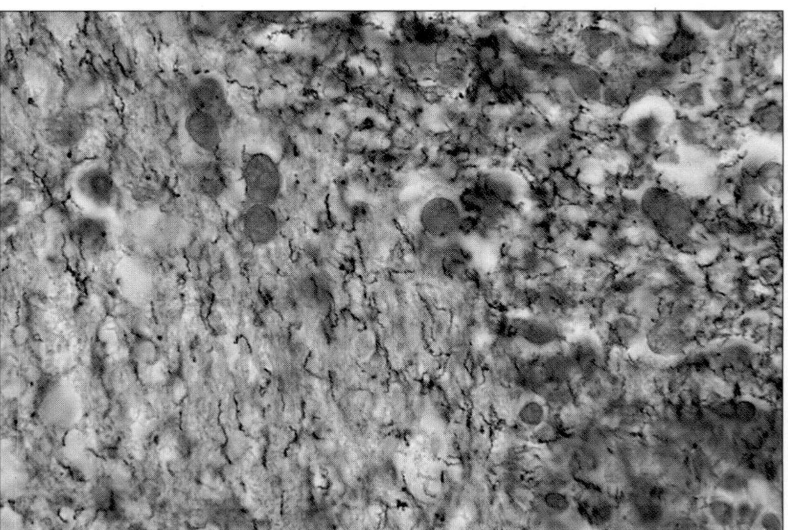

FIGURE 1-72 Neurosyphilis. Both neurosyphilis and HIV may result in chronic meningitis, dementia, cranial neuropathies, and myelopathies. Additionally, both are associated with similar cerebrospinal fluid (CSF) abnormalities, particularly a persistent pleocytosis. Although a positive CSF Venereal Disease Research Laboratories (VDRL) test is diagnostic of neurosyphilis, this assay has a sensitivity of only 30% to 70%. In an HIV-infected patient with symptoms consistent with neurosyphilis, even in the absence of a positive CSF VDRL, a reactive CSF profile justifies treatment with intravenous penicillin. HIV infection may alter the natural history of syphilis, with an increased incidence of neurologic disease and possibly a worsened clinical course. In the untreated autopsied case demonstrated here, a fulminant encephalitis with numerous treponemes was seen (modified Steiner's stain with tangles of black-appearing organisms) [88].

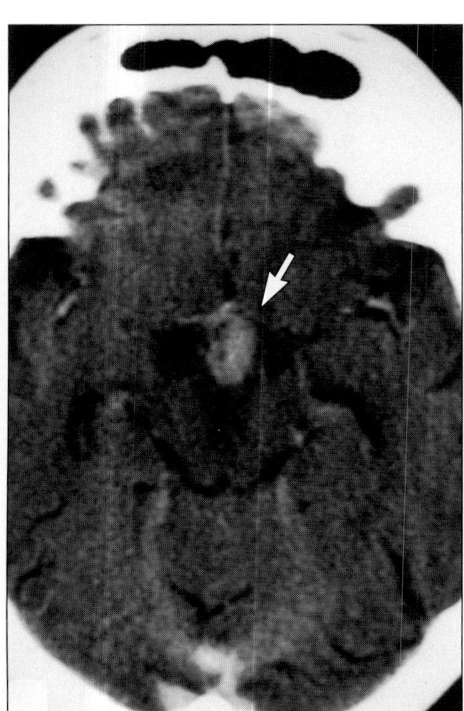

FIGURE 1-73 Primary central nervous system (CNS) lymphoma. Brain magnetic resonance imaging of lymphoma reveals a hyperintense lesion in the hypothalamic region (*arrow*). It may be difficult to differentiate between lymphoma and toxoplasmosis on clinical and radiologic grounds. Definitive diagnosis is achieved in most cases with stereotactic brain biopsy. Although the prognosis of AIDS-associated CNS lymphoma is poor, radiation therapy improves quality of life and survival. The addition of chemotherapy is under investigation in controlled trials [89].

Metabolic Manifestations

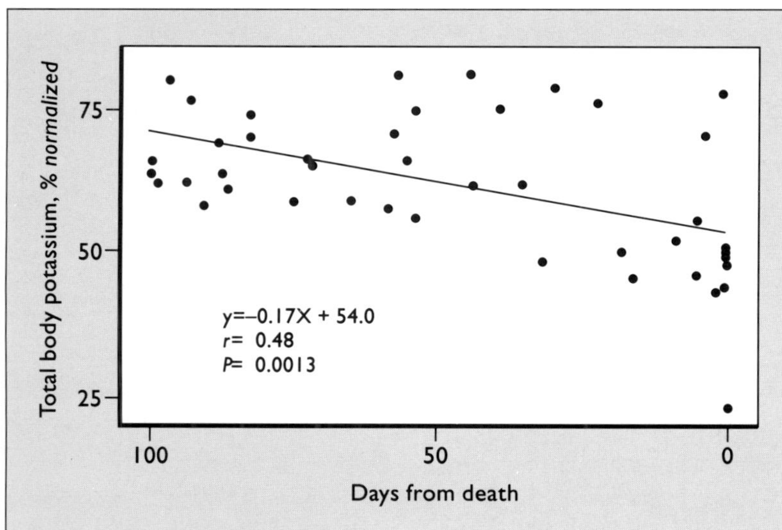

Figure 1-74 Body cell mass as measured by total body potassium in 43 patients with AIDS who died with the wasting syndrome. Total body potassium is plotted against the days before death on which the measurement was made. These values extrapolate to a body cell mass at the time of death at 54% of normal. Projected body weight at death was 66% of ideal body weight, a percentage that is similar to that seen during death from starvation. (*Adapted from* Kotler *et al.* [90].)

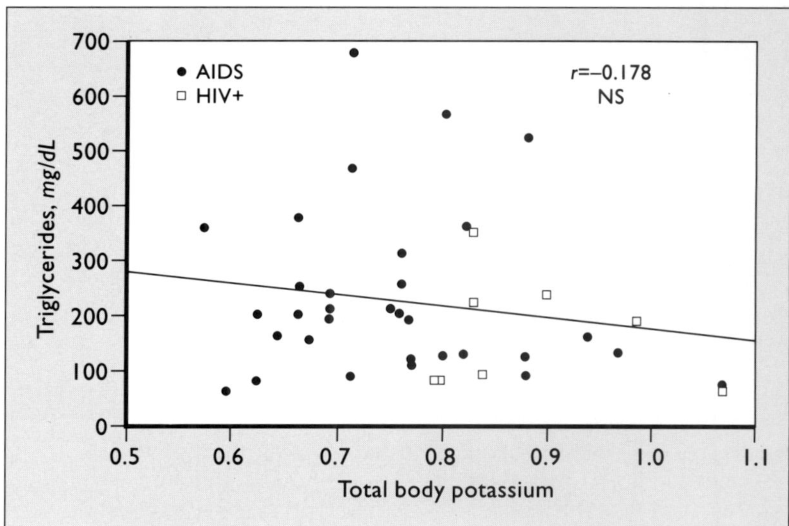

Figure 1-75 There is no correlation between the presence of hypertriglyceridemia and wasting as detected by measurement of body cell mass using total body potassium (normalized to 1.0). It had previously been speculated that certain metabolic disturbances, in particular those of triglyceride metabolism, directly caused weight loss. Studies in animal models and in patients with AIDS indicate that there is no direct relationship between hypertriglyceridemia and wasting. Patients with hypertriglyceridemia can have long periods of stable weight and body cell mass (total body potassium). (*Adapted from* Grunfeld *et al.* [91].)

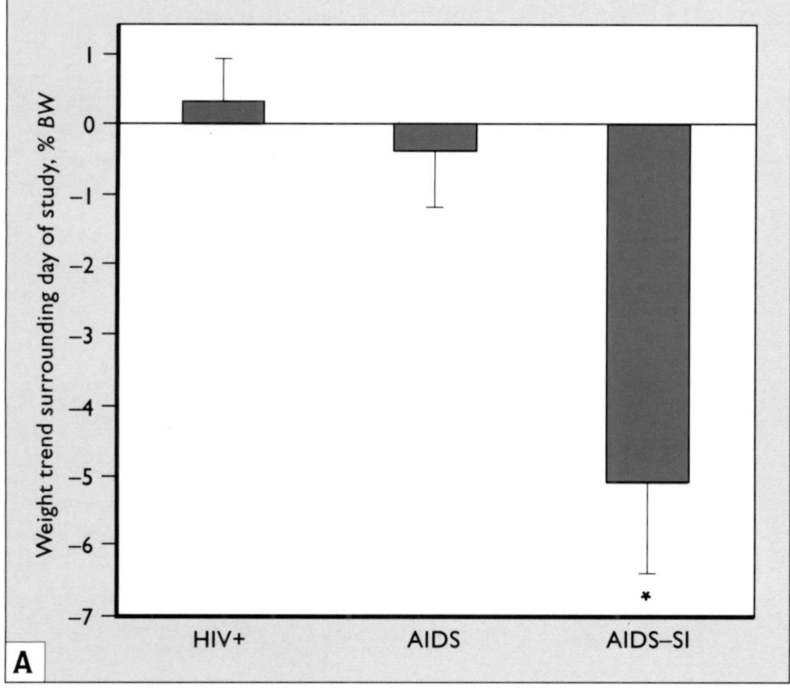

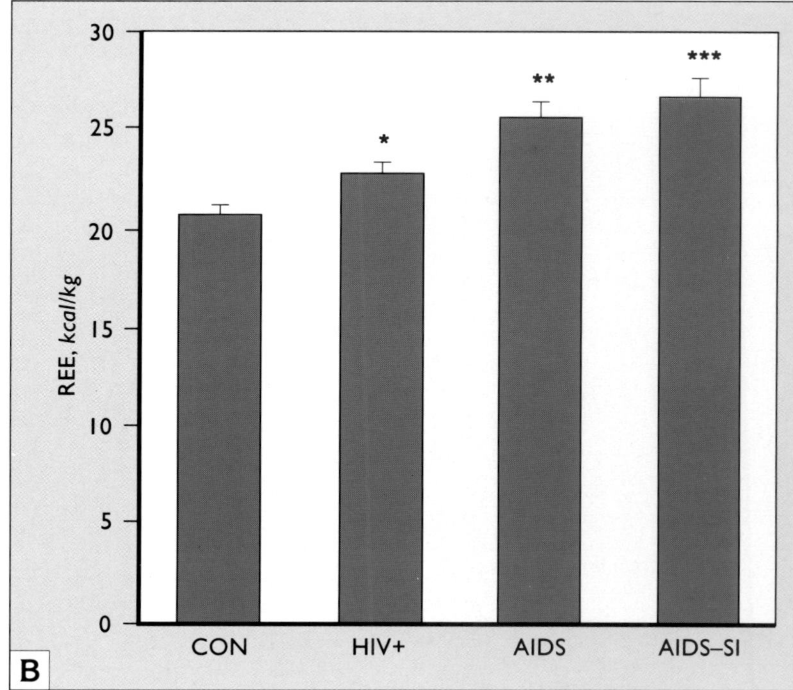

Figure 1-76 Decreased caloric intake not increased resting energy expenditure drives weight loss in AIDS. **A**, Average weight change in selected cohorts of patients with HIV infection and AIDS. Weight change during a 28-day period surrounding a metabolic study was determined for patients with early HIV infection (HIV+), patients with AIDS in the absence of opportunistic or secondary infection (AIDS), and patients with AIDS during the course of an acute opportunistic or secondary infection (AIDS-SI). Although some patients in the HIV+ and AIDS cohort gained weight and others lost weight, patients in the AIDS-SI cohort consistently showed a rapid weight loss, averaging 5% of body weight in 4 weeks (*$P < 0.002$ vs HIV+; $P = 0.02$ vs AIDS). Patients with significant diarrhea (> five bowel movements/day) were excluded from this study. **B**, Resting energy expenditure (REE) is significantly elevated in persons with HIV infection and AIDS. Previous theories had suggested that excess energy expenditure, particularly due to increased REE, was a major cause of weight loss. (*continued*)

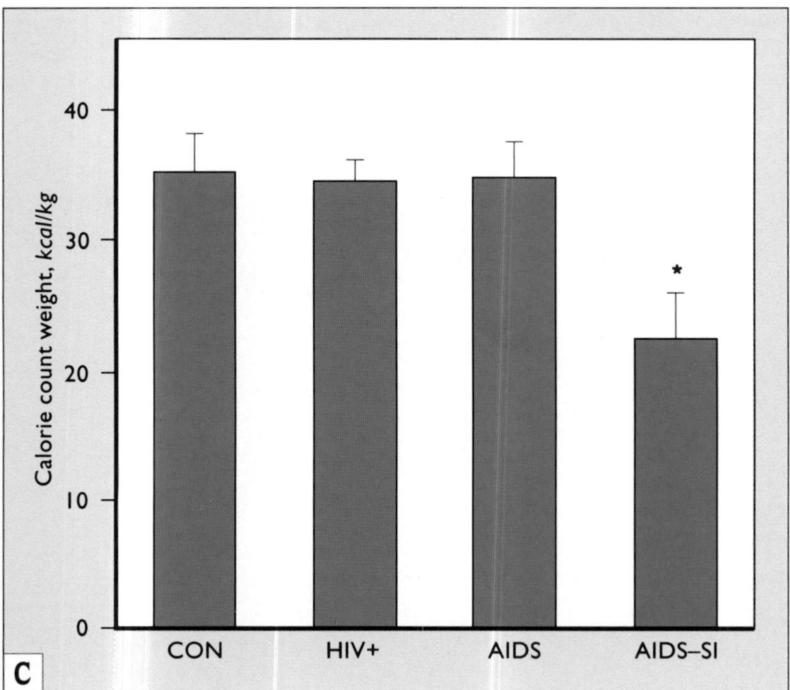

FIGURE 1-76 (*continued*) However, in AIDS (without known active secondary infection), REE is elevated nearly to the same extent as in AIDS-SI (with active secondary infection), yet only the latter group consistently shows weight loss. There was no correlation between REE and weight change (*$P < 0.025$ vs control [CON]; **$P < 0.0001$ vs control, $P < 0.025$ vs HIV+; ***$P < 0.0001$ vs control, $P < 0.01$ vs HIV+). **C**, Caloric intake in HIV infection and AIDS. Caloric intake was normal in HIV+ and AIDS (without secondary infection), whereas caloric intake was markedly reduced in AIDS-SI (with active secondary infection) (*$P < 0.01$ vs control and HIV+, $P < 0.02$ vs AIDS). In fact, caloric intake in AIDS-SI was only 83% of REE, a level that would lead to weight loss even if these patients were bedridden. Caloric intake was measured during a metabolic ward admission at the time of studying REE. (*Adapted from* Grunfeld *et al.* [92].)

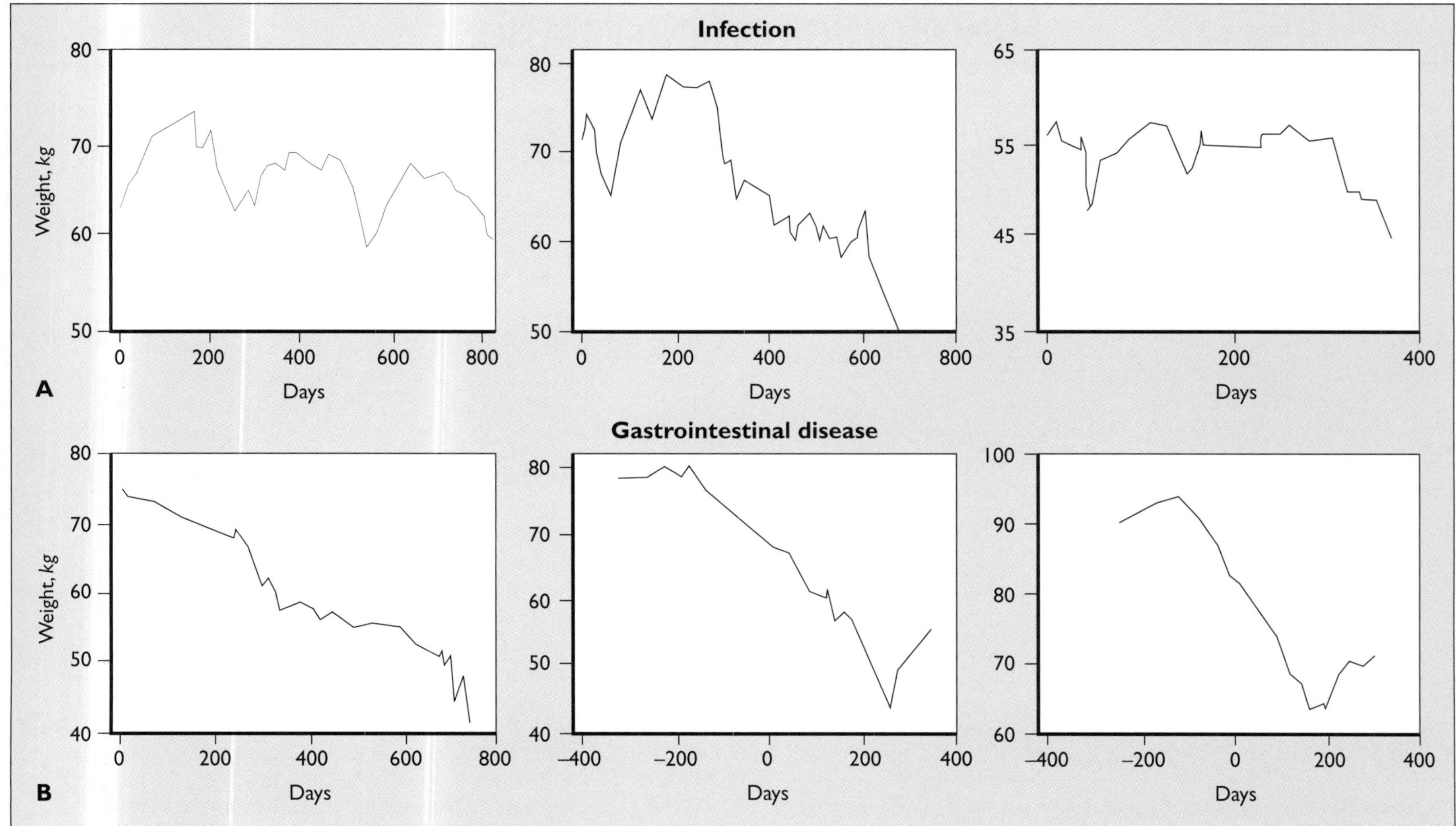

FIGURE 1-77 Rapid weight loss is associated with secondary infection, whereas slow weight loss is associated with gastrointestinal disease in AIDS. **A**, Acute weight loss pattern accompanying secondary infection in AIDS. In a prospective study of weight change in HIV infected patients, it was noted that episodes of rapid weight loss (> 4 kg in < 4 months) were frequently (82%) associated with acute infection. The patterns presented for these three patients are notable both for the periods of rapid weight loss and the fact that weight was often not fully regained after successful treatment of secondary infection. A wide variety of secondary infections have been associated with weight loss, including *Pneumocystis carinii* pneumonia, *Mycobacterium avium* complex infection, tuberculosis, sinusitis, urosepsis, bronchitis, cryptococcosis, salmonellosis, cytomegalovirus infection, and indwelling catheter infection. **B**, Slow pattern of weight loss seen in HIV infection and AIDS. Compared with the patients in *panel 77A*, other patients showed a slower, more progressive period of weight loss. These patients frequently (65%) had gastrointestinal disorders often accompanied by diarrhea. Gastrointestinal disorders and infections associated with slow weight loss include severe refractory diarrhea, malabsorption, candidiasis, cryptosporidiosis, giardiasis, herpes simplex and other forms of esophagitis, and anogenital disease. Day 0 notes the day of diagnosis of stage-IV AIDS. (*Adapted from* Macallan *et al.* [93].)

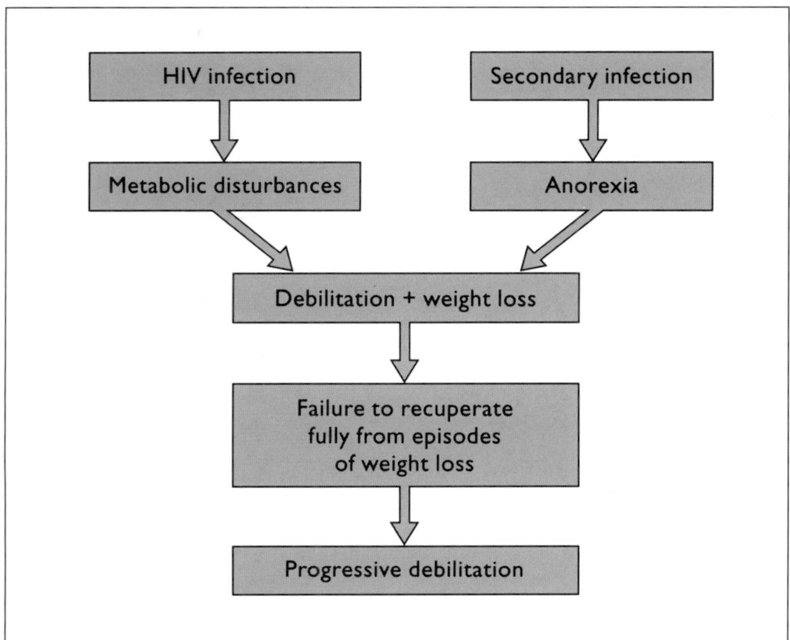

FIGURE 1-78 The mechanisms and consequences of weight loss in AIDS. HIV infection (and to a certain extent, secondary infection) leads to metabolic disturbances that contribute to debilitation. Secondary infection (and to a lesser extent primary HIV infection itself) leads to anorexia, which in the presence of the metabolic disturbances leads to rapid weight loss. Because the underlying metabolic disturbances cause debilitation, patients often fail to recuperate fully from episodes of weight loss. The net consequence is progressive debilitation and, in the extreme, death from inanition. (*Adapted from* Grunfeld and Feingold [94].)

HEMATOLOGIC MANIFESTATIONS

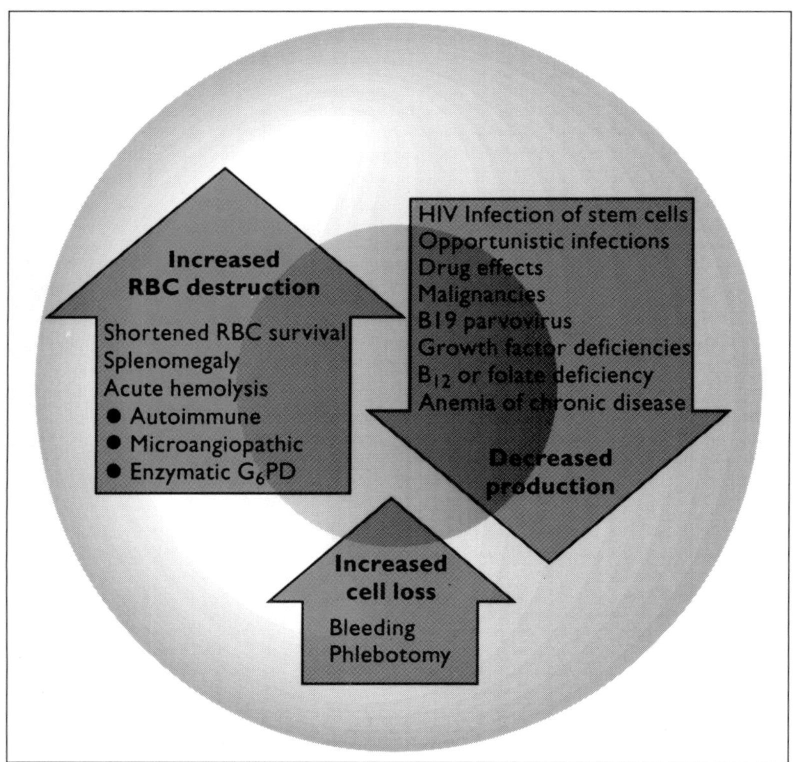

FIGURE 1-79 Anemia. Anemia has many possible causes in HIV-infected subjects, and these causes can be divided into those causing decreased production of red blood cells (RBCs), increased destruction of RBCs, and increased RBC loss. Most HIV-infected subjects develop anemia during the course of their illness, which is typically a hypoproliferative anemia (decreased production with a low reticulocyte count). Accelerated RBC destruction or loss can also contribute to the anemia. Although acute hemolysis is rare, patients with congenital glucose-6-phosphate dehydrogenase (G_6PD) deficiency can develop acute hemolysis when given some medications, such as dapsone or trimethoprim/sulfamethoxazole.

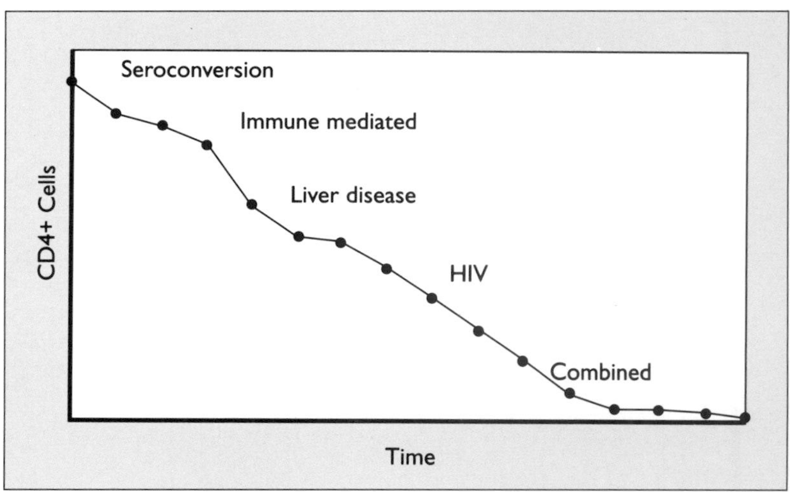

FIGURE 1-80 Possible causes of thrombocytopenia during the course of HIV infection. Some patients become thrombocytopenic during the acute viral illness, which results in seroconversion. As CD4 counts decline, B-cell derangement may produce one of the forms of immune-mediated thrombocytopenia. In hemophiliacs with chronic liver disease caused by hepatitis C virus infection, thrombocytopenia may be caused either by the liver disease or the subsequent portal hypertension and splenomegaly. Later in the course of HIV infection, megakaryocytes may become infected with HIV, leading to a hypoproliferative thrombocytopenia. It is this form of thrombocytopenia that may respond to treatment with zidovudine. As patients develop severe immune deficiency, opportunistic infections and the drugs used to treat them impair platelet production.

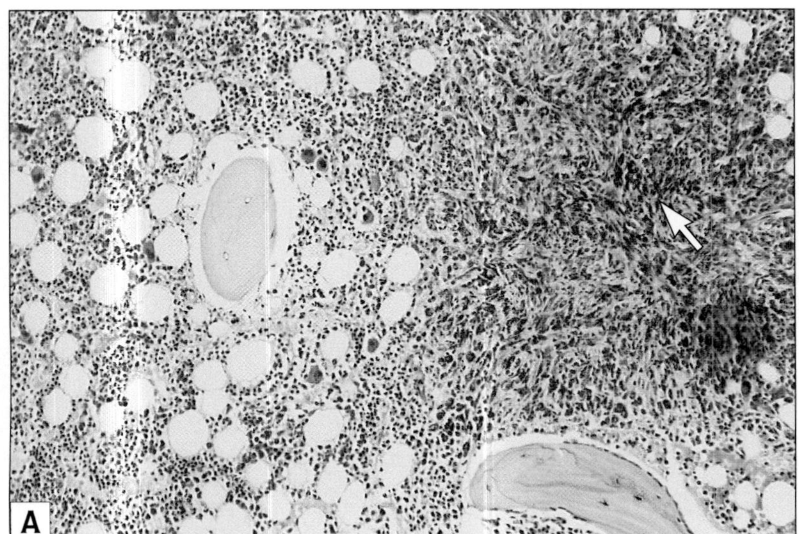

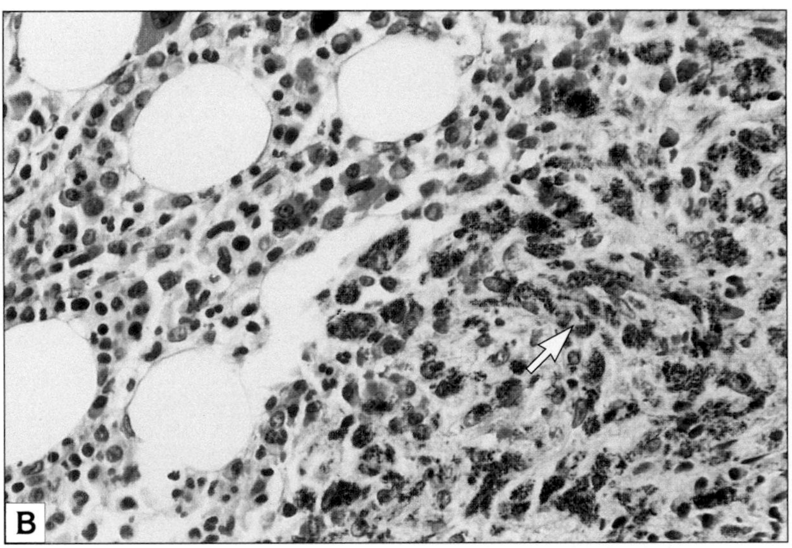

FIGURE 1-81 Bone marrow biopsies. A range of abnormalities are seen on bone marrow biopsy specimens of HIV-infected subjects. **A** and **B**, The typical heavy growth of acid-fast bacilli (AFB) in a granuloma (*panel 81A, arrow*) is shown when the specimen is stained with a Ziehl-Neelsen stain. (*Panel 81A*, × 100; *panel 81B*, × 400.) The AFB (*panel 81B, arrow*) stain red on a blue background. Subsequent culture identified these organisms as *Mycobacterium avium* complex (MAC).

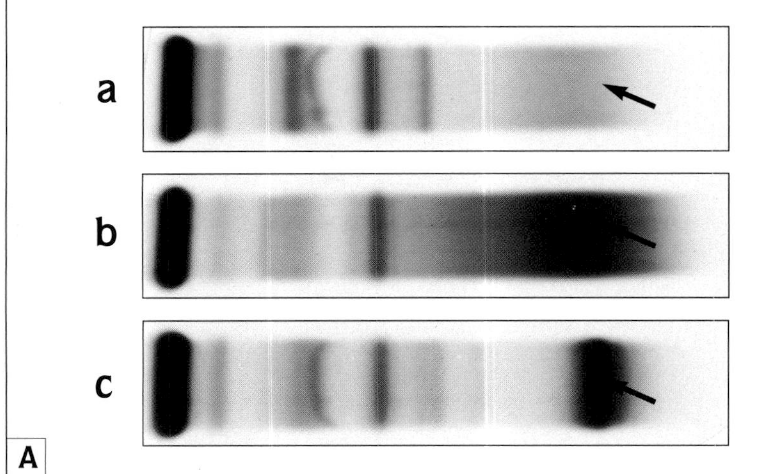

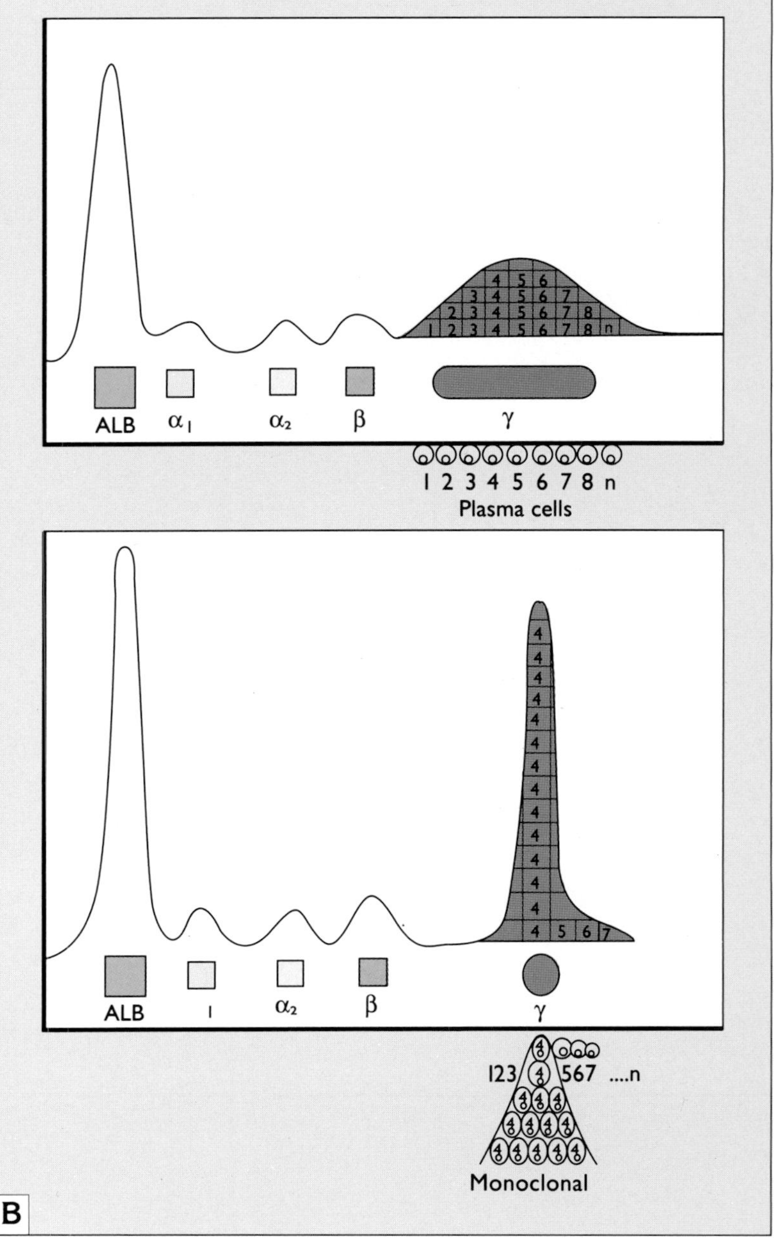

FIGURE 1-82 Immunoglobulins in HIV infection. **A**, Serum electrophoresis demonstrates a normal pattern (*lane a*, for comparison), a polyclonal gammopathy (*lane b*), and a monoclonal gammopathy (*lane c*). Immunoglobulins (*arrows*) migrate toward the negatively charged electrode (to the right of the gel) and demonstrate a light staining diffuse pattern in normals, a heavy broad band in those with a polyclonal gammopathy, and a discrete heavy staining band in those with a monoclonal gammopathy. HIV-infected subjects often have a polyclonal gammopathy, which may be a manifestation of B-cell dysregulation occurring early in HIV infection. Polyclonal gammopathies may be responsible for some of the autoimmune phenomena that accompany HIV infection, such as a positive antinuclear antibody test or a positive direct Coombs' test. **B**, A polyclonal gammopathy is the result of immunoglobulin secretion from many different plasma cells (*upper panel*). In contrast, a monoclonal gammopathy is the result of immunoglobulin secretion from a single clone of plasma cells, all secreting the same immunoglobulin with the same electrophoretic mobility, resulting in a narrow band on the gel (*lower panel*). (ALB—albumin.) (*Adapted from* Paraskevas and Foerster [95]; with permission.)

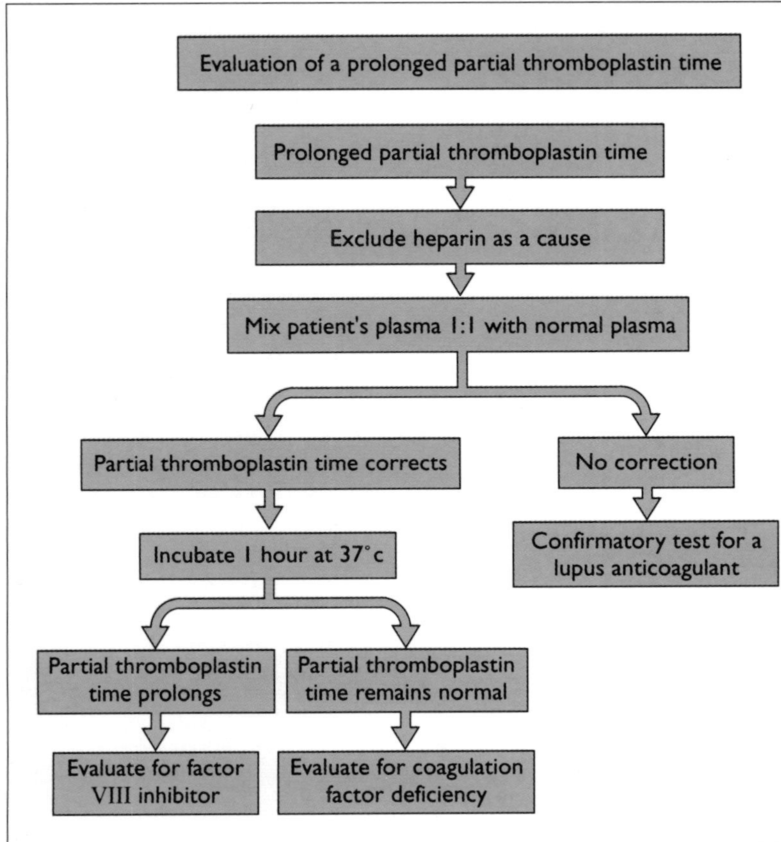

FIGURE 1-83 Coagulation abnormalities in HIV infection. Evaluation of a prolonged partial thromboplastin time (PTT). Many HIV-infected subjects have lupus anticoagulants, which appear as patients become more acutely ill and disappear as they recover. These antibodies react with the phospholipid used in the PTT test. Although they prolong the PTT, they probably have no clinical significance [96].

Effects of antiretroviral drugs on cellular elements

	Red blood cells	White blood cells	Platelets	Comments
Nucleoside analog reverse transcriptase inhibitors				
Zidovudine	↓↓↓	↓↓	↑, ↓	Macrocytic anemia common Platelets usually increased, occasionally decreased
Didanosine	±	↓	↓	Leukopenia approximately one half as common as with zidovudine
Zalcitibine	±	↓	↓	Less effect on white blood cells and platelets than didanosine
Stavudine	±	↓	↓	
Lamivudine	±	↓	↓	
Nonnucleoside reverse transcriptase inhibitors				
Nevirapine	±	±	±	Little hematologic toxicity in this class
Protease inhibitors				
Saquinavir	±	↓	±	
Retonavir	±	±	±	
Indinavir	±	↓	±	

↑ to ↑↑↑↑—Increase in likelihood.
↓ to ↓↓↓↓—Decrease in likelihood.
±—Little or no effect (seen in ≤ 1% of subjects).

FIGURE 1-84 Hematologic toxicities of the antiretroviral drugs currently available. Generally, these toxicities become likely in advanced HIV infection. Drugs should be combined cautiously because toxicities may be additive or synergistic.

Microbiology of Opportunistic Infections

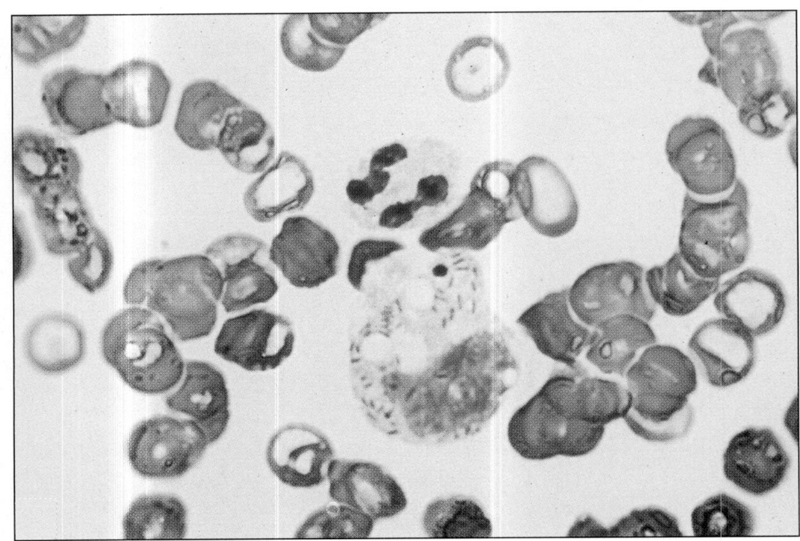

Figure 1-85 *Salmonella* species. A bone marrow aspirate shows macrophages containing numerous intracellular bacilli, which on culture proved to be *Salmonella enteritidis* serovar *tymphimurium*.

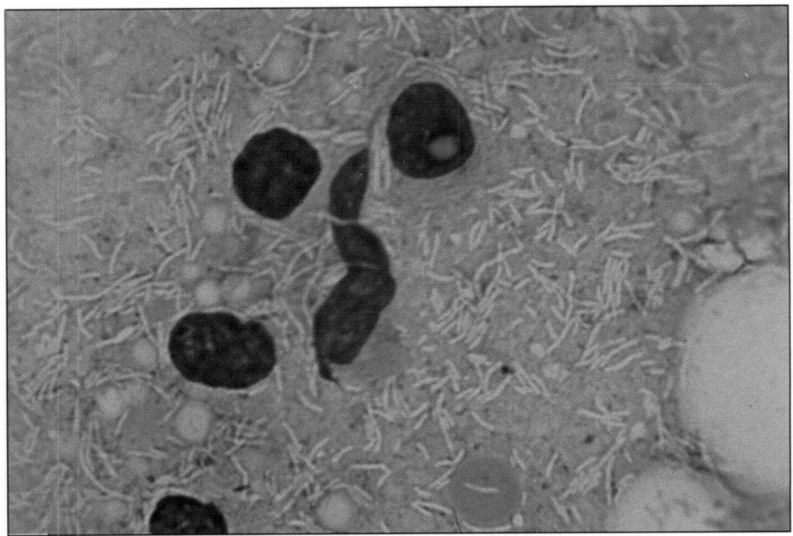

Figure 1-86 *Myocbacterium avium-intracellulare*. A touch preparation of lymph node biopsy shows innumerable unstained bacillary forms of *M. avium-intracellulare*. These were subsequently confirmed by Kinyoun acid-fast stain of companion smears and by culture. (Giemsa stain, × 1000.)

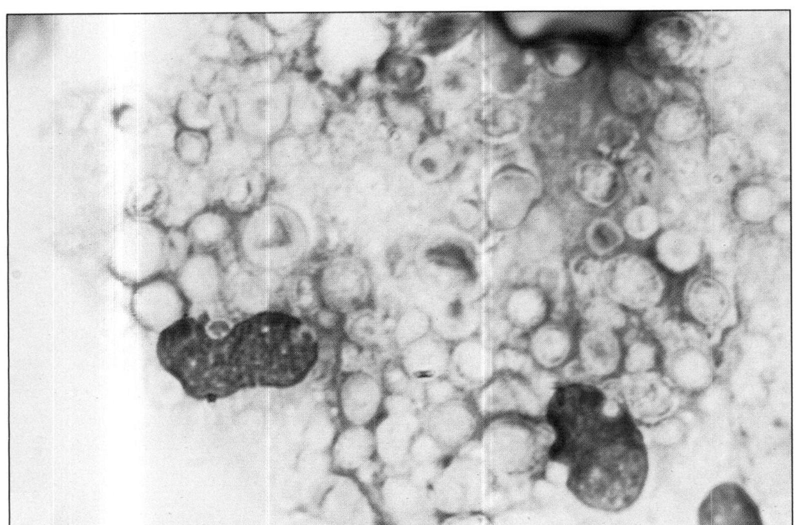

Figure 1-87 *Cryptococcus neoformans*. Bronchoalveolar lavage (BAL) fluid shows dense clusters of encapsulated yeast cells of *C. neoformans*. (Giemsa stain, × 1000.) The diagnosis of pulmonary cryptococcosis may be advanced by assaying for cryptococcal capsular polysaccharide antigen in BAL fluid, in which fluid is reacted to an endpoint titration with latex particles coated with anticryptococcal antibody. Confirmation of *C. neoformans* infection rests on isolation of the mycotic agent.

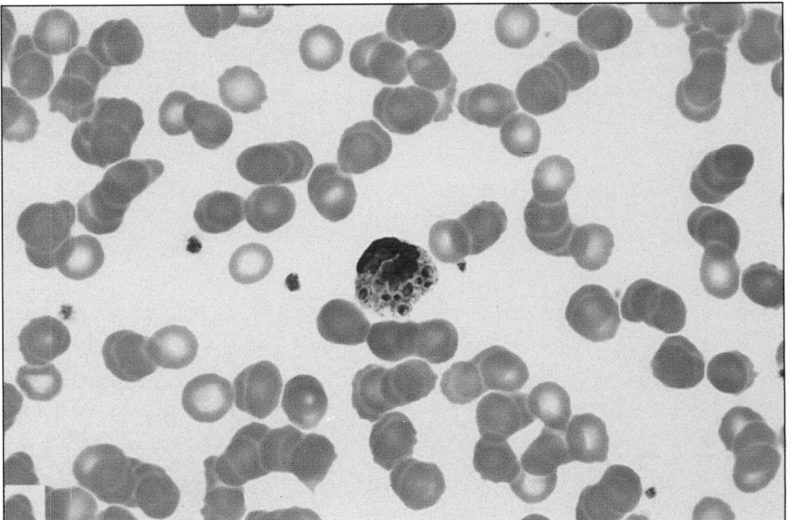

Figure 1-88 *Histoplasma capsulatum*. Peripheral blood smear of a patient with disseminated histoplasmosis showing several yeast cells of *H. capsulatum* within a polymorphonuclear leukocyte. Examination of peripheral blood smears in cases of suspected disseminated histoplasmosis may lead to diagnosis prior to other modalities such as culture.

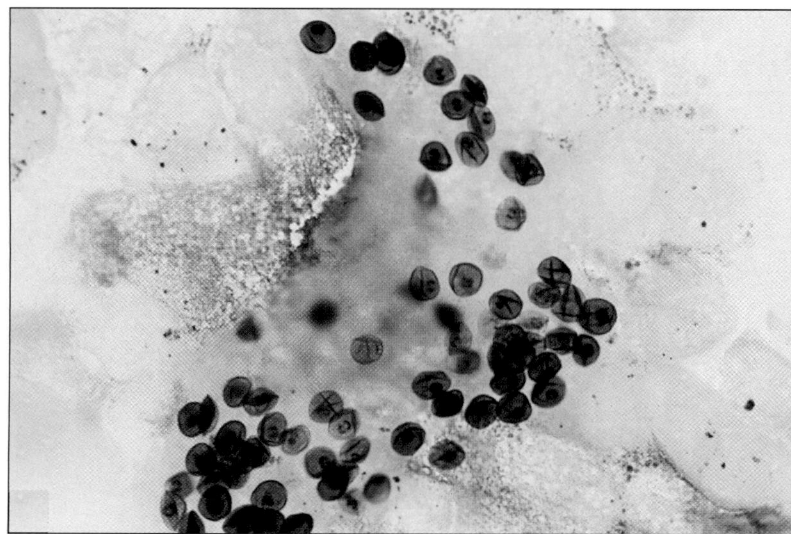

Figure 1-89 *Pneumocystis carinii.* Methenamine silver stain of BAL fluid showing cysts of *P. carinii*, which are often characterized by the presence of parenthesis- or comma-shaped collapsed cell wall material. (× 1000.)

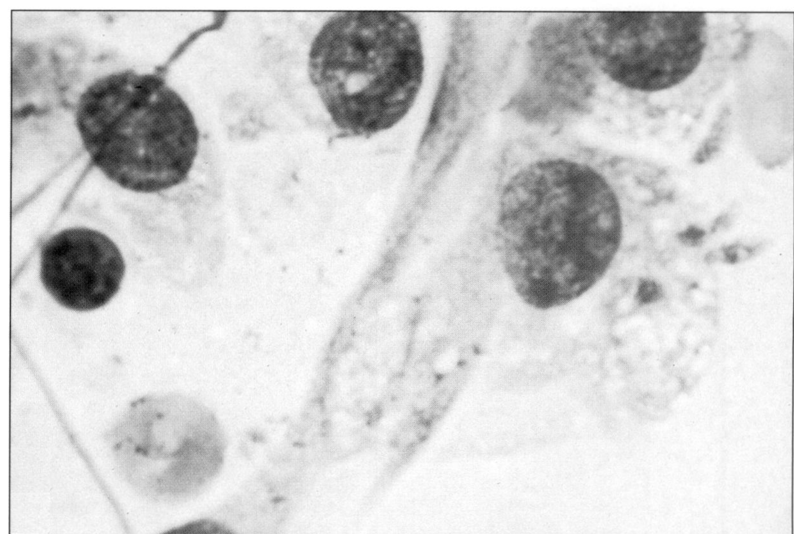

Figure 1-90 *Toxoplasma gondii.* A bronchoalveolar lavage smear shows crescent-shaped tachyzoites of *T. gondii* within, penetrating, and adjacent to pulmonary epithelial cells. The tachyzoite is distinguished by its arc-shape, with one end tapered more than the other. The tachyzoite cytoplasm stains light blue with a reddish or purplish nucleus. (Giemsa stain, × 1000.) The tachyzoite of *Toxoplasma* is the invasive form and can enter phagocytic and nonphagocytic cells with subsequent destruction of these cells as a consequence of internal multiplication. The invasion process takes 15 to 45 seconds.

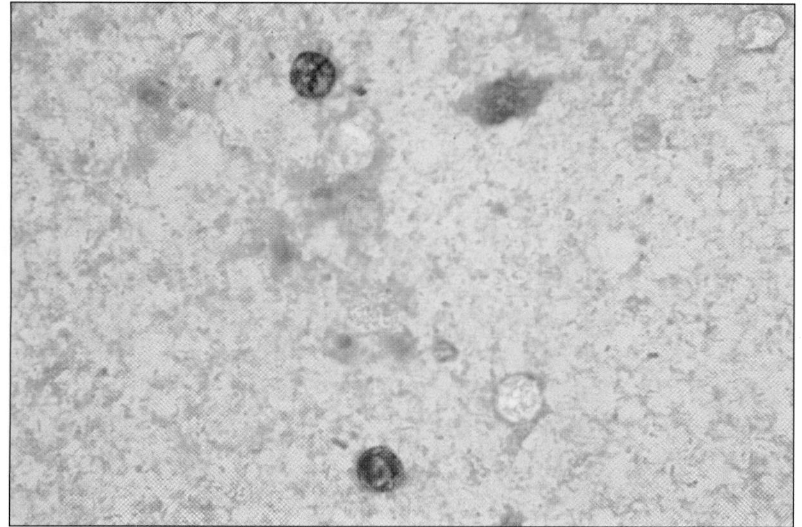

Figure 1-91 *Cyclospora* species. Modified Kinyoun acid-fast stain of fecal specimen showing variably staining oocysts of *Cyclospora* ranging from unstained, oval transparent spheres to faint staining (pink) and intensely red staining oocysts. Granular inclusions may be observed in stained and unstained oocysts.

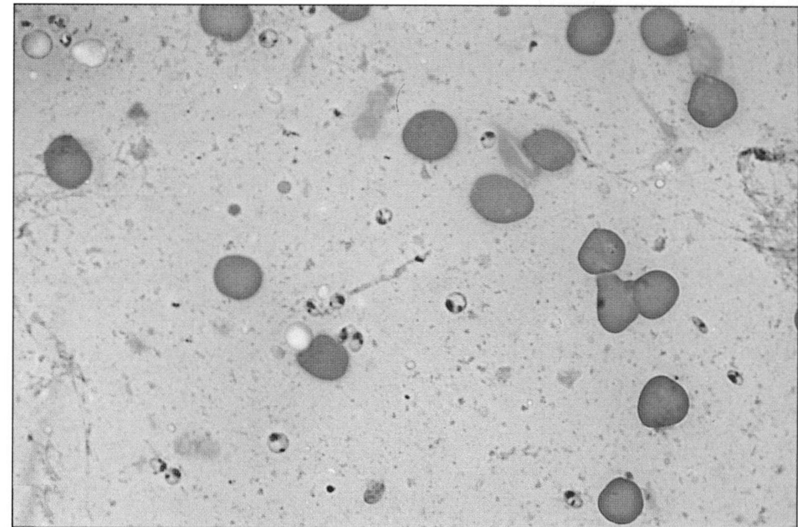

Figure 1-92 *Leishmania* species. Smear of forearm lesion shows numerous oval amastigotes of *Leishmania*, which are characterized and differentiated from *Histoplasma capsulatum* by the presence of rod-shaped kinetoplast opposite the nucleus. (Giemsa stain, × 1000.)

Clinical Manifestations of Opportunistic Infections

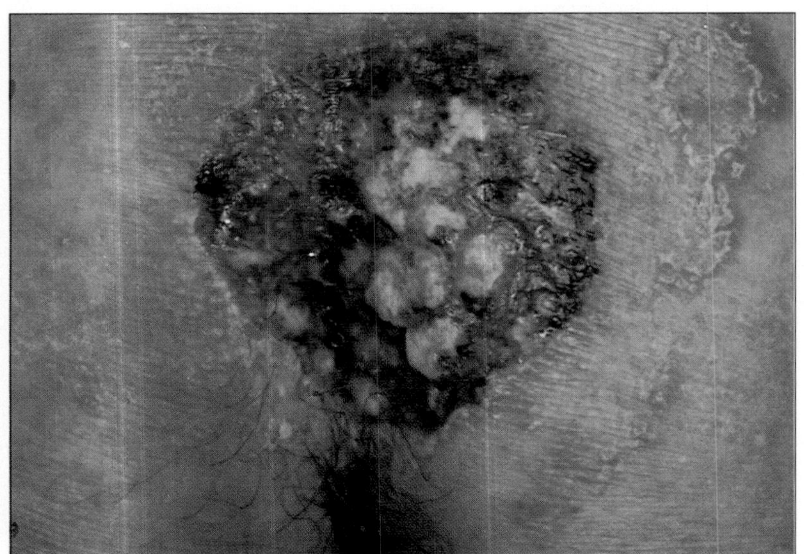

Figure 1-93 Chronic mucocutaneous herpes simplex infection. Recurrent mucocutaneous herpes simplex virus (HSV) infections are common in the general population. In the immune competent host, these recurrences are self-limited, but in patients with severe immune suppression, such as those with advanced HIV disease, recurrences may be progressive. These herpetic lesions are nonhealing and expand relentlessly over time if not treated with effective antiviral therapy. The drug of choice for these infections is acyclovir. In some patients with advanced immune suppression who have received repeated courses of acyclovir, an acyclovir-resistant mutant population of virus may emerge. The exact incidence of this complication in patients with AIDS is unknown, but it appears to be relatively uncommon, given the common occurrence of HSV infections in patients with AIDS and their frequent treatment with acyclovir. The patient in this figure had chronic mucocutaneous herpes simplex type 2 infection of the sacrum, which was unresponsive to oral and intravenous acyclovir. The lesion healed completely with intravenous foscarnet therapy, which is active against acyclovir-resistant strains of HSV.

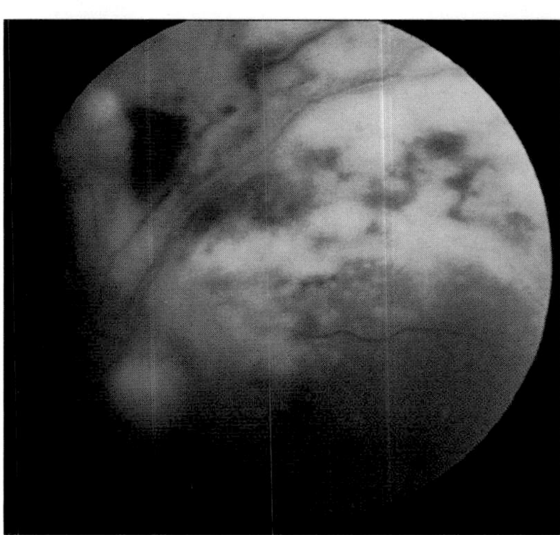

Figure 1-94 Cytomegalovirus (CMV) retinitis. CMV disease occurs in approximately 20% of CMV-infected AIDS patients per year, with the most common target organ for reactivation of CMV disease being the retina. CMV retinitis has a very characteristic appearance, as demonstrated in this figure. Inflammatory sheathing of retinal blood vessels and associated hemorrhage are pathognomonic of the disease.

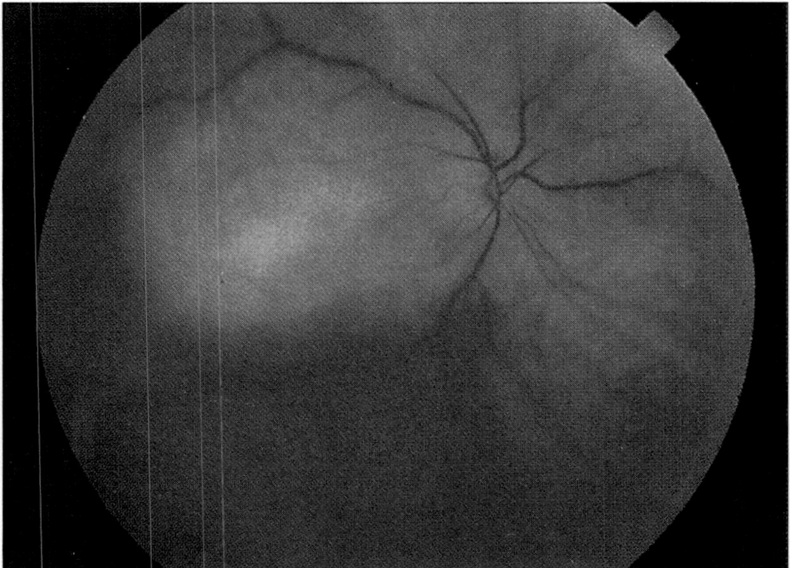

Figure 1-95 Acute retinal necrosis syndrome due to varicella-zoster virus. Varicella-zoster (herpes zoster) virus infections are more common in patients with HIV infection under 50 years of age than in similar age-matched persons from the general population. Acute herpes zoster in a patient under age 50 is recommended by some experts to be an indication for testing for HIV infection, in the absence of other causes of immune suppression. Herpes zoster usually presents as a typical dermatomal rash but can occasionally affect the eye. The acute retinal necrosis syndrome due to varicella-zoster virus has been reported in patients with AIDS and is a devastating infection frequently resulting in loss of vision. This patient presented with a complete retinal detachment with minimal vasculitis of the right fundus due to acute retinal necrosis; the central aspect of the macula is whitened. (*From* Hellinger *et al.* [97]; with permission.)

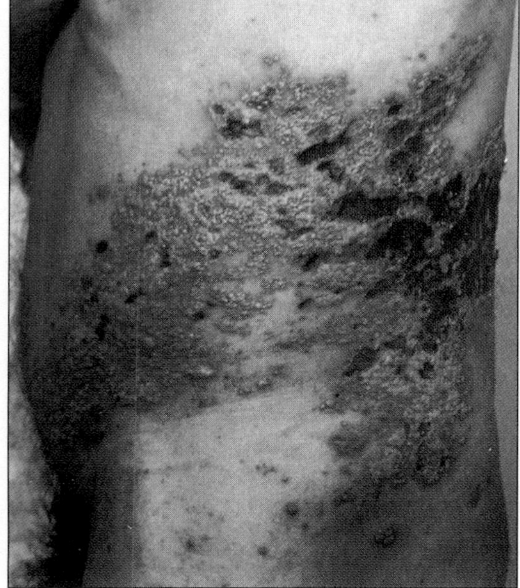

Figure 1-96 Disseminated herpes zoster. Multidermatomal herpes zoster in a patient with HIV infection is considered to be an AIDS-defining event. This patient has herpes zoster infection involving the left L1–L3 dermatomes with additional lesions scattered over the remainder of the body indicative of disseminated disease. (*From* Cohen *et al.* [98]; with permission.)

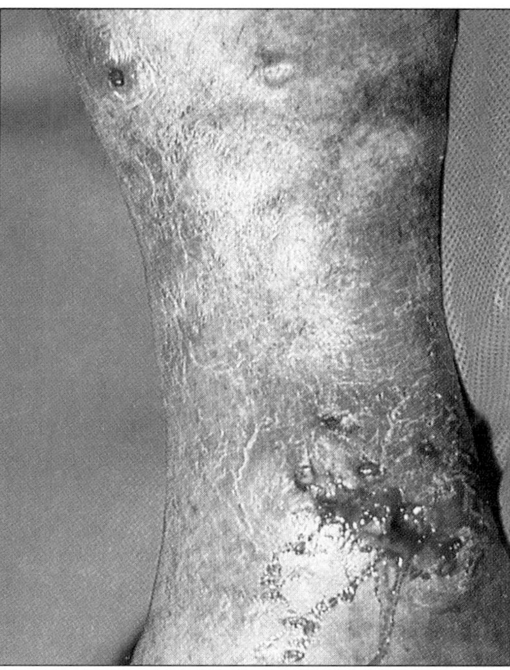

Figure 1-97 Cutaneous *Mycobacterium kansasii* infection affecting the lower extremity in association with disseminated disease. The ulcerating nodules are nonspecific and require biopsy and culture for diagnosis. (*From* Cockerell [99]; with permission.)

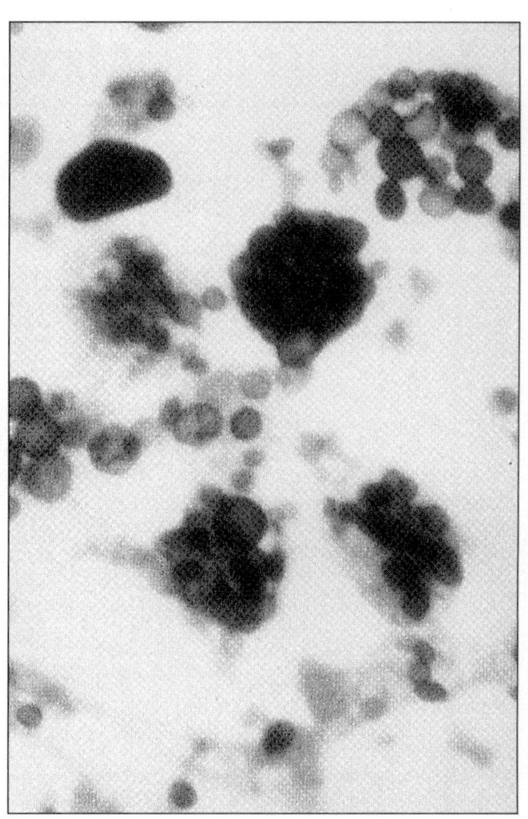

Figure 1-98 *Histoplasma capsulatum* in a bronchoalveolar lavage specimen. Abundant intracellular forms of *H. capsulatum* in alveolar macrophages are demonstrated by Gomori's methenamine stain. (× 75.) (*From* Pottage and Sha [100]; with permission.)

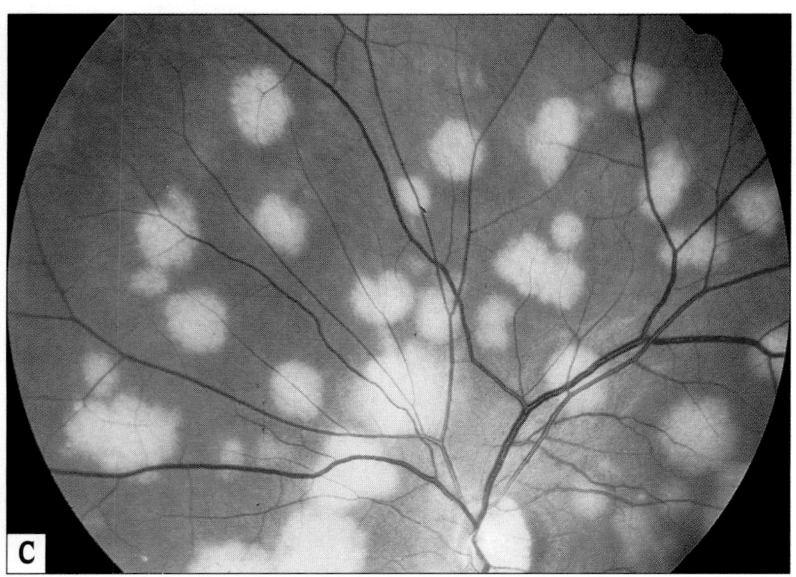

Figure 1-99 Disseminated *Pneumocystis carinii* infection. *P. carinii* has been the most common opportunistic pulmonary pathogen associated with AIDS. Infection outside the lungs has been reported most commonly in association with aerosolized pentamidine prophylaxis, presumably due to the uneven distribution of the aerosolized pentamidine in the lungs, which allows pneumocystis to persist in the upper lung fields and become invasive. Disseminated *P. carinii* infection can affect almost any organ. This retinal photograph of the patient shows choroiditis typical of disseminated *P. carinii* infection. The lesions appear as discrete yellowish-white exudates, which are differentiated from the chorioretinitis of cytomegalovirus by the lack of involvement of retinal blood vessels. These lesions are deep to the retina, and therefore the retinal vessels appear to run through the lesions.

Treatment and Prophylaxis of Opportunistic Infections

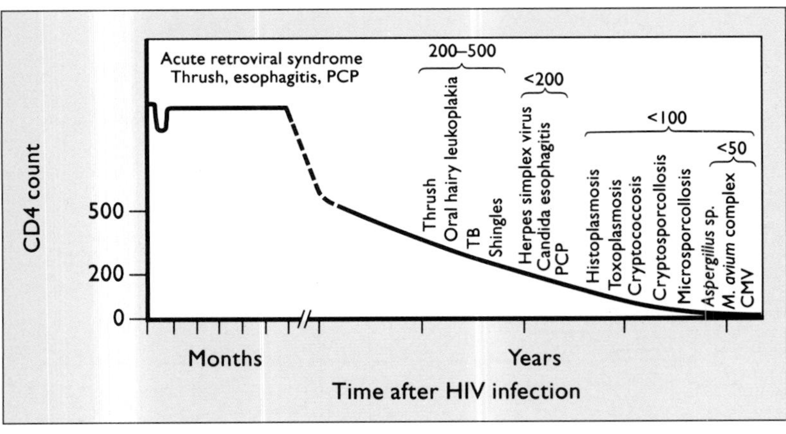

Figure 1-100 Opportunistic infections in HIV disease. The appearance of opportunistic infections in the course of HIV disease is primarily a function of declining CD4+ cell counts. The spectrum of opportunistic infections, however, is also dependent on the prevalence of a given infection in a given area, with an increased prevalence of some diseases being seen in hyperendemic areas, such as histoplasmosis in the Ohio and Mississippi River valleys, coccidioidomycosis in the southwest, and tuberculosis in New York City. Because of improved survival and increased use of primary prophylaxis, many opportunistic infections seem to be appearing at lower CD4+ counts now than they did in the mid-1980s. Because the immunosuppression of AIDS is chronic and progressive, lifelong suppressive therapy is generally required once a patient has had a serious opportunistic infection. (CMV—cytomegalovirus; PCP—*Pneumocystis carinii* pneumonia; TB—tuberculosis.)

A. Standard treatment for acute *Pneumocystis carinii* pneumonia

Trimethoprim/sulfamethoxazole: 15–20 mg/kg/d of trimethoprim component IV or orally in 3–4 divided doses
Pentamidine: 4 mg/kg/d as a single IV dose
Duration: 21 days
Treatment-limiting toxicity is common to both

B. Drug-associated adverse effects of TMP/SMX vs pentamidine

	TMP-SMX, %	Pentamidine, %
Fever (> 37° C)	78	82
Hypotension	0	27
Nausea, vomiting	25	24
Rash	44	15
Anemia	39	24
Leukopenia	72	47
Thrombocytopenia	3	18
Azotemia	14	64
Alanine aminotransferase	22	15
Alkaline phosphatase	11	18
Hypoglycemia	0	21
Hypocalcemia	0	3

TMP/SMX—trimethoprim/sulfamethoxazole.

Figure 1-101 **A**, Standard treatment for acute *Pneumocystis carinii* pneumonia (PCP). Trimethoprim/sulfamethoxazole (TMP/SMX, co-trimoxazole; oral or parenteral) and pentamidine (parenteral) are the mainstays of treatment for acute PCP. TMP/SMX acts by providing sequential blockage of folate metabolism, with TMP inhibiting the dihydrofolate reductase enzyme and SMX blocking the dihydropteroate synthesis enzyme. In recent studies, TMP/SMX is effective (as measured by survival) in up to 99% of patients with mild to moderate disease and in up to 84% with a moderately severe episode; unfortunately, a significant proportion of patients (30%–50%) experience dose-limiting toxicity. Pentamidine is generally reserved for patients who cannot tolerate or do not respond to TMP/SMX. Some investigators advocate a lower dose of pentamidine, 3 mg/kg/d, as effective and less toxic [101]. Pentamidine must be given as a slow infusion over 1 hour to avoid hypotension; intramuscular administration can cause painful sterile abscesses. Treatment-limiting toxicity is common with both agents. Unlike other immunocompromised patients, AIDS patients require a longer duration of therapy to be effectively treated, 21 days rather than 14 [102]. **B**, Drug-related toxicities of TMP/SMX and pentamidine. Toxicity is rarely life-threatening; one approach may be dosage reduction and aggressive supportive care, as described by Sattler and colleagues [103]. They found that rash and fever subsided with continued therapy, lasting on average 2 to 7 days, and could be made tolerable with acetaminophen or diphenhydramine. Leukopenia and thrombocytopenia were the most serious adverse affects associated with TMP/SMX and appeared to be dosage-dependent. The potentially serious reactions of nephrotoxicity, hypotension, and hypoglycemia occured more often with pentamidine and may relate to blood and tissue concentrations of this agent. The length of treatment did not appear to increase the frequency of adverse effects.

A. Adjunctive corticosteroids in antipneumocystis therapy
Indicated in patients with PaO_2 < 70 mm Hg or A–a gradient > 35 mm Hg on room air
Corticosteroids begun within 72 hrs of initiating *Pneumocystis carinii* pneumonia treatment improve clinical outcome and reduce mortality by 50%
No benefit shown for milder episodes or salvage therapy
Recommended approach: oral prednisone given
40 mg twice daily × 5 days, then
40 mg once daily × 5 days, then
20 mg once daily × 11 days

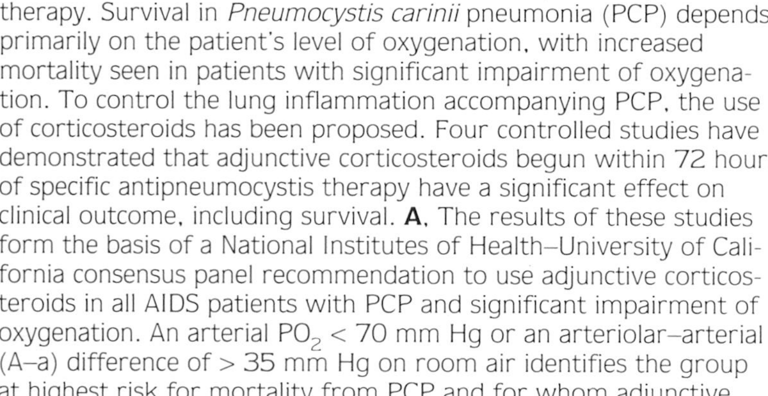

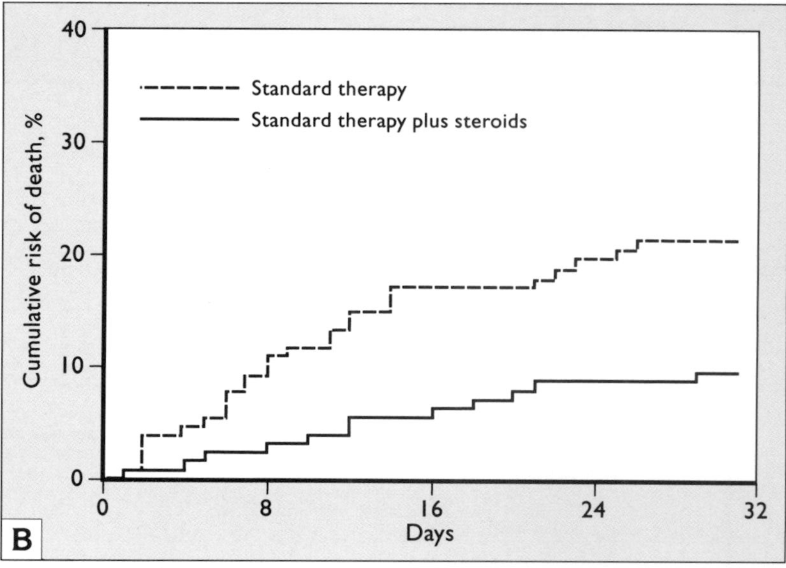

Figure 1-102 Adjunctive corticosteroids in antipneumocystis therapy. Survival in *Pneumocystis carinii* pneumonia (PCP) depends primarily on the patient's level of oxygenation, with increased mortality seen in patients with significant impairment of oxygenation. To control the lung inflammation accompanying PCP, the use of corticosteroids has been proposed. Four controlled studies have demonstrated that adjunctive corticosteroids begun within 72 hours of specific antipneumocystis therapy have a significant effect on clinical outcome, including survival. **A**, The results of these studies form the basis of a National Institutes of Health–University of California consensus panel recommendation to use adjunctive corticosteroids in all AIDS patients with PCP and significant impairment of oxygenation. An arterial PO_2 < 70 mm Hg or an arteriolar–arterial (A–a) difference of > 35 mm Hg on room air identifies the group at highest risk for mortality from PCP and for whom adjunctive corticosteroids are indicated. Because steroids can have a detrimental effect in patients with tuberculosis, fungal pneumonia, or pulmonary Kaposi's sarcoma, caution should be exercised in these patients and vigorous attempts to confirm a diagnosis of PCP should be made rather than initiating adjunctive corticosteroids empirically. **B**, A Kaplan-Meier plot from the largest and most compelling of the four studies demonstrates a 50% improvement in survival for patients given early adjunctive prednisone as compared with standard therapy alone for moderate to severe episodes of PCP. A regimen of oral prednisone, as employed by Bozzette and colleagues [104], is recommended because of its ease of use and low cost; no further tapering of dosage is needed after the 20-mg dose segment is completed [105]. (*Adapted from* Bozzette *et al.* [104].)

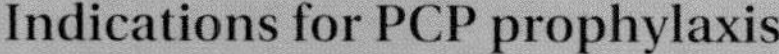

Indications for PCP prophylaxis
Prior episode of PCP
CD4⁺ count < 200/mm³
Earlier initiation warranted for patients with:
Oral candidiasis
Unexplained fever > 100° F for ≥ 2 wks
Rapid fall in CD4⁺ count
PCP—*Pneumocystis carinii* pneumonia.

Figure 1-103 Indications for *Pneumocystis carinii* pneumonia (PCP) prophylaxis. The Multicenter AIDS Cohort Study has provided the best information on the population at risk for developing PCP [106]. Individuals with HIV infection are at greatest risk for an initial episode of PCP when their absolute $CD4^+$ count drops below 200 cells/mm^3 (although the risk is not zero at counts above 200). Additional factors that are independently associated with PCP development and warrant earlier prophylaxis include unexplained fever and thrush (the predictive value of vaginal candidiasis in women is unknown). Patients with a recent rapid decline in $CD4^+$ count also should be monitored closely for initiation of prophylaxis. All patients with a prior documented episode are at increased risk of recurrence and should receive prophylaxis. PCP prophylaxis should be continued for life. These guidelines are the updated recommendations of the US Public Health Service Task Force on Antipneumocystis Prophylaxis [107,108].

A. Standard therapy for candidiasis
Mucocutaneous (pharyngitis, vaginitis)
Topical: Nystatin, clotrimazole
Oral: Ketoconazole, fluconazole, itraconazole
Esophagitis
Oral: Fluconazole, 100 mg/d, is superior to ketoconazole, 200 mg/d

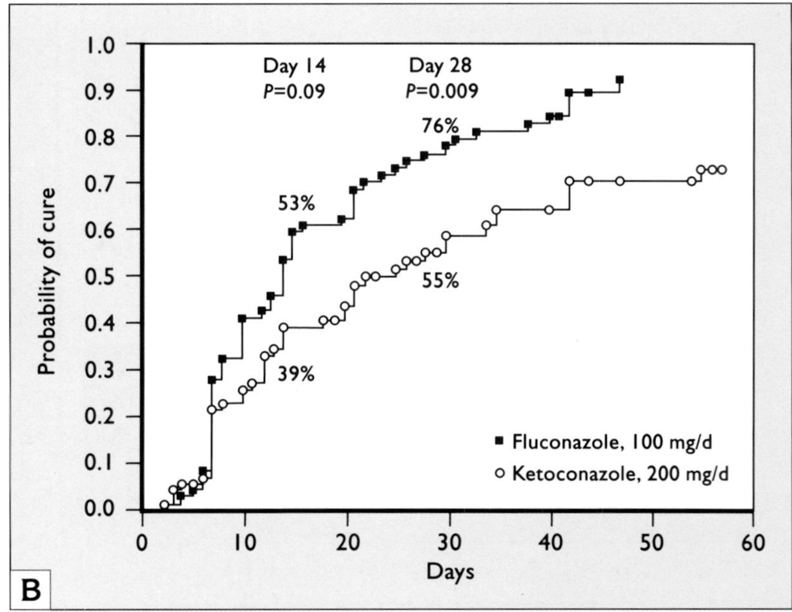

FIGURE 1-104 Standard therapy for candidiasis. Candida is the most common opportunistic pathogen in HIV disease. **A**, Many drugs are effective for management of mucocutaneous candidiasis. Oral azoles are comparable or superior to topical agents. Because of the growing problem of fluconazole resistance, topical agents should probably be used preferentially for thrush and vaginitis. **B**, Oral agents are clearly preferred for esophagitis, and fluconazole has been shown to be superior to ketoconazole for this indication. The role of itraconazole in esophagitis is less clear. Achlorhydria noted in many patients with advanced HIV disease may impair absorption of ketoconazole, which requires an acid environment for bioavailability; administration with acidic foods such as orange juice may be helpful. (*Adapted from* Laine *et al.* [109].)

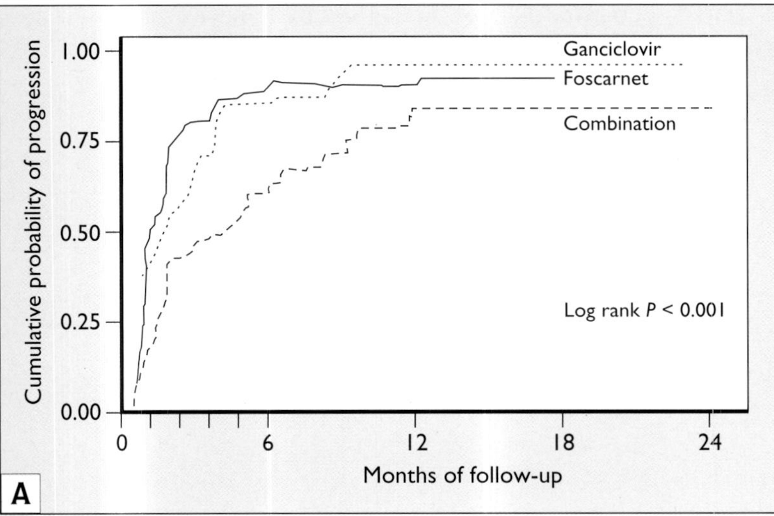

B. Immediate vs deferred cidofovir for newly diagnosed cytomegalovirus retinitis

	Immediate (n=25)	Deferred (n=23)	P value
CD4⁺	6	9	—
Bilateral disease	27%	36%	—
Time to progression (median)	120 days	22 days	< 0.001

*5 mg/kg/wk × 2 wks, then 5 mg/kg every other wk.

FIGURE 1-105 New approaches to the treatment of cytomegalovirus (CMV) retinitis. Both intravenous ganciclovir and foscarnet previously have been shown to delay the time to retinitis progression in two small immediate vs deferred treatment trials of peripheral retinitis and to have equivalent impact on disease progression in a head-to-head comparison. **A**, Recent advances in the management of CMV retinitis include the demonstration that combination therapy with ganciclovir and foscarnet for patients experiencing disease progression after initial management with either drug as monotherapy significantly delays the time to retinitis progression [110]. Median time to first progression was 2.0 months for the ganciclovir arm, 1.9 months for the foscarnet arm, and 4.3 months for the combination therapy arm (P<0.001), although the quality of life was significantly diminished for the combination group, which also had a higher rate of therapy discontinuation for toxicity. **B**, Intermittent intravenous (IV) cidofovir also significantly delays the time to progression in an immediate vs deferred trial of peripheral retinitis [111]. In this study, IV cidofovir induction and maintenance therapy (a 2-week induction of 5 mg/kg IV once a week, followed by once every other week maintenance, together with IV saline hydration and probenecid to promote drug excretion) resulted in a sixfold increase in time to progression (120 days vs 22 days, P<0.001). An advantage is that cidofovir tends to be active against ganciclovir-resistant CMV and acyclovir-resistant herpes simplex, although it can cause nephrotoxicity in the form of proximal renal tubular injury. Oral ganciclovir, in a dose of 1 g three times a day, can be used for the chronic maintenance phase of retinitis therapy [112]. Retinitis progression was significantly shorter among participants randomized to oral ganciclovir maintenance compared with those who received IV drug according to the treating ophthalmologist, but this statistically significant difference did not hold up when retinal photographs were reviewed independently. Many clinicians reserve oral maintenance therapy for patients with unilateral, non–sight-threatening disease.

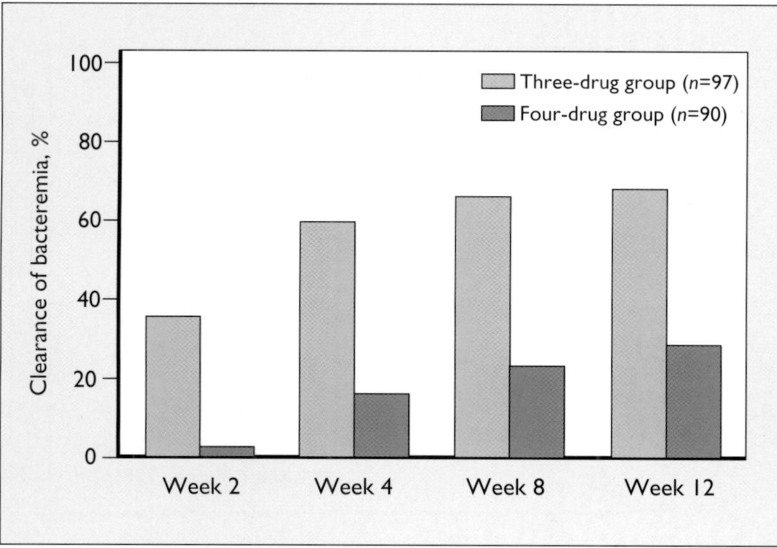

Figure 1-106 Clearance of *Mycobacterium avium* complex (MAC) over time. The new macrolides, clarithromycin and azithromycin, have proven to be the single most active agents against MAC bacteremia and are recommended by the US Public Health Service to serve as the cornerstone of a multidrug regimen [113]. Because resistance develops rapidly to use of these agents alone, one or more additional drugs active against MAC must be added, such as rifabutin, rifampin, clofazimine, ciprofloxacin, and ethambutol. Several trials have shown that various combinations of these orally administered drugs may be effective. The most recent study, a three-drug regimen consisting of rifabutin (initially 600 mg daily and later lowered to a dose of 300 mg daily), clarithromycin (1000 mg twice a day) and ethambutol (approximately 15 mg/kg daily) was significantly more effective than a four-drug regimen consisting of ethambutol (dose as above), rifampin (600 mg daily), clofazimine (100 mg daily), and ciprofloxacin (750 mg twice a day) with regard to both survival and time to clearance of MAC bacteremia [114]. The rifabutin dose was decreased in midtrial because of the increased incidence of uveitis at the higher dose.

AIDS-Associated Malignancies

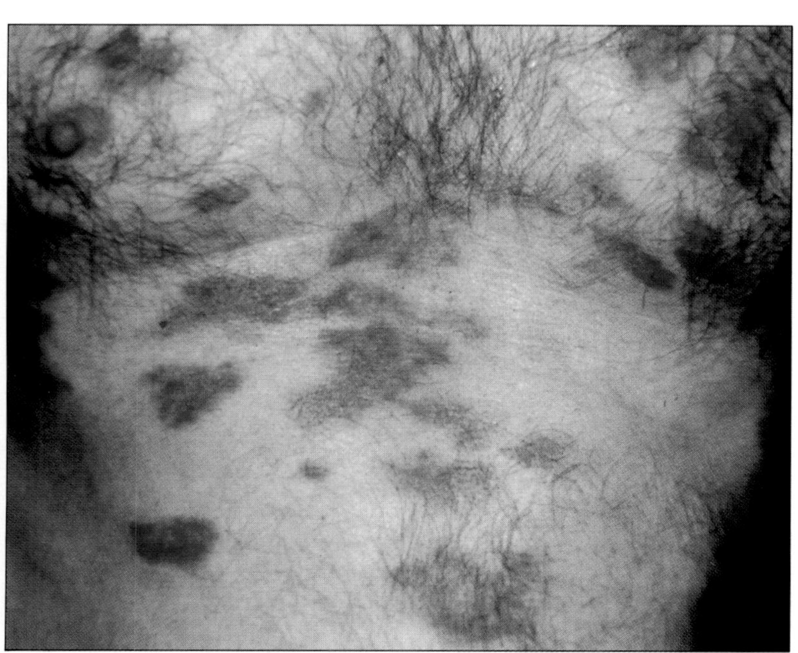

Figure 1-107 Kaposi's sarcoma is, by far, the most common HIV-associated neoplasm. Skin lesions caused by Kaposi's sarcoma may be few and small or may be widespread and large.

Chemotherapeutic agents used to treat Kaposi's sarcoma

Single agents	Combination regimens	Alternating regimens
Doxorubicin	Bleomycin + vincristine	Vincristine/vinblastine
Bleomycin	Doxorubicin + bleomycin + vincristine	Doxorubicin + bleomycin + vinblastine/vincristine + actinomycin D + dacarbazine
Vinblastine	Doxorubicin + bleomycin + vinblastine	Bleomycin/vinblastine
Vincristine	Vinblastine + methotrexate	Doxorubicin/bleomycin + vincristine
Etoposide	Doxorubicin + bleomycin + vinblastine + etoposide	
Teniposide		
Liposomal anthracyclines		
Doxorubicin (Doxil)		
Daunorubicin (Daunoxome)		

Figure 1-108 Chemotherapeutic agents in the treatment of Kaposi's sarcoma (KS). Chemotherapy is the most widely used approach to the systemic treatment of KS. A variety of chemotherapeutic agents are available (single agents or multidrug combinations administered every 2 to 4 weeks), which can induce tumor regression and provide effective and often long-term KS palliation, although this therapy is not curative. To decrease toxicity, some investigators have used alternating sequences of drugs, giving one or more drugs at one time and a different drug or drug combination at weekly or longer intervals [115].

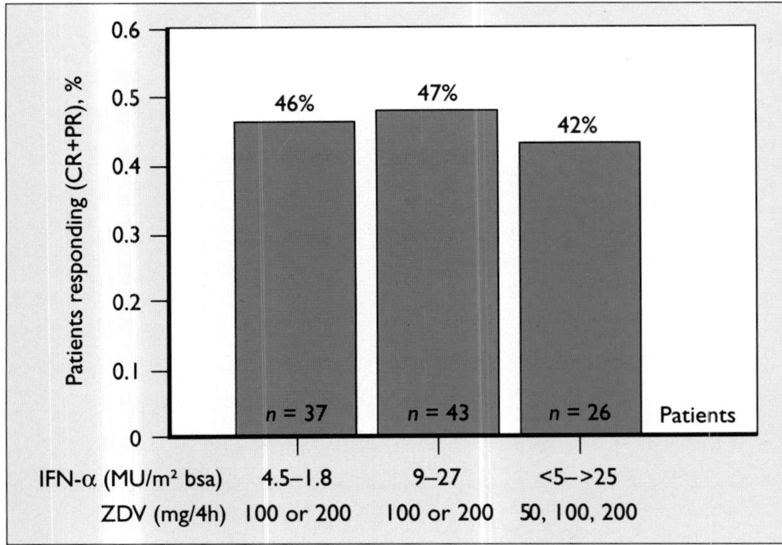

FIGURE 1-109 Phase I studies of the interferon-α (IFN-α) and zidovudine combination in patients with Kaposi's sarcoma have all documented tumor response rates > 40%. Responses have been observed in some patients with CD4 counts < 200/mm^3 and in patients treated with interferon doses < 10×10^6 U/m^2. The optimal dosage combination and the minimal effective doses have yet to be defined [116–118]. (ZDV—zidovudine.)

Therapy for non-Hodgkin's lymphoma

Increased hematologic toxicity with full-dose, standard chemotherapy regimens
Reduced-dose regimens better tolerated
- 46% complete response rate with reduced-dose m-BACOD

Dose-intensification possible with hematopoietic CSF
- Standard-dose m-BACOD tolerated with GM-CSF support
- 5 of 8 complete responses at standard-dose m-BACOD, 3 with sustained remission at 19, 22, and 23 mos

Randomized, prospective study comparing low-dose m-BACOD vs standard-dose m-BACOD + GM-CSF (ACTG 142)
- CR rate of 46% vs 50%
- Reduced toxicity profile with low-dose therapy

Continuous-infusion chemotherapy

GM-CSF—granulocyte-macrophage colony-stimulating factor; m-BACOD—methotrexate, bleomycin, doxorubicin, cyclophosphamide, vincristine, dexamethasone.

FIGURE 1-110 Treatment of systemic AIDS-associated non-Hodgkin's lymphomas (NHLs) has been complicated by the poor tolerance of many patients to chemotherapeutic regimens considered standard for treatment of NHLs in the general population. Modified-dose chemotherapeutic regimens have been reasonably well tolerated and have induced complete tumor regression in close to 50% of patients. The availability of myeloid colony-stimulating factors (CSF) made it possible to safely administer standard chemotherapeutic dosage regimens to the majority of patients with AIDS-associated NHLs. A prospective, randomized trial that directly compared standard regimen with the use of CSFs with the modified-dose chemotherapeutic regimen resulted in no difference with respect to complete response (CR) rate (50% vs 46%), relapse after CR, time to progression, overall median survival, death from lymphoma, and death from AIDS. The only difference between the two groups was in their toxicity, with grade 4 neutropenia occurring with significantly higher frequency and more rapidly in patients receiving the standard regimen with the use of CSFs. This study suggests that low-dose therapy with its reduced toxicity profile may be a better choice for the immunocompromised AIDS patient. Although some reports also have suggested that very high complete response rates and long survival durations can be achieved in AIDS patients with NHL using intensive chemotherapeutic regimens, it remains to be seen whether these regimens are superior to less intensive regimens or whether their utility will be confined to limited good-risk patient subgroups [119–120].

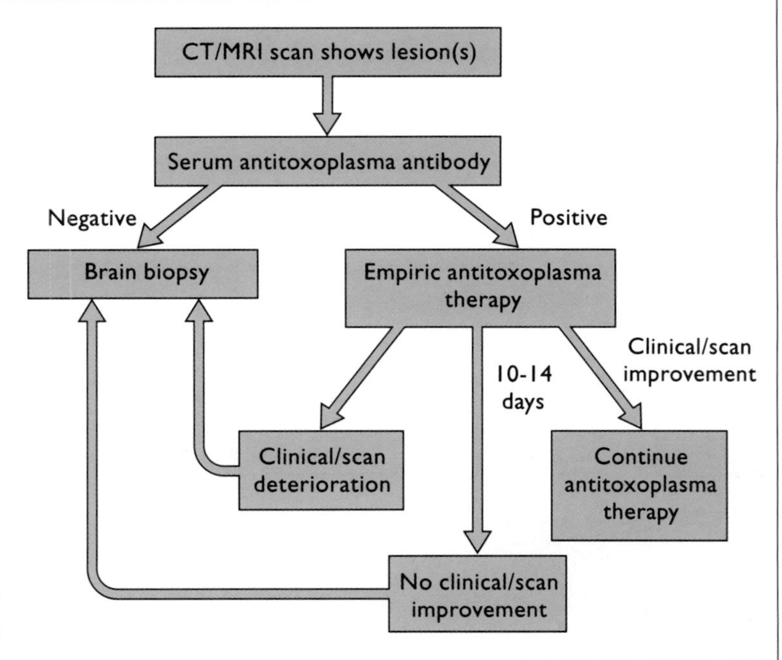

FIGURE 1-111 Evaluation of a patient with ring-enhancing brain lesions. In such patients, empiric antitoxoplasma therapy may be attempted before proceeding with brain biopsy, which can often be obtained through computed tomography (CT)-guided stereotactic methods. Patients who deteriorate or in whom no improvement occurs after a 10 to 14-day course of treatment should be referred promptly for biopsy. The use of corticosteroids to treat brain edema may lead to temporary clinical and radiographic improvement of primary central nervous system lymphoma in a toxoplasma-seropositive individual, obscuring the true diagnosis. It should also be kept in mind that coexistent primary central nervous system lymphoma and toxoplasmosis has been reported. (MRI—magnetic resonance imaging.)

Hodgkin's disease in association with HIV infection
Increased incidence in association with HIV is controversial
High incidence of advanced-stage (III or IV) disease
Frequent bone marrow involvement
Predominance of mixed cellularity phenotype
Median survival <1 year
Decreased response rates to standard chemotherapy
50% complete response to MOPP or MOPP/ABVD
Decreased duration of complete response
ABVD—doxorubicin, bleomycin, vinblastine, and dacarbazine; MOPP—mechlorethamine, vincristine, procarbazine, and prednisone.

FIGURE 1-112 Increasing evidence suggests that the incidence of Hodgkin's disease has increased among HIV-infected patients, with injection drug users most likely to develop the disease. Patients with HIV-associated Hodgkin's disease most often present with high incidence of advanced-stage extranodal disease, frequent bone marrow involvement (40%–50%), a predominance of mixed cellularity phenotype, short survival with complete remissions of approximately 50%, and a median response duration of only 18 months. These features are all unusual among non–HIV-infected patients with Hodgkin's disease.

Screening for anogenital neoplasia in HIV-infected individuals
Cervical neoplasia
Annual Papanicolaou smear every 6 months for women at high risk for HPV infection (CD4 < 200/mm^3, multiple sexual partners, partners with HIV infection)
Consider colposcopy, especially in women at high risk for human papillomavirus
Anal neoplasia
Anal Papanicolaou smear
Anoscopy and anal biomicroscopy (colposcopy) with biopsy of abnormal areas, with follow-up abnormalities every 3–6 mos

FIGURE 1-113 Given the poor results of treatment of invasive anogenital neoplasia in HIV-infected people and the possibility of cure if lesions are detected at a preinvasive stage, regular screening is recommended. For all HIV-infected women, an annual Papanicolaou (Pap) smear should be performed. Some investigators advocate routine colposcopy, as the routine Pap smear may not detect cervical neoplasia in some patients. Although there are no general agreed-upon guidelines for screening for anal neoplasia, techniques are available to perform anal Pap smears, and some investigators advocate their use in conjunction with routine anoscopy. The frequency of Pap smears should probably be increased in women and men who are at high risk for dysplasia and human papillomavirus infection (every 3–6 months) [121].

PEDIATRIC HIV INFECTION

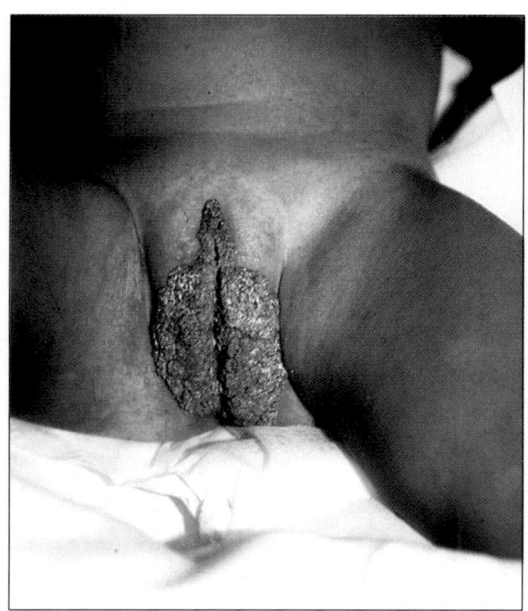

FIGURE 1-114 Large lesion of condyloma acuminata in the genital area occurring without severe depletion of CD4$^+$ cells in the peripheral blood. (*Courtesy of* J. Oleske, MD.)

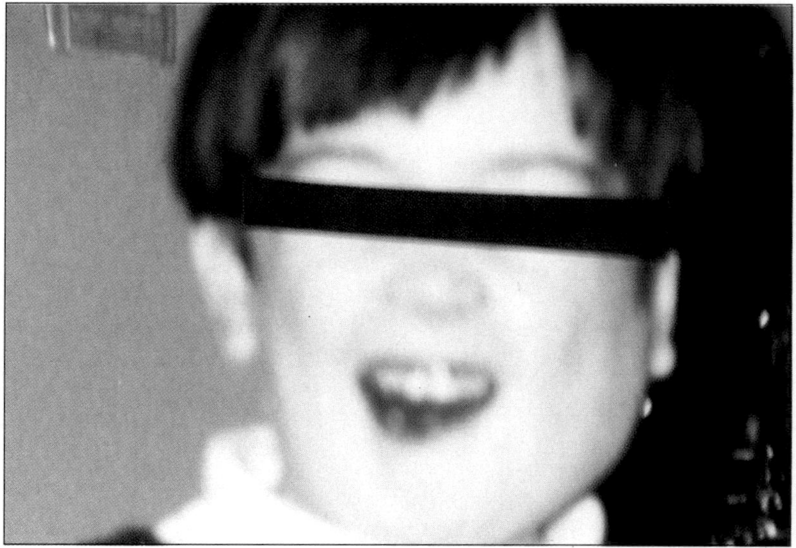

FIGURE 1-115 Parotid gland enlargement. The incidence rate is 10% to 15% in symptomatic HIV-infected children. Although the parotid gland is diffusely swollen, as seen here on the child's left side, there is no tenderness to touch or evidence of inflammation. Histologically, the gland is infiltrated with lymphocytes. The differential diagnosis includes acute suppurative parotitis, mumps, other viral infections (*eg*, parainfluenza, coxsackie, or influenza), tumors, and heavy metal or drug toxicity (*eg*, sulfisoxazole, iodides, etc.). Usually the HIV parotitis is chronic and painless. Treatment with zidovudine causes a rapid resolution in many patients, but the parotitis may recur when zidovudine is discontinued [122].

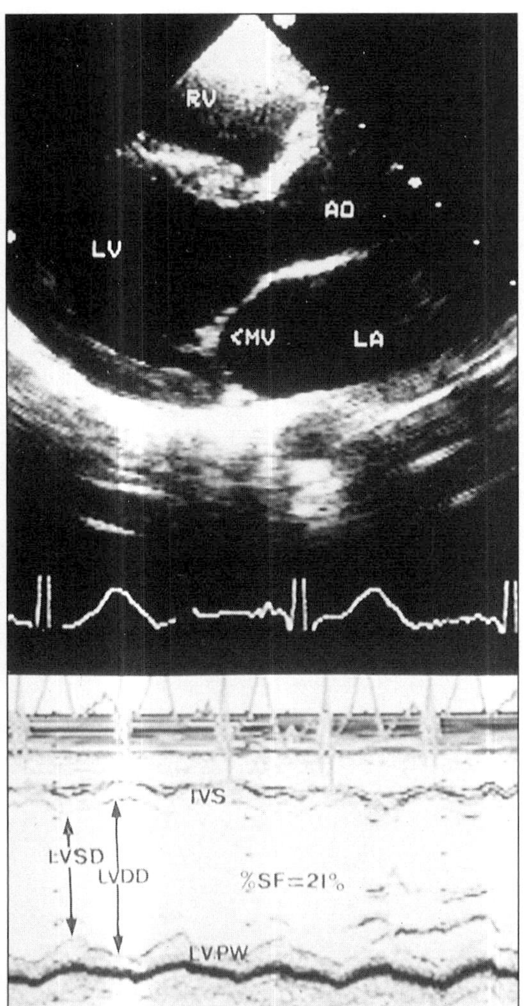

Figure 1-116 Echocardiogram of a patient with HIV cardiomyopathy. The *top panel* shows a parasternal long axis view of the heart, demonstrating dilatation of the left ventricle (LV) and left atrium (LA). (AO—aorta; MV—mitral valve.) The *bottom panel* is an M-mode tracing in the same patient from the same view, quantifying the dilated left ventricle and decreased contractility. Contractility is measured as the difference between the left ventricle diastolic dimension (LVDD) and left ventricular systolic dimension (LVSD), resulting in a shortening fraction (%SF) of 21% (normal is > 29%). (IVS—interventricular septum; LVPW—left ventricular posterior wall.)

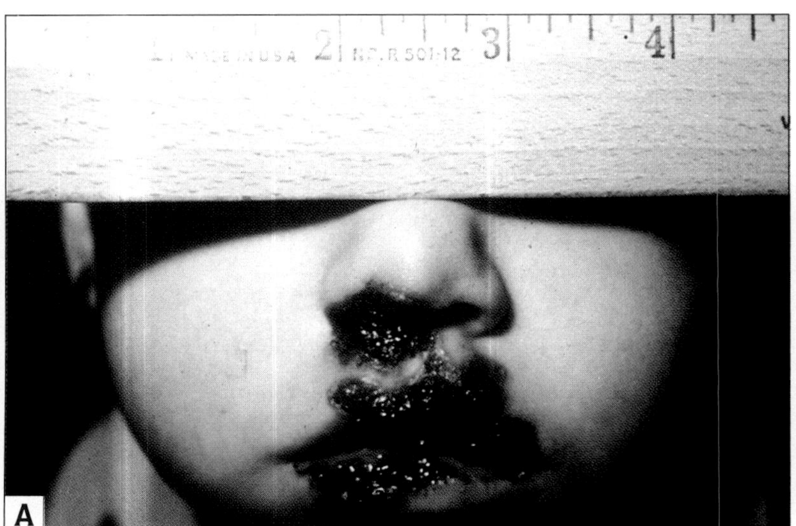

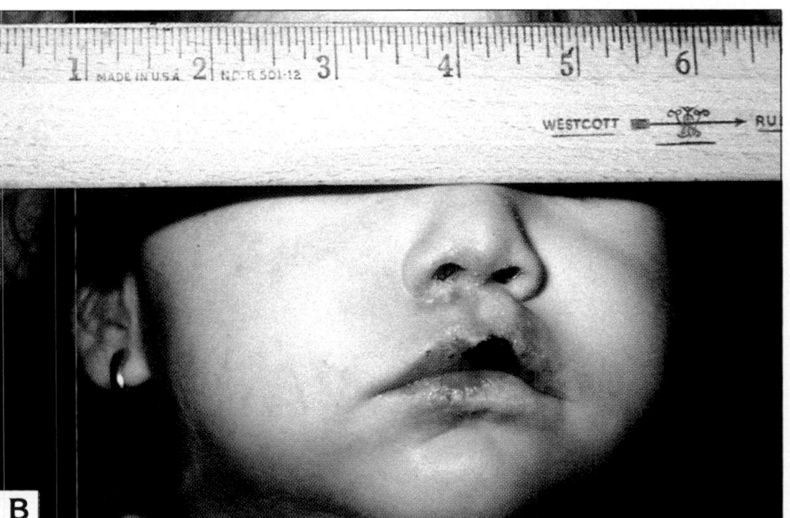

Figure 1-117 Herpes stomatitis (two or more episodes within a year). Oral lesions due to herpes simplex virus occur commonly in HIV-infected children and have a tendency to recur. The frequency of the recurrences increases as the HIV disease progresses. Although in many patients, the lesions heal within 7 to 10 days, chronic infections that continue for weeks occur. Clinical diagnosis is usually easy, but atypical lesions should be scraped and examined for intranuclear inclusions and multinucleated giant cells (Tzank smear). Oral acyclovir (750–1000 mg/m^2/day in divided doses every 6 or 8 hrs) or foscarnet for acyclovir-resistant strains will reduce morbidity and potential serious complications. Intravenous therapy is required for more severe infections. In patients with frequent recurrences, chronic suppressive therapy with acyclovir is recommended. **A**, Extension of herpes simplex stomatitis to the nares. **B**, The same patient following therapy with foscarnet for an acyclovir-resistant strain. (*Courtesy of* C. Diaz, MD.)

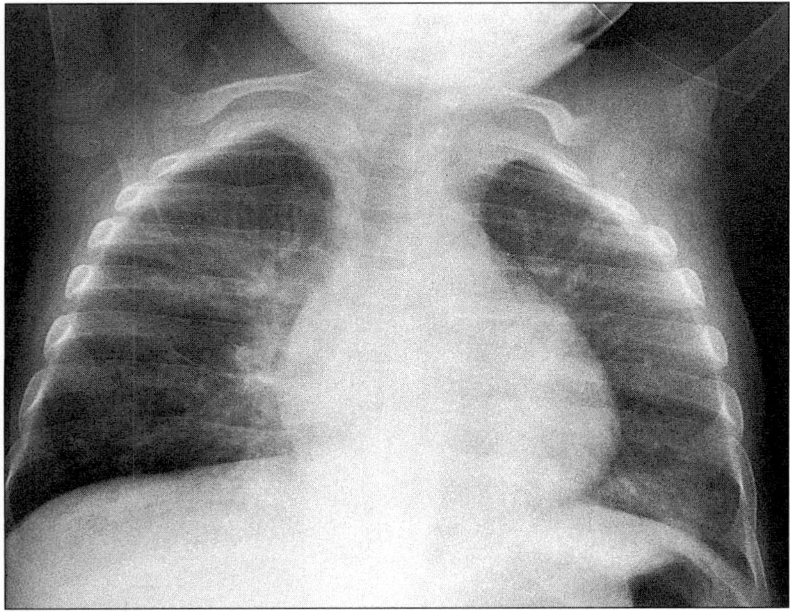

FIGURE 1-118 Lymphoid interstitial pneumonitis (LIP). A chest radiograph in an 8-month-old child shows prominent interstitial infiltrates, despite the lack of respiratory symptoms. The etiologic agent of LIP is not known. Some evidence suggests that Epstein-Barr virus may play a role in the pathogenesis, either by itself or by enhancing replication of HIV. The usual course of LIP is that of a slowly progressive, chronic pulmonary disease with intercurrent respiratory decompensation as the result of pulmonary infections. Serial cutaneous oxygen saturation determinations help in following the progression of LIP and development of hypoxemia. Children with LIP have a good prognosis compared with children with other AIDS-defining events (*eg*, *Pneumocystis carinii* pneumonia, encephalopathy). The use of steroids is associated with rapid improvement in respiratory symptoms and oxygenation. The usual dose is 2 mg/kg/day for 2 to 3 weeks followed by a tapering dose according to the O_2 saturation [123].

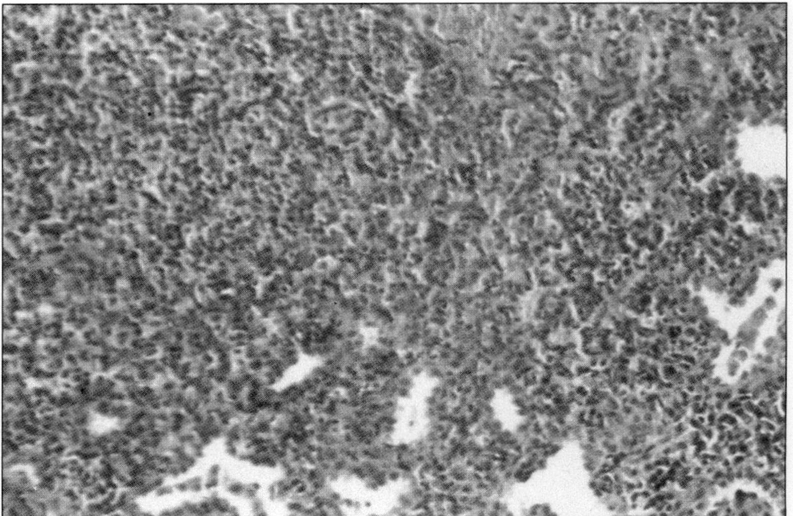

FIGURE 1-119 Hematoxylin-eosin staining of a lung biopsy specimen demonstrating lymphoid interstitial pneumonitis. Diffuse infiltration of alveolar space by lymphocytes and plasma cells. The infiltrated lymphocytes are both B cells and T cells with predominance of T-suppressor cells. (*Courtesy of* J. Oleske, MD.)

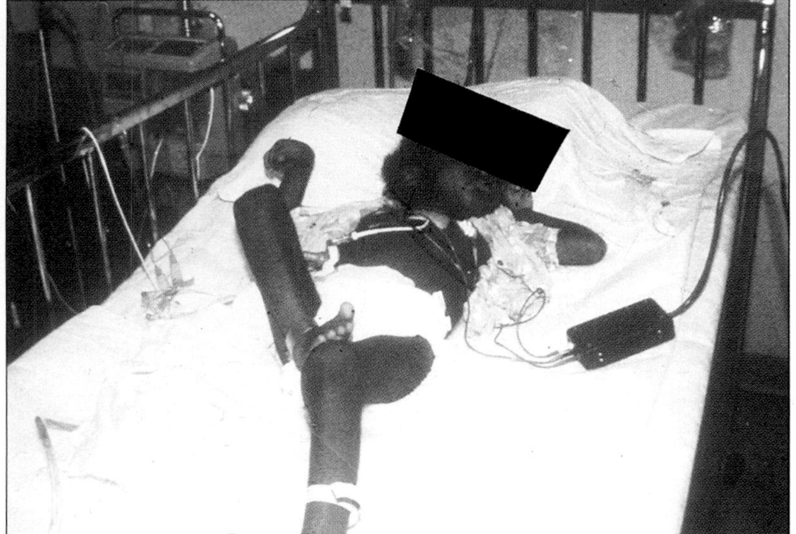

FIGURE 1-120 Central nervous system (CNS) dysfunction occurs in 20% to 30% of HIV-infected children. In symptomatic children, the incidence is even higher (> 40%). Some infants develop encephalopathy as their first AIDS-defining illness, whereas most children have deterioration of CNS function as part of the systemic progression of the disease. Severely affected infants present with progressive deterioration in their motor, language, and cognitive abilities. Loss of acquired developmental milestones is common. With more advanced disease, paresis, hypertonicity, and spasticity (as seen in this patient) appear with or without extrapyramidal dysfunction signs (*ie*, rigidity and dystonia). Cerebral atrophy with enlargement of the ventricles and bilateral calcifications, especially in the basal ganglia (*see* Fig. 1-121), are some of the manifestations of impaired brain growth. (*Courtesy of* J. Oleske, MD.)

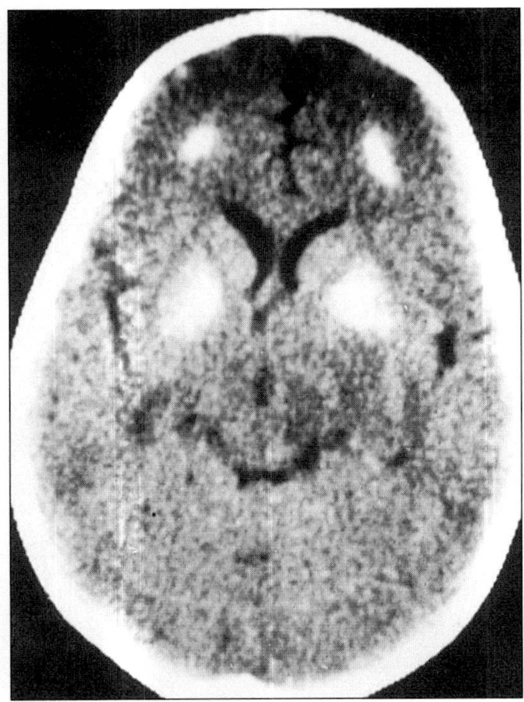

Figure 1-121 Computed tomography scan showing bilateral symmetrical calcification of the basal ganglia. (*Courtesy of* J. Oleske, MD.)

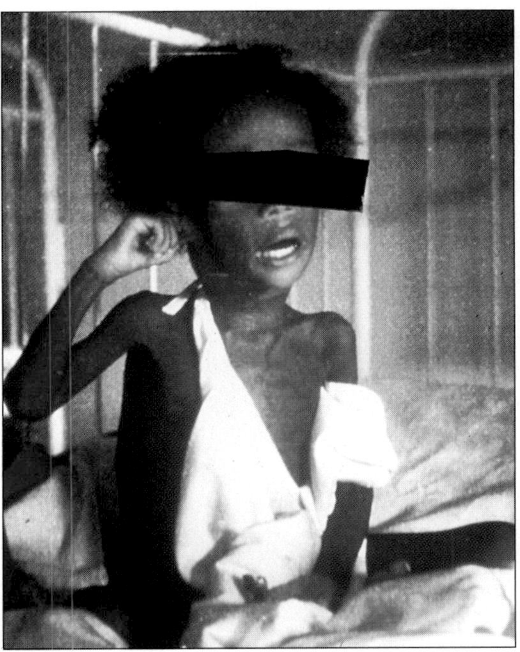

Figure 1-122 Severe failure to thrive. The incidence of this condition ranges from 25% to 75% in symptomatic HIV-infected children. The hypermetabolic state during fever and infections, gastrointestinal malabsorption and accelerated losses (*eg*, diarrhea), limited caloric intake, central nervous system impairment (which affects appetite or swallowing), and abnormalities of the endocrine system are some of the multiple factors that contribute to failure to thrive. Treatment should include optimization of nutritional status through the use of high caloric supplements and appetite stimulants (*eg*, megestrol acetate). If oral feeding is insufficient, enteral tube feeding (nasogastric or gastrostomy) should be done, and as a last resort, total parenteral nutrition should be considered. Severe failure to thrive is part of the HIV wasting syndrome. (*Courtesty of* J. Oleske, MD.)

HIV Infection in Women

Possible factors related to maternal transmission of HIV
Zidovudine (preventive)
Impaired clinical status of mother
Impaired immunologic status of mother
HIV seroconversion during pregnancy
Shortened duration of pregnancy
Chorioamnionitis
Vaginal delivery
Prolonged complicated delivery
Breastfeeding
Maternal viral load

Figure 1-123 Maternal–infant transmission of HIV. Possible factors related to maternal–infant transmission. Zidovudine administered to women during pregnancy, labor, and delivery, as well as to the newborn, can *reduce* the risk of perinatal transmission by two thirds [124,125]. Factors that increase the exposure of the baby *in utero* or intrapartum to maternal blood or other HIV-infected body fluids increase transmission. Breastfeeding provides an additional risk of infection. The passive transfer of maternal antibodies to all newborns makes it difficult to accurately determine which infants are truly infected until maternal antibodies wane at approximately 15 to18 months [126,127].

Women with AIDS: 10 most common AIDS-indicator diseases in the United States

Rank	Disease	Patients, %*
1	*Pneumocystis carnii* pneumonia	43
2	HIV wasting syndrome	21
3	Candidiasis, esophageal	21
4	HIV encephalopathy	6
5	Herpes simplex	6
6	Toxoplasmosis (brain)	6
7	*Mycobacterium avium* complex	6
8	Cryptococcus (extrapulmonary)	4
9	Cytomegalovirus disease	3
10	Cytomegalovirus retinitis	3

*Some women were reported with multiple diagnoses.

Figure 1-124 Common AIDS-indicator diseases in women. In 1992, the most common AIDS-indicator disease in women in the United States was *Pneumocystis carinii* pneumonia, which was diagnosed in approximately 40% of women reported with AIDS. Both HIV wasting syndrome and esophageal candidiasis were diagnosed in approximately 20% of women reported with AIDS, whereas each of the other diseases was diagnosed in < 7% of the women with AIDS. The percentages of conditions listed are based primarily on information from women recently diagnosed with AIDS, and some women with AIDS were reported with multiple diagnoses. Accordingly, this list probably underestimates AIDS-indicator diseases that occur later in the course of AIDS. (*Courtesy of* Centers for Disease Control and Prevention.)

Women with AIDS: Transmission category of race/ethnic group reported in the US

Transmission category	White, *n* (%)	Black, *n* (%)	Hispanic, *n* (%)	Total, *n* (%)*
Intravenous drug use	617(42)	1600(47)	581(43)	2815(45)
Heterosexual contact	535(37)	1328(39)	549(41)	2437(39)
Transfusion	143(10)	78(2)	49(4)	279(4)
Other/undetermined	163(11)	388(11)	158(12)	724(12)
	1458(100)	3394(100)	1337(100)	6255(100)

*Includes 66 women of unknown or other race/ethnic groups.

Figure 1-125 Mode of transmission for women with AIDS in the United States by race/ethnicity. In 1992, the overall percentages of women with AIDS who were white, black, or Hispanic tended to be similar for each transmission category. Injection drug use was the most common means of transmission for all three groups, followed by heterosexual contact, undetermined route, and finally transfusion. (*Courtesy of* Centers for Disease Control and Prevention.)

Cervical cancers in HIV-infected women

Author	Country	HIV+	Cervical cancer
Provencher	US	213	–
Carpenter	US	100	–
Vermund	US	47	–
Schafer	Germany	111	5
Kreiss	Kenya	42	–
Wright	US	398	–
Laga	Zaire	41	–
Maggwa	Kenya	205	–

Figure 1-126 Cervical cancers in HIV-infected women. Many studies have used either cytology or a combination of cytology and colposcopy to screen HIV-infected women for cervical cancer. For the most part, these studies have failed to detect invasive cervical cancers in the women screened. The only exception is a study of Schafer from Berlin. However, this study enrolled women from the inpatient gynecologic service of a Berlin teaching hospital, which might explain the large number of invasive cancers detected [128–135].

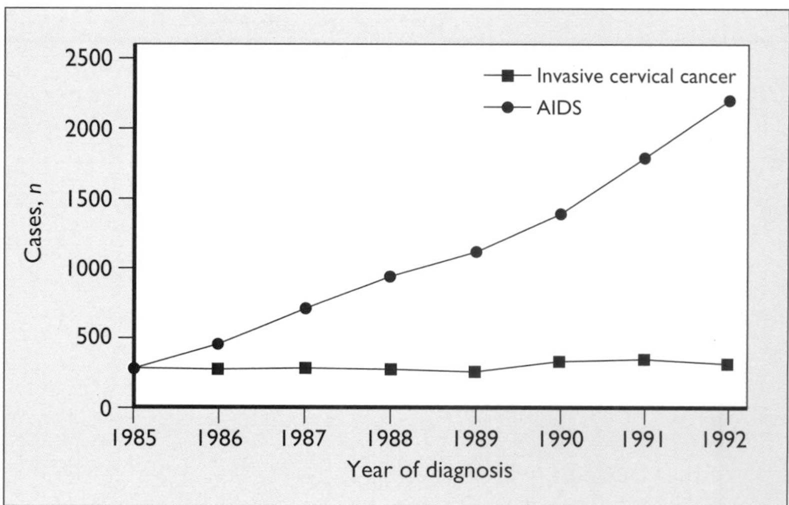

Figure 1-127 A comparison of the incidence of AIDS and the incidence of invasive cervical cancer in women < 55 years of age in New York City. Despite the dramatic increase in the number of women diagnosed with AIDS in New York City since 1985, there has been no concomitant overall increase in the number of invasive cervical cancer cases reported in the city. However, the incidence of invasive cervical cancer in HIV-infected women may be approximately two times higher than that expected in the general population [136]. Thus far, 107 of 16,612 women with AIDS from New York City have been reported to have invasive cervical cancer [137].

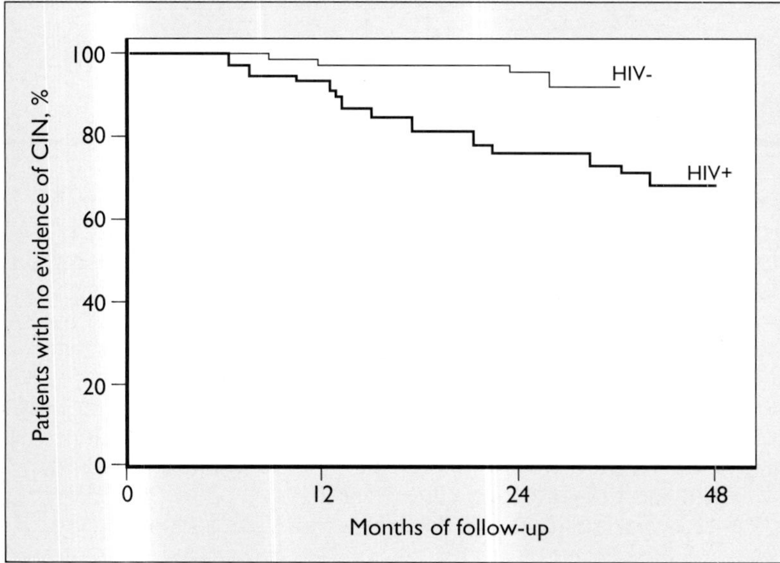

FIGURE 1-128 Increased incidence of cervical intraepithelial neoplasia (CIN) in HIV-infected women. Not only is the prevalence of CIN elevated in HIV-infected women, but these women also are more likely to develop new disease. In a study of 353 HIV-infected and 367 HIV-uninfected women, who were disease-free at baseline and followed at 6-month intervals, the annual incidence of biopsy-confirmed CIN was 8.1% among the HIV-infected women compared with only 1.1% among the uninfected women [138].

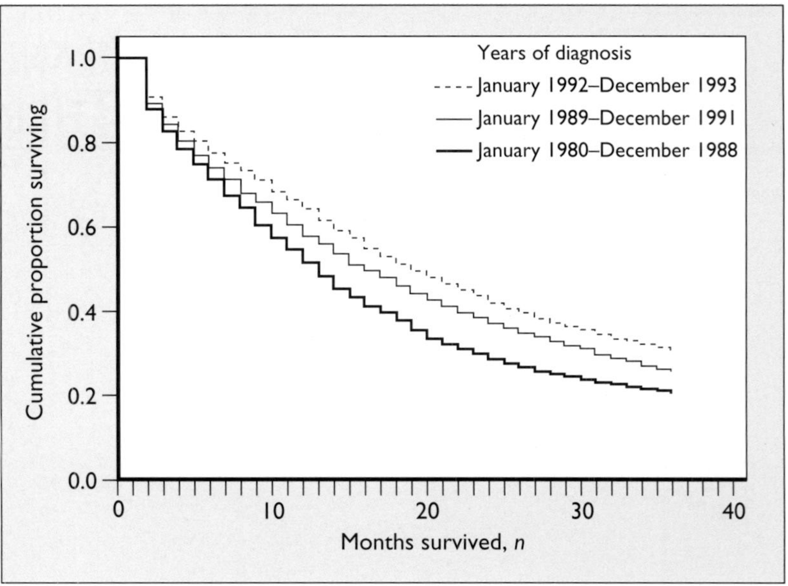

FIGURE 1-129 Survival trends for 2402 women diagnosed with AIDS in New York City from the beginning of the epidemic through December 1988, 3468 diagnosed from January 1989 through December 1991, and 2392 diagnosed from January 1992 through December 1993 are compared. (Women meeting only the 1993 expanded AIDS case definition were excluded from this analysis.) Both median survival and the proportion of women surviving > 3 years after a diagnosis of AIDS have increased over time. Among women diagnosed most recently, approximately 30% of those surviving at least 1 month after diagnosis are expected to survive at least 3 years.

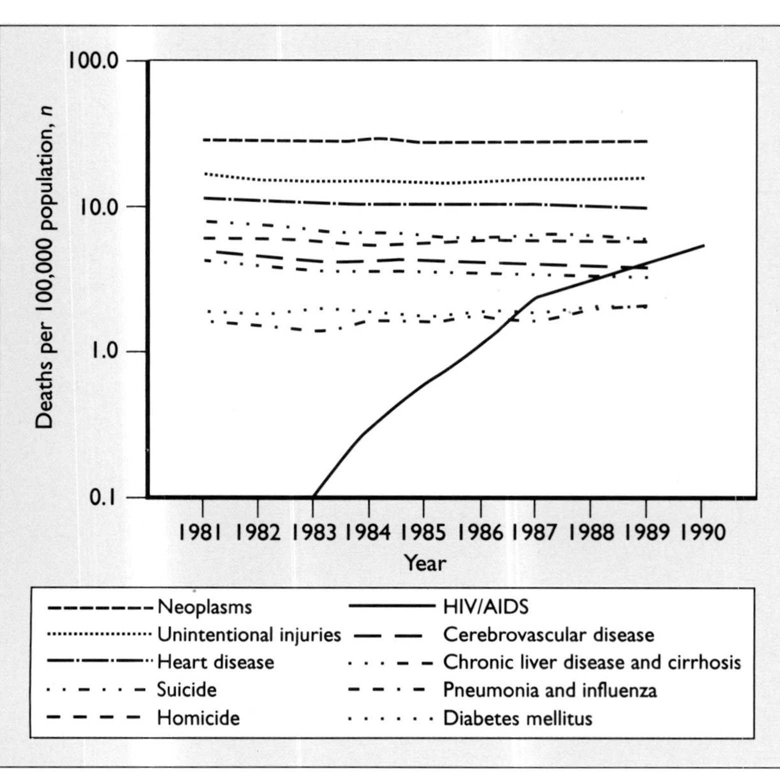

FIGURE 1-130 Death rates for HIV/AIDS and other leading causes in women in the United States, 1981 to 1990. HIV infection has emerged as an important cause of mortality in young women (aged 25–44 years) in the United States. The *solid line* represents the death rate due to HIV infection in women, which has increased rapidly since 1983, whereas the rates for other leading causes of mortality have remained relatively stable. In 1989, HIV infection was the sixth leading cause of death among women 25 to 44 years of age. By 1994, HIV/AIDS rose to the third leading cause of death for this age group. (*Courtesy of* Centers for Disease Control and Prevention.)

Rationale and Strategies for Antiretroviral Therapy in HIV-1 Infection

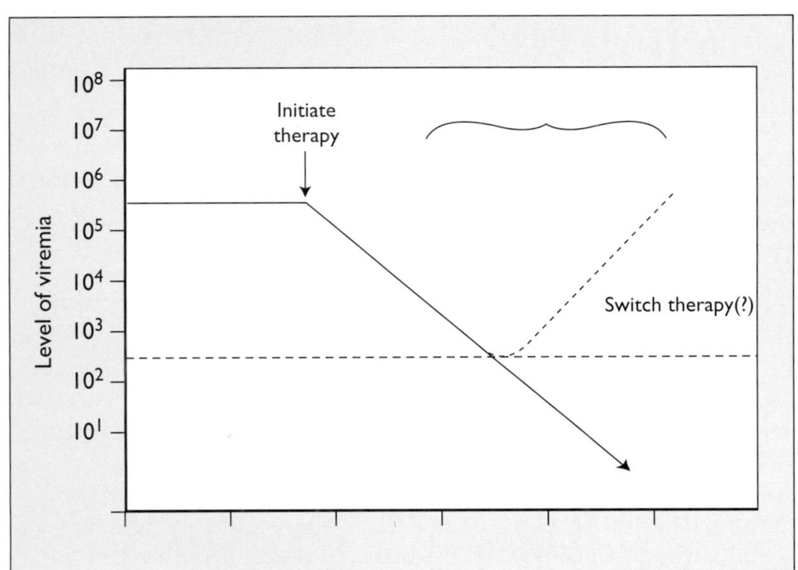

Figure 1-131 Plasma RNA levels as markers of antiretroviral activity. The idealized clinical application of viral load assays is depicted in this figure, which shows plasma HIV-1 RNA concentrations, quantitated as $\log_{10}$ copy numbers/mL, displaying with excellent sensitivity the effects of antiretroviral treatment. Levels decline rapidly on initiation of active therapy and reapproximate the baseline as therapeutic activity wanes. The lower limit of detection for the reverse transcriptase polymerase chain reaction, branched DNA, and nucleic acid sequence–based amplification assays varies from 200 to 500 copies/mL; with newer modifications, the limit of detection can be reduced to 10 to 25 copies/mL. Intra-assay variability is low for all methods. As a major advantage, the assays can be performed on batched stored samples or in real time, making them practical for clinical use. (*Courtesy of* B. McCreedy, Laboratory Corporation of America.)

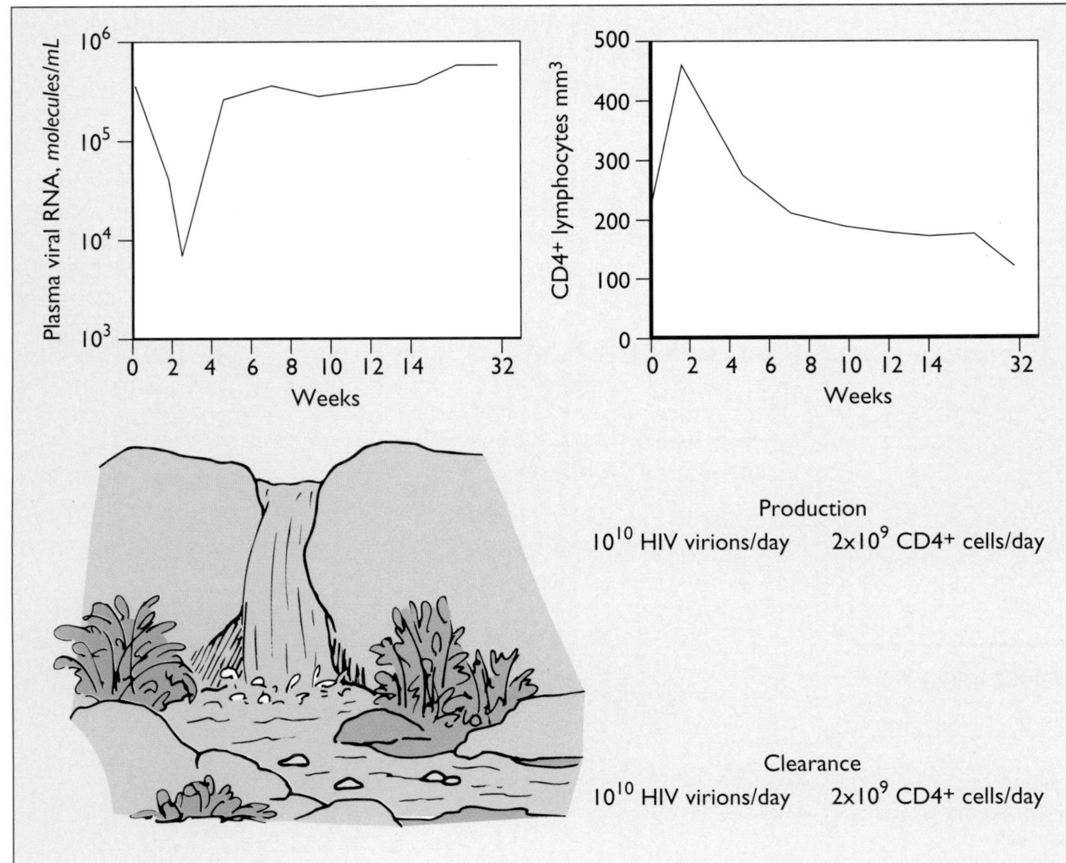

Figure 1-132 A dynamic infectious process. Viral production and $CD4^+$ cell production is balanced by viral clearance and $CD4^+$ cell destruction, representing a steady state. Pivotal studies to characterize the rate of HIV-1 and $CD4^+$ cell turnover used highly active antiretroviral agents to perturb the steady state of plasma viremia. These investigations estimated plasma virion turnover to be approximately 10 billion viral particles per day. A similarly rapid turnover is estimated for $CD4^+$ cells, with approximately 1.8 billion cells produced and destroyed daily. The life span of plasma virions is estimated at 0.3 days and that of virus-producing $CD4^+$ cells at 2.2 days [139–142]. (*Adapted from* Wei *et al.* [140].)

Viral dynamics: Implications for treatment
1. All stages of infection
2. Advantage of early intervention
3. Limitations of monotherapy
4. Rationale for combination therapy

FIGURE 1-133 Viral dynamics: implications for treatment. The stunning findings on viral dynamics have the following broad implications for treatment: 1) All patients should be considered for antiretroviral therapy, regardless of $CD4^+$ cell count or stage of disease, as long as viremia is detected. 2) Because viral burden and degree of immunodeficiency are lowest in early HIV infection, it is anticipated that aggressive treatment undertaken at this time will achieve the best results. 3) Given the magnitude of viral turnover, resistance to a *single* antiretroviral agent is expected, as long as selective pressure is exerted but is insufficient to suppress viral replication completely. 4) Combination therapy will be required for maximal suppression of viral replication to avoid breakthrough and development of drug resistance.

Antiretroviral agents

Agent	Brand name (abbreviation)	Manufacturer
Approved agents		
Nucleoside reverse transcriptase inhibitors		
Zidovudine	Retrovir (ZDV)	Glaxo Wellcome
Didanosine	Videx (ddI)	Bristol-Myers Squibb
Zalcitabine	Hivid (ddC)	Hoffmann-La Roche
Stavudine	Zerit (d4T)	Bristol-Myers Squibb
Lamivudine	Epivir (3TC)	Glaxo Wellcome
Nonnucleoside reverse transcriptase inhibitors		
Nevirapine	Viramune (NVP)	Boehringer Ingelheim
Delavirdine*	Rescriptor	Pharmacia & Upjohn
Protease inhibitors		
Saquinavir	Invirase	Hoffmann-La Roche
Ritonavir	Norvir	Abbott
Indinavir	Crixivan	Merck
Additional agents with anti-HIV activity		
Interferon-α	Roferon-A	Hoffmann-La Roche
	Intron-A	Schering Plough
Foscarnet	Foscavir	Astra

*In compassionate use.

FIGURE 1-134 Antiretroviral agents approved for use in HIV-1 infection, and other agents with anti–HIV-1 activity.

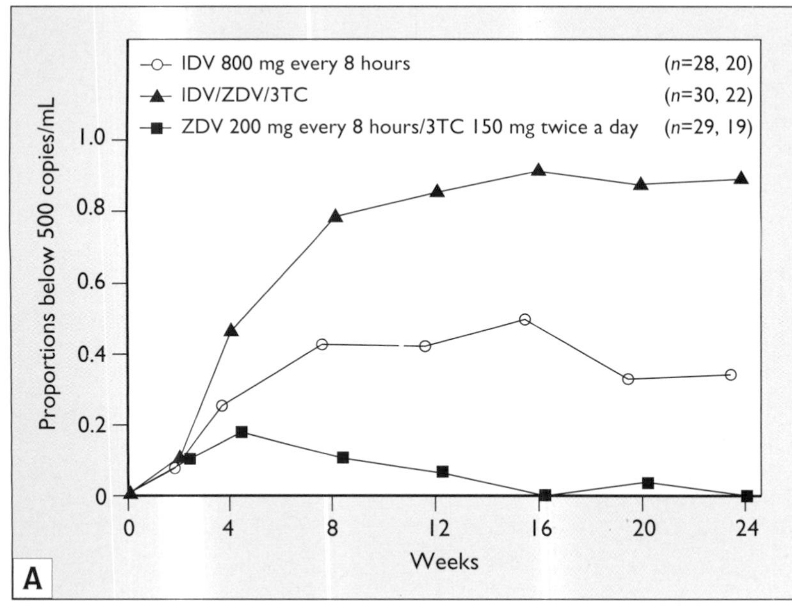

FIGURE 1-135 Changing the paradigm. Studies have begun to address the possibilities for complete viral suppression and will even focus on the question of eradication of HIV in infected persons. **A**, In patients with ≥ 6 months of prior zidovudine (ZDV), 50 to 400 $CD4^+$ cells/mm^3, and ≥ 20,000 copies/mL serum HIV RNA (Merck Protol 035), indinavir plus ZDV plus lamivudine (3TC) is a potent antiretroviral regimen that suppressed HIV-1 RNA in 80% to 90% of treated subjects to values that were below the level of detection of the assay (< 500 copies/mL) [143,144]. (*continued*)

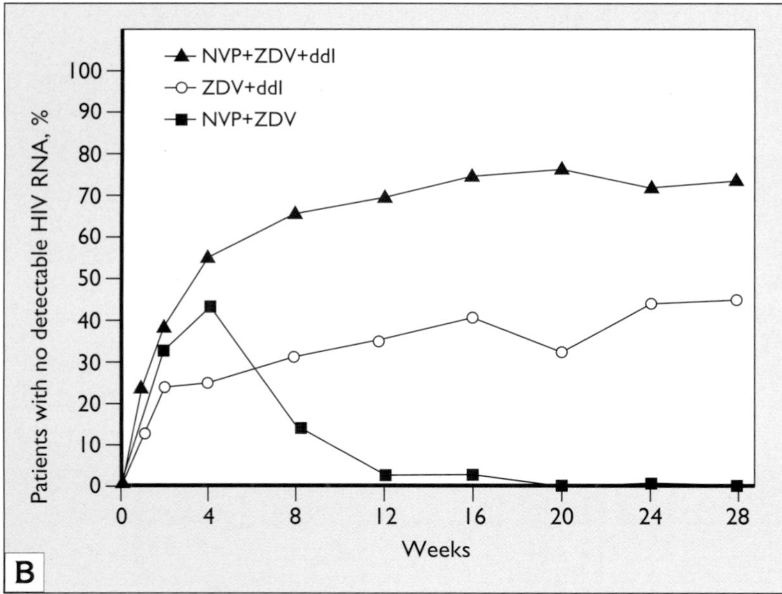

Figure 1-135 *(continued)* **B**, Superior viral load suppression occurs with ZDV/didanosine (ddI)/nevirapine, compared with either ZDV/nevirapine or ZDV/ddI, when administered to antiretroviral naive patients with CD4+ cell counts between 200 and 600 cells/mm^3. Approximately 70% of patients on the triple combination suppressed viral replication to below the level of detection of the Roche assay at 28 weeks. Compliance appeared to be an important contributor in those patients who did not achieve maximal suppression. **C**, Aggressive triple combination therapy (ZDV/3TC/ritonavir) in 12 subjects treated within 90 days of acquisition of HIV-1 infection resulted in negative cultures in peripheral blood mononuclear cells, undetectable RNA concentrations by branched DNA assay (< 500 copies/mL), and CD4 cell count increases. The advantage of potent treatment at the earliest stage of infection relates to the intactness of the immune system and the relative homogeneity of the virus, reducing the likelihood of accumulation of multiple resistance mutations. (Panel 135A *adapted from* Gulick *et al.* [144]; panel 135B *adapted from* Myers *et al.* [145]; panel 135C *adapted from* Markowitz *et al.* [146].)

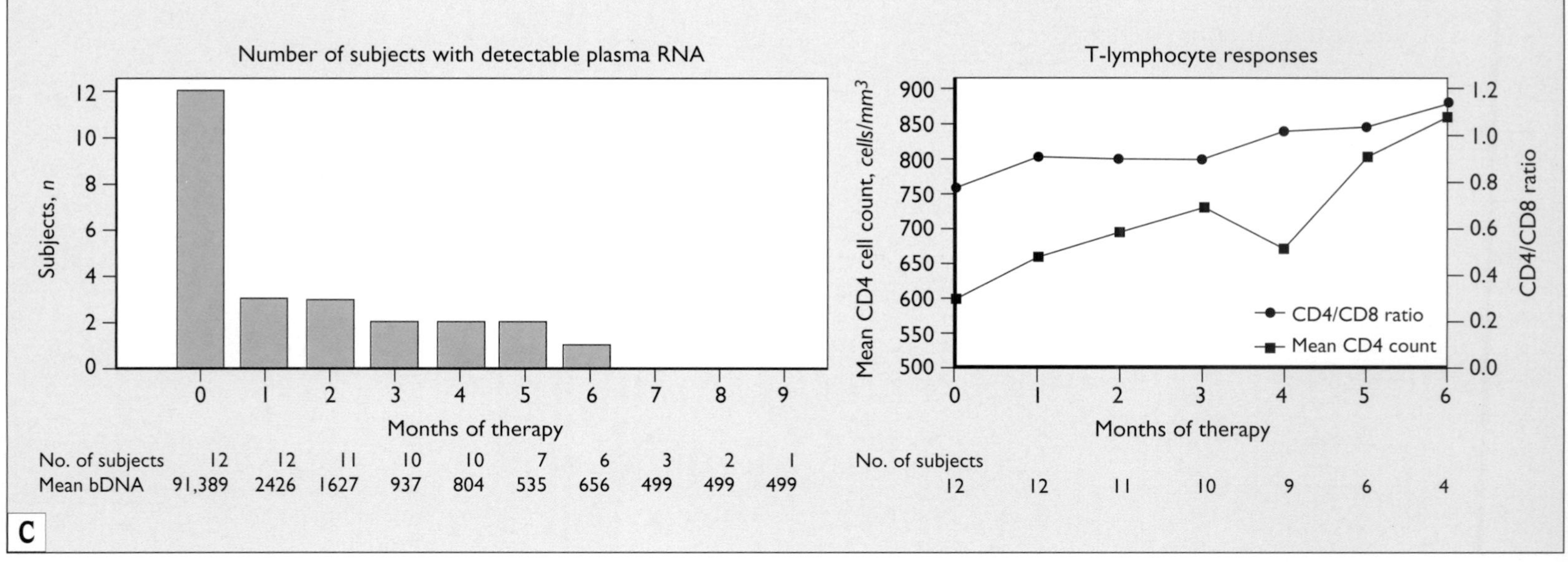

Antiviral Treatments

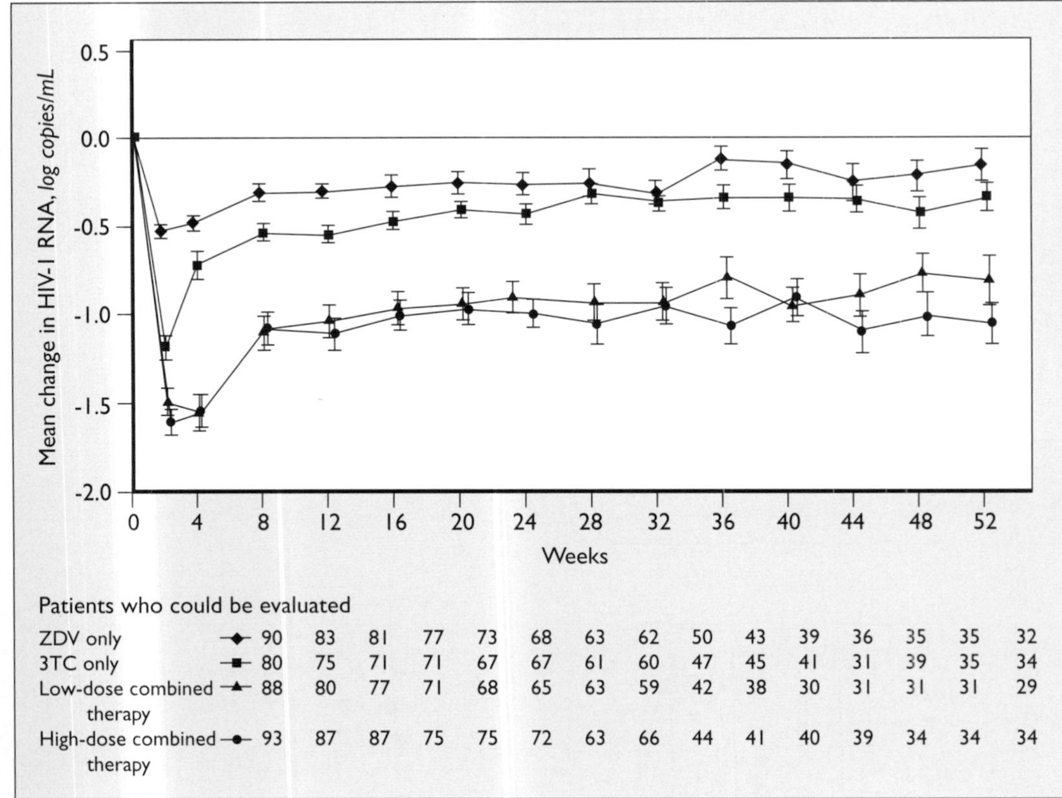

Figure 1-136 Changes in log concentration of HIV RNA, low-dose and high-dose lamivudine (3TC) and zidovudine (ZDV) vs 3TC or ZDV. Mean reductions in HIV RNA levels of 1.12±0.0.7 log for the low-dose combination group and 1.15±0.07 log for the high-dose combination group were noted compared with mean reductions of 0.31±0.03 log for the ZDV group ($P<0.001$ each) and 0.59±0.04 log for the 3TC group ($P<0.001$ each). (*Adapted from* Eron *et al.* [147].)

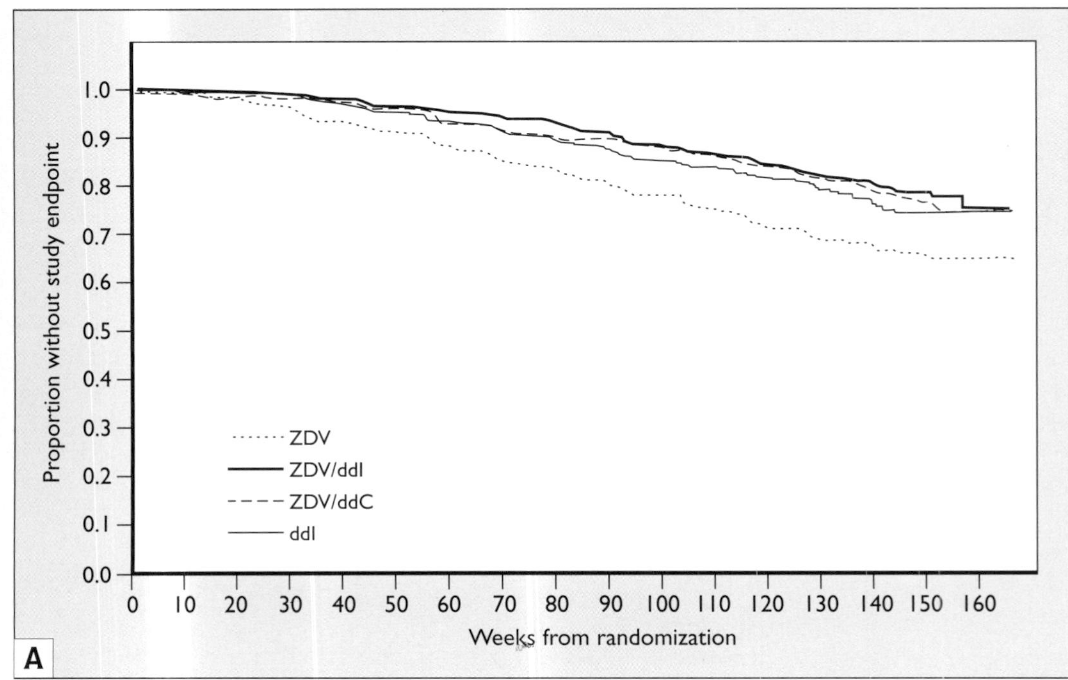

Figure 1-137 Cumulative study endpoint-free and AIDS-free survivals, zidovudine (ZDV) or didanosine (ddI) monotherapy vs the combination of ZDV and ddI or zalcitabine (ddC). A total of 2467 patients with HIV infection and 200 to 500 CD4 cells/mm^3 who received < 1 week or > 1 week of prior antiretroviral therapy were randomized to ZDV (600 mg/d), ddI (400 mg/d), or ZDV (600 mg/d) and either ddI (400 mg/d) or ddC (2.25 mg/d). **A**, After a mean of 143 weeks, CD4 cell count declined and AIDS or deaths (whichever occurred first) were higher with ZDV (32%) compared with ddI (22%, $P<0.001$), combination with ddI (18%, $P<0.001$) and combination with ddC (20%, $P<0.001$). (*continued*).

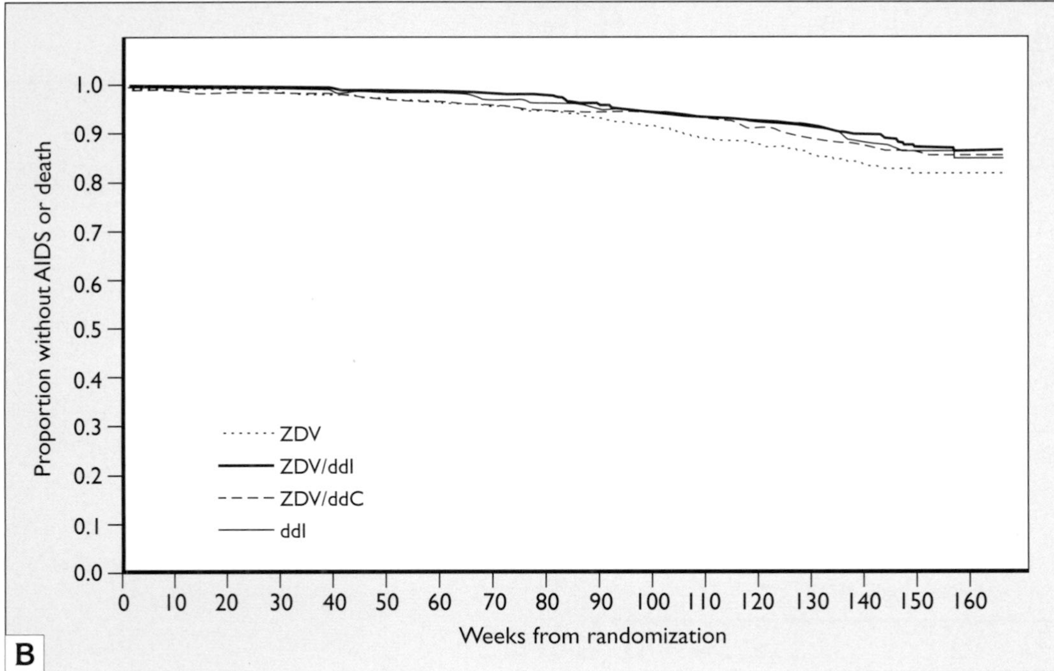

FIGURE 1-137 (*continued*) **B**, The relative hazards for AIDS-free survival compared with ZDV were 0.69, 0.64, and 0.77, respectively. (*Adapted from* Hammer *et al.* [148].)

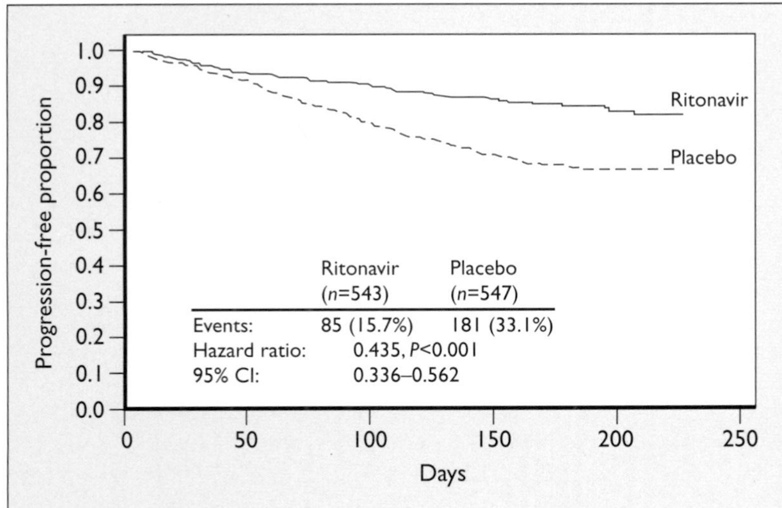

FIGURE 1-138 Cumulative disease-free survival, ritonavir vs placebo plus approved nucleoside antiretrovirals. A total of 1090 patients with ≤ 100 CD4 cells/mm^3 who had > 9 months of previous antiretroviral therapy and concurrent use of no more than two approved drugs received either ritonavir (600 mg twice a day) or placebo. Eighty-five patients (15.7%) in the ritonavir group and 181 (33.1%) in the placebo group developed AIDS or died (P<0.001). (*Adapted from* Cameron *et al.* [149].)

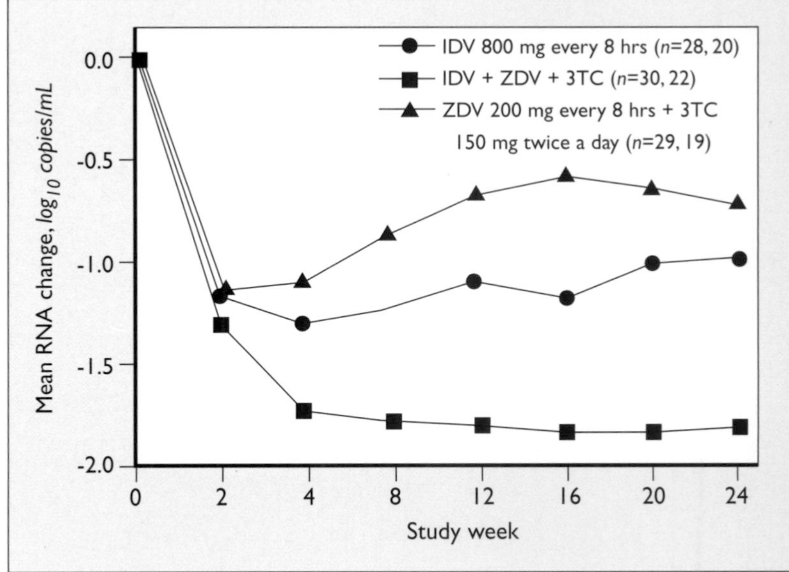

FIGURE 1-139 Changes in log concentration of HIV RNA, indinavir (IDV), zidovudine (ZDV), and lamivudine (3TC). A total of 97 patients with 50 to 400 CD4 cells/mm^3, plasma RNA levels ≥ 20,000 copies/mL, and ≥ 6 months of prior ZDV were randomized to IDV (800 mg three times a day), ZDV (200 mg three times a day), and 3TC (150 mg twice a day) vs IDV (800 mg three times a day) vs ZDV (200 mg three times a day) and 3TC (150 mg twice a day). Median HIV RNA levels decreased by 2.2 $\log_{10}$ for the triple combination group, 0.7 $\log_{10}$ for the IDV group, and 0.6 $\log_{10}$ for the ZDV plus 3TC group at 24 weeks. At 32 weeks, 19 (83%) patients on triple therapy, eight (36%) on IDV, and 0 (0%) patients on ZDV and 3TC had HIV RNA levels below assay detection (< 500 copies/mL). (*Adapted from* Gulick *et al.* [144].)

Antiretroviral drugs

Drug name (trade name)	Tablet/capsule size, *mg*	Recommended dosage
Nucleoside analogues		
Zidovudine (Retrovir)	100	200 mg TID 300 mg BID*
Didanosine (Videx)	25, 50, 100, 150	200 mg BID (fasting)† 125 mg BID‡
Zalcitabine (HIVID)	0.375, 0.750	0.75 mg TID
Stavudine (Zerit)	15, 20, 30, 40	40 mg BID 30 mg BID‡
Lamivudine (Epivir)	150	150 mg BID
Nonnucleosides		
Nevirapine (Viramune)	200	200 mg BID§
Protease inhibitors		
Saquinavir (Invirase)	200	600 mg TID (with food)
Ritonavir (Norvir)	100	600 mg BID¶ (with food)
Indinavir (Crixivan)	200, 400	800 mg TID (fasting)

*Alternate dose schedule.
†Alternate formulation: pediatric powder (4 g): 25 mL (250 mg) BID.
‡< 60 kg.
§200 mg every day for 14 days, then 200 mg BID.
¶Dose escalates over 7–10 days: 400 mg BID, then 500 mg BID, then 600 mg BID.
BID—twice a day; TID—three times a day.

FIGURE 1-140 Antiretroviral drugs for the treatment of HIV infection. Eight drugs have been approved for the treatment of HIV infection. For adult patients with HIV infection, monotherapy zidovudine is no longer recommended. Several combination regimens, including zidovudine and either didanosine, zalcitabine, or lamivudine, are clinically useful at all stages of HIV disease as first-line therapies. For more advanced disease or patients with high RNA levels, combination regimens that include protease inhibitors should be chosen. When protease inhibitors should be used (early vs late disease) is under evaluation. Nivera-pine recently has been approved by the Food and Drug Administration and can be used in combination regimens with nucleoside analogues, as first-line therapy. Similar strategies can be used when switching therapy. However, when changing therapy for treatment failure or relapse, at least two new drugs should be chosen.

Toxicities associated with nucleoside analogues

	Zidovudine	Didanosine	Zalcitabine	Stavudine	Lamivudine
Constitutional					
Fever	+	+	++++	+	+
Malaise	++++	++++	++++	++++	++++
Myalgias	++++	+	+	++++	++++
Headache	++++	++++	++++	++++	++++
Fatigue	++++	++++	+	++++	++++
Altered taste	+	++++	+	NR	NR
Insomnia	++++	NR	NR	NR	NR
Gastrointestinal					
Nausea	++++	++++	+	++++	++++
Vomiting	+	+	+	+	+
Diarrhea	+	++++	+	+	+
Abdominal pain	+	++++	+	+	+
Pancreatitis	NR	++++	+	+	+
Elevated transaminase	++++	++++	+	++++	++++
Stomatitis	NR	NR	++++	NR	NR
Hematologic					
Anemia	++++	+	+	++	++
Neutropenia	++++	+	+	++	++
Thrombocytopenia	NR	+	+	+	+
Neuromuscular					
Myopathy	++++	+	+	+	+
Peripheral neuropathy	NR	++++	++++	++++	+
Metabolic					
Hyperuricemia	NR	++++	NR	NR	NR
Hypertriglyceridemia	NR	++++	NR	NR	NR
Hyperamylasemia	NR	++++	+	++++	+
Allergic					
Rash	+	+	++++	+	+
Fever	+	+	++++	+	+

+—rare; ++++—more common; NR—not reported.

FIGURE 1-141 Toxicities with nucleoside analogues. The more common toxicities noted with zidovudine therapy include headache, malaise, myalgias, anemia, and neutropenia and longer-term myopathy. The more common toxicities seen with didanosine therapy include palatability of the current formulation (the pediatric powder may be substituted), pancreatitis, hyperamylasemia, and peripheral neuropathy. The more common toxicities noted with zalcitabine initially include rash, fever and stomatitis (rarely esophagitis), and longer-term peripheral neuropathy. The most common toxicities noted with stavudine therapy include peripheral neuropathy and less commonly headache, anemia, pancreatitis, and elevation in serum transaminases. The toxicities associated with lamivudine include headache, myalgia, dizziness, restlessness, nausea, and neutropenia and less commonly altered mood, anemia, and elevation in serum transaminases. Liver toxicity as manifested by steatosis has been described with this class of drugs, as well as rare cases of cardiomyopathy.

REFERENCES

1. World Health Organization: *The HIV/AIDS Pandemic*: 1993 Overview. Geneva: WHO; 1993.
2. Centers for Disease Control and Prevention: US HIV and AIDS cases reported through December 1995. In *HIV/AIDS Surveillance Report*. 1995, 7(2):1–36.
3. Selik RM, Chu SY, Buehler JW: HIV infection as leading cause of death among young adults in US cities and states. *JAMA* 1993, 263:2991–2994.
4. Vermund SH: Rising HIV-mortality in young Americans. *JAMA* 1993, 269:3034–3035.
5. Centers for Disease Control and Prevention: 1993 revised classification system for HIV infection and expanded surveillance case definition for AIDS among adolescents and adults. *MMWR* 1992, 41[RR-17]:1–19.
6. Saag MS, Holodniy M, Kuritzkes DR, *et al.*: HIV viral load markers in clinical practice. *Nature Med* 1996, 2:625–629.
7. Pantaleo G, Graziosi C, Fauci AS: New concepts in the immunopathogenesis of human immunodeficiency virus infection. *N Engl J Med* 1993, 328:327–335.
8. Elias CJ, Heise L: *The Development of Microbicides: A New Method of HIV Prevention for Women*. New York: The Population Council, 1993, Programs Division Working Paper no. 6.
9. Grosskurth H, Mosha F, Todd J, *et al.*: Impact of improved treatment of sexually transmitted diseases on HIV infection in rural Tanzania: Randomized controlled trial. *Lancet* 1995, 346:530–536.
10. Minkoff H, Burns DN, Landesman S, *et al.*: The relationship of the duration of ruptured membranes to vertical transmission of human immunodeficiency virus. *Am J Obstet Gynecol* 1995, 173:585–589.
11. Biggar RJ, Miotti PG, Taha TE, *et al.*: Perinatal intervention trial in Africa: Effect of a birth canal cleansing intervention to prevent HIV transmission. *Lancet* 1996, 347:1647–1650.
12. Connor EM, Spering RS, Gilber R, *et al.*: Reduction of maternal-infant transmission of human immunodeficiency virus type 1 with zidovudine treatment. Pediatric AIDS Clinical Trials Group Protocol 076 Study Group. *N Engl J Med* 1994, 331:1173–1180.
13. Kaplan EH: Needle exchange or needless exchange? *Infect Agents Dis* 1992, 1:92–98.
14. Flier JS, Underhill LH, Crumpacker CS: Molecular targets of antiviral therapy. *N Engl J Med* 1985, 321:163–172.
15. Cullen BR: Mechanism of action of regulatory proteins encoded by complex retroviruses. *Microbiol Rev* 1992, 56:375–394.
16. Hahn BH: Viral genes and their products. *In* Broder S, Merigan TC, Bolognesi D (eds.): *Textbook of AIDS Medicine*. Baltimore: Williams & Wilkins; 1994:21–44.
17. Saag MS, Hahn BS, Gibbons J: Extension variation of HIV-1 *in vivo*. *Nature* 1988, 334:440–444.
18. Saag MS: AIDS testing now and in the future. *In* Sande MA, Volberding PA (eds.): *Medical Management of AIDS*, 4th ed. Philadelphia: W.B. Saunders; 1994.
19. Brock TD, Madigan MT: *Biology of Microorganisms*, 5th ed. Englewood Cliffs, NJ: Prentice Hall; 1988:454.
20. Meyer UB, Paulker SG: Screening for HIV: Can we afford the false-positive rate? *N Engl J Med* 1987, 317:238–241.
21. Saag MS, Holodniy M, Kuritzkes DR, *et al.*: HIV viral load markers in clinical practice. *Nature Med* 1996, 2(6):625–629.
22. Weiss RA: How does HIV cause AIDS? *Science* 1993, 260:1273–1279.
23. Pantaleo G, Graziosi C, Fauci AS: New concepts in the immunopathogenesis of human immunodeficiency virus infection. *N Engl J Med* 1993, 328:327–335.
24. Cao Y, Qin L, Zhang L, *et al.*: Virologic and immunologic characterization of long-term survivors of human immunodeficiency virus type 1 infection. *N Engl J Med* 1995, 332:201–208.
25. Pantaleo G, Menzo S, Vaccarezza M, *et al.*: Studies in subjects with long-term nonprogressive human immunodeficiency virus infection. *N Engl J Med* 1995, 332:209–216.
26. Kirchhoff F, Greenough TC, Brettler DB, *et al.*: Brief report: Absence of intact *nef* sequences in a long-term survivor with nonprogressive HIV-1 infection. *N Engl J Med* 1995, 332:228–232.
27. Baltimore A: Lessons from people with nonprogressive HIV infection [editorial]. *N Engl J Med* 1995, 332:259–260.
28. Bryson YJ, Pang S, Wei LS, *et al.*: Clearance of HIV infection in a perinatally infected infant. *N Engl J Med* 1995, 332:833–838.
29. McIntosh K, Burchett SK: Clearance of HIV—Lessons from newborns. *N Engl J Med* 1995, 332:883–884.
30. Gougeon MI: Apoptosis in AIDS. *Science* 1993, 260:1269–1270.
31. Ameisen JC: Programmed cell death and AIDS: From hypothesis to experiment. *Immunol Today* 1992, 13:388.
32. Cohen JJ: Apoptosis: The physiologic pathway of cell death. *Hosp Pract* 1993, (Dec):35.
33. Matsuyama T, Kobayashi N, Yamamoto N: Cytokines and HIV infection: Is AIDS a tumor necrosis factor disease? *AIDS* 1991, 5:1405–1417.
34. Fauci AS: Multifactorial nature of human immunodeficiency virus disease: Implications for therapy. *Science* 1993, 262:1011–1018.
35. Centers for Disease Control and Prevention: 1993 Revised classification system for HIV infection and expanded surveillance case definition for AIDS. *MMWR* 1992, 41[RR-17]:1–19.
36. Pedersen C, Lindhart BO, Jensen BL, *et al.*: Clinical course of primary HIV infection: Consequences for subsequent course of infection. *BMJ* 1989, 299:154–157.
37. Tindall B, Barker S, Donovan B, *et al.*: Characterization of the acute clinical illness associated with human immunodeficiency virus infection. *Arch Intern Med* 1988, 148:945–949.
38. Gaines H, von Sydow, Pehrson PO, *et al.*: Clinical picture of primary HIV infection presenting as a glandular-fever-like illness. *BMJ* 1988, 297:1363–1368.
39. Hulsebosch HJ, Claessen FAP, van Ginkel CJW, *et al.*: Human immunodeficiency virus exanthem. *J Am Acad Dermatol* 1990, 23:483–485.
40. Rabeneck L, Popovic M, Gartner S, *et al.*: Acute co-infection with human immunodeficiency virus (HIV) and esophageal ulcers. *JAMA* 1990, 263:2318–2332.
41. Centers for Disease Control and Prevention: Classification system for human T-lymphotropic virus type III/lymphadenopathy-associated virus infection. *MMWR* 1986, 35:334–339.
42. Gherardi R, Belec L, Mhiric C, *et al.*: The spectrum of vasculitis in human immunodeficiency virus-infected patients. *Arthritis Rheum* 1993, 36:1164–1174.
43. Berman A, Espinoza LR, Diaz JD, *et al.*: Rheumatic manifestations of human immunodeficiency virus infection. *Am J Med* 1988, 85:59–64.
44. Seifert M: *The Rheumatology of HIV Infection (Topical Reviews, no 11)*. Arthritis and Rheumatism Council for Research, Jan. 1989.
45. Davis P, Stein M, Latif S, Emmanuel J: HIV and polyarthritis. *Lancet* 1988, i:356.
46. Schwartz JJ, Myskowski PL: Molluscum contagiosum in patients with human immunodeficiency virus infection: A review of twenty-seven patients. *J Am Acad Dermatol* 1992, 27:583–588.
47. Robinson MR, Udell IJ, Garber PF, *et al.*: Molluscum contagiosum of the eyelids in patients with acquired immune deficiency syndrome. *Ophthalmology* 1992, 99:1745–1747.
48. Sandor EV, Millman A, Croxson TS, Mildvan D: Herpes zoster ophthalmicus in patients at risk for the acquired immune deficiency syndrome (AIDS). *Am J Ophthalmol* 1996, 101:153–155.
49. Sellitti TP, Huang AJ, Schiffman J, Davis JL: Association of herpes zoster ophthalmicus with acquired immunodeficiency syndrome and acute retinal necrosis. *Am J Ophthalmol* 1993, 116:297–301.
50. Litoff D, Catalano RA: Herpes zoster optic neuritis in human immunodeficiency virus infection. *Arch Ophthalmol* 1990, 108:782–783.
51. McLeish W, Pflugfelder SC, Crouse C, *et al.*: Interferon treatment of herpetic keratitis in a patient with acquired immunodeficiency syndrome. *Am J Ophthalmol* 1990, 109:93–95.
52. Young TL, Robin JB, Holland GN, *et al.*: Herpes simplex keratitis in patients with acquired immune deficiency syndrome. *Ophthalmology* 1989, 96:1476–1479.
53. Nanda M, Pflugfelder SC, Holland S: Fulminant pseudomonal keratitis and scleritis in human immunodeficiency virus–infected patients. *Arch Ophthalmol* 1991, 109:503–505.
54. Spaide RF, Vitale AT, Toth IR, Oliver JM: Frosted branch angiitis associated with cytomegalovirus retinitis. *Am J Ophthalmol* 1992, 113:522–528.
55. Jabs DA, Enger C, Bartlett JG: Cytomegalovirus retinitis and acquired immunodeficiency syndrome. *Arch Ophthalmol* 1989, 107:75–80.
56. The Ocular Complications of AIDS Study Group: Mortality in patients with the acquired immunodeficiency syndrome treated with either foscarnet or ganciclovir for cytomegalovirus retinitis. *N Engl J Med* 1992, 326:213–220.

57. Jabs DA, Enger C, Haller J, de Bustros S: Retinal detachments in patients with cytomegalovirus retinitis. *Arch Ophthalmol* 1991, 109:794–799.

58. Iannucci AA, Hart LL: Clindamycin in the treatment of toxoplasmosis in AIDS. *Ann Pharmacother* 1992, 26:645–647.

59. Kovacs JA: Efficacy of atovaquone in treatment of toxoplasmosis in patients with AIDS. The NIAID-Clinical Center Intramural AIDS Program. *Lancet* 1992, 340:637–638.

60. Elkins BS, Holland GN, Opremcak EM, *et al.*: Ocular toxoplasmosis misdiagnosed as cytomegalovirus retinopathy in immunocompromised patients. *Ophthalmology* 1994, 101:499–507.

61. Ficarra G, Person AM, *et al.*: Kaposi's sarcoma of the oral cavity: A study of 134 patients with a review of the pathogenesis, epidemiology, clinical aspects, and treatment. *Oral Surg Oral Med Oral Pathol* 1988, 66:543–550.

62. Epstein JB, Scully C: Intralesional vinblastine for oral Kaposi's sarcoma in HIV infection. *Lancet* 1989, 2:1100–1101.

63. Greenspan D, Greenspan JS, *et al.*: *AIDS and the Mouth.* Copenhagen, Munksgaard, 1990.

64. Greenspan D, Greenspan JS, *et al.*: Oral "hairy" leukoplakia in male homosexuals: Evidence of association with both papillomavirus and a herpes-group virus. *Lancet* 1984, 2:831–834.

65. Feigal DW, Katz MH, *et al.*: The prevalence of oral lesions in HIV-infected homosexual and bisexual men: Three San Francisco epidemiological cohorts. *AIDS* 1991, 5:519–525.

66. Greenspan D, Greenspan JS: The significance of oral hairy leukoplakia. *Oral Surg Oral Med Oral Pathol* 1992, 73:151–154.

67. Katz MH, Greenspan D, Westenhouse J, *et al.*: Progression to AIDS in HIV-infected homosexual and bisexual men with hairy leukoplakia and oral candidiasis. *AIDS* 1992, 6:95–100.

68. Zambon JJ, Reynolds H, Smutko J, *et al.*: Are unique bacterial pathogens involved in HIV-associated periodontal disease? In *Oral Manifestations of HIV Infection: Proceedings of the Second International Workshop.* Carol Stream, IL: Quintessence Publishing Co., 1995.

69. Palmer GD: Periodontal therapy for patients with HIV infection. In *Oral manifestations of HIV Infection: Proceedings of the Second International Workshop.* Carol Steam, IL: Quintessence Publishing Co., 1995.

70. Masur H: Prevention and treatment of pneumocystis pneumonia. *N Engl J Med* 1992, 326:1853–1860.

71. Maxfield RA, Sorkin B, Fazzini EP, *et al.*: Respiratory failure in patients with acquired immunodeficiency syndrome and *Pneumocystis carinii* pneumonia. *Crit Care Med* 1986, 14:443–449.

72. Pitchenik AE, Rubinson HA: The radiologic appearance of tuberculosis in patients with the acquired immune deficiency syndrome (AIDS) and pre-AIDS. *Am Rev Respir Dis* 1985, 131:393–396.

73. Laine L, Dretler RH, Conteas CN, *et al.*: Fluconazole compared with ketoconazole for the treatment of candidal esophagitis in AIDS: A randomized trial. *Ann Intern Med* 1992, 117:655–660.

74. Gillin JS, Urmacher C, West R, Shike M: Disseminated *Mycobacterium avium-intracellulare* infection in acquired immunodeficiency syndrome mimicking Whipple's disease. *Gastroenterology* 1983, 85:1187–1191.

75. Kemper CA, Meng TC, Nussbaum J, *et al.*: Treatment of *Mycobacterium avium* complex bacteremia in AIDS with a four-drug oral regimen: Rifampin, ethambutol, clofazimine, and ciprofloxacin. *Ann Intern Med* 1992, 116:466–472.

76. Weber R, Bryan RT, Juranek DD: Improved stool concentration procedure for detection of *Cryptosporidium* oocysts in fecal specimens. *J Clin Microbiol* 1992, 30:2869–2873.

77. Wurtz RM, Kocka FE, Peters CS, *et al.*: Clinical characteristics of seven cases of diarrhea associated with a novel acid-fast organism in the stool. *Clin Infect Dis* 1993, 16:136–138.

78. Simon D, Weiss LM, Tanowitz HB, *et al.*: Light microscopic diagnosis of human microsporidiosis and variable response to octreotide. *Gastroenterology* 1991, 100:271–273.

79. Goodgame RW: Gastrointestinal cytomegalovirus disease. *Ann Intern Med* 1993, 119:924–935.

80. Janoff EN, Orenstein JM, Manischewitz JF, Smith PD: Adenovirus colitis in the acquired immunodeficiency syndrome. *Gastroenterology* 1991, 100:976–979.

81. Safrin S, Crumpacker C, Chatis P, *et al.*: A controlled trial comparing foscarnet with vidarabine for acyclovir-resistant mucocutaneous herpes simplex in the acquired immunodeficiency syndrome. *N Engl J Med* 1991, 325:551–555.

82. Mayer HB, Wanke CA: Enteroaggregative *Escherichia coli* as a possible cause of diarrhea in an HIV infected patient. *N Engl J Med* 1995, 332:273–274.

83. Kotler DP, Giang TT, Thiim M, *et al.*: Chronic bacterial enteropathy in patients with AIDS. *J Infect Dis* 1995, 171:552–558.

84. Johnson RD, McArthur JC, Narayano C: The neurobiology of human immunodeficiency virus infections. *FASEB J* 1988, 2:2970–2981.

85. Navia BA, Cho ES, Petito CK, Price RW: The AIDS dementia complex: II. Neuropathology. *Ann Neurol* 1986, 19:525–535.

86. Schaumburg HH, Spencer PS, Thomas PK (eds.): Anatomical classification of PNS disorder. In *Disorders of Peripherals Nerves.* Philadelphia: FA Davis, Co; 1983.

87. Luft B, Hafner R, Korzun A, *et al.*: Toxoplasmic encephalitis in patients with acquired immunodeficiency syndrome. *N Engl J Med* 1993, 329:995–1000.

88. Morgello S, Laufer H: Quaternary neurosyphillis in a Haitian man with human immunodeficiency virus infection. *Hum Pathol* 1989, 20:805–811.

89. Baumgarten J, Rachlin J, Beckstead J, *et al.*: Primary central nervous system lymphomas: Natural history and response to radiation therapy in 55 patients with acquired immunodeficiency syndrome. *J Neurosurg* 1990, 73:206–211.

90. Kotler DP, Tierney AR, Wang J, Pierson RN Jr: Magnitude of body-cell-mass depletion and timing of death from wasting in AIDS. *Am J Clin Nutr* 1989, 50:444–447.

91. Grunfeld C, Kotler DP, Hamadeh R, *et al.*: Hypertriglyceridemia in the acquired immunodeficiency syndrome. *Am J Med* 1989, 86:27–31.

92. Grunfeld C, Pang M, Shimizu, *et al.*: Resting energy expenditure, caloric intake, and short-term weight change in human immunodeficiency virus infection the acquired immunodeficiency syndrome. *Am J Clin Nutr* 1992, 55:455–460.

93. Macallan DC, Noble C, Baldwin C, *et al.*: Prospective analysis of weight changes in IV human immunodeficiency virus infection. *Am J Clin Nutr* 1993, 58:417–424.

94. Grunfeld C, Feingold KR: Metabolic disturbances and wasting in the acquired immunodeficiency syndrome. *N Engl J Med* 1992, 327:329–337.

95. Paraskevas F, Foerster J: Immunodiagnostics. *In* Lee GR, Bithell TC, Foerster J (eds.): *Wintrobe's Clinical Hematology*, 9th ed. Philadelphia: Lea & Febiger; 1993:488.

96. Cohen AJ, Phillips TM, Kessler CM: Circulating coagulation inhibitors in the acquired immunodeficiency syndrome. *Ann Intern Med* 1986, 104:175–180.

97. Hellinger WC, Bolling JP, Smith TF, Campbell RJ: Varicella-zoster virus retinitis in a patient with AIDS-related complex: Case report and brief review of the acute retinal necrosis syndrome. *Clin Infect Dis* 1993, 16:208–212.

98. Cohen PR, Beitrani VP, Grossman ME: Disseminated herpes zoster in patients with human immunodeficiency virus infection. *Am J Med* 1988, 84:1076–1080.

99. Cockerell CJ: Human immunodeficiency virus and the skin: A crucial interface. *Arch Intern Med* 1991, 151:1295–1303.

100. Pottage JC Jr, Sha BE: Development of histoplasmosis in a human immunodeficiency virus-infected patient receiving fluconazole [letter]. *J Infect Dis* 1991, 164:622–623.

101. Conte JE Jr, Hollander H, Golden JA: Inhaled or reduced-dose intravenous pentamidine for *Pneumocystis carinii* pneumonia: A pilot study. *Ann Intern Med* 1987, 107:495–498.

102. Kovacs JA, Hiementz JW, Macher AM, *et al.*: *Pneumocystis carinii* pneumonia: A comparison between patients with the acquired immunodeficiency syndrome and patients with other immunodeficiencies. *Ann Intern Med* 1984, 100:633–641.

103. National Institutes of Health-University of California Expert Panel for Corticosteroids as Adjunctive Therapy for Pneumocystis Pneumonia: Consensus statement on the use of corticosteroids as adjunctive therapy for pneumocystis pneumonia in the acquired immunodeficiency syndrome. *N Engl J Med* 1990, 323:1500–1504.

104. Bozzette SA, Sattler FR, Chiu J, *et al.*: A controlled trial of early adjunctive treatment with corticosteroids for *Pneumocystis carinii* pneumonia in the acquired immunodeficiency syndrome. *N Engl J Med* 1990, 323:1451–1457.

105. National Institutes of Health-University of California Expert Panel for Corticosteroids as Adjunctive Therapy for Pneumocystis Pneumonia: Consensus statement on the use of corticosteroids as adjunctive therapy for pneumocystis pneumonia in the acquired immunodeficiency syndrome. *N Engl J Med* 1990, 323:1500–1504.

106. Phair J, Muòoz A, Detels R, *et al.*: The risk of *Pneumocystis carinii* pneumonia among men infected with human immunodeficiency virus type 1. *N Engl J Med* 1990, 322:161–165.

107. Centers for Disease Control and Prevention: USPHS/IDSA guidelines for the prevention of opportunistic infections in persons infected with human immunodeficiency virus: A summary. *MMWR* 1995, 44(RR-8):1–34.

108. Masur H, Feinberg J, *et al.*: Guidelines for prophylaxis of *Pneumocystis carinii* pneumonia for persons with the human immunodeficiency virus. *J Acquir Defic Syndr* 1993, 6:46–55.

109. Laine L, Dretier RH, Conteas CN, *et al.*: Fluconazole compared with ketoconazole for the treatment of esophagitis in AIDS: A randomized trial. *Ann Intern Med* 1992, 117:655–660.

110. The Studies of Ocular Complications of AIDS with the AIDS Clinical Trials Group: Combination foscarnet and ganciclovir therapy vs monotherapy for the treatment of relapsed cytomegalovirus retinitis in patients with AIDS. *Arch Ophthalmol* 1996, 114:23–33.

111. Lalezari J, Stagg R, Kuppermann B, *et al.*: A phase II/III randomized study of immediate versus deferred cidofovir for the treatment of peripheral CMV retinitis in patients with AIDS [abstract LB18]. Presented at the Second National Conference on Human Retroviruses and Related Infections. Washington, DC, 1995.

112. Drew WL, Ives D, Lalezari JP, *et al.*: Oral ganciclovir as maintenance treatment for cytomegalovirus retinitis in patients with AIDS. *N Engl J Med* 1995, 333:615–620.

113. Masur H and the Public Health Service Task Force on Prophylaxis and Therapy for *Mycobacterium avium* Complex: Recommendations on prophylaxis and therapy for disseminated *Mycobacterium avium* complex disease in patients infected with the human immunodeficiency virus. *N Engl J Med* 1993, 329:898–904.

114. Shafran SD, Singer J, Zarowny DP, *et al.*: A comparison of two regimens for the treatment of *Mycobacterium avium* bacteremia in AIDS: Rifabutin, ethambutol, and clarithromycin versus rifampin, ethambutol, clofazimine, and ciprofloxacin. *N Engl J Med* 1996, 335:377–383.

115. Krown SE, Myskowski PL, Paredes J: Kaposi's sarcoma: Management of Kaposi's sarcoma in HIV-infected patients. *Med Clin North Am* 1992, 76:235–252.

116. Krown SE, Gold JWM, Niedzwiecki D, *et al.*: Interferon-alpha with zidovudine: Safety, tolerance, and clinical and virologic effects in patients with Kaposi's sarcoma associated with the acquired immunodeficiency syndrome (AIDS). *Ann Intern Med* 1990, 112:812–821.

117. Fischl MA, Uttamchandani RB, Resnick L, *et al.*: A phase I study of recombinant human interferon-alpha-2a or human lymphoblastoid interferon alpha-n1 and concomitant zidovudine in patients with AIDS-related Kaposi's sarcoma. *J Acquir Immune Defic Syndr* 1991, 4:1–10.

118. Kovacs JA, Deyton L, Davey R, *et al.*: Combined zidovudine and interferon-alpha therapy in patients with Kaposi sarcoma and the acquired immunodeficiency syndrome (AIDS). *Ann Intern Med* 1989, 111:280–287.

119. Levine AM, Wernz JC, Kaplan, *et al.*: Low dose chemotherapy with CNS prophylaxis and zidovudine maintenance in AIDS-related lymphomas: A prospective multi-institutional trial. *JAMA* 1991, 266:84–88.

120. Kaplan L, Straus D, Testa M, *et al.*: Randomized trial of standard dose m-BACOD with GM-CSF vs. reduced dose m-BACOD for systemic HIV-associated lymphoma: ACTG 142 [abstract]. *Proc Am Assoc Clin Oncol* 1995, 14:818.

121. Maiman M, Tarricons N, Viera J, *et al.*: Colposcopic evaluation of human immunodeficiency virus seropositive women. *Obstet Gynecol* 1991, 78:84–88.

122. Rubinstein A: Pediatric AIDS. *Curr Probl Pediatr* 1986, 16:361–409.

123. Scott GB, Hutto C, Markuch RW, *et al.*: Survival in children with perinatally acquired human immunodeficiency virus type 1 infection. *N Engl J Med* 1989, 321:1971–1976.

124. Connor EM, Sperling RS, Gelber R, *et al.*: Reduction of the material–infant transmission of human immunodeficiency virus type 1 with zidovudine treatment. *N Engl J Med* 1994, 331:1173–1180.

125. Centers for Disease Control and Prevention: Recommendations for the use of zidovudine to reduce perinatal transmission of human immunodeficiency virus. *MMWR* 1994, 43(RR-11).

126. Dabis F, Msellati P, Dunn D, *et al.*: Estimating the rate of mother-to-child transmission of HIV: Report of a workshop of methological issues, Ghent [Belgium]. *AIDS* 1993, 7:1139–1148.

127. Dickover RE, Garratty EM, Herman SA, *et al.*: Identification of levels of maternal HIV-1 RNA associated with risk of perinatal transmission: Effect of maternal zidovudine treatment on viral load. *JAMA* 1996, 275:599–605.

128. Provencher D, Valme B, Averette HE, *et al.*: HIV status and positive Papanicolaou screening: Identification of a high-risk population. *Gynecol Oncol* 1988, 31:184–188.

129. Carpenter CCJ, Mayer KH, Stein MD, *et al.*: Human immunodeficiency virus infection in North American women: Experience with 200 cases and a review of the literature. *Medicine* 1991, 70:307–325.

130. Vermund SH, Kelly KE, Klein RS, *et al.*: High risk of human papillomavirus infection and cervical squamous intraepithelial lesions among women with symptomatic human immunodeficiency virus infection. *Am J Obstet Gynecol* 1991, 165:392–400.

131. Shafer A, Friedman W, Mielke M, *et al.*: The increased frequency of cervical dysplasia-neoplasia in women infected with the human immunodeficiency virus is related to the degree of immunosuppression. *Am J Obstet Gynecol* 1991, 164:593–599.

132. Kreiss JK, Kiviat NB, Plummer FA, *et al.*: Human immunodeficiency virus, human papillomavirus, and cervical intraepithelial neoplasia in Nairobi prostitutes. *Sex Trans Dis* 1992, 19:54–59.

133. Wright TC, Ellerbrock TV, Chiasson MA, *et al.*: Cervical intraepithelial neoplasia in women infected with human immunodeficiency virus: Prevalence, risk factors, and validity of Papanicolaou smears. *Obstet Gynecol* 1994, 84:591–597.

134. Laga M, Icenogle JP, Marsella R, *et al.*: Genital papillomavirus infection and cervical dysplasiaóopportunistic complications of the HIV infection. *Int J Cancer* 1992, 50:45–48.

135. Maggwa BN, Hunter DJ, Mbungua S, *et al.*: The relationship between HIV infection and cervical intraepithelial neoplasia among women attending two family planning clinics in Nairobi, Kenya. *AIDS* 1993, 7:733–738.

136. Chiasson MA, Kelley KF, Williams R, *et al.*: Invasive cervical cancer in HIV+ women in New York City. Presented at the 3rd Conference on Retroviruses and Opportunistic Infections, Washington, DC, 1996.

137. New York City Department of Health: *AIDS Case Surveillance Report*, January 1996.

138. Wright TC, Ellerbrock TV, Chiasson MA, *et al.*: Incidence and risk factors for cervical intraepithelial neoplasia (CIN) in HIV-infected women. Presented at the 2nd National Conference on Human Retroviruses and Related Infections. Washington, DC, 1995.

139. Saag MS, Holodny M, Kuritzkes DR, *et al.*: HIV viral load markers in clinical practice. *Nature Med* 1996, 2:625–629.

140. Wel X, Ghosh SK, Taylor ME, *et al.*: Viral dynamics in human immunodeficiency virus type 1 infection. *Nature* 1995, 373:117–122.

141. Ho DD, Neumann AU, Perelson AS, *et al.*: Rapid turnover of plasma virions and $CD4^+$ lymphocytes in HIV-1 infection. *Nature* 1995, 373:123–126.

142. Perelson AS, Neumann AU, Markowitz M, *et al.*: HIV-1 dynamics in vivo: Virion clearance rate, infected cell life-span, and viral generation time. *Science* 1996, 271:1582–1586.

143. Emini EA: HIV-1 protease inhibitors [abstract LB7]. Presented at the Third Conference on Retroviruses and Opportunistic Infections. Washington, DC, 1996.

144. Gulick RM, Mellors J, Havir D, *et al.*: Potent and sustained antiretroviral activity of indinavir (IDV), zidovudine (ZDV) and lamivudine (3TC) [Abstract ThB.931]. In the Program and Abstracts of the XI International Conference on AIDS. Vancouver, BC, 1996.

145. Meyers MW, Montaner JG, The Incas Study Group: A randomized, double-blinded comparative trial of the effects of zidovudine, didanosine and nevirapine combinations in antiviral naive, AIDS-free, HIV-infected patients with $CD4^+$ counts 200–600/mm^3 [abstract Mo.B.294]. Presented at the 11th International Conference on AIDS. Vancouver, BC, 1996.

146. Markowitz M, Cao Y, Hurley A, *et al.*: Triple therapy with AZT, 3TC, and ritonavir in 12 subjects newly infected with HIV-1 [abstract Th.B.933]. Presented at the 11th International Conference on AIDS. Vancouver, BC, 1996.

147. Eron JJ, Benoit SJ, Jemsek J, *et al.*: Treatment with lamivudine, zidovudine, or both in HIV-positive patients with 200 to 500 $CD4^+$ cells per cubic millimeter. *N Engl J Med* 1995, 333:1662–1669.

148. Hammer S, Katzenstein D, Hughes M, *et al.*: Nucleoside monotherapy (MT) vs combination therapy (CT) in HIV infected adults: A randomized, double-blind, placebo-controlled trial in persons with CD4 cell counts 200-500/mm^3 [Abstract LB7]. In the Program and abstracts of the 35th Interscience Conference on Antimicrobial Agents and Chemotherapy, San Francisco, 1995.

149. Cameron B, Health-Chiozzi M, Kravick S, *et al.*: Prolongation of life and prevention of AIDS in advanced HIV immunodeficiency with ritonavir [Abstract LB6a]. In the Program and Abstract of the 3rd Conference on Retroviruses and Opportunistic Infections, Washington, DC, 1996.

Chapter 2

Skin, Soft Tissue, Bone, and Joint Infections

Editor

Dennis L. Stevens

Contributors

Rodolfo M. Abalos
Jason Calhoun
Roland V. Cellona
Michael J. Chiu
Clay J. Cockerell
E. Dale Everett
Tranquilino T. Fajardo
Julie S. Francis
Robert Gelber
Bruce C. Gilliland
Ellie J.C. Goldstein
Ricardo S. Guinto
Jan Hirschmann
Karen R. Houpt
Elaine C. Jong
Rajendra Kumar
Jon T. Mader
John Neff
Justin D. Radolf
Gregory J. Raugi
David Simmons
Dennis L. Stevens
Milan Trpis
Gerald P. Walsh
Mark H. Wener
Herman Zaiman

Introduction

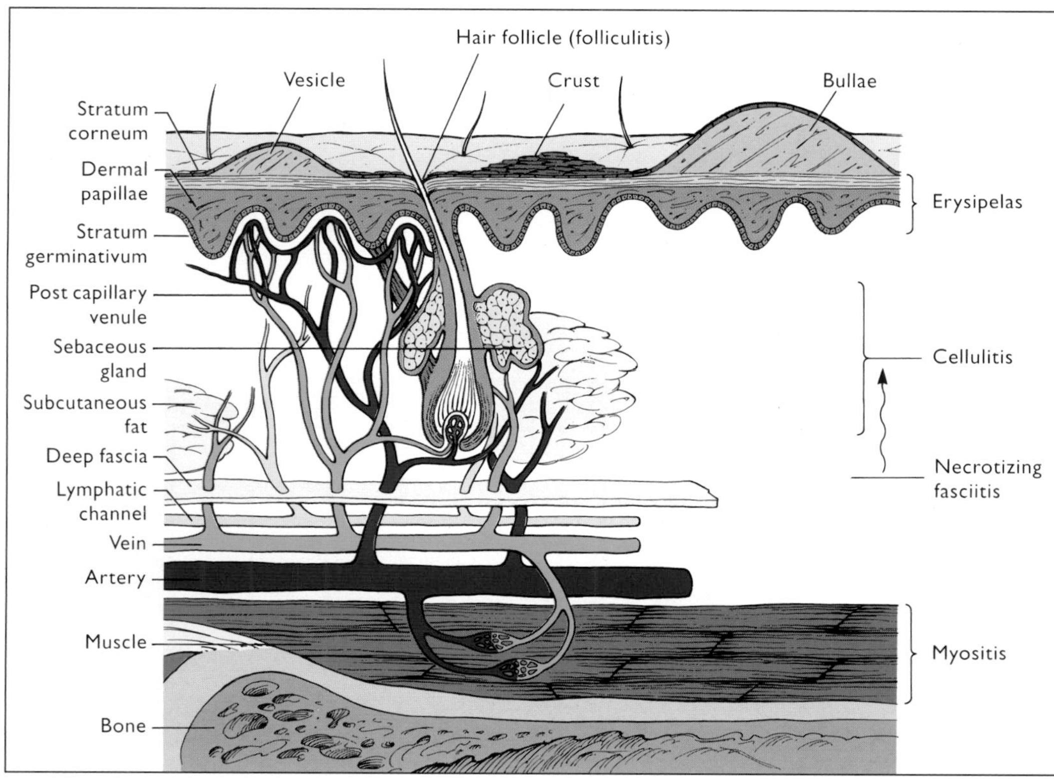

Figure 2-1 The structural components of the skin and soft tissue are illustrated on the left of the figure. Superficial infections are depicted on the top of the figure, and infections of the deeper structures of the soft tissue are located on the right edge of the figure. The rich capillary network beneath the dermal papillae plays a key role in localizing infection and in the development of the acute inflammatory reaction. (Illustration by Michael Wyett.)

Anatomical approach to soft-tissue infections

Infections associated with vesicles	Infections associated with bullae	Infections associated with crusted lesions	Etiologies of folliculitis
Variola (smallpox) Varicella (chickenpox) Herpes zoster (shingles) Herpes simplex types 1 and 2 Coxsackie A-16 (hand, foot, and mouth disease) Orf	Staphylococcal scalded skin syndrome Necrotizing fasciitis Gas gangrene Halophilic vibrio infection	Impetigo Superficial dermatophyte infection Systemic dimorphic fungal infection Cutaneous leishmaniasis Cutaneous tuberculosis Nocardiosis	*Staphylococcus aureus* *Pseudomonas aeruginosa* (hot tub folliculitis) *Schistosoma* (swimmer's itch) Acne vulgaris
Ulcers with or without eschars	**Causes of necrotizing fasciitis**	**Myositis**	
Anthrax Cutaneous diphtheria Ulceroglandular tularemia Bubonic plague Mycobacterial infections Syphilis Chancroid Miscellaneous	*Streptococcus pyogenes* Mixed aerobic/anaerobic infection	Pyomyositis Streptococcal necrotizing myositis Gas gangrene Nonclostridial (crepitant) myositis Synergistic nonclostridial anaerobic Myonecrosis	

Figure 2-2

Staphylococcal Soft Tissue Infections

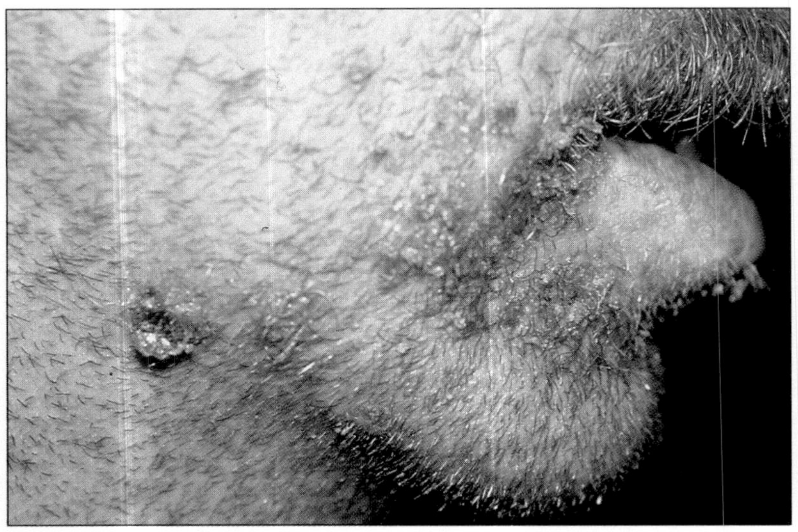

Figure 2-3 Impetigo. Thick, adherent, golden ("honey-colored") crusts surmounting an erythematous base are present around the mouth and on the jaw. These findings are characteristic of nonbullous impetigo, which typically occurs on the face or extremities. More common in children than adults, impetigo often follows minor trauma, such as abrasions and insect bites, and is more prevalent in tropical climates, crowded living conditions, and circumstances of poor hygiene. Cultures of impetigo most frequently yield *Staphylococcus aureus* alone, less commonly a mixture of *S. aureus* and *Streptococcus pyogenes* (group A streptococci), and, least often, streptococci alone. Treatment is topical mupirocin or an oral antistaphylococcal antibiotic.

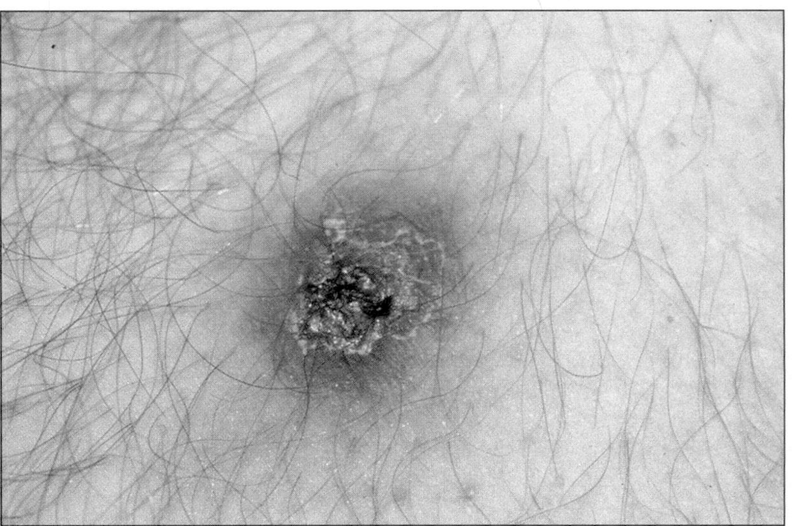

Figure 2-4 Ecthyma. Erythematous ulcerations with adherent crusts, most commonly on the lower extremities, characterize ecthyma. It begins as vesicles or bullae, which rupture to form scabs. Unlike impetigo, the infection penetrates to the dermis to produce ulcerations below the crust and heals with scarring. As in nonbullous impetigo, ecthyma often follows skin trauma in patients with poor hygiene, and the cause may be *Staphylococcus aureus*, *Streptococcus pyogenes*, or both. Treatment is topical mupirocin or an oral antistaphylococcal antibiotic.

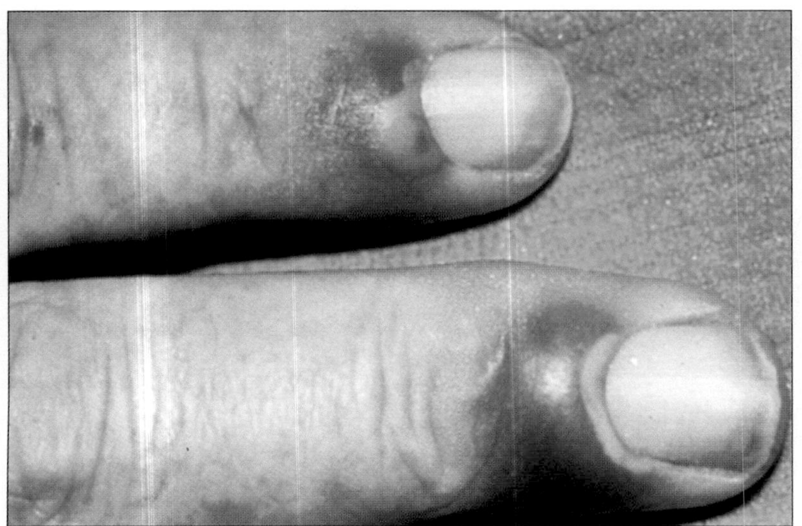

Figure 2-5 Paronychia. Erythema, swelling, and accumulated pus are present proximal to the nail plates on these fingers. *S. aureus* is the isolate in about 60% of finger paronychia. Predisposing factors include trauma, finger sucking, and protracted or repeated exposure to water. Streptococci and mouth anaerobes are frequent isolates in those not due to *Staphylococcus aureus*. Gentle separation of the cuticle from the underlying nail plate with a scalpel blade provides drainage of the pus. Topical or systemic antimicrobials are rarely necessary.

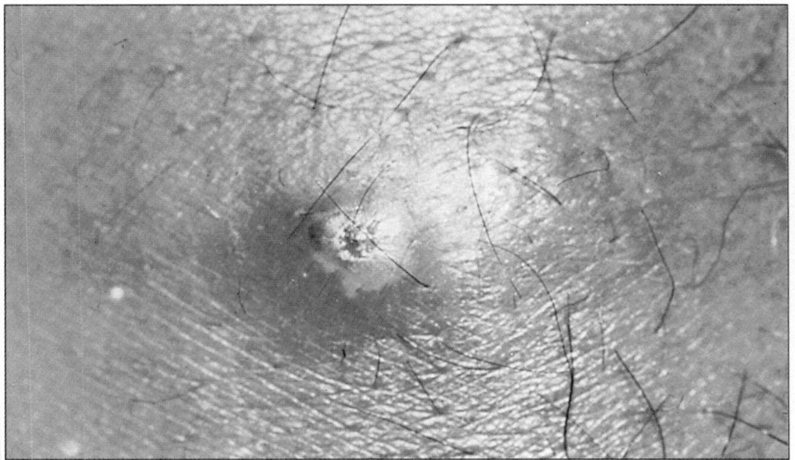

Figure 2-6 Furuncle. A furuncle (boil) is a deeper infection of the hair follicle than folliculitis and consists of an inflammatory nodule with a pustular center through which a hair emerges. By contrast, a carbuncle (*see* Fig. 2-7) involves several adjacent hair follicles, creating an inflammatory mass with pus discharging from several follicular orifices. Furuncles commonly occur on the face, neck, upper extremities, and buttocks. Treatment is incision and drainage, with oral antistaphylococcal antibiotics reserved for those with numerous lesions, substantial surrounding cellulitis, or fever. Some patients develop recurrent episodes of furunculosis. Occasionally, a white cell disorder such as Job's syndrome may be responsible, but most victims are otherwise healthy and have colonization of the anterior nares with *Staphylococcus. aureus*, as does about 30% of the general population. Why some nasal carriers develop skin infections and others do not is unknown, but trauma to the skin is often an important factor.

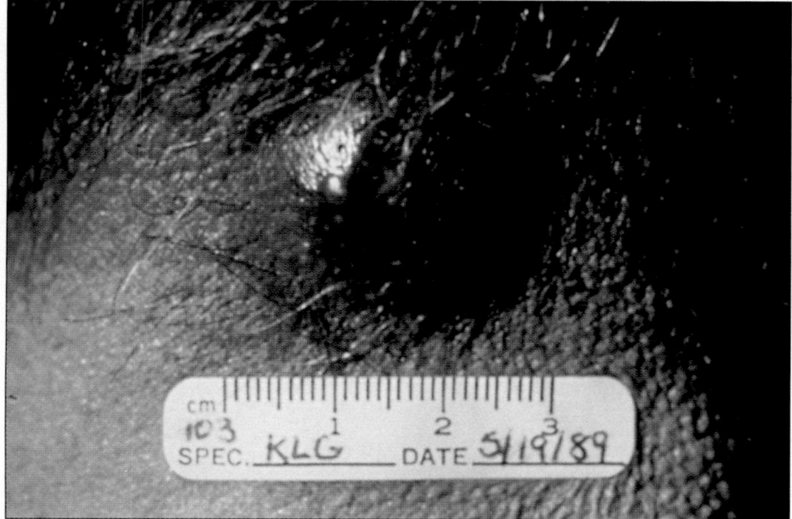

FIGURE 2-7 Carbuncle. A large violaceous nodule has formed on the back of the neck with a pustule near its left border. A carbuncle is a staphylococcal infection involving several adjacent hair follicles. It typically occurs on the posterior neck, especially in diabetics, and begins as a nodule that enlarges to form an inflammatory mass with pus discharging from several follicular openings. Other common sites are the shoulders, hips, and thighs. Treatment consists of incision and drainage. Systemic antibiotics are unnecessary unless substantial surrounding cellulitis or fever is present.

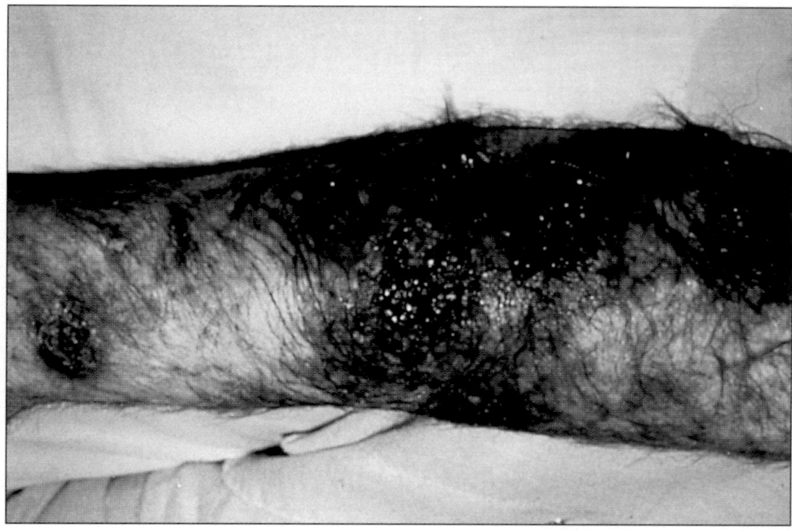

FIGURE 2-8 Infected superficial trauma. Abrasions to the forearm incurred in a fall preceded this infection, which consists of areas of erythema, crusting, ulcerations, and pustules. *S. aureus* is a common cause of infection in diffusely damaged skin, as well as in small areas of trauma. Treatment is an antistaphylococcal antibiotic given orally or parenterally, depending on the severity of infection.

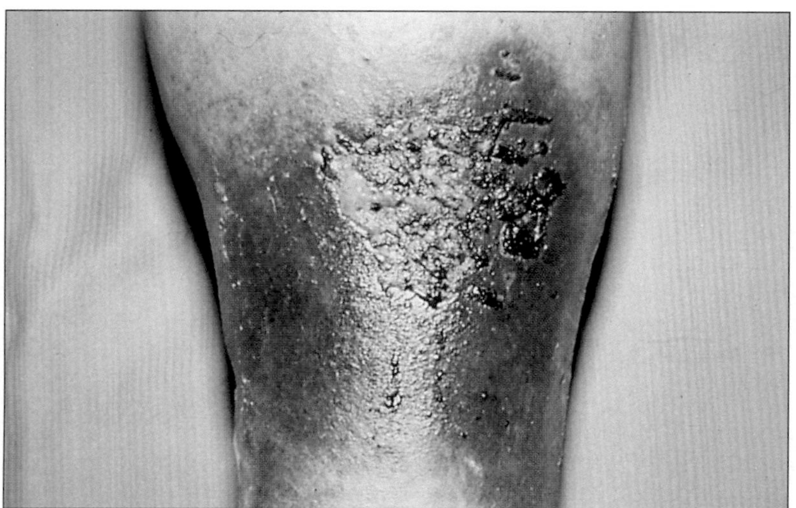

FIGURE 2-9 Staphylococcal cellulitis. A dusky, edematous erythema extends from purulent erosions on the shin of this patient. Most cases of substantial cellulitis are due to *Streptococcus pyogenes* or other streptococci, which produce enzymes that allow infection to spread widely along tissue planes. *S. aureus*, on the other hand, tends to produce localized pus and abscesses with a small amount of circumferential cellulitis, rather than diffuse soft tissue inflammation. Staphylococcal cellulitis, therefore, is most commonly associated with cutaneous abscesses, open wounds, or damaged skin, where it appears as a relatively small area of erythema and edema surrounding the suppurative focus.

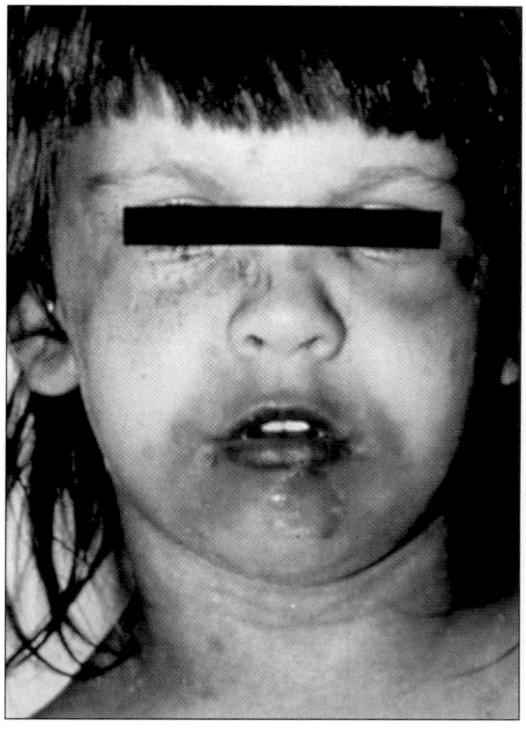

FIGURE 2-10 Staphylococcal scalded skin syndrome. Erythema is prominent on the neck and around the eyes and mouth. Crusting is also apparent in the periorificial areas. Over the chin, a bulla has ruptured, leaving a moist erosion. The usual sequence of this disease is cutaneous erythema, the development of superficial vesicles and bullae, and, finally, skin separation in sheets and ribbons, leaving a moist red base that dries quickly. The toxins responsible for this disease cause intraepidermal cleavage, typically at the granular layer. Toxic epidermal necrolysis, a rare complication of therapy with certain medications, also causes diffuse blistering and skin separation, but the split occurs lower, at the dermal–epidermal junction. Furthermore, target lesions and mucous membrane involvement are characteristic of toxic epidermal necrolysis but are absent in the staphylococcal scalded skin syndrome.

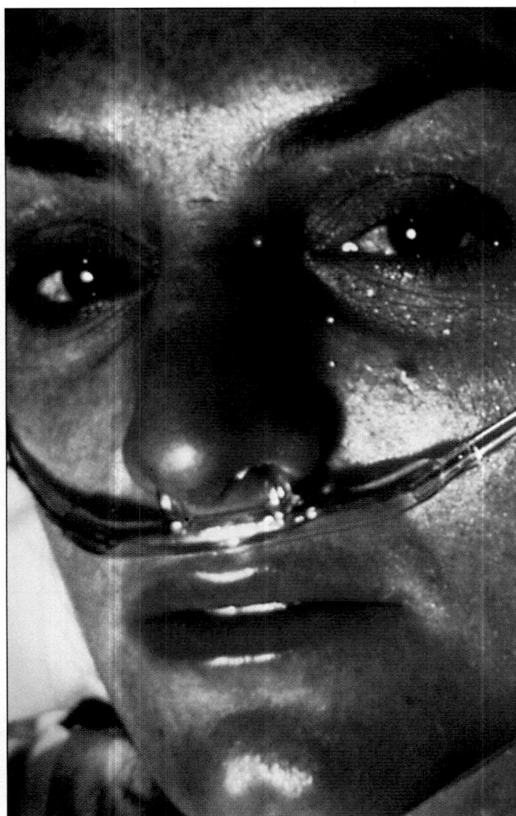

FIGURE 2-11 Staphylococcal toxic shock syndrome. The bulbar conjunctivae are reddened in this young woman with menstrual-related toxic shock syndrome. Hyperemia of the mucous membranes, including the vagina, pharynx, and conjunctivae is common in this disorder. Sometimes, subconjunctival hemorrhages occur, and erosions can develop in the oral cavity and vagina.

STREPTOCOCCAL INFECTIONS OF SKIN AND SOFT TISSUES

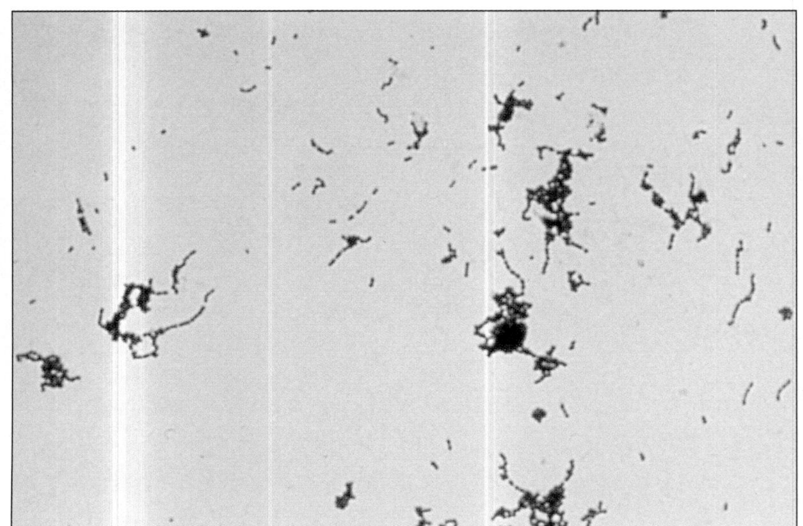

FIGURE 2-12 Gram stain of *Streptococcus pyogenes* grown in Todd-Hewitt broth, showing characteristic chains of Gram and cocci.

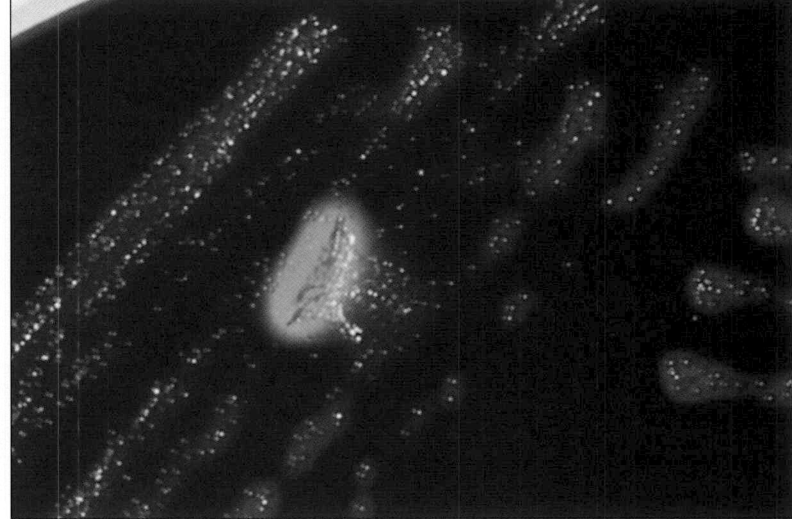

FIGURE 2-13 β-Hemolysis can be accentuated by "stab" inoculation. This enhancement is due to increased production or stability of the oxygen-labile streptolysin O.

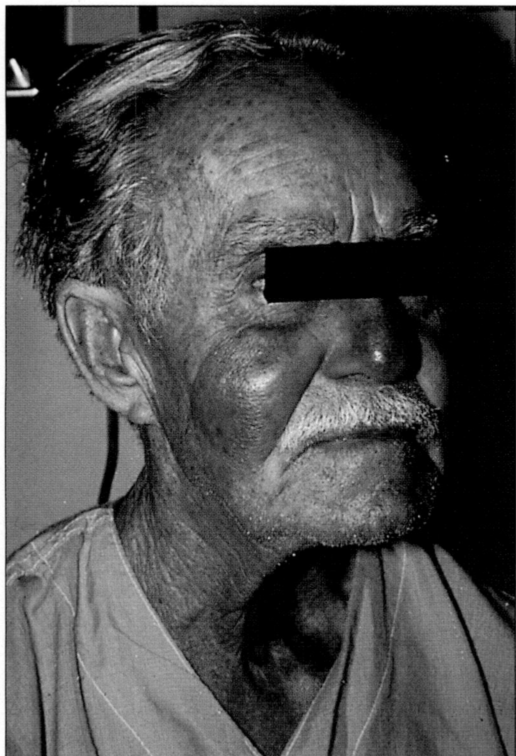

Figure 2-14 Erysipelas. In the characteristic appearance of erysipelas, a brilliant red or salmon red, painful confluent erythema in a "butterfly" distribution involves the nasal eminence, cheeks, and nose with abrupt borders along the nasolabial fold. The erythema increases over a course of 3–6 days and usually re-solves in 7–10 days. Erysipelas has been associated with high fevers, bacteremia, and possible death, even in modern times. The fluctuation in severity may reflect cyclical changes in the virulence of group A-β hemolytic streptococci.

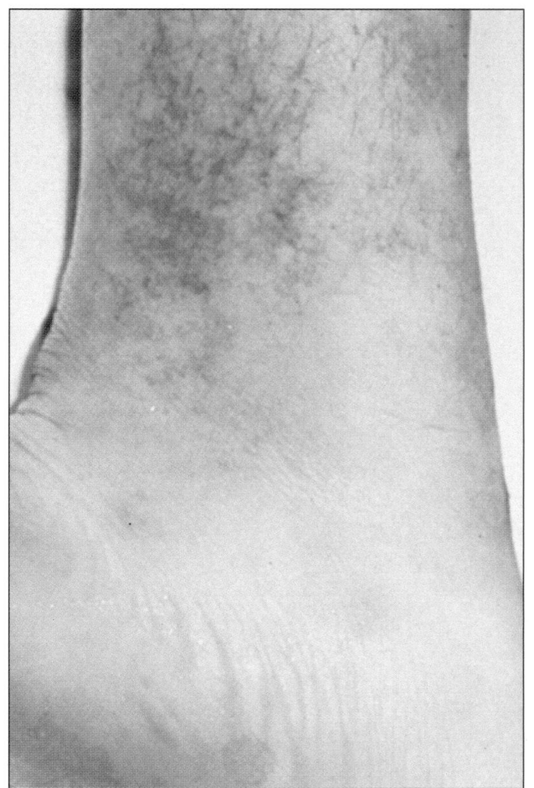

Figure 2-15 Cellulitis of the skin. Erythema, swelling, heat, and pain are cardinal features of cellulitis. The erythema may be pink or red but lacks the intense, fiery-red or salmon-colored appearance of erysipelas. Small breaks in the skin are associated with streptococcal infection, whereas staphylococcal cellulitis is often associated with larger wounds, ulcers, or abscesses. Fever is suggestive of streptococcal infection.

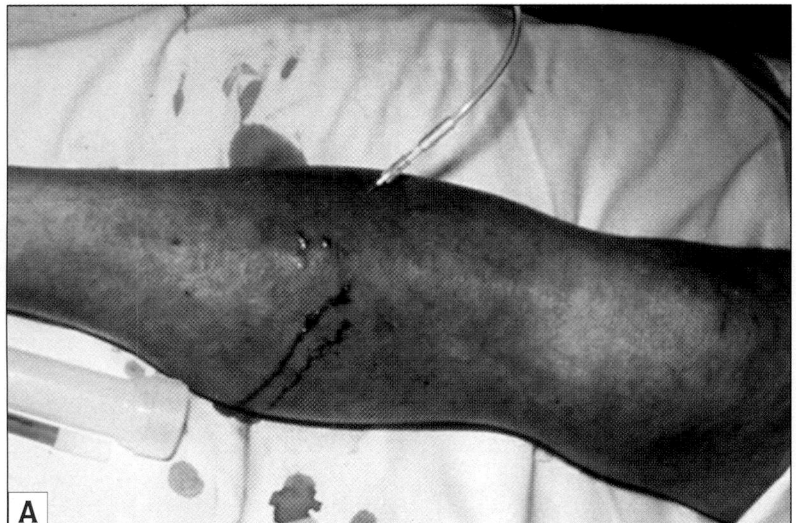

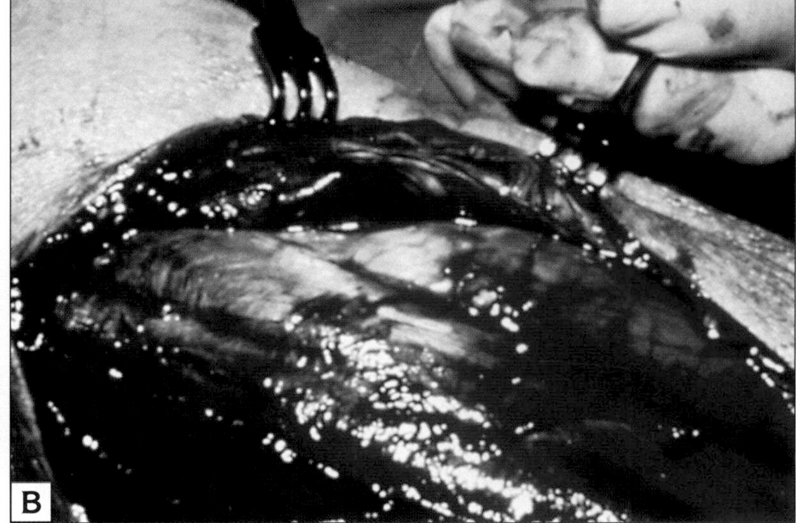

Figure 2-16 Necrotizing fasciitis and myositis. The patient had sudden onset of excruciating pain and signs of systemic toxicity. **A**, Note the swelling of the leg and two small purple or violaceous bullae on the anterior shin, whereas the adjacent skin appears healthy. The pressures in the anterior and lateral compartments were measured by placing a needle in the deep tissue (hence the blood at the sampling site). Pressures were elevated and surgical exploration was performed. **B**, The fascia overlying the deep musculature was friable and brownish to dishwater-gray in appearance, establishing a diagnosis of necrotizing fasciitis. Deeper exploration of muscle compartments is warranted in such cases.

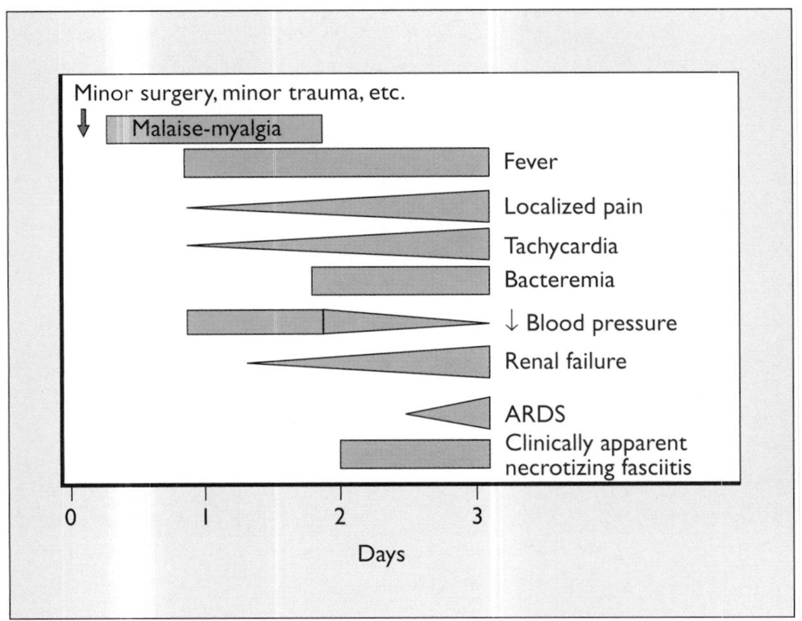

Figure 2-17 Clinical signs and symptoms of streptococcal toxic shock syndrome. (ARDS—adult respiratory distress syndrome.)

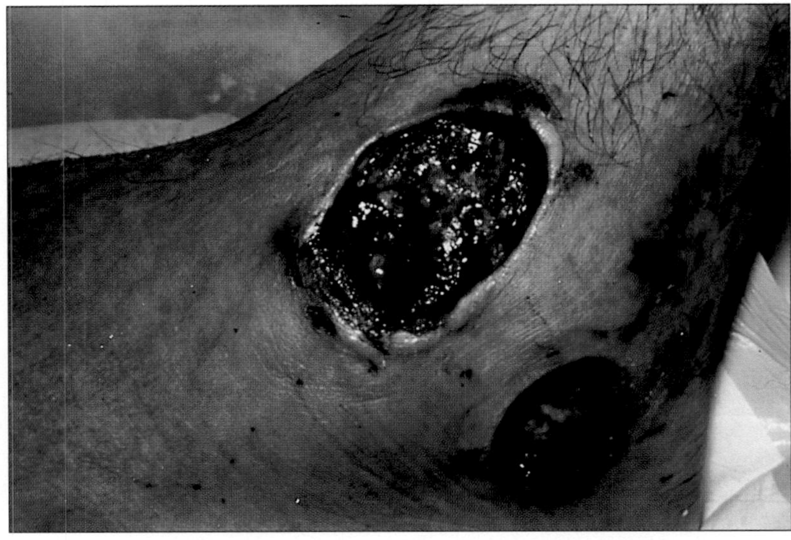

Figure 2-18 Localized cutaneous gangrene in a patient with group A streptococcal bacteremia. The well-circumscribed necrotic areas are likely due to vascular occlusion and tissue infarction.

Animal Bite Infections

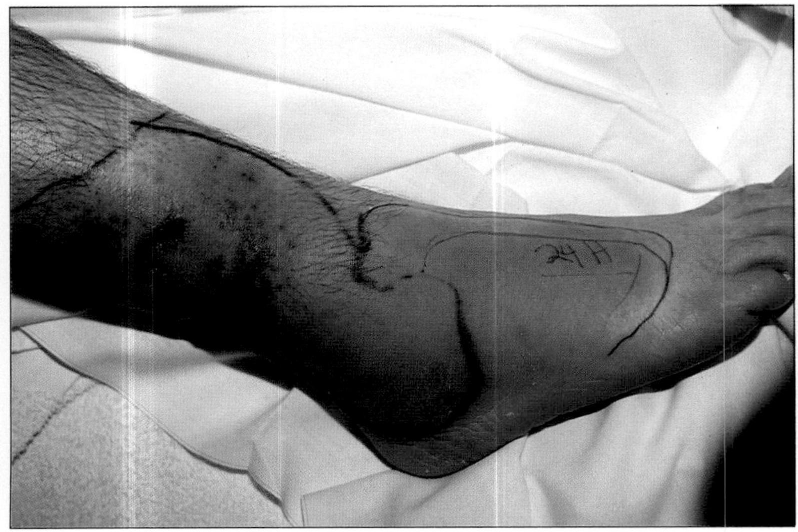

Figure 2-19 Leg wound infection, which developed during ampicillin therapy. Despite ampicillin therapy, the cellulitis extended (note marks on leg). *Staphylococcus aureus* was grown from this wound and is present in approximately 25% of dog bite wounds as a secondary invader. *Staphylococcus intermedius* is an animal-infecting species, which can be coagulase-positive and mistaken for *S. aureus*, though it is often penicillin-susceptible.

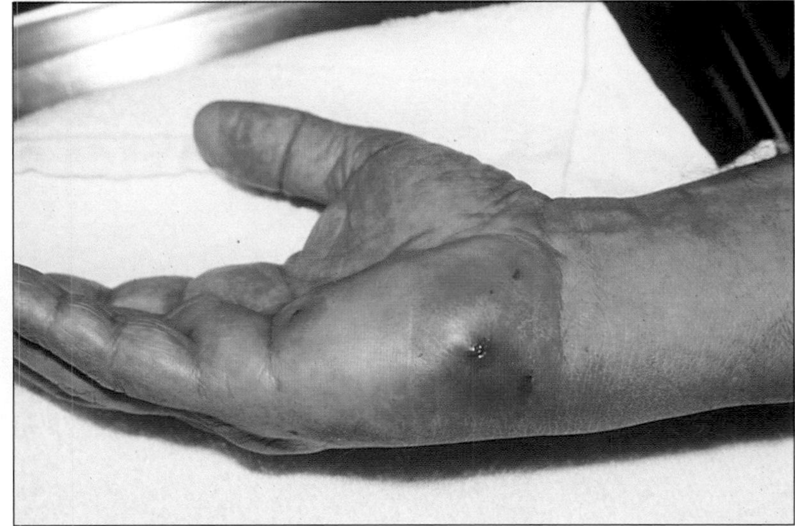

Figure 2-20 Dog bite wound to the hand. Two days after injury, the hand shows swelling of the hypothenar eminence with surrounding cellulitis and underlying abscess formation. This patient's wound grew seven isolates: α-streptococci, EF-4, *Pasteurella multocida*, *Moraxella* sp., *Fusobacterium nucleatum*, *Prevotella oralis*, and *Peptostreptococcus* sp.

Bacteriology of dog bite wounds

Aerobes	Anaerobes
α-Streptococci	*Actinomyces* sp.
β-Streptococci, group A and others	*Bacteroides* sp.
γ-Streptococci, including enterococci	*Bacteroides fragilis*
Actinobacillus actinomycetemcomitans	*Clostridium perfringens*
Capnocytophaga canimorsus (DF-2)	*Eubacterium lentum*
Capnocytophaga cynodegmi	*Eubacterium moniliforme*
Eikenella corrodens	*Fusobacterium nucleatum*
Haemophilus aphrophilus	*Fusobacterium russii*
Micrococcus sp.	*Leptotrichia buccalis*
Neisseria canis	*Porphyromonas asaccharolytica*
Neisseria weaveri (M-5)	*Prevotella bivia*
Pasteurella multocida	*Prevotella intermedia*
Pseudomonas aeruginosa	*Prevotella melaninogenica*
Staphylococcus aureus	*Prevotella oris*
Staphylococcus epidermidis	*Prevotella oris-buccae*
Staphylococcus intermedius	*Peptostreptococcus* sp.
	Peptostreptococcus anaerobius
	Peptococcus magnus
	Veillonella parvula

FIGURE 2-21 Bacteriology of dog bite wounds.

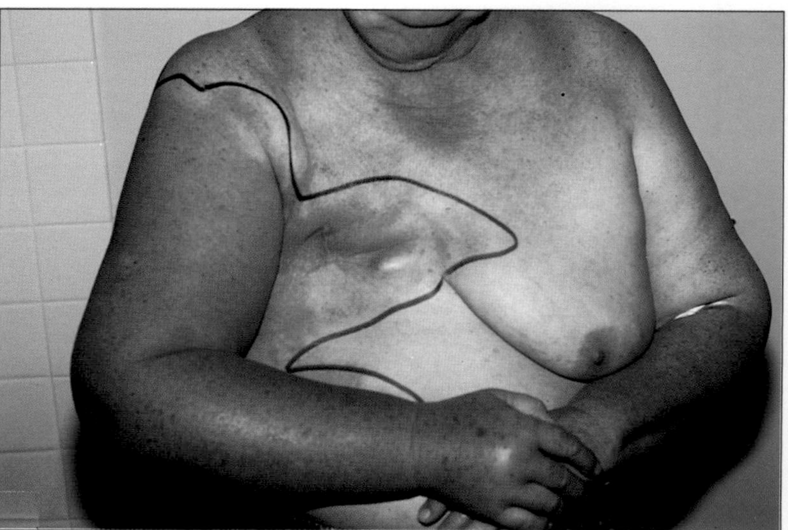

FIGURE 2-22 A woman with a cat bite and cephalexin failure. This patient had a previous mastectomy with resultant chronic edema of the arm. After being bitten by her cat, she developed a fever and cellulitis and was treated with oral cephalexin. After 72 hours of therapy, the infection spread all over her torso, and she became septic due to *Pasteurella multocida*.

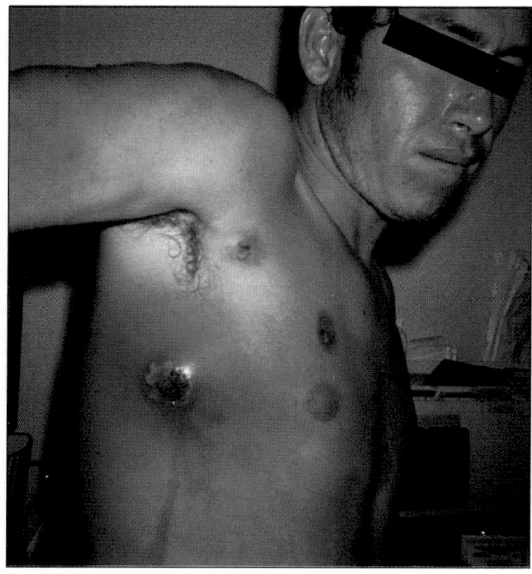

FIGURE 2-23 Multiple occlusional human bites to the torso. This patient stated he was walking on the street, minding his own business, when someone came up to him and bit him in multiple locations. Obviously, the stories given by patients are not always true. Approximately, 60 mL of pus was drained from the axillary wound and yielded a pure growth of *Streptococcus pyogenes* (group A). (From Goldstein [1];with permission.)

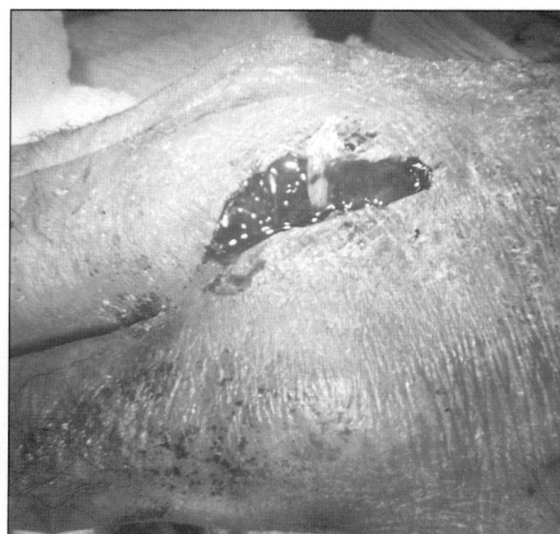

FIGURE 2-24 Clenched fist injury with osteomyelitis. The patient had undergone several operations and had been on 6 weeks of intravenous antibiotic therapy when this photograph was taken. Routine aerobic culture had yielded only a coagulase-negative staphylococcus. Anaerobic culture yielded *Eikenella corrodens*, which when treated appropriately led to healing. (*From* Goldstein [2]; with permission.)

Antibiotic activity: Animal bites

	P. multocida	*S. aureus*	*S. intermedius*	*Capnocytophaga*	Anaerobes
Penicillin	+	–	V	++	V
Dicloxacillin	–	+	+	–	–
Amoxicillin/clavulanate, Ampicillin/sulbactam	+	+	+	+	+
First-generation cephalosporins	–	+	+	V	–
Cefuroxime	+	+	+	+	–
Cefoxitin	+	+	+	+	+
Quinolones	+	V	+	+	–
Erythromycin	–	V	+	+	–
Azithromycin	+	V	+	+	V
Clarithromycin	+	V	+	+	V
Tetracycline	+	V	U	V	V

Figure 2-25 Susceptibilities of animal bite wound pathogens to antimicrobial agents. (+ —active; – —not active; U—unknown; V—variable activity.)

Antibiotic activity: Human bites

	S. aureus	*Eikenella*	*Haemophilus*	Anaerobes
Penicillin	–	+	–	–
Dicloxacillin	+	–	–	–
Amoxicillin/clavulanate Ampicillin/sulbactam	+	+	+	+
First-generation cephalosporins	+	–	–	–
Cefuroxime	+	+	+	–
Cefoxitin	+	+	V	+
Quinolones	V	+	+	–
Erythromycin	V	–	+	–
Azithromycin	V	+	+	V
Clarithromycin	V	+	V	V

Figure 2-26 Susceptibilities of human bite wound pathogens to antimicrobial agents. (+ —active; – —not active; V—variable activity.)

Infections Associated With Animal Contact

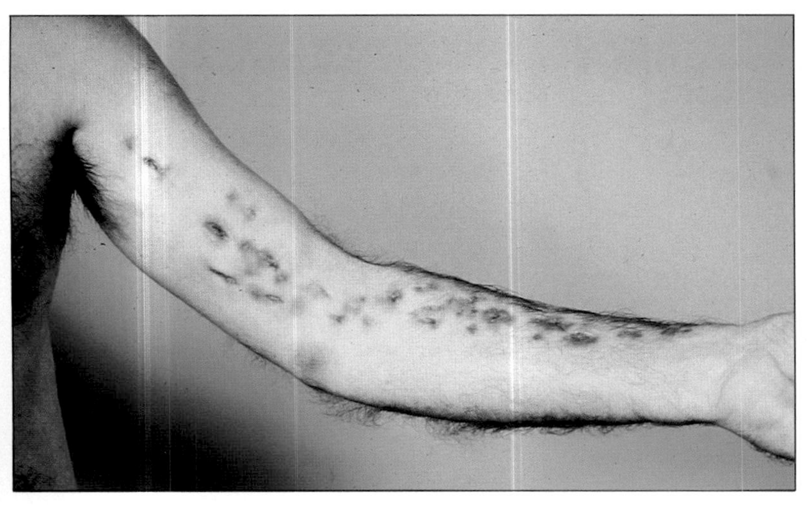

Figure 2-27 Sporotrichosis. Lymphocutaneous sporotrichosis, the most common clinical syndrome caused by *Sporothrix schenckii*, usually begins with a solitary lesion followed by red nodules ascending along superficial lymphatics. The disease, which is acquired most commonly from the soil, but occasionally from animals, especially cats, has no systemic symptoms. Diagnosis is by culture; the organism is rarely seen in biopsy material. Saturated solution of potassium iodide administered orally or itraconazole is considered effective therapy.

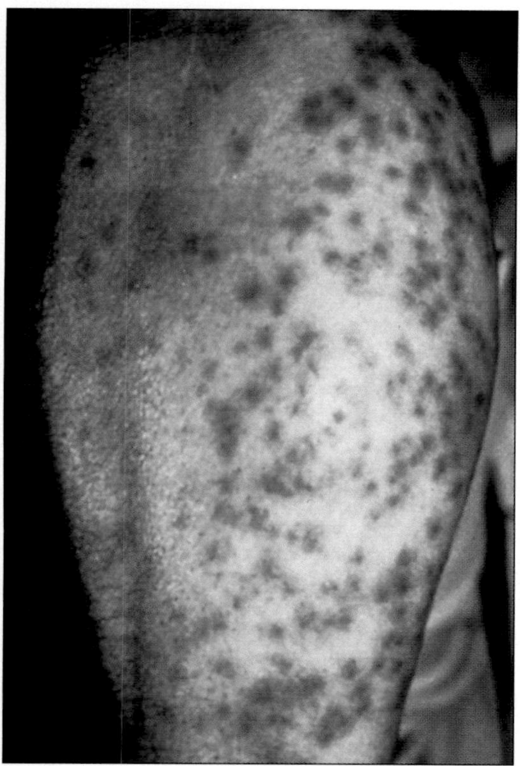

Figure 2-28 Swimmer's itch. A pruritic, erythematous, papular rash is acquired by exposure to water contaminated by avian schistosomal species. It usually occurs in swimmers or fishermen. A rash occurs 5–14 days after water exposure and is caused by an allergic response to disintegration of cercariae in the skin. The rash is self-limited.

Fungal and Yeast Infections of the Skin, Appendages, and Subcutaneous Tissues

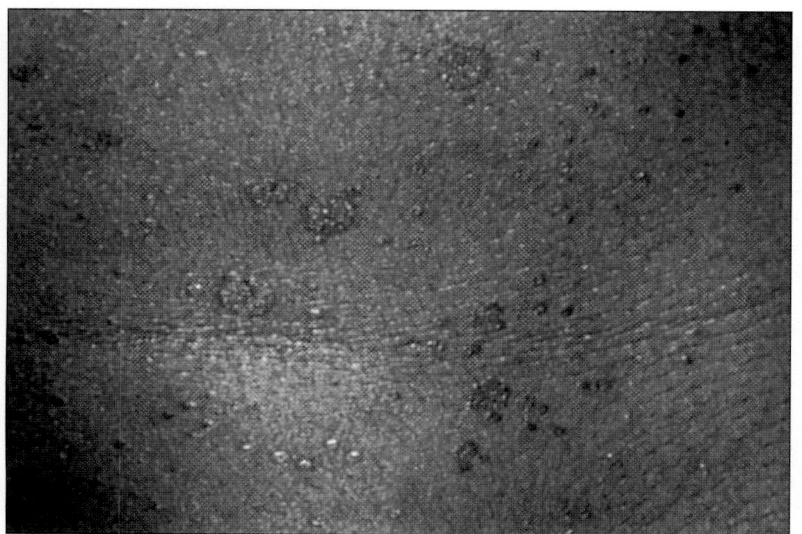

Figure 2-29 Hyperpigmented tinea versicolor (Latin *versicolor*, of many colors). Round, hyperpigmented, barely palpable plaques and some perifollicular patches are evident on the upper abdomen.

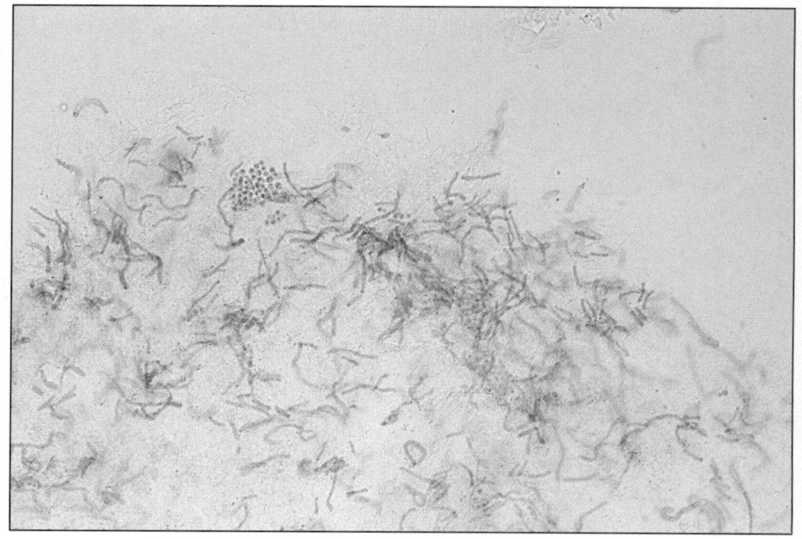

Figure 2-30 KOH wet mount of tinea versicolor. Adding a small amount of Parker's blue-black ink to the KOH stains *Pityrosporon* organisms blue and facilitates their identification from skin scrapings.

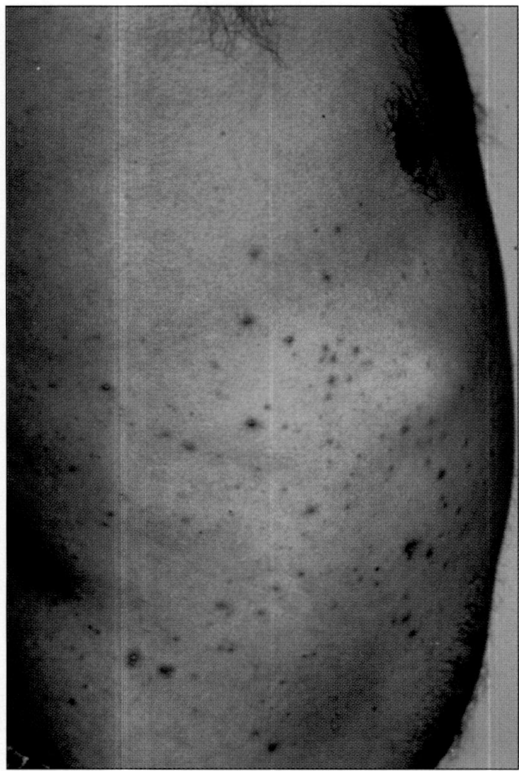

Figure 2-31 *Pityrosporon* folliculitis. This variant often occurs in young or middle-aged patients. Sometimes, tinea versicolor or seborrheic dermatitis coexists, but usually this fine follicular, pustular eruption occurs on the upper back and chest in isolation. Differential diagnosis includes miliaria pustulosa, bacterial folliculitis, mild acne vulgaris, or pustular drug eruption. Diagnosis is easily made by Gram stain of pus. Because *Pityrosporon* is a normal inhabitant of the hair follicle, clinicopathologic correlation is required to make the diagnosis from a skin biopsy.

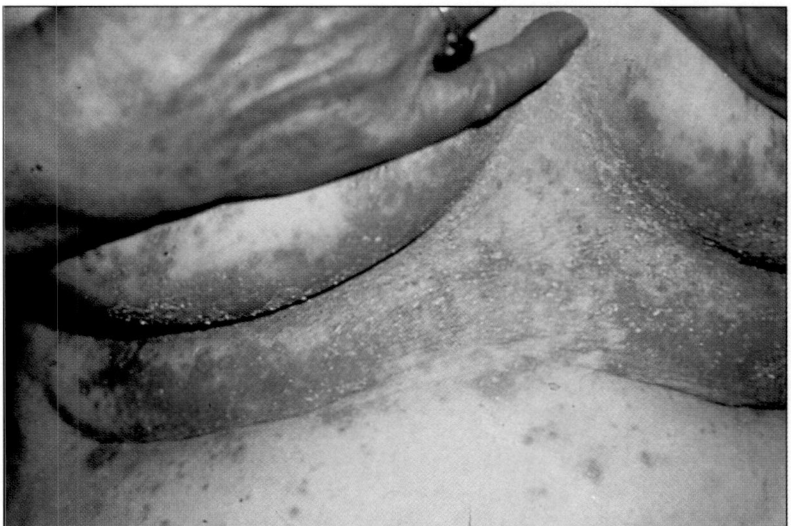

Figure 2-32 Intertriginous candidiasis. The typical appearance of candidiasis is with bright red erythema and satellite papules and pustules, occurring in the axillae, groin, or other skin folds, as beneath pendulous breasts in this woman. The vigorous neutrophilic response is thought to be due to release of complement-derived chemotactic factors by fungal polysaccharides.

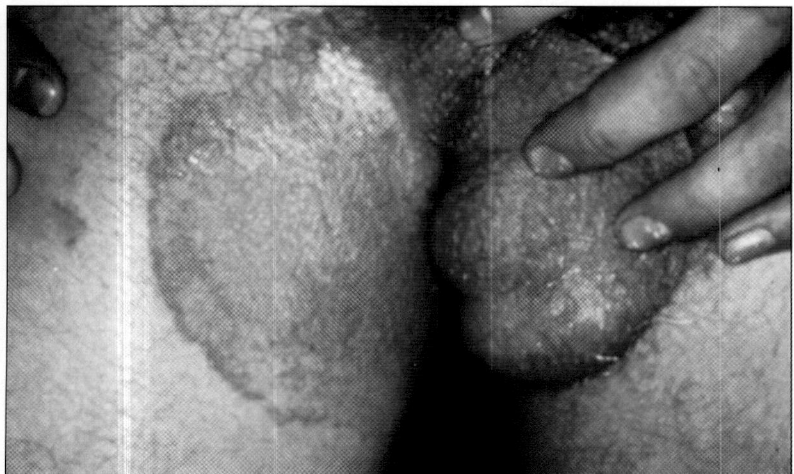

Figure 2-33 Chronic tinea cruris. Asymmetrical distribution on the medial thighs, lack of scrotal skin involvement, and the papular erythematous border are characteristic of chronic tinea cruris. The best area to sample for a wet mount is the scaling just central to the papular erythematous border. Extension of tinea cruris to the buttock area occurred in this patient. Little inflammation accompanies this chronic stable infection.

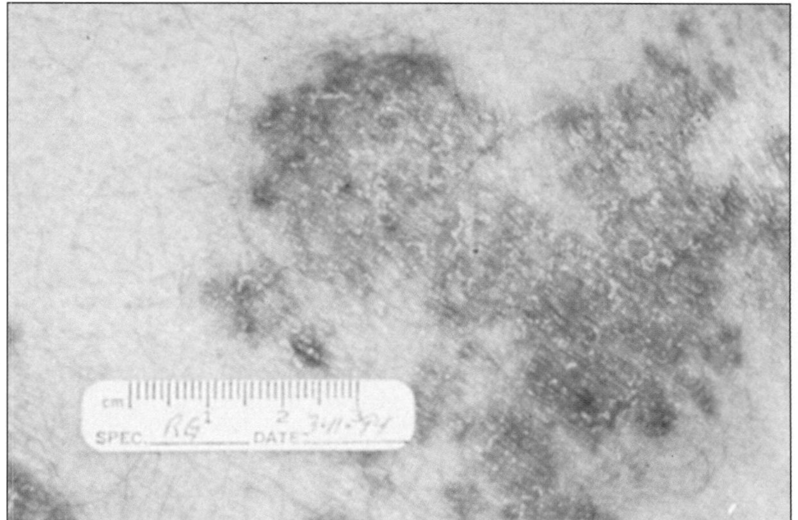

Figure 2-34 Tinea corporis modified by topical corticosteroid treatment. The lesion on the leg is an indolent, patchy, erythematous, papular dermatitis. These characteristics, together with an absence of central clearing and indistinct borders define "tinea incognito." Wet mounts from the lesion showed abundant fungal elements.

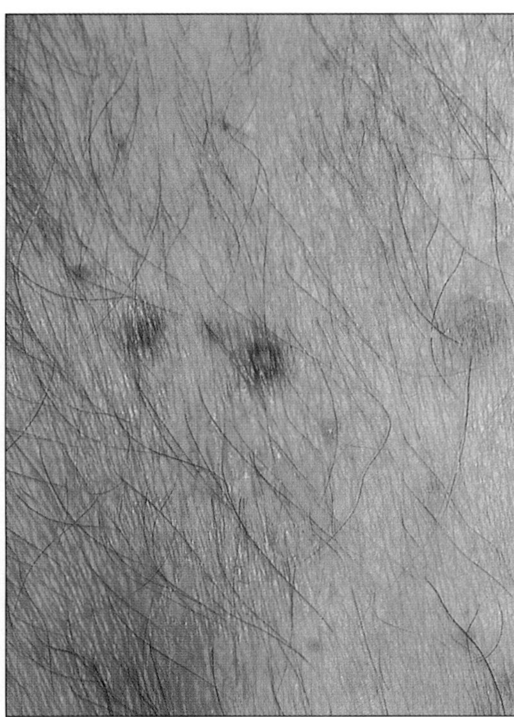

FIGURE 2-35 Disseminated candidiasis. A patient whose neutrophil count was recovering developed a rash with tiny central pustules, indicating an early neutrophilic response.

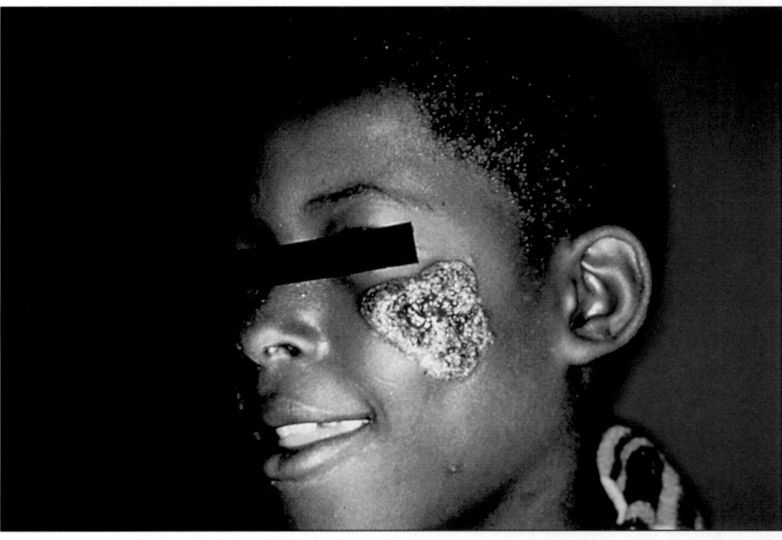

FIGURE 2-36 Blastomycosis. Skin lesions occur after systemic dissemination of *Blastomyces dermatitidis* from a primary pulmonary focus. Skin lesions occur in about 70% of patients with systemic blastomycosis and are usually vegetating plaques with slowly advancing, raised, hyperkeratotic, or verrucous borders with central healing and scarring. Small pustules are present in the verrucous border, and thrombosed dermal capillaries are present in the central scar. In this patient, *Blastomyces* was recovered from the darkly pigmented ulcerated plaque with verrucous indurated borders. (*Courtesy of* K. Abson, MD.)

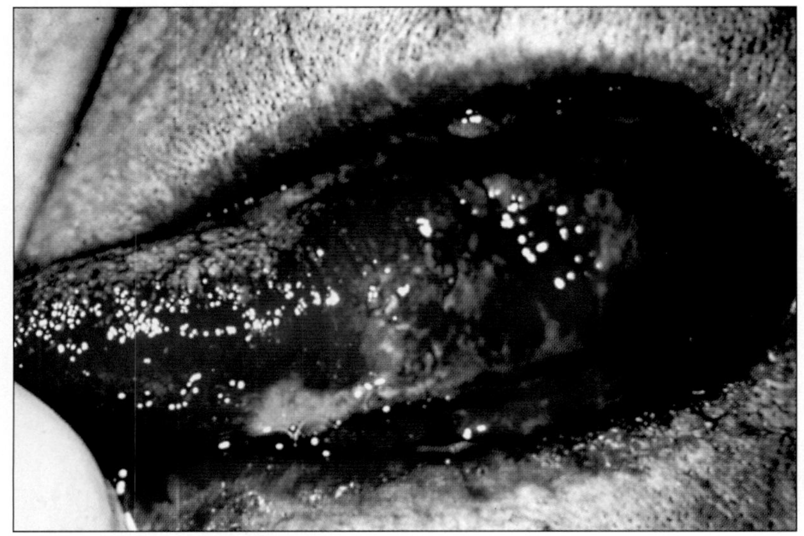

FIGURE 2-37 Histoplasmosis. Infection with *Histoplasma capsulatum* occurs when microconidia are inhaled into the lungs. Most cases go unrecognized or asymptomatic; the severity of illness depends on the size of the inoculum, whether the host had experienced previous infection, the presence of underlying chronic obstructive pulmonary disease, and the general immune status of the host. Dissemination from the primary pulmonary focus occurs only in about 1 in 2000 cases, but over half develop oropharyngeal ulcers. In this patient, the indurated ulcer on the tongue was shown to contain *Histoplasma* in stained sections and by culture. (*Courtesy of* E.D. Everett, MD.)

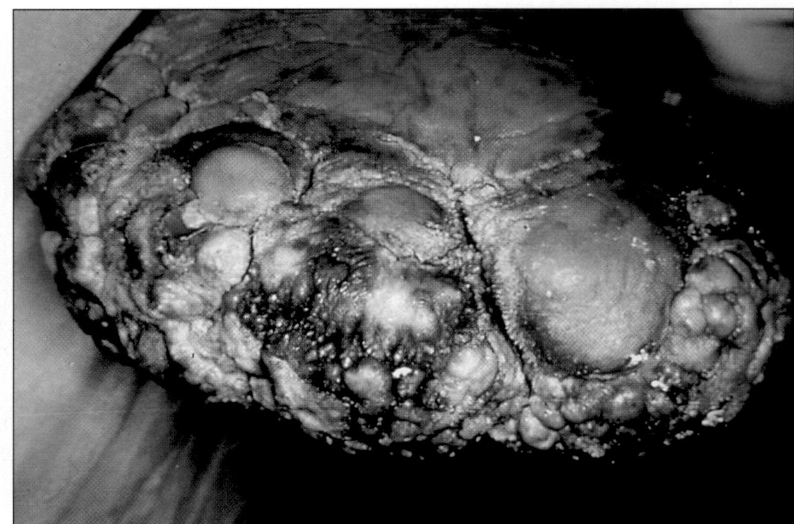

FIGURE 2-38 Mycetoma (Madura foot). This indolent and usually painless local infection is characterized by induration and tumefaction, with sinus tract formation and drainage of granule-containing pus. Late in the course of the disease, the bones may become involved. Two groups of organisms may cause this clinical presentation. Actinomycetoma is caused by filamentous bacteria, including *Nocardia* and *Actinomyces* species. Eumycetoma is caused by a group of true fungi, including *Petriellidium* and *Madurella* species. Gram stain is useful in distinguishing those cases caused by filamentous bacteria (gram positive) from those caused by the true fungi (not stained), whereas periodic acid–Schiff and methenamine silver reagents stain both. This view of a patient's foot shows the grotesque deformity (maduramycosis) that accompanies long-standing infection. (*Courtesy of* K. Abson, MD.)

Viral Infections of the Skin and Soft Tissues

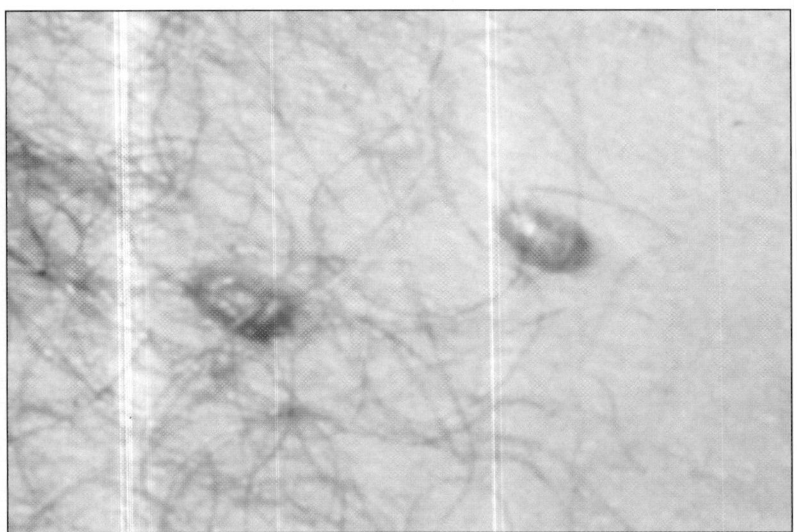

Figure 2-39 Molluscum contagiosum. Molluscum is a common, benign viral infection of the skin and mucous membranes, which can occur at any age but is most common in children. It is characterized by distinct single or multiple, dome-shaped papules, which are flesh or pink-colored. Lesions generally range in size from 1–5 mm, although larger papules measuring 10–15 mm are occasionally seen. With time, central umbilication of the papules can occur. (*Courtesy of* G. Raugi, MD.)

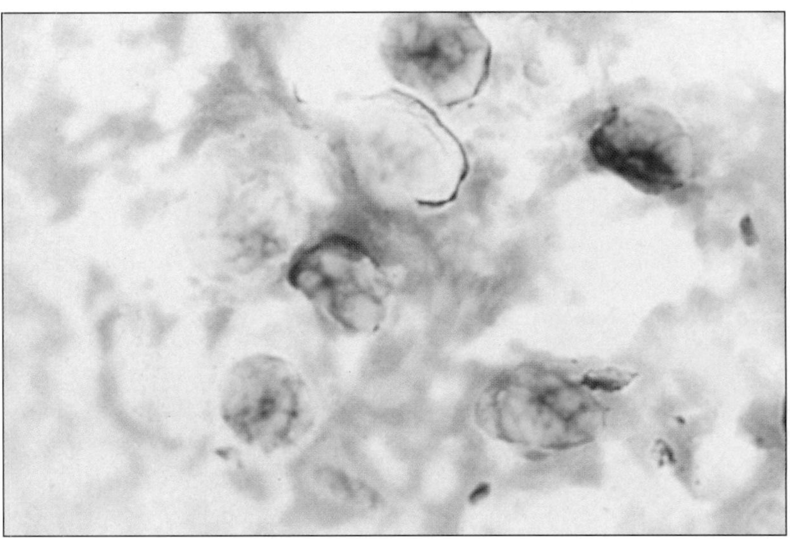

Figure 2-40 Wright's stain of the extruded contents of a molluscum papule. Note the blue-stained viral inclusions (known as molluscum bodies) within the cytoplasm of epidermal cells. Molluscum contagiosum is caused by a DNA pox virus, the largest virus to infect humans. The infection is limited to the skin and mucous membranes; there are no systemic manifestations. Considered moderately contagious, molluscum is spread via autoinoculation and direct contact. (*Courtesy of* G. Raugi, MD.)

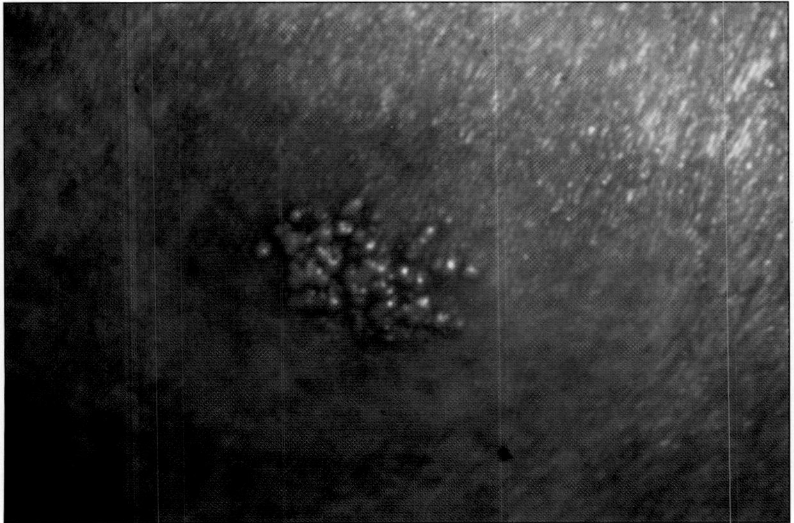

Figure 2-41 Herpes simplex virus (HSV). *Herpesvirus hominis* is the causative agent in herpes simplex infections and is characterized by two major serologic types. Type I HSV (HSV-1) usually causes infections on the head, neck, and upper torso. Type 2 HSV (HSV-2) usually causes recurrent genital herpes infections and is primarily responsible for neonatal herpes. Both types of HSV cause primary and recurrent infections. This figure illustrates a classic example of recurrent HSV-1 infection. Note the grouped vesicles and pustules on an erythematous base. (*Courtesy of* M. Welch, MD.)

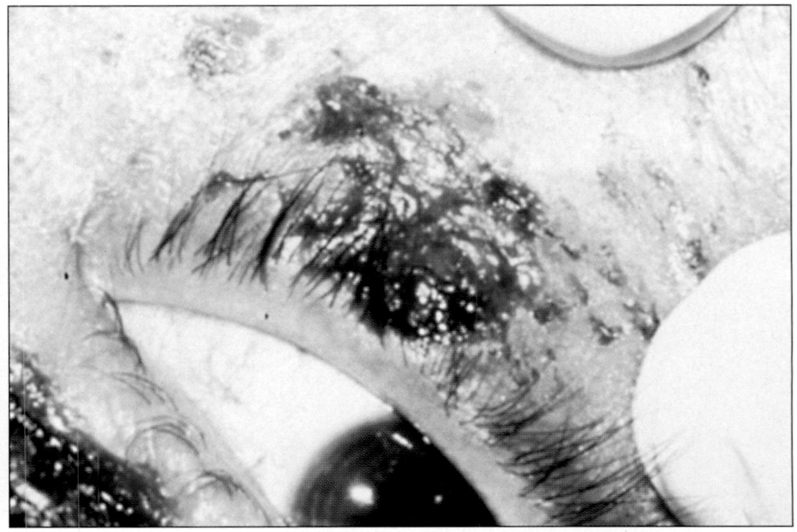

Figure 2-42 Chronic cutaneous herpes simplex infection. In immunocompromised hosts, recurrent herpes simplex virus (HSV) infections can be more severe. This patient with AIDS has chronic HSV-1 infection of the skin around the eye, with ulceration, crusting, and pain. (*Courtesy of* G. Raugi, MD.)

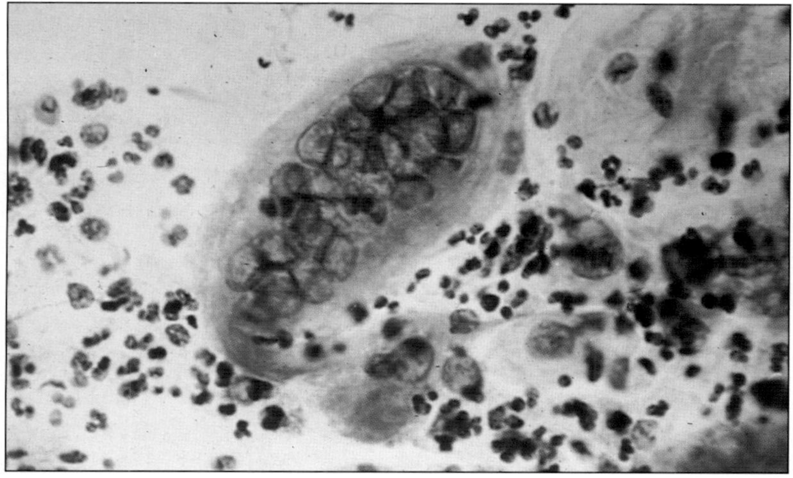

FIGURE 2-43 Tzanck stain of a herpetic vesicle. Note the large multinucleated giant cell. The preparation is obtained by scraping the base of a new, freshly opened vesicle and staining with Giemsa stain or toluidine blue. (*Courtesy of* D. Benjamin, MD.)

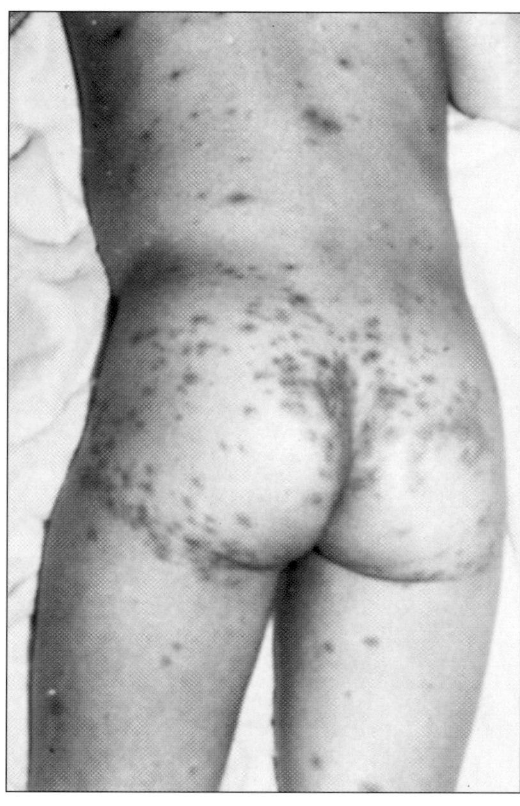

FIGURE 2-44 Varicella in a child. The eruption generally begins on the trunk or head and spreads centrifugally. New lesions generally begin to crust within 1–2 days. It is common to find various-sized papules, vesicles, pustules, and crusts all present on the skin at the same time. (*Courtesy of* D. Stevens, MD.)

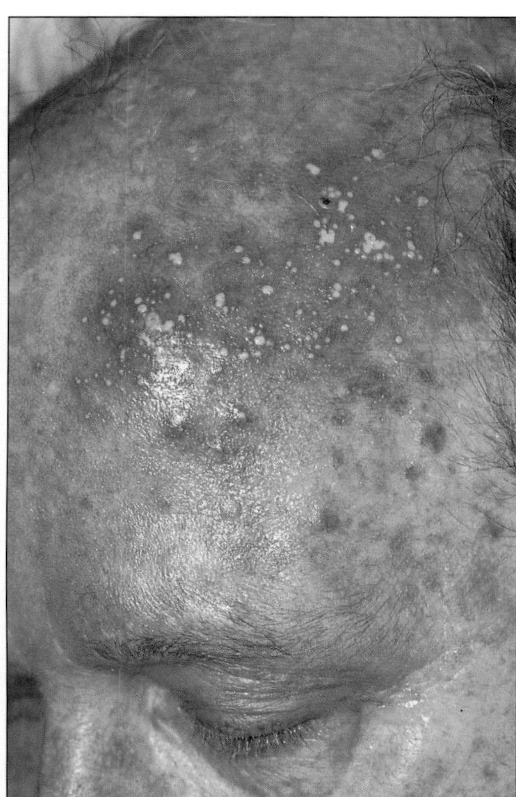

FIGURE 2-45 Acute herpes zoster. After primary varicella-zoster virus infection, the virus persists in a latent form and can be reactivated, resulting in herpes zoster or "shingles." Herpes zoster is characterized by papules, vesicles, and pustules on an inflammatory base in a dermatomal distribution, frequently associated with burning pain and tenderness. (*Courtesy of* G. Raugi, MD.)

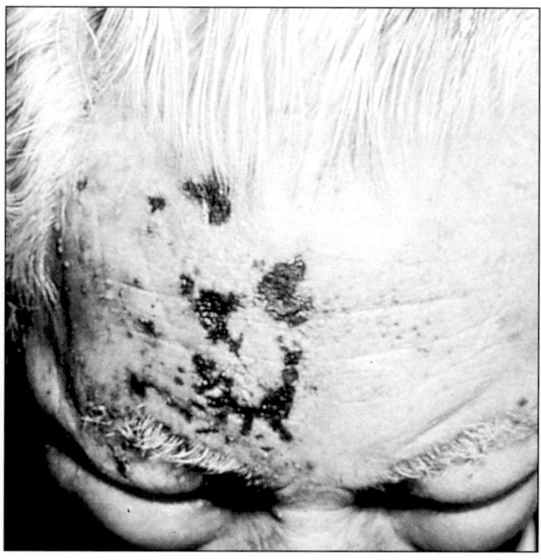

FIGURE 2-46 Resolving herpes zoster. Crops of vesicles appear for about 1 week and then dry out and crust over. The infection usually lasts 1–3 weeks. Other than mild fever, systemic symptoms are usually absent. (*Courtesy of* G. Raugi, MD.)

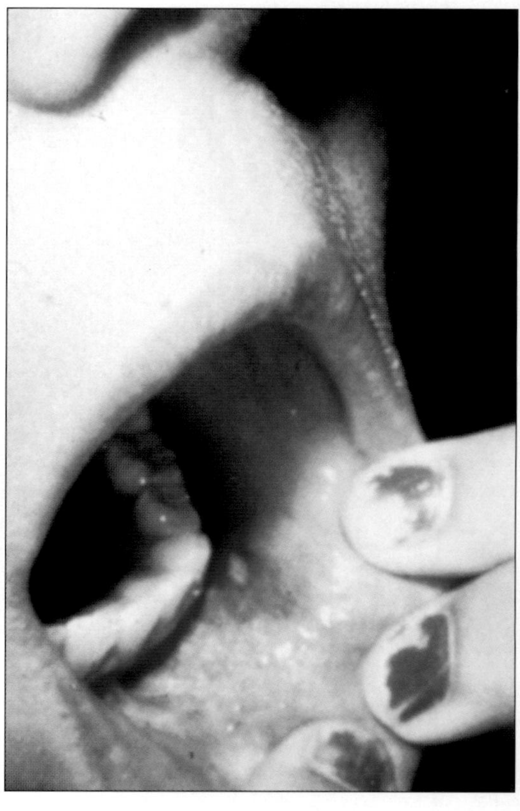

FIGURE 2-47 Hand, foot, and mouth disease. Coxsackievirus A16 is the most common cause of hand, foot, and mouth disease. The illness begins with a prodrome of fever, malaise, anorexia, and sore mouth. The enanthem occurs 1–2 days after the onset of fever, and the exanthem appears shortly after. The oral lesions appear as various-sized erosions and ulcerations on an erythematous base. The tongue and buccal mucosa are the areas most frequently affected.

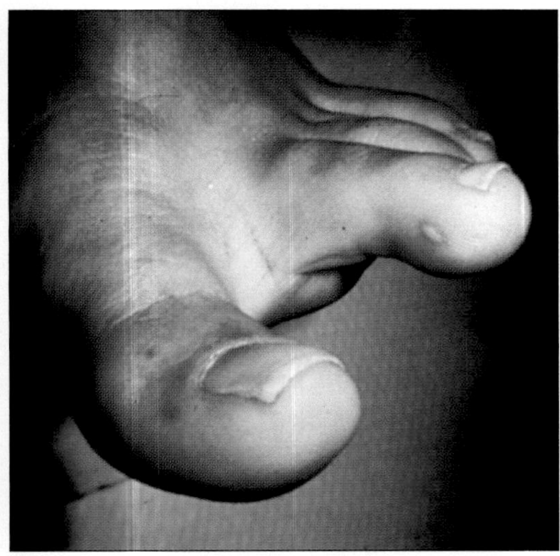

Figure 2-48 Hand, foot, and mouth disease. The exanthem characteristically involves the hands and feet but may involve the buttocks as well. The lesions on the hands and feet consist of 3–7-mm gray-white vesicles on an erythematous base. They frequently have an elliptical or "football-shaped" appearance. (*Courtesy of* G. Raugi, MD.)

Ectoparasitic Diseases of the Skin

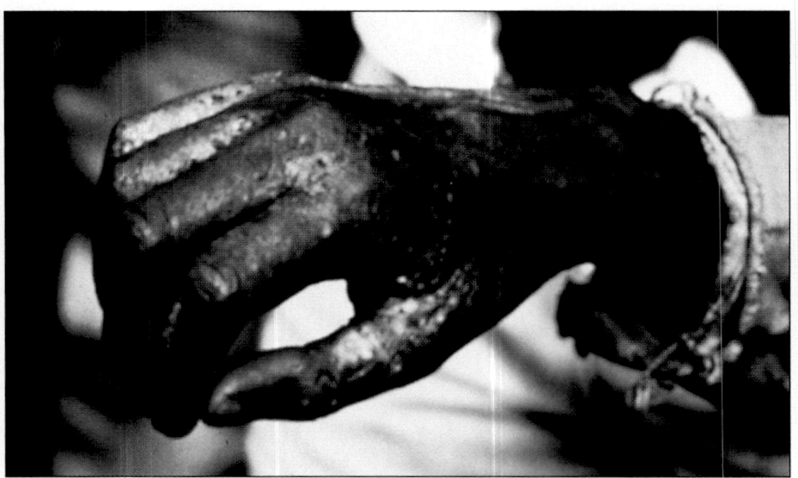

Figure 2-49 The hand of a person infested with the scab mite *Sarcoptes scabiei*. Female mites burrow in the skin, make corridors in the upper layer of the skin, and feed on dermal tissue and oozing lymph. Mating takes place on the skin. Inseminated females make new corridors as they burrow into the skin and lay their eggs there. Lymph oozing from injured skin forms scabs that grow progressively thicker. To remove the scabies condition, mites must be removed from infested areas by treatment with acaricides.

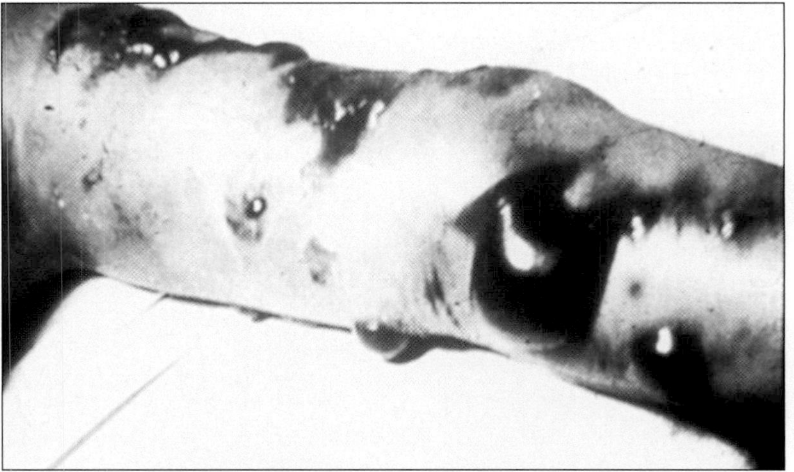

Figure 2-50 Multiple necroses on the arm caused by bites of the recluse spider, *Loxosceles reclusa*. The bites are not painful and usually unnoticeable. However, after 2–6 hrs, a blue-white circle is formed at the site of the bite, which changes into a blister that becomes red and later black. The affected area becomes necrotic, and dermal and subdermal tissue are destroyed. Regeneration of the necrotic tissue is limited and often needs surgical repair by skin grafting. (*From* Scott [3]; with permission.)

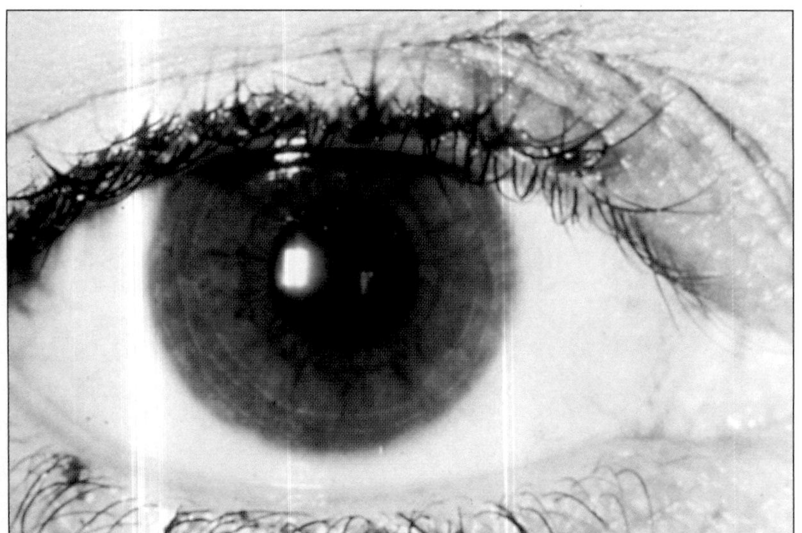

Figure 2-51 Pubic or crab louse. Heavy infestation of a woman s eye lashes with pubic lice, acquired most probably during sexual activity. Redness of the eyelids results from lice feeding. The louse prefers the pubic area, where it finds suitable temperature and humidity, but it may occasionally be found on a moustache, eyebrow, or eyelashes.

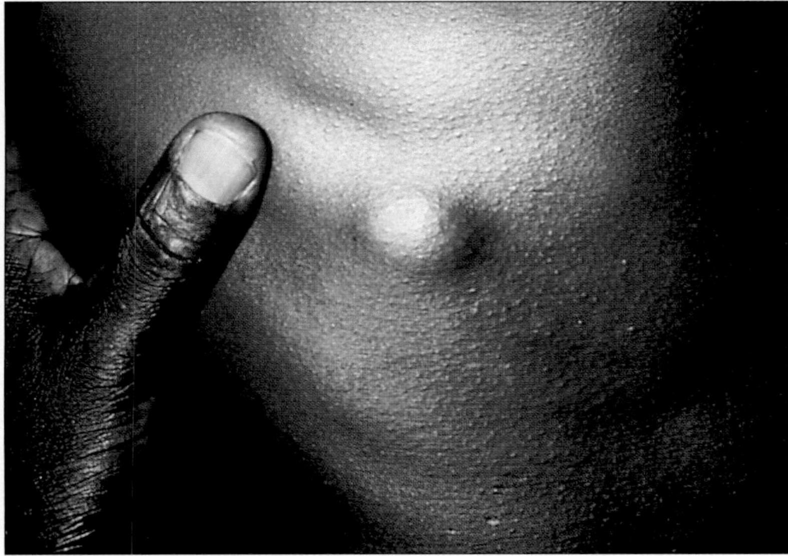

Figure 2-52 Onchocerciasis nodule. *Onchocerca* nodule on the trunk of a male from Sierra Leone. Several males and females of *O. volvulus* live in one nodule. Females produce hundreds of embryos daily. The embryos free themselves from shells and penetrate the ectodermal tissue, and many may remain trapped in the eye, where they eventually die.

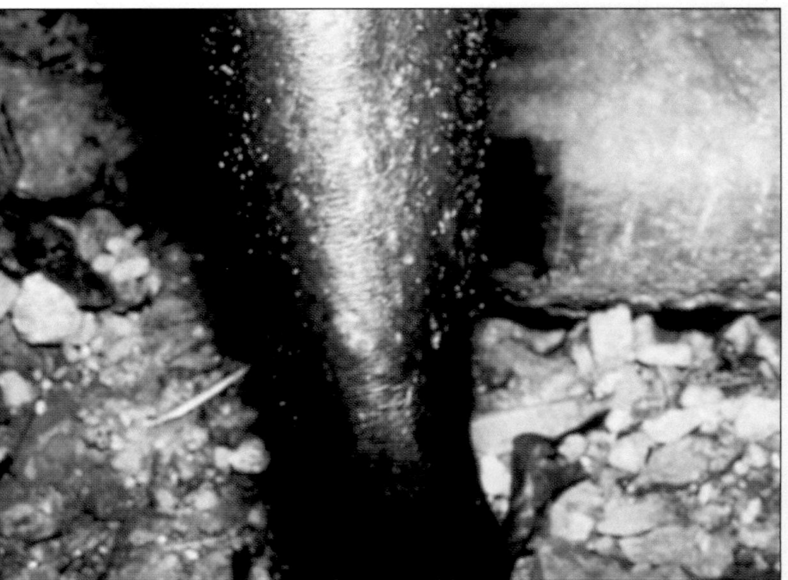

Figure 2-53 Onchoceriasis skin depigmentation. Depigmentation of skin (leopard skin) on an onchocercal patient. The skin loses its elasticity and has a scaly appearance. The dead filarial bodies cause itching.

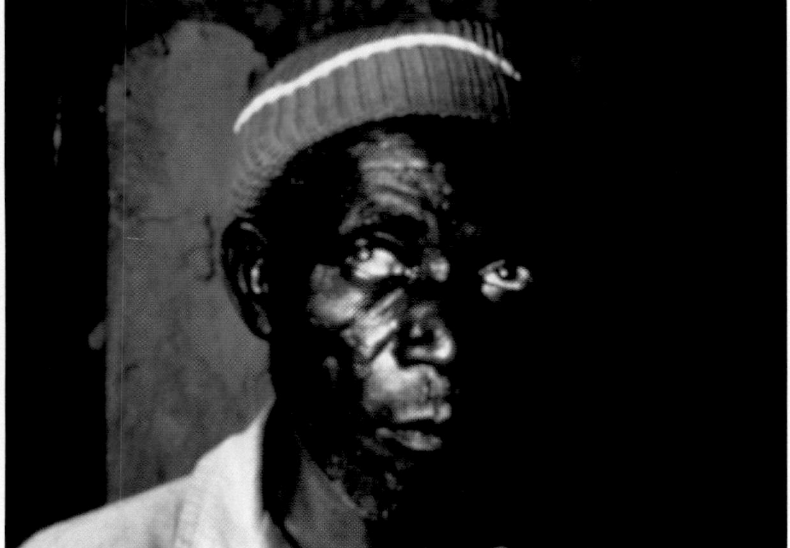

Figure 2-54 Onchocerciasis. This man is completely blind in the right eye and has blurry vision in the left eye. River blindness is a progressive chronic disease. The eye damage is irreversible even after removal of adult worms and microfilariae from the tissues.

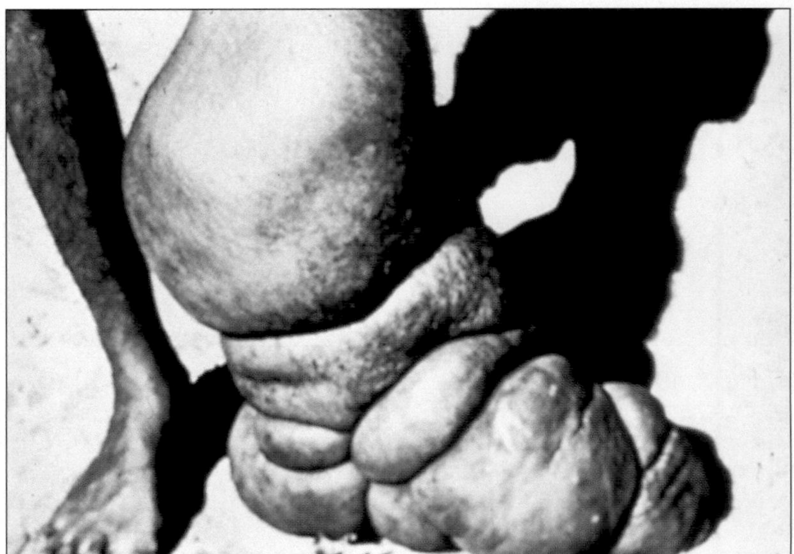

Figure 2-55 Elephantiasis. Elephantiasis of the left leg of a patient from India, caused by *Wuchereria bancrofti*. The vector in urban filariasis in India is *Culex pipiens* breeding in highly polluted water. Disfigurement of elephantoid limbs is irreversible. Filariasis is a chronic disease that poses a tremendous economic burden in affected countries. (*Courtesy of* the Indian Commission on Filariasis.)

PARASITIC DISEASES OF THE SKIN AND SOFT TISSUE

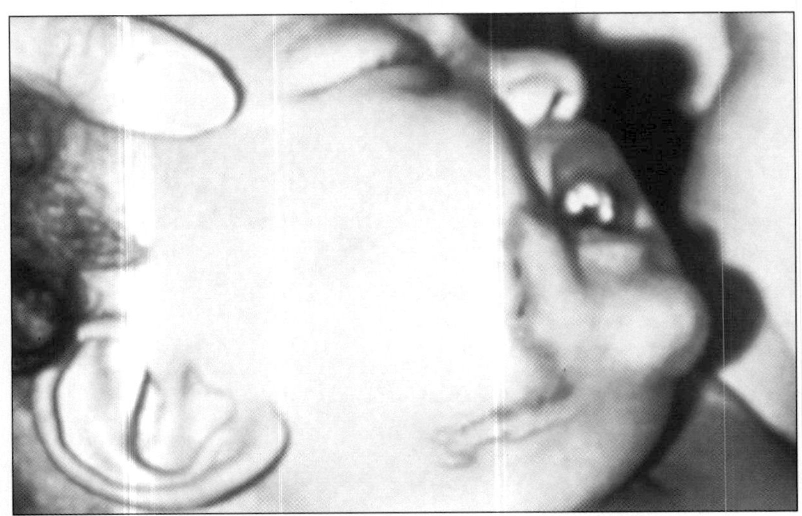

FIGURE 2-56 Cutaneous larva migrans. The face of a 2-year-old boy from Venezuela is shown. This infection is acquired from direct skin contact with soil contaminated by dog or cat feces containing hookworm eggs. These develop into infective larvae that penetrate skin they contact. Such larvae are usually limited to the skin because they are in an inappropriate host. (*Courtesy of* F. Battistini, MD.)

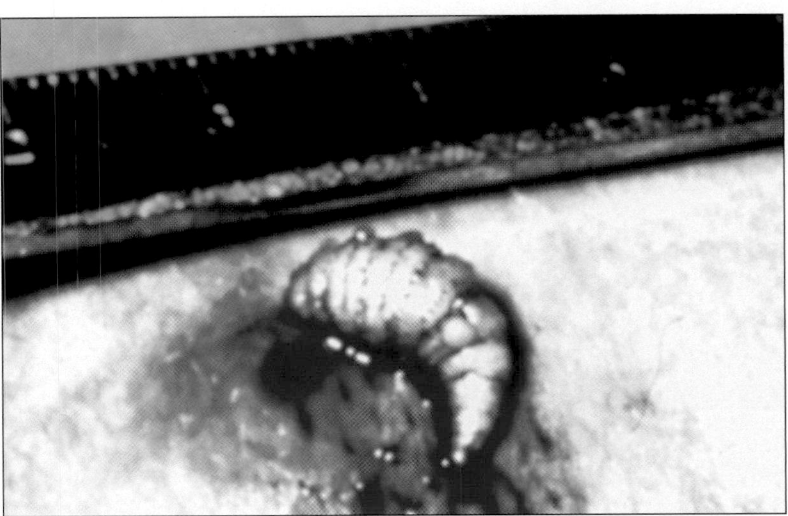

FIGURE 2-57 Cutaneous myiasis. A larva of *Dermatobia hominis* is shown emerging from the skin. Female flies of the genus *Dermatobia* use mosquites to transport their eggs. When such a mosquito bites, the fly eggs are deposited on the victim's skin. The larvae hatch and rapidly penetrate the skin, inciting the development of a small nodule around each larva. (*Courtesy of* H. Rosen, MD.)

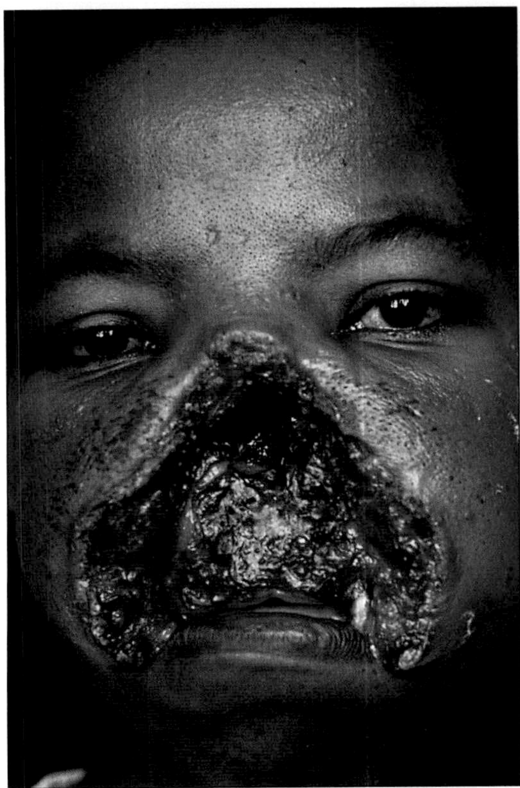

FIGURE 2-58 Mucocutaneous leishmaniasis destruction of the nose and mouth due to leishmaniasis in a patient from Colombia, South America. (*Courtesy of* F. Etges, PhD.)

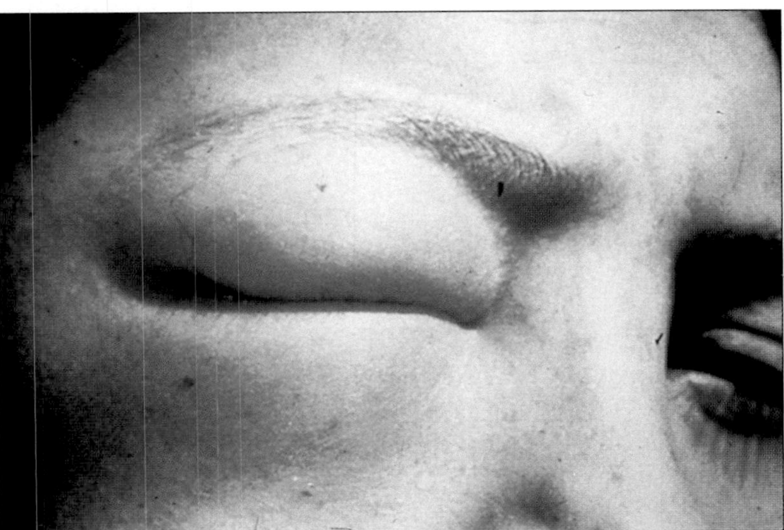

FIGURE 2-59 Chagas' disease. A woman from Argentina shows Romaña's sign, a unilateral swelling about the eye, which is a typical early finding in Chagas' disease. The causative parasite *Trypanosoma cruzi* is transmitted in the feces of a reduviid bug. (*Courtesy of* E. Kuschnir, MD.)

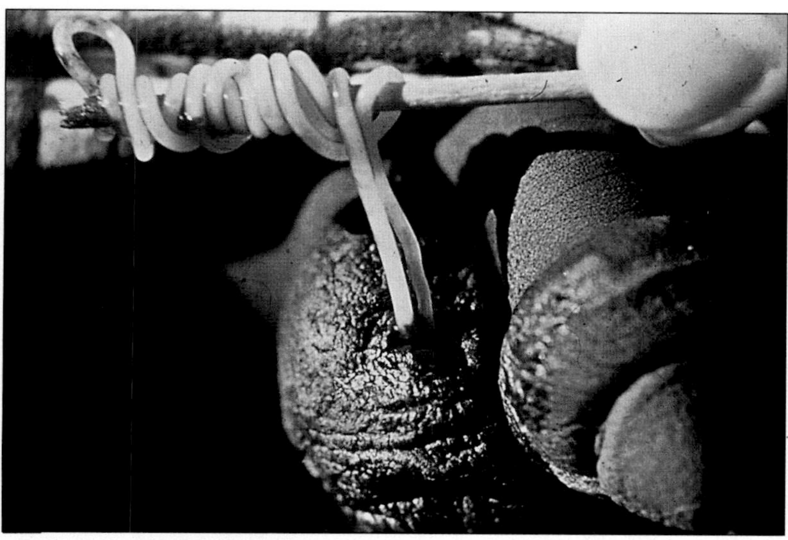

Figure 2-60 Dracunculiasis. A migrating adult female nematode, *Dermatobia medinensis*, is present in the scrotum. The classical matchstick recovery technique used in extracting the adult female worm is demonstrated. (*Courtesy of* J. Donges, MD.)

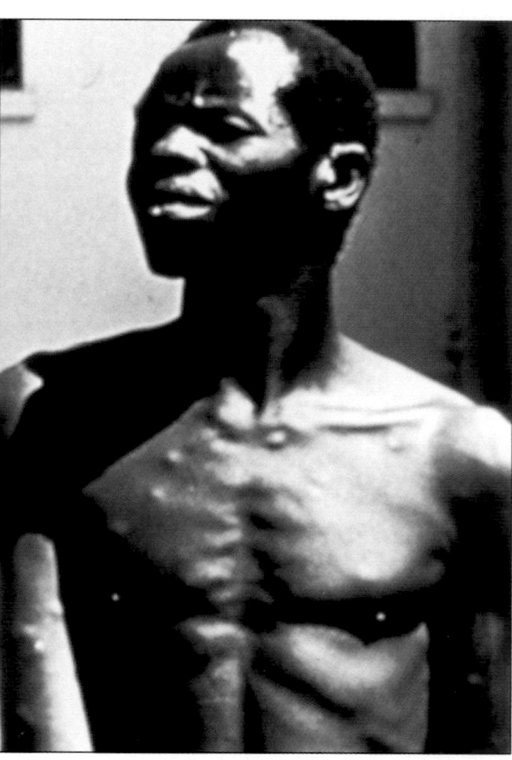

Figure 2-61 Cysticercosis. An adult African man shows numerous subcutaneous nodules of larval *Taenia solium* (*Cysticercus cellulosae*). Nodular lesions may also be found in the brain—*eg*, neurocysticereosis; and their presence may cause seizure activity. (*Courtesy of* M. King, MD.)

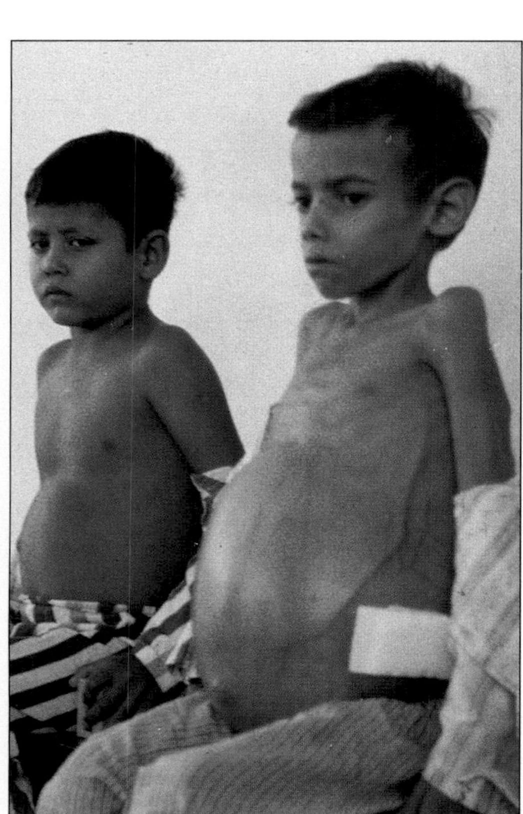

Figure 2-62 Hepatosplenic schistosomiasis. These two boys have end-stage hepatosplenic schistosomiasis. The child on the right shows massive ascites, with tremendous engorgement of the enlarged collateral venous structures. He died soon after the photograph was taken. (*Courtesy of* F. Etges, PhD.)

LEPROSY (HANSEN'S DISEASE)

Ridley-Jopling classification of leprosy

Clinical and histologic features	Tuberculoid (TT)	Borderline tuberculoid (BT)	Borderline (BB)	Borderline lepromatous (BL)	Lepromatous (LL)
Skin lesions	Up to 3 in number. Sharply defined asymmetric plaques with tendency for central clearing, elevated borders.	Smaller or larger than in TT. Potentially more numerous than in TT. Usually annular lesions with sharp margination on exterior and interior borders. Borders not as elevated as in TT.	Dimorphic lesions intermediate between BT and BL.	LL type lesions. Ill-defined plaques with an occasional sharp margin. Few or many in number, shiny appearance.	Symmetric. Poorly marginated, multiple infiltrated nodules and plaques or diffuse infiltration. Xanthoma-like or dermatofibroma papules. Leonine facies and eyebrow alopecia.
Nerve lesions	Skin lesions anesthetic early. Nerve near lesion may be enlarged.	Skin lesions anesthetic early. Nerve trunk palsies asymmetric. Nerve abscesses most common in BT.	Anesthetic skin lesions. Nerve trunk palsies.	Skin lesions usually hypoesthetic, may be anesthetic. Nerve trunk palsies common and frequently symmetric.	Hyperesthesia a late sign. Nerve palsies variable. Acral, distal, symmetric anesthesia common.
Lepromin skin test	Positive	Usually positive (80% to 90%).	Negative	Negative	Negative
Lymphocytes	Dense peripheral infiltration about epithelioid tubercle. Infiltration into epidermis well developed.	Less numerous than in TT. Peripheral infiltration about granuloma. Variable epidermal infiltration usually focal.	Lymphopenic	Moderately dense and in the same distribution as macrophages.	Scant, diffuse, or focal in distribution.
Macrophage differentiation	Epithelioid	Epithelioid	Epithelioid	Usually undifferentiated. Epithelioid foci may be present. May show foamy change.	Foamy change the rule. May be undifferentiated in early lesions.
Langhans' giant cells	Present, well developed.	May be present. Usually few in number.	Absent	Absent	Absent
Acid-fast bacilli (AFB)	Rare, < 1/100 OIF or BI=0 (paucibacillary)	Rare, usually BI=0 (paucibacillary). If AFB present, consider a reversal reaction.	1–10/OIF or BI=3–4.	10–100/OIF or BI=4–5.	10–1000/OIF or BI=4–6. Globi present.

FIGURE 2-63 The Ridley-Jopling classification of leprosy. This classification scheme provides a very useful clinical/pathologic framework for understanding the broad spectrum of immune-mediated reactions in leprosy. Possible reactional states, complications, and prognosis are indicated for each form of leprosy. Leprosy has a broad range of clinical manifestations marked by a variable immune response and inflammatory reaction within infected tissues. At one end of the spectrum is tuberculoid (TT) leprosy, in which only a single area of skin and possibly its associated nerve supply are affected. At the opposite end of the spectrum is lepromatous (LL) leprosy, with massive skin infection plus involvement of nerves, nasopharynx, testes, and lymphoreticular system. The intermediate forms are less stable clinically and often progress to the lepromatous form, although regression toward the tuberculoid forms occurs with therapy or sometimes spontaneously. These "upward" and "downward" shifts depend on gains or losses in host resistance. (OIF—oil immersion field; BI—bacteriologic index.) (*From* Gelber [4]; with permission.)

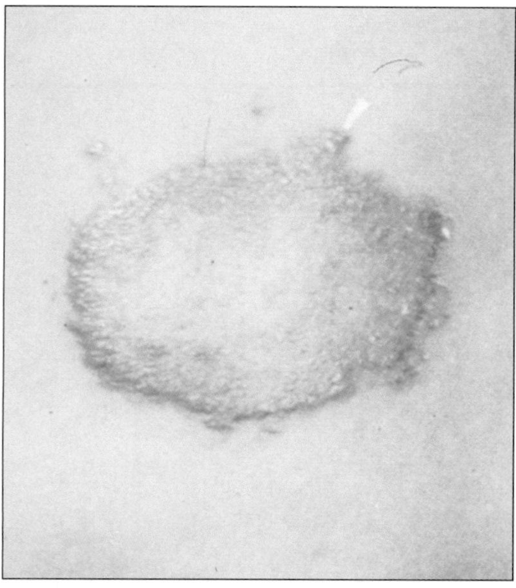

FIGURE 2-64 A single borderline tuberculoid (BT) leprosy lesion in a patient with several BT lesions. The lesion is anesthetic, has a sharp edge, and is largely erythematous with a fairly thick granular margin, which is associated with small satellite lesions. In BT leprosy, lesions may be few or numerous. Although they may be red or brown, most commonly they are hypopigmented macules with raised, well-defined borders or elevated plaques. Lesions are generally hypoesthetic or anesthetic. Patients with BT leprosy may develop lepra type-1 reactions associated with signs of inflammation in preexisting lesions and peripheral nerves, with "satellite" inflamed new lesions at times developing.

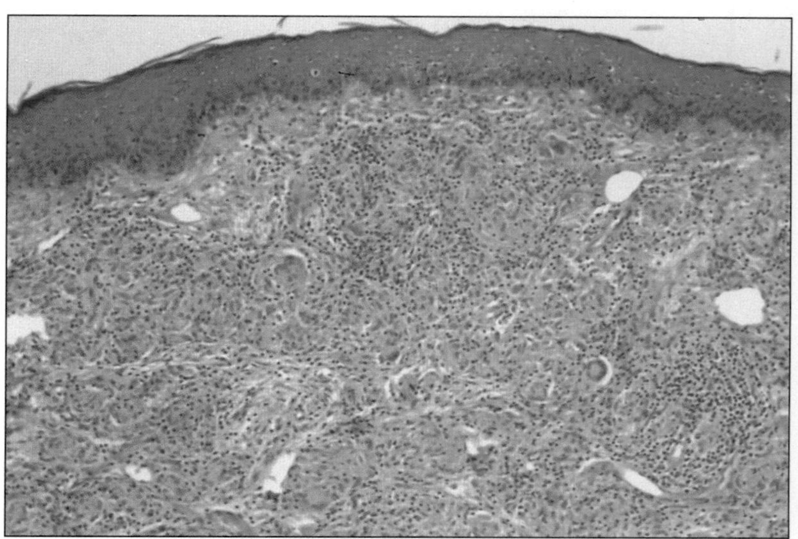

FIGURE 2-65 A hematoxylin-eosin–stained section of the skin from a patient with borderline tuberculoid (BT) leprosy, showing an epithelioid cell granuloma, occasional Langhans' giant cells, and a moderate number of lymphocytes occupying the superficial dermis. As is characteristic in BT leprosy, there is a clear subepidermal zone without pathology. In BT leprosy, there may be a few acid-fast bacilli which, when present, can be demonstrated mostly within nerves.

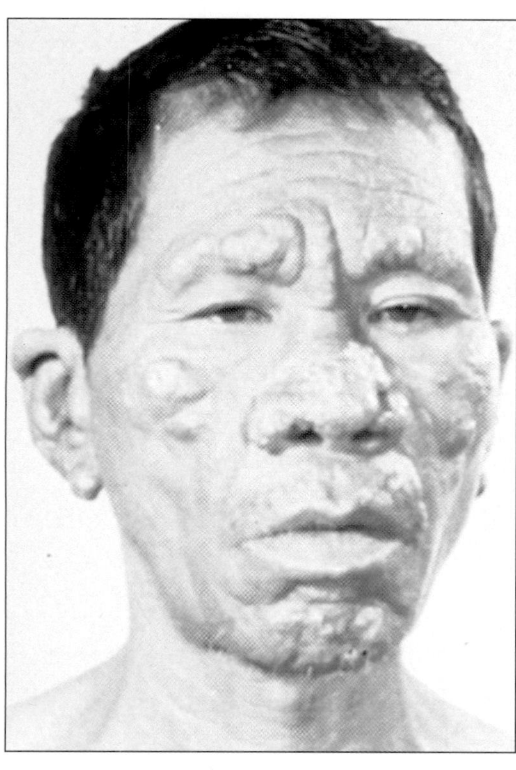

FIGURE 2-66 A man with far-advanced, nodular lepromatous (LL) leprosy. Diffuse infiltration coupled with nodules over the eyebrows, cheeks, ear lobes, nose, and chin are observed. Patients demonstrate *Mycobacterium leprae*–specific anergy (cell-mediated responses) but have high levels of circulating antibody to *M. leprae* and a diffuse polyclonal hyperglobulinemia, which may lead to a variety of false-positive serologic tests, including VDRL, antinuclear antibodies, and rheumatoid factor.

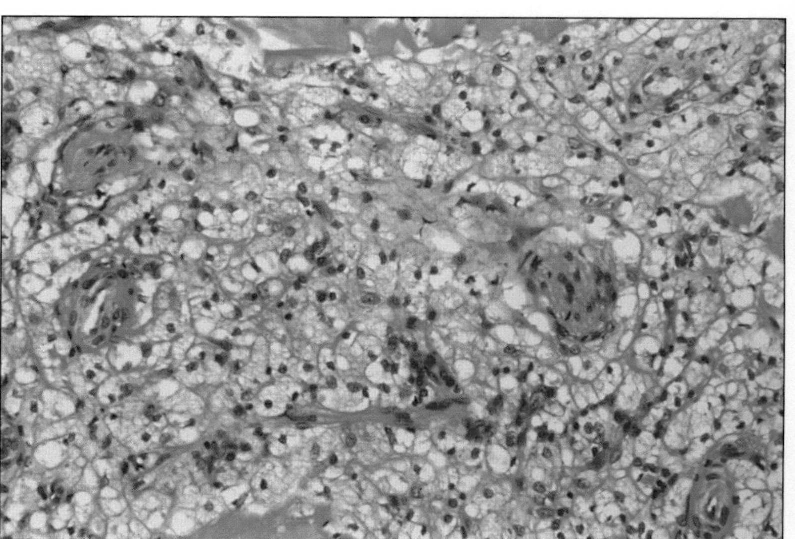

FIGURE 2-67 A hematoxylin-eosin–stained section of skin is typical of a patient with active lepromatous leprosy and demonstrates highly vacuolated foam cells, normal-appearing nerves, and a histiocytic granuloma. In the dermis, nerves may appear normal, hyalinized, with pathology of the perineurium, or fibrosed. Lymphocytes, if present, are usually scanty.

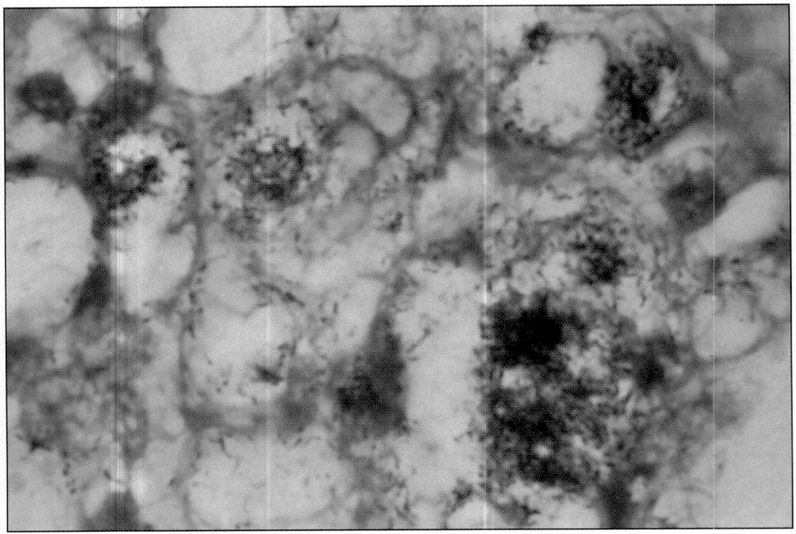

Figure 2-68 Lepromatous leprosy patients have enormous numbers of acid-fast bacilli, often in huge clumps, termed *globi.* It has been estimated that at times 10% of the dry weight of the skin in these patients may be bacilli. In lepromatous patients, acid-fast bacilli are most plentiful in the skin, peripheral nerves, upper airways, and anterior chamber of the eye, but they are also present in every organ system except the central nervous system and lungs.

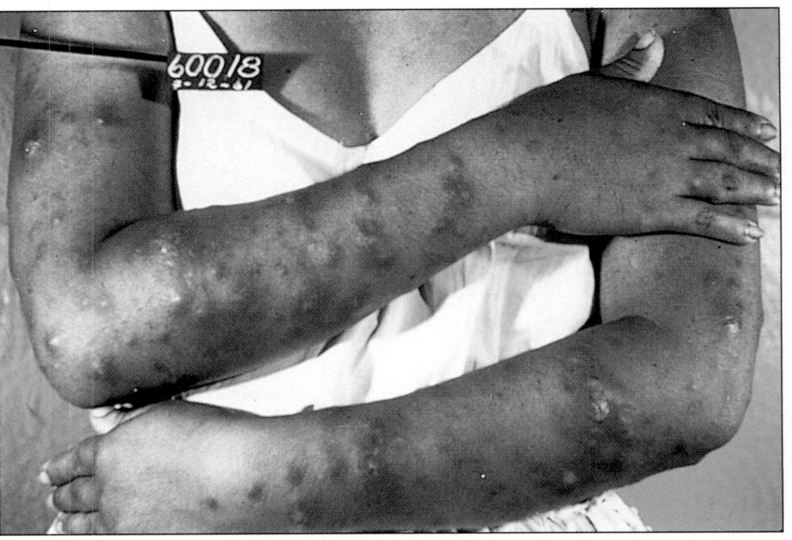

Figure 2-69 A patient with several cutaneous and subcutaneous inflammatory erythema nodosum leprosum (ENL) lesions. As in this patient, at times these lesions may pustulate and ulcerate. ENL appears to be caused by circulating immune complexes. It is associated with elevated levels of tumor necrosis factor (TNF) and a local increase in cell-mediated immunity, as manifested by increased numbers of T-helper cells, interleukin-2, interferon-γ, and a loss of suppressor T-cell activity. Corticosteroids or thalidomide is effective therapeutically, with thalidomide acting by inhibiting TNF synthesis.[5]

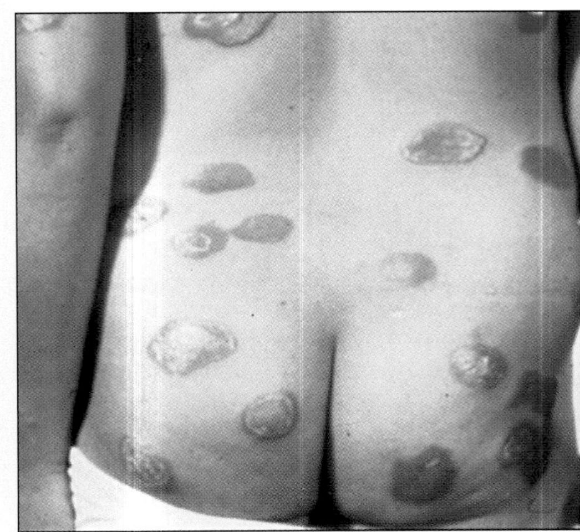

Figure 2-70 Lepra type-1 reaction (reversal reaction): multiple, moderately inflamed, sharply demarcated, subsiding reactional lesions are seen in a patient with borderline tuberculoid leprosy. Lepra type-1 reactions may occur prior to therapy as patients are becoming more lepromatous (downgrading reactions), or during therapy as the histopathologic picture is shifting toward the tuberculoid end of the spectrum (reversal reaction). Symptoms of lepra type-1 reactions are confined to skin inflammation (generally in old borderline lesions, but new "satellite" lesions may also appear), neuritis, and occasionally low-grade fever. If neuritis is untreated for as little as 24 hours, irreversible sensory or motor defects may occur.

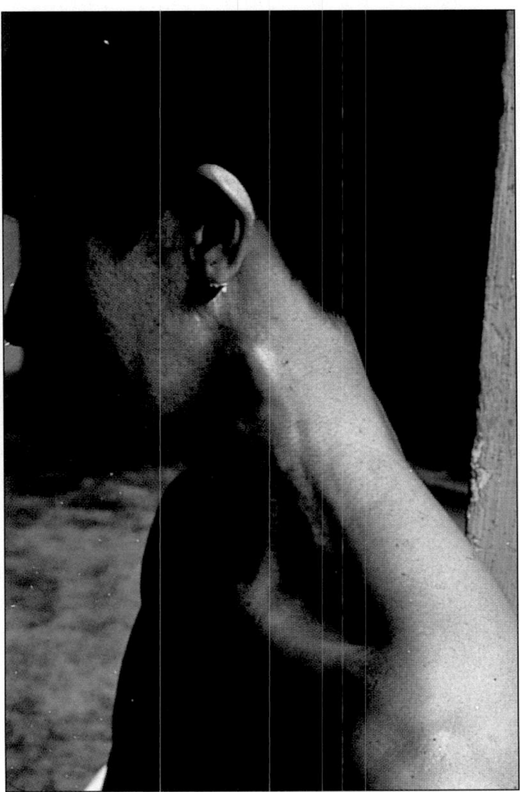

Figure 2-71 Large peripheral nerves in leprosy. The swelling in the neck is a huge posterior auricular nerve, this nerve generally being neither visible nor palpable. Leprosy is the only disease (except for a few rare hereditary neuropathies) that results in enlarged peripheral nerves. Almost all the morbidity of leprosy is due to *M. leprae's* unique tropism, among bacteria, for peripheral nerves and its resultant peripheral neuropathy. In leprosy, large nerve trunks, small superficial nerve twigs, and microscopic dermal nerves may be pathologically enlarged. The most commonly involved and enlarged peripheral nerve trunks include the ulnar nerve at the elbow, superficial radial nerve at the wrist, peroneal nerve just below the knee, sural nerve in the posterior calf, and posterior tibial nerve just behind the medial malleolus at the ankle.

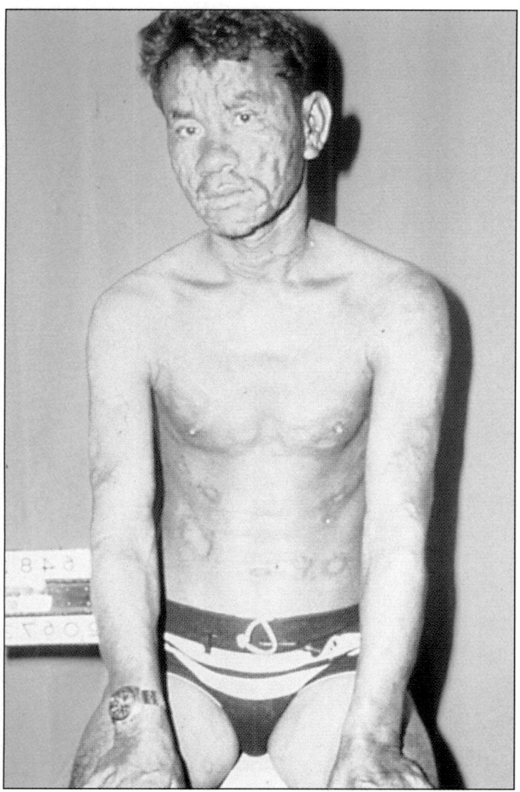

FIGURE 2-72 Response to therapy. A patient with borderline lepromatous leprosy; his face is infiltrated and, indeed, as in lepromatous leprosy, "leonine," whereas the trunk has a more borderline appearance. After several months of effective antimicrobial therapy, there is a dramatic reduction of the dermal infiltration of the face. Indeed, lepromatous nodules and plaques regularly resolve with effective treatment, whereas tuberculoid lesions may resolve entirely, partially, or change little on therapy.

SPIROCHETAL INFECTIONS OF THE SKIN

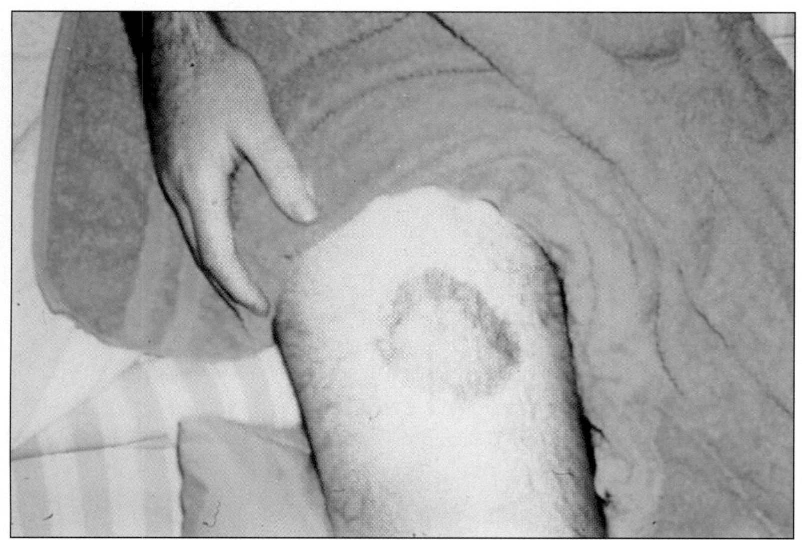

FIGURE 2-73 Erythema migrans. A burning sensation, itching, or pain may be noted over the lesion. Approximately 75% of patients with Lyme disease manifest this pathognomonic skin finding. Constitutional symptoms, such as fever, chills, headache, myalgias, arthralgias, fatigue, and lymphadenopathy, are often seen in association with erythema migrans and probably represent hematogenous dissemination of *Borrelia burgdorferi* and systemic release of cytokines. A small percentage of untreated patients experience recurrences of erythema migrans from 1–14 months after the original lesion.

Clostridial Infections

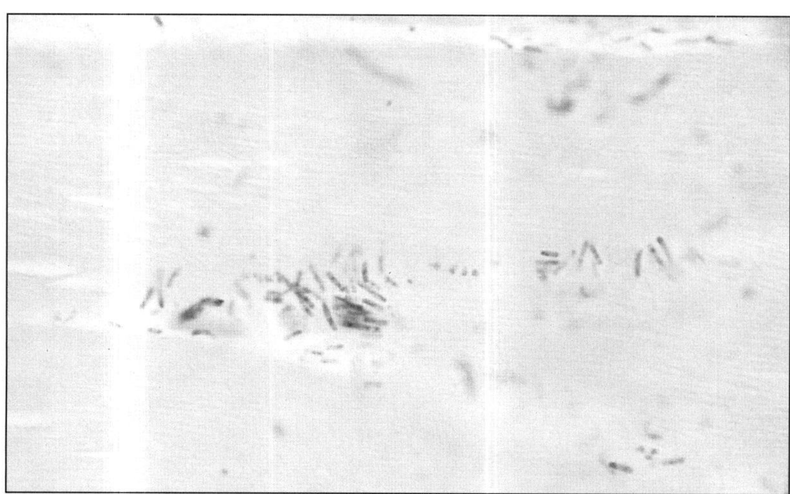

Figure 2-74 Tissue Gram stain showing slender rods with subterminal spores. Note that *in vivo Clostridium perfringens* are gram-variable and may be confused with gram-negative rods.

Types of *Clostridium*-associated gas gangrene

Traumatic
- Caused by *C. perfringens*, *C. septicum*, and *C. histolyticum*
- Trauma is usually crush injury or associated with compromise of blood supply

Spontaneous
- More commonly due to *C. septicum*
- Often associated with metastatic seeding from bowel portal
- Predisposing factors are intra-abdominal tumor, acute leukemia, neutropenia, cancer chemotherapy, or radiation therapy

Recurrent
- More than one episode of gas gangrene

Figure 2-75 Gas gangrene caused by *Clostridium* species can occur in three different settings. Traumatic is clearly the most common type of gas gangrene.

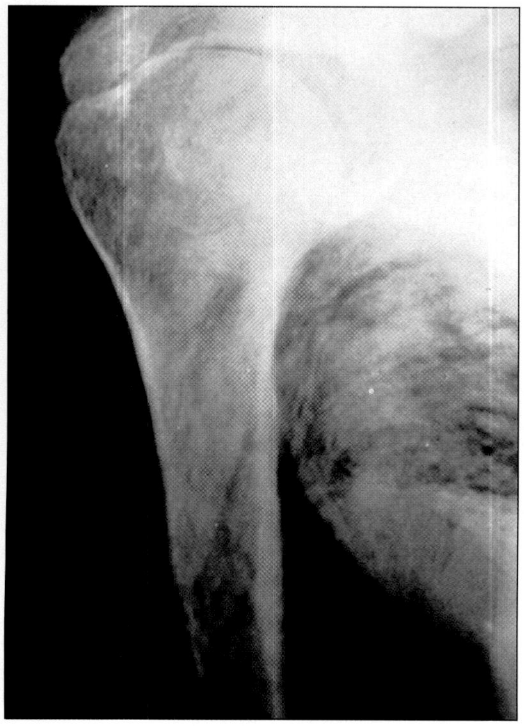

Figure 2-76 Spontaneous gas gangrene. Radiograph shows gas in tissue. The patient developed spontaneous gas gangrene of the hand, which spread rapidly up the arm and onto the thorax. *Clostridium septicum* was grown from blood and necrotic tissue of the arm.

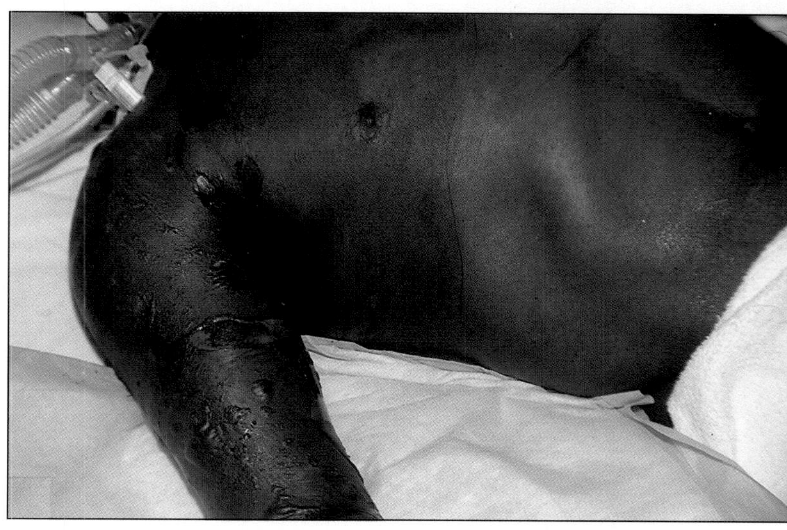

Figure 2-77 The line of demarcation in the patient shown in Fig. 2-76. The causative organism was *Clostridium septicum.* The patient received hyperbaric oxygen therapy, antibiotics, and aggressive surgical debridement with disarticulation of the arm at the shoulder. Two months after recovery, a barium enema demonstrated carcinoma of the colon. (Courtesy of J. Mader, MD.)

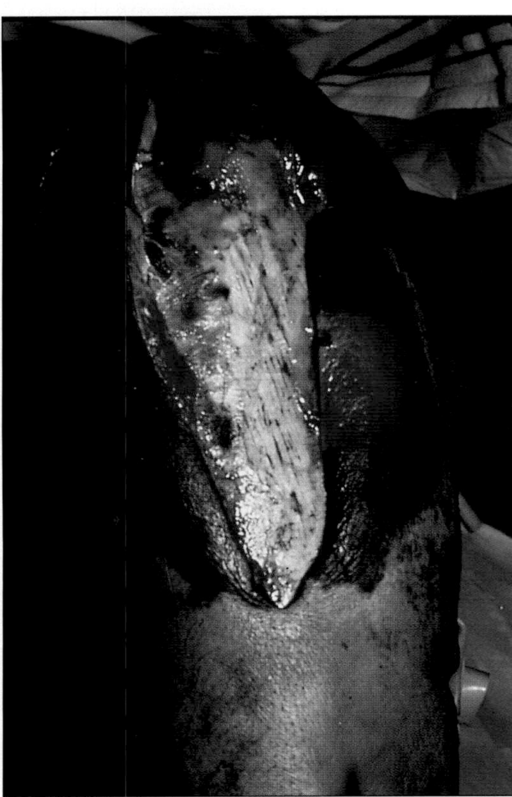

Figure 2-78 Spontaneous necrotizing fasciitis due to *C. septicum* in a patient with known carcinoma of the colon. Note the maroon/violaceous color of the skin. This photograph was taken immediately after fasciotomy.

Nonclostridial necrotizing soft tissue infections
Gram-negative aerobic infections
Pasteurella multocida
Pseudomonas
Streptococcal gangrene
Mixed staphylococcal/streptococcal infection
Halophilic *Vibrio* infection
Mixed aerobic/anaerobic infections
Diabetic gangrene
Postsurgical gangrene
Fournier's gangrene

Figure 2-79 Possible causes of necrotizing soft tissue infections other than *Clostridium* species.

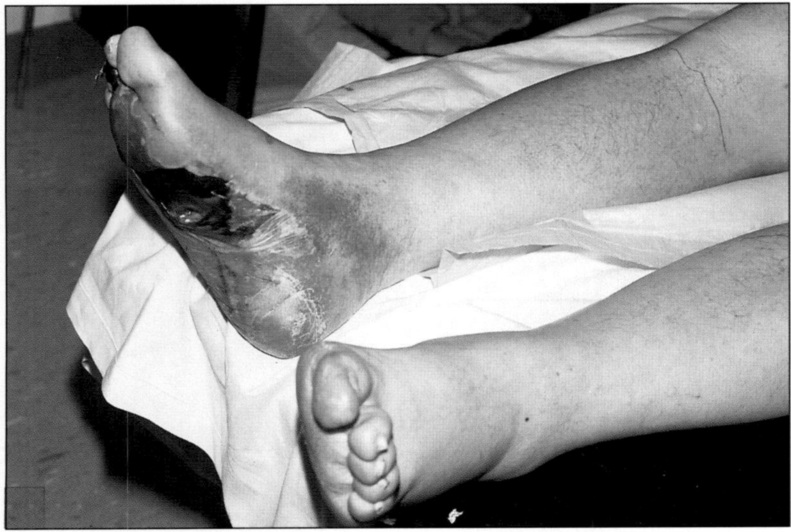

Figure 2-80 Mixed aerobic/anaerobic infection occurred in this diabetic patient with peripheral neuropathy and peripheral vascular disease. Emergent surgical debridement was performed. *Escherichia coli*, group B streptococcus, *Enterococcus faecalis*, *Bacteroides fragilis*, and *Proteus mirabilis* were grown from the biopsy specimen.

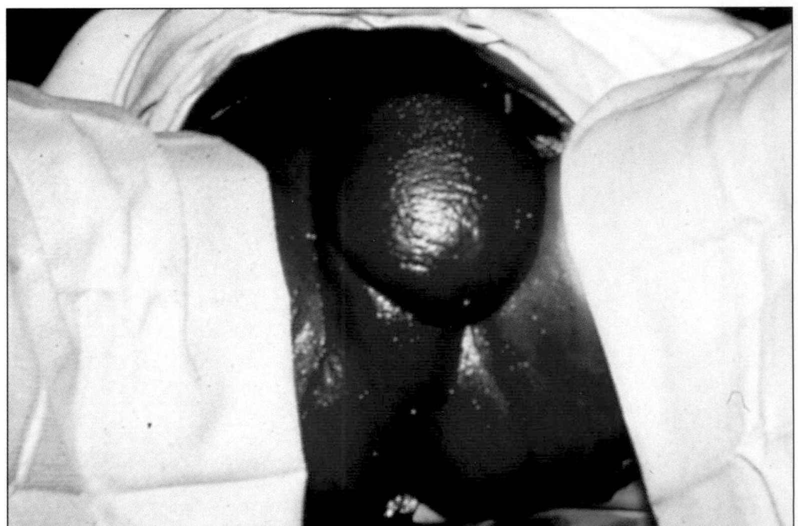

Figure 2-81 Fournier's gangrene. Scrotal swelling in a young man with Fournier's gangrene. The brown color is due to povidone-iodine surgical preparation. Gram stain of the scrotal fluid demonstrates many types of gram-positive and gram-negative bacteria. Cultures grew *Enterococcus faecalis*, *Bacteroides* sp., *Escherichia coli*, and anaerobic streptococci. After 3 weeks of antibiotic therapy (gentamicin, ampicillin, and clindamycin), the infection has resolved. However, in many cases of Fournier's gangrene, aggressive radical surgery may be indicated.

OSTEOMYELITIS

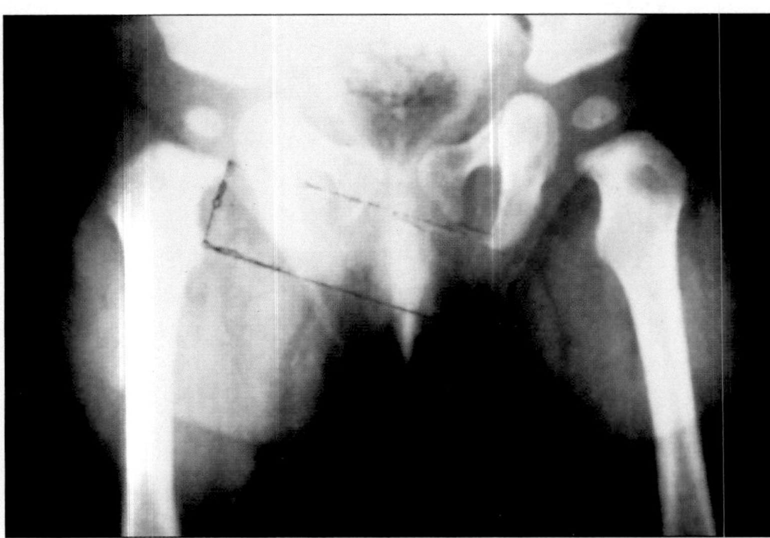

FIGURE 2-82 Hematogenous osteomyelitis of the hip. Anteroposterior radiograph of the pelvis in a 4-year-old child shows a lytic lesion with minimal sclerosis in the metaphysis of the left proximal femur.

Cierry-Mader staging system
Disease
I. Medullary
II. Superficial
III. Localized
IV. Diffuse
Host
A. Good immune system and delivery
B. Compromised locally or systemically
C. Requires no or merely suppressive treatment

FIGURE 2-83 Cierny-Mader classification. Four major factors influence treatment and prognosis of osteomyelitis: Disease factors include (1) the degree of necrosis and (2) the site and extent of involvement; host factors include (3) the condition of the host and (4) the disabling effects on the host of the disease itself. These factors must be considered when assessing treatment results and efficacy of treatment alternatives. The Cierny-Mader classification includes these factors and stages the infection and host using four anatomic types (I–IV) and three physiologic classes (A–C) [6].

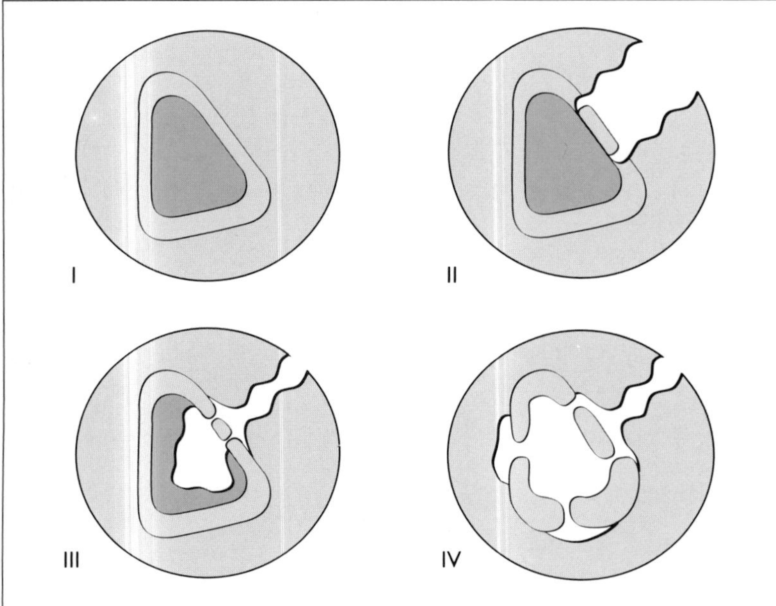

FIGURE 2-84 Disease classification (anatomic types of osteomyelitis). Medullary osteomyelitis (I) denotes infection confined to the intramedullary surfaces of the bone. Superficial osteomyelitis (II), a true contiguous-focus infection of bone, occurs when an exposed infected necrotic surface of bone lies at the base of a soft-tissue wound. Localized osteomyelitis (III) is usually characterized by a full-thickness cortical sequestration, which can be removed surgically without compromising bony stability. Diffuse osteomyelitis (IV) is a through-and-through process that usually requires an intercalary resection of the bone for cure. Diffuse osteomyelitis includes those infections associated with a loss of bony stability either before or after debridement surgery [6].

Host factors that affect treatment

Local compromise	Systemic compromise
Chronic lymphoedema	Malnutrition
Venous stasis	Immune deficiency
Major vessel disease	Immunosuppressive therapy
Arteritis	Malignancy
Extensive scarring	Diabetes mellitus
Radiation fibrosis	Extremes of age
Extensive small vessel	Renal failure
Compromise	Hepatic failure
Insensate region	Active cigarette abuse

FIGURE 2-85 Host classification. The patient is classified as an A, B, or C host according to the status of his or her physiologic, metabolic, and immunologic capabilities. The A host represents a patient with normal capabilities. The B host is either systemically or locally compromised, or both; coexistent diseases and factors compromising the host's status are listed. When the morbidity of treatment is worse than that imposed by the disease itself, the patient is given the C host classification. The terms acute and chronic osteomyelitis are not used in this staging system because areas of macronecrosis must be removed regardless of the acuity or chronicity of an uncontrolled infection. The stages are dynamic and interact according to the pathophysiology of the disease; they may be altered by successful therapy, host alteration, or treatment [6].

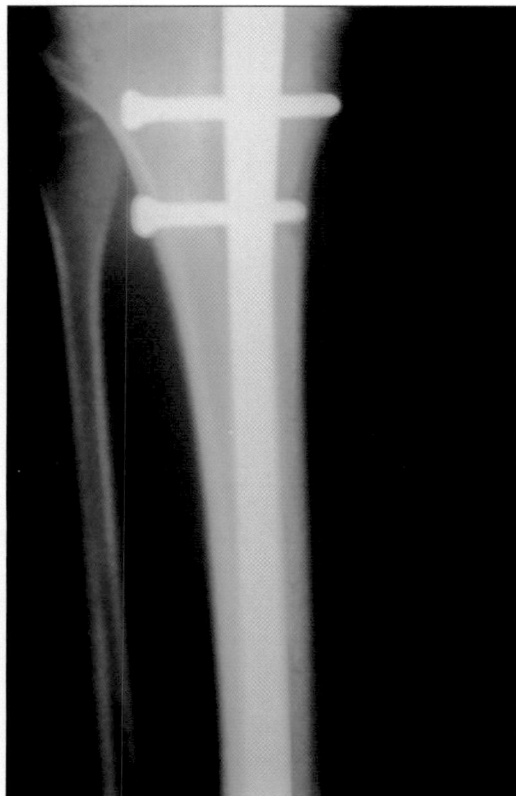

Figure 2-86 Stage I osteomyelitis of the proximal tibia. Anteroposterior radiograph of a 24-year-old man shows an infected intramedullary rod in place in the tibia. Note the lucencies surrounding the proximal rod and around the distal ends of the two screws.

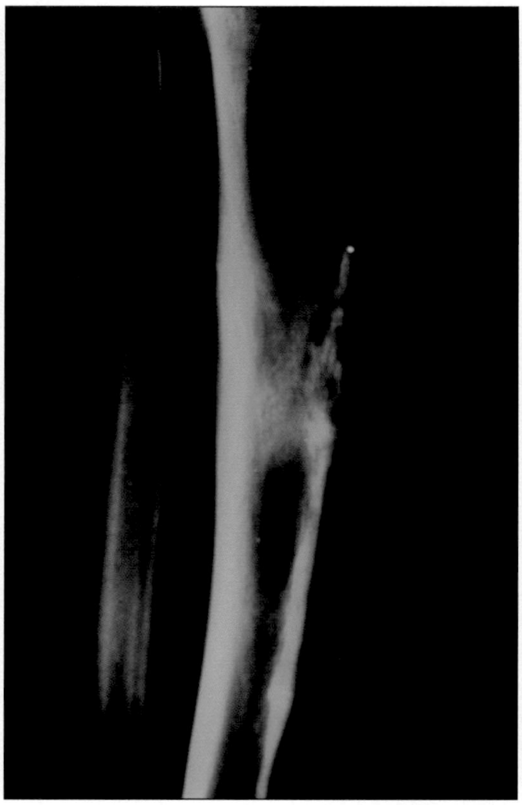

Figure 2-87 Stage II or superficial osteomyelitis of the proximal tibia. A 66-year-old man had developed a medial draining lesion following a tick bite 30 years prior to admission. Because of the persistent, purulent foul-smelling discharge, he or his wife had to change the dressing several times a day. His wife became tired of the dressing changes and requested that he be treated. Lateral radiograph shows superficial involvement of the tibia. The patient was taken to surgery for superficial debridement and a local muscle flap. Following surgery and antibiotic therapy, the osteomyelitis was arrested.

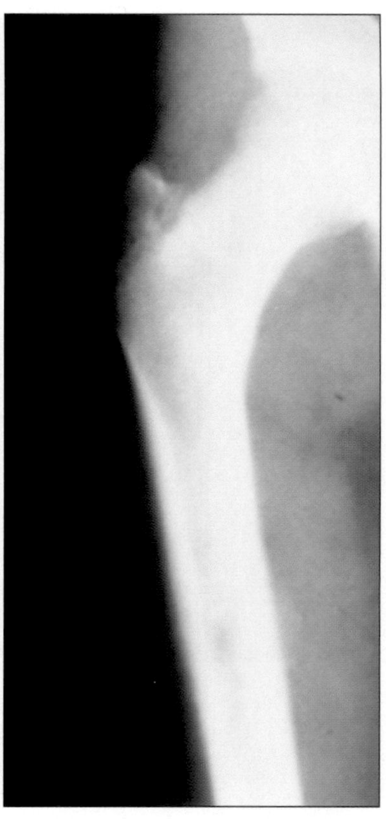

Figure 2-88 Stage III or localized osteomyelitis of the femur. An anteroposterior radiograph of a 48-year-old man shows a lytic lesion in the proximal femur. A 3-hour ^{99m}Tc-methyl-diphosphonate scan demonstrates increased uptake in the proximal femur. The patient was treated with surgical saucerization of the osteomyelitis and 4 weeks of parenteral antibiotic therapy. The osteomyelitis was arrested.

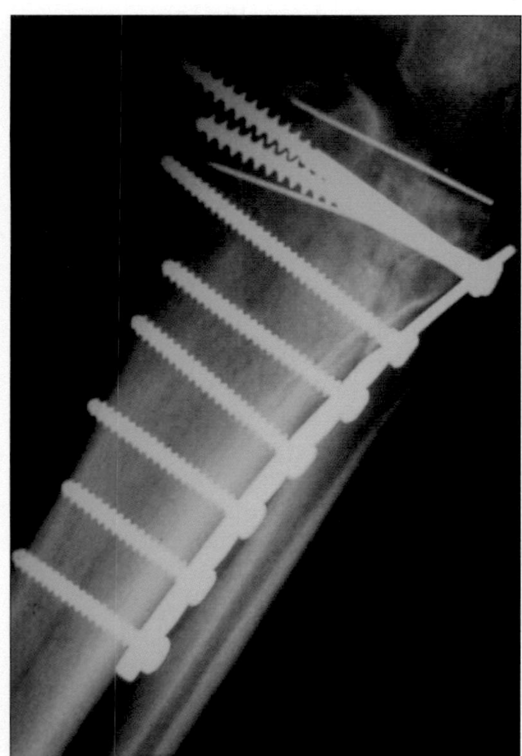

Figure 2-89 Stage III or localized osteomyelitis of the tibial plateau. Anteroposterior radiograph of the left upper leg of a 35-year-old man. The fracture of the left upper leg is well healed, but there is a lucency under the tibial plate and around the proximal pin. The hardware was removed, and the cultures were positive for methicillin-sensitive *Staphylococcus aureus*. The osteomyelitis was arrested. Hardware infection in a healed and stable bone is an example of Stage III osteomyelitis.

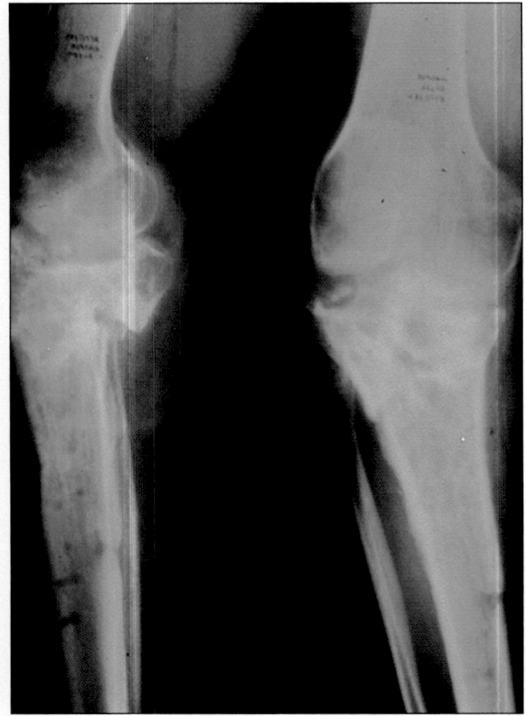

Figure 2-90 Stage IV or diffuse osteomyelitis of the proximal tibia and distal femur. Anteroposterior radiograph of the right knee of a 45-year-old man shows bony destructive changes about the joints and a healed proximal tibial fracture. The osteomyelitis developed after an open fracture of the tibia. *Pseudomonas aeruginosa* was isolated on multiple occasions from the bone. The patient had undergone multiple surgical procedures previously.

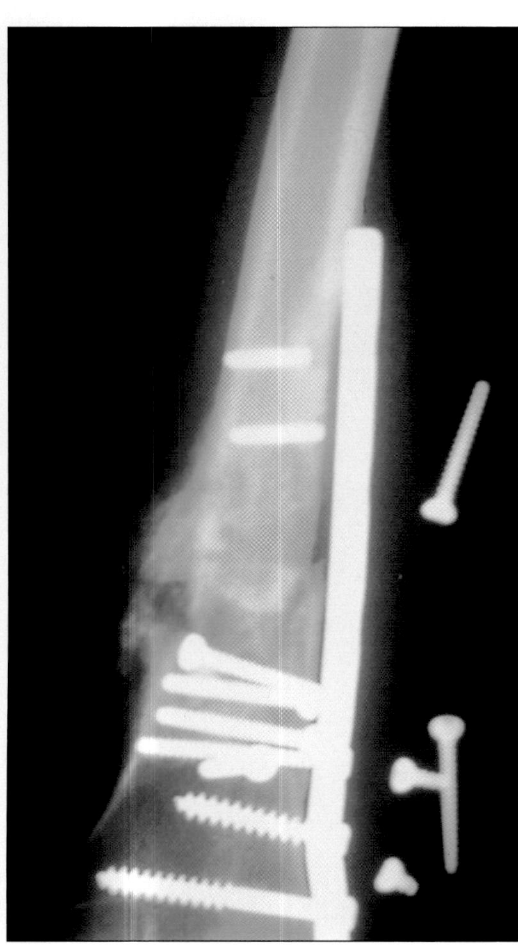

Figure 2-91 Stage IV or diffuse osteomyelitis of the femur. The plate affixing the nonunited fracture is infected and loose with screws lying freely in the soft tissues.

Stage I
(Medullary osteomyelitis)

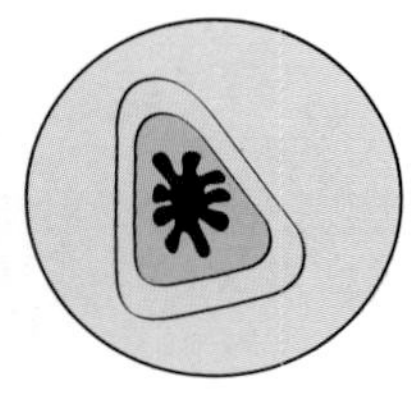

Necrosis limited to medullary contents and endosteal surfaces
Etiology: Hematogenous
Treatment:
Early: Antibiotics / host alteration
Late: Unroofing, intramedullary reaming

Stage II
(Superficial osteomyelitis)

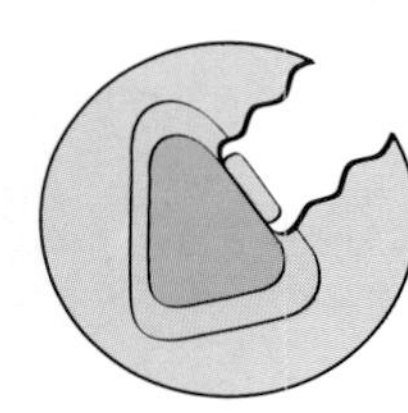

Necrosis limited to exposed surfaces
Etiology:
Early: Antibiotics / host alteration
Late: Superficial debridement / coverage, possible ablation

Stage III
(Localized osteomyelitis)

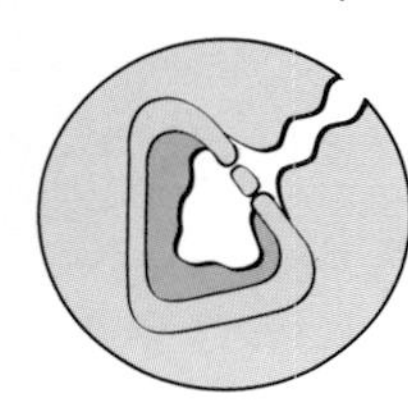

Well marginated and stable before and after debridement
Etiology: Trauma, evolving stages I and II, latrogenic
Treatment:
Antibiotics / host alteration
Debridement, dead space management
Temporary stabilization, bone graft optional

Stage IV
(Diffuse osteomyelitis)

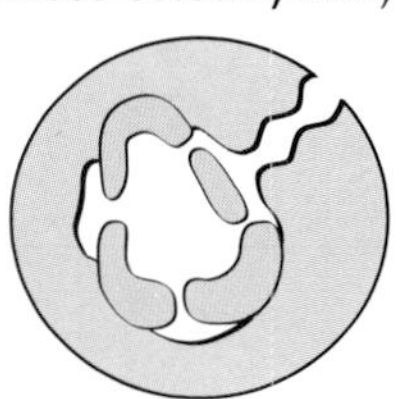

Circumferential and/or permeative
Unstable prior to or after debridement
Etiology: Trama, evolving stages I and II and III, latrogenic
Treatment:
Antibiotics / host alteration
Stabilization-ORIF, external fixation (Ilsizarov)
Deabridement, dead space management
Possible ablation

Figure 2-92 Treatment summary of the Cierny-Mader staging system.

Joint Infections and Rheumatic Manifestations of Infectious Diseases

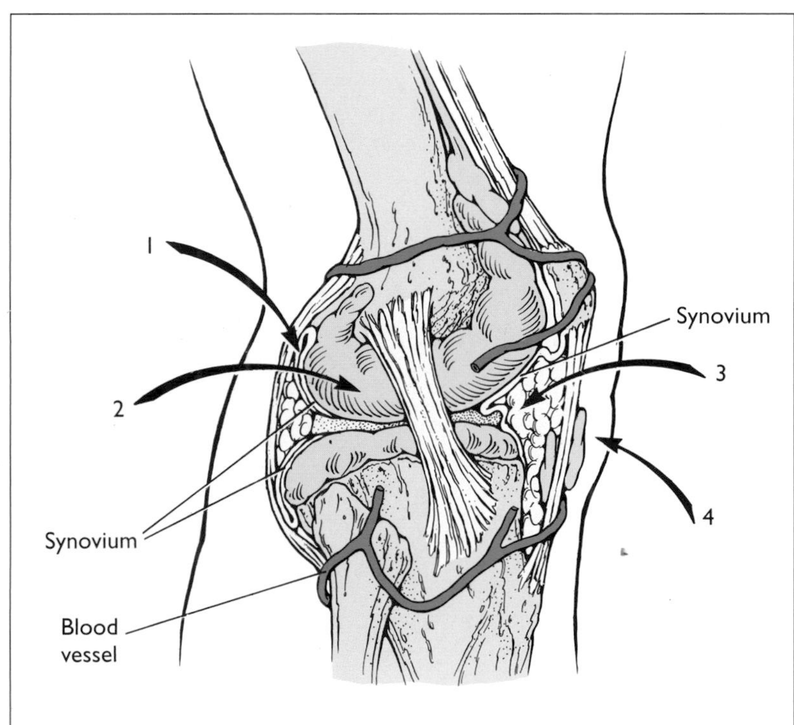

Figure 2-93 Routes of microbial invasion of the joint. Microorganisms can be carried by the circulation from a distant site of infection to the synovial membrane and then enter the joint cavity (*1*). They are deposited from the circulation into the subchondral bone with extension into the joint cavity (*2*). Microorganisms also can spread from an adjacent soft-tissue infection into the joint cavity (*3*). Microorganisms can be directly introduced into the joint by penetration through the skin (*4*).

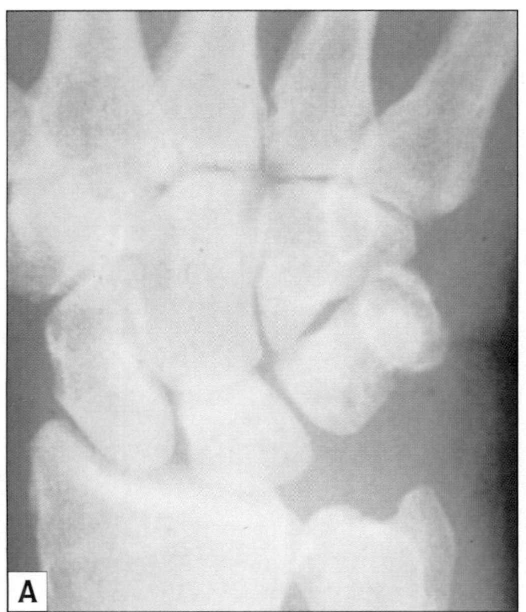

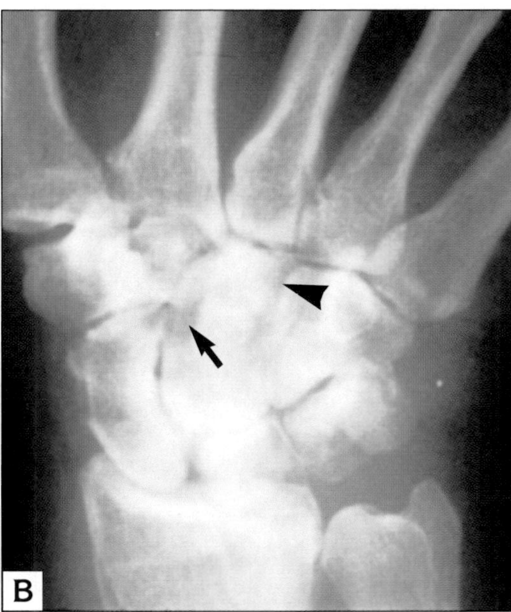

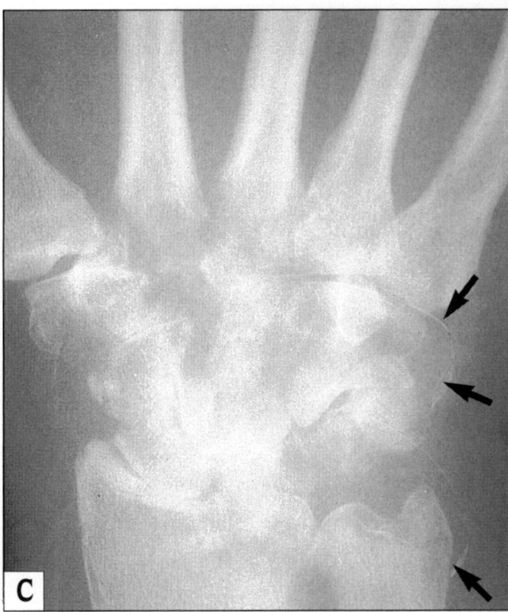

Figure 2-94 Septic arthritis of the wrist. Serial radiographs show progression of septic arthritis caused by *Staphylococcus aureus* infection of the wrist. This infection was hematogenously spread; however, a portal of entry could not be identified. The first sign of a septic joint is pain, quickly followed by swelling and redness of the overlying skin. The patient may experience fever and chills. The joint is exquisitely tender and painful. Arthrocentesis reveals cloudy fluid with cell counts of 50,000 to 100,000/mm^3 or greater that are predominantly polymorphonuclear leukocytes. **A**, A radiograph on admission shows only soft-tissue swelling. **B**, Four weeks later, there is osteopenia of the carpal bones and proximal metacarpals. Joint space narrowing of the carpal articulations is present (*arrowhead*) and erosions can be seen (*arrow*). **C**, At 2.5 weeks later, diffuse destruction of the carpals and proximal metacarpals with extensive erosions is evident (*arrows*). There is loss of joint space at the radial carpal, midcarpal, and common carpometacarpal articulations. (*Courtesy of* T. Gillespy, MD.)

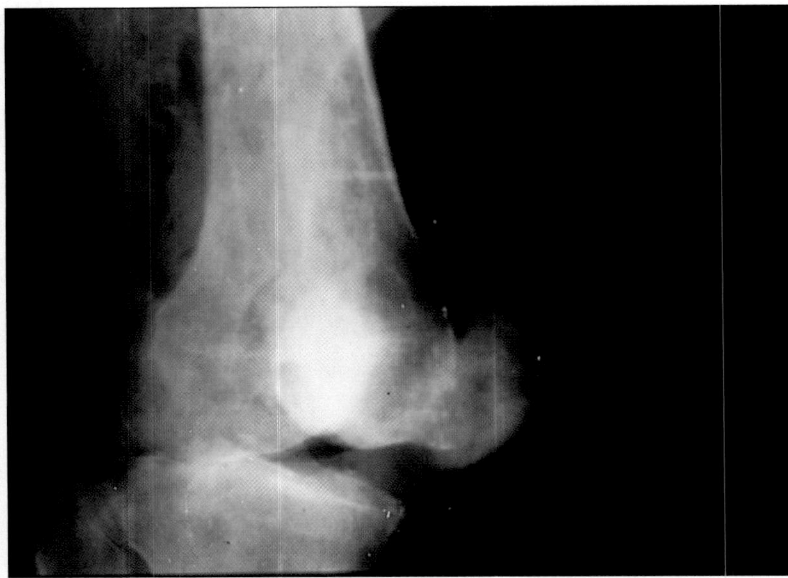

FIGURE 2-95 Septic arthritis of the knee. Lateral view of the knee showing intra-articular gas. Cultures from the joint, blood, and urine grew a gas-forming *Escherichia coli*. Erosions have not yet developed. There is underlying osteoarthritis manifested by joint-space narrowing, subchondral sclerosis, and osteophytes at the joint margins. Septic arthritis caused by gram-negative bacilli represents only 5% of joint infections and occurs most commonly in patients with chronic debilitating illness or those on immunosuppressive agents. Joint infection tends to affect previously damaged joints, as occurred in this patient. (*From* Gilliland and Caldwell [7]; with permission.)

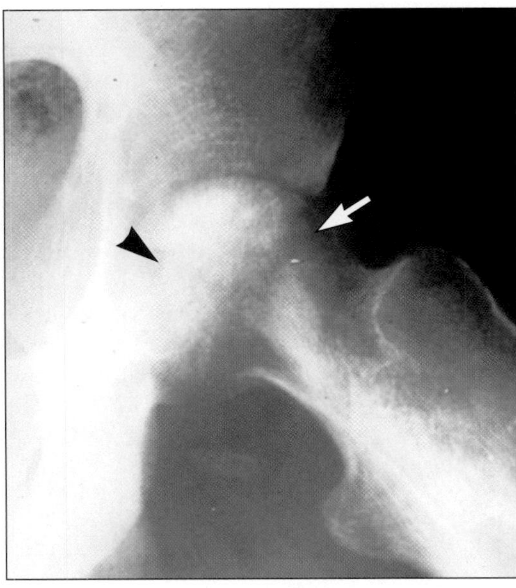

FIGURE 2-96 Septic arthritis and osteonecrosis of the right hip in a 25-year-old African-American man with sickle cell disease. The infection in this case was caused by *Staphylococcus aureus*. Patients with sickle cell disease are prone both to osteonecrosis and osteomyelitis. Septic arthritis is less common. Evidence for septic arthritis on this radiograph includes a bone erosion (*arrow*), joint-space narrowing, osteopenia and an effusion. A range of microorganisms have been described in septic arthritis, including *Salmonella*, *Staphylococcus*, *Streptococcus*, *Escherichia coli*, and *Enterobacter*. Of note, over half of the cases of osteomyelitis in patients with sickle cell disease are due to salmonellae, and in the remainder, gram-negative organisms predominate. Features of osteonecrosis in this radiograph are patchy sclerosis and lucency of the femoral head (*arrowhead*). Decreased blood flow secondary to sickling of red cells may result in a poor response to antibiotic therapy in some patients. (*Courtesy of* T. Gillespy, MD.)

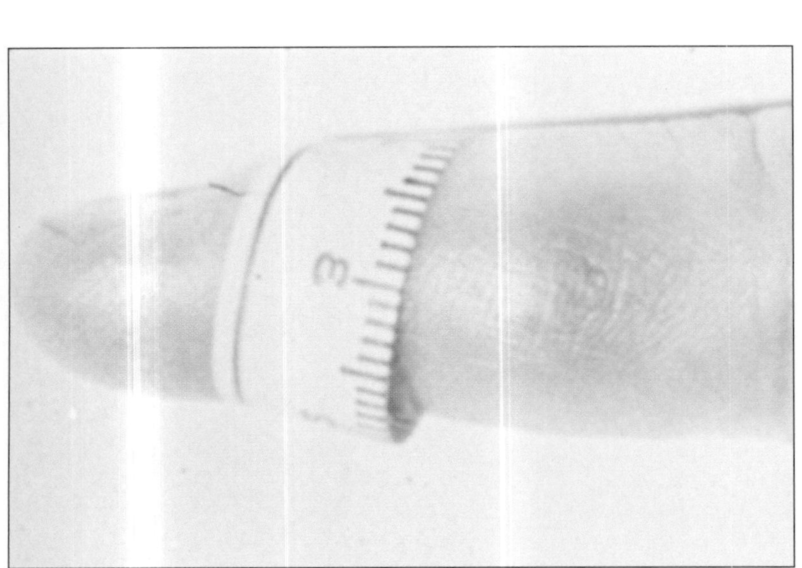

FIGURE 2-97 Arthritis and skin lesions in disseminated gonococcal and meningococcal infection. Patients with disseminated gonococcal infection (DGI) present with fever, skin lesions, tenosynovitis, and migratory polyarthritis, and a similar clinical picture is seen in patients with disseminated meningococcal infection. Skin lesions occur in about two thirds of patients with DGI and can appear as pustules, hemorrhagic macules or papules, vesicles, bullae, erythema multiforme, or erythema nodosum. This figure shows a hemorrhagic papule on finger. Tenosynovitis most often involves the wrist, ankles, and digits and helps to distinguish DGI from other forms of bacterial arthritis in which tenosynovitis is unusual. Suppurative arthritis develops in about 50% of patients with DGI and involves one or only a few joints. Arthritis is less common in disseminated meningococcal disease. Knees, ankles, and wrists are most often affected. Synovial fluid leukocyte counts range from 25,000–100,000/mm^3 with predominantly polymorphonuclear leukocytes. Unlike in other bacterial arthritis, Gram stains of synovial fluid show microorganisms in less than 25% of effusions. Blood and joint fluid cultures are positive in only about one third of patients. Cultures of the genitourinary track offer the best yield, and when positive along with clinical features of DGI, a presumptive diagnosis can be made. Cultures should also be obtained from the rectum and pharynx. Patients with DGI should be hospitalized and treated with parenteral antibiotics and adequate joint drainage. The antibiotic of choice is ceftriaxone, which should be continued until resolution of the disease. Individuals with hereditary deficiency of a complement component, particularly a late-acting C5, 6, 7, or 8 component, are susceptible to *Neisseria* infections. Patients with acquired complement deficiency, especially those with systemic lupus erythematosus, are also at risk for *Neisseria* infections.

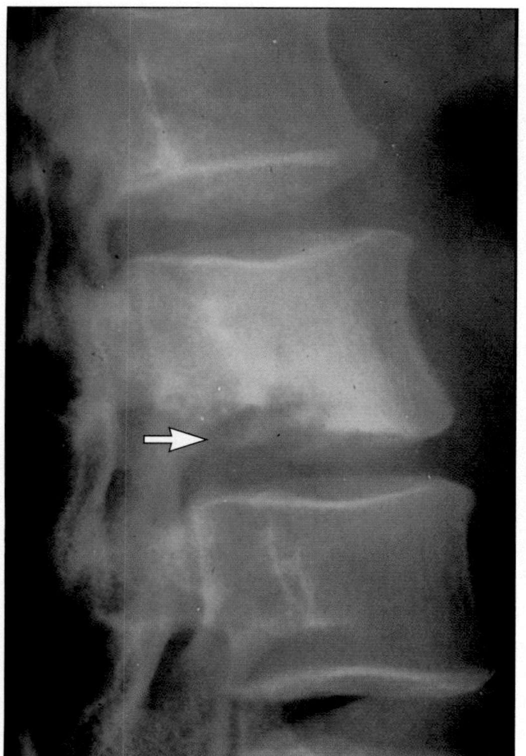

FIGURE 2-98 Tuberculosis of the spine. A radiograph shows osteolytic destruction in the body of L3 (*arrow*) extending into the disk and posteriorly into the isthmus of the inferior articular process. The adjacent disk space is narrowed. This patient experienced low back pain and low-grade fevers for the previous 2 months. Pain was aggravated by bending, straining, and lifting heavy objects. The patient was PPD positive, and a chest film did not show evidence of tuberculosis. The needle biopsy from the L3 area was nondiagnostic by microscopic examination but subsequently grew *Mycobacterium tuberculosis* on culture. Approximately 50% of skeletal tuberculosis involves the spine, with the thoracolumbar spine being the most common site. Active or even inactive pulmonary tuberculosis is not present in most cases; almost all patients are PPD positive. Mycobacteria reach the vertebral body by the hematogenous route. Infection initially involves the subchondral bone of the vertebral body, but may spread to other vertebrae beneath the anterior and/or posterior longitudinal ligaments or into the adjacent disk leading to disk space narrowing. Collapse of vertebrae and destruction of the disk may result in the development of kyphosis or a gibbous deformity and can cause cord compression and paraplegia. Infection can spread to the paraspinal tissue, forming a psoas abscess, which may extend into the groin and thigh. Paraspinal abscesses can also invade internal organs, such as the esophagus, bronchus, lung, and even aorta. Other sites of axial involvement include the sacroiliac joints and ribs.

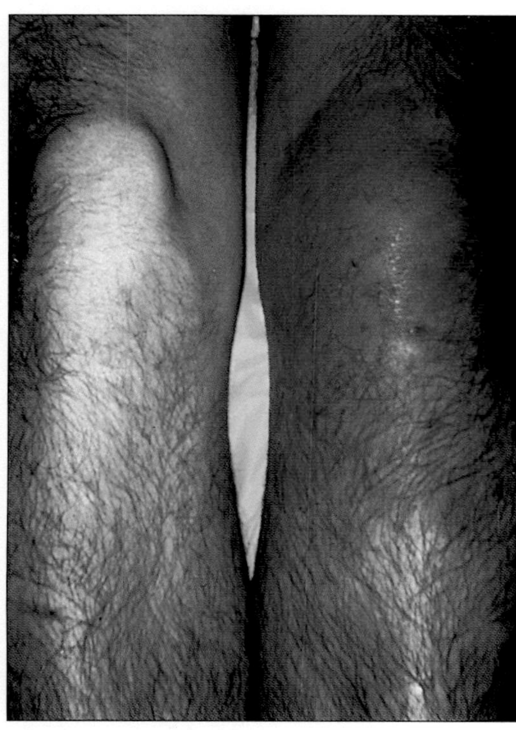

FIGURE 2-99 Acute prepatellar bursitis with cellulitis. Signs of acute inflammation can be seen in and around the knee. In > 50% of patients with septic bursitis an overlying skin infection is present, which may be an infected laceration, abrasion, or cellulitis. Distinguishing bursitis around the knee from septic arthritis or gout may be difficult. Useful distinguishing features include the anatomic localization of the signs of inflammation, including the amount and location of effusions, erythema, and tenderness. An inflamed bursa requires aspiration and examination for microorganisms and crystals. (*Courtesy of* the American College of Rheumatology.)

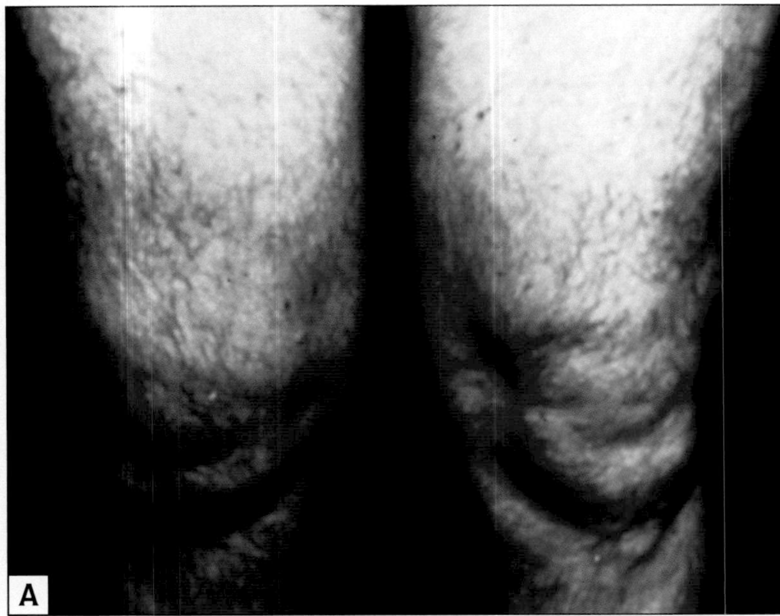

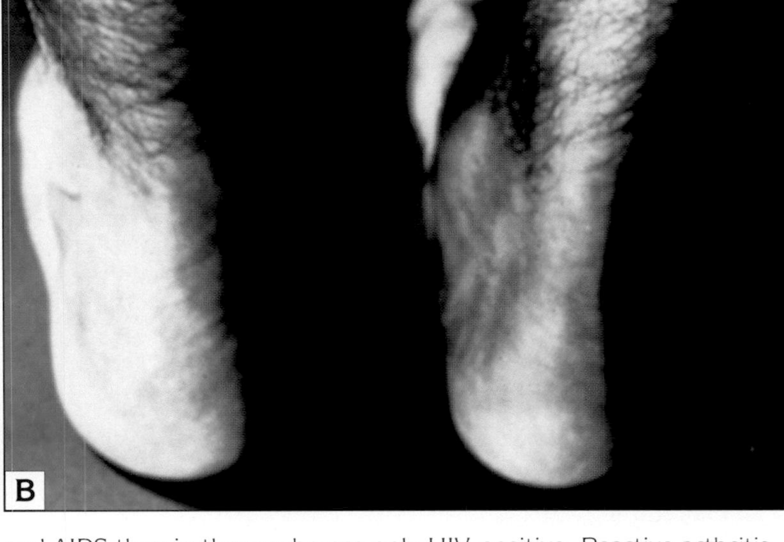

FIGURE 2-100 Reiter's syndrome and reactive arthritis. Reiter's syndrome is characterized by arthritis, urethritis, conjunctivitis, and mucocutaneous lesions, which are expressed in varying combinations and times. Reiter's syndrome is a reactive arthritis, which is defined as an acute immune-mediated inflammatory arthritis closely related to a preceding nonarticular infection caused by various organisms. The extra-articular features of Reiter's syndrome may not be present in reactive arthritis. Both are associated with HLA-B27, which is present in 60% to 80% of patients. Infectious agents that may trigger Reiter's syndrome/reactive arthritis include *Shigella, Yersinia, Salmonella, Campylobacter, Chlamydia, Ureaplasma*, and HIV. In the latter infectious agent, reactive arthritis and Reiter's syndrome appear to be more common in patients with AIDS-related complex and AIDS than in those who are only HIV-positive. Reactive arthritis follows *Streptococcus* group A infections and is considered to be an incomplete form of acute rheumatic fever. **A**, Acutely swollen knee in a patient with reactive arthritis. Typically, arthritis is an inflammatory, oligoarticular, asymmetric disorder, often beginning in the lower extremities before involving upper extremities. Sacroiliac joint and mild spinal involvement may occur. (*Courtesy of* the American College of Rheumatology.) **B**, Swelling over the posterior calcaneus at the insertion of the Achilles' tendon in a patient with Reiter's syndrome. Inflammation at sites of ligamentous and tendinous insertions into bone is referred to as *enthesopathy* or *enthesitis* and is characteristic of the spondyloarthropathies, which include Reiter's syndrome, ankylosing spondylitis, and psoriatic arthritis. (*Courtesy* of the American College of Rheumatology.) Patients with Reiter's syndrome may also have circinate balanitis of the penis and deratoderma blenorrhagica involving the sole of the foot.

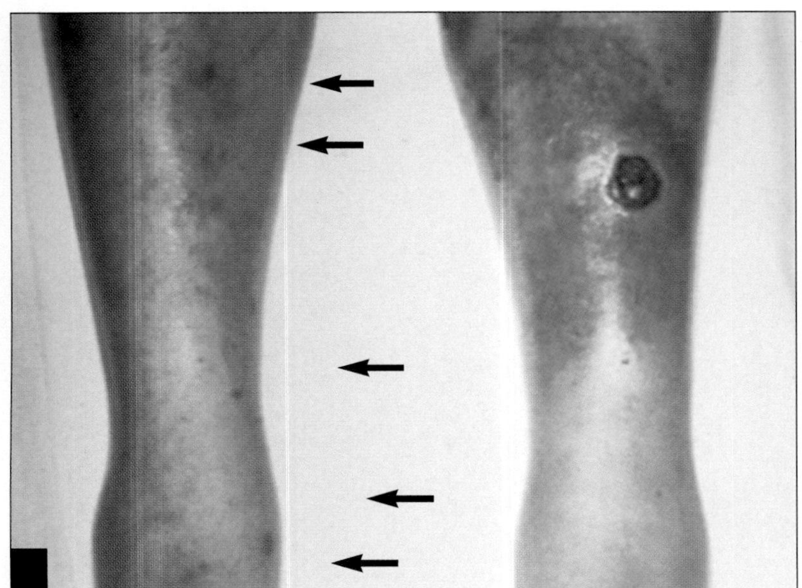

FIGURE 2-101 Mixed cryoglobulinemia due to hepatitis C. Vasculitic ulcers and cutaneous vasculitis. Confluent petechiae surround the large cutaneous ulcer on the left leg. Note also the scattered petechial rash on the right leg (*arrows*). Both legs are somewhat edematous, and the erythematous, swollen area surrounding the ulcer resembles cellulitis. This patient had mixed cryoglobulinemia associated with hepatitis C as documented by both serology and the presence of circulating hepatitis C virus RNA. Clinical features included arthralgias, vasculitic rash, rheumatoid factor, and a mixed monoclonal IgM/polyclonal IgG cryoglobulin, but she lacked evidence of the glomerulonephritis frequently associated with mixed cryoglobulinemia.

References

1. Goldstein EJC: Infections following human bite. *Infect Surg* 1985, 4:849–852.
2. Goldstein EJC: Clenched-fist injury infections. *Infect Surg* 1986; 5(Jul):384–390.
3. Scott HG: Envenomization. *In* Tipton VJ (ed.): *Medical Entomology.* Salt Lake City: Entomological Society of America and Brigham Young University; 1970:257–269.
4. Gelber RH: Leprosy. *In* Arnedt K, Dover JS *et al* (eds.): *Cutaneous Medicine and Surgery: Self-Assesment and Review.* Philadelphia: W.B. Saunders; 1995.
5. Sampaio EP, Sarno EN, Galilly R, *et al.*: Thalidomide selectively inhibits tumor necrosis factor alpha production by stimulated human monocytes. *J Exp Med* 1991, 173:669–703.
6. Cierny G, Mader JT, Pennick H: A clinical staging system of adult osteomyelitis. *Contemp Orthop* 1985, 10:17–37.
7. Gilliland BC, Caldwell JH: A splash in the joint. *West J Med* 1975, 123:58–59.

Chapter 3

Central Nervous System and Eye Infections

Editor
Thomas P. Bleck

Contributors
Sebastian R. Alston
Joseph R. Berger
Thomas P. Bleck
Jose M. Bonnin
David G. Brock
Sidney E. Croul
Thomas A. Deutsch
Jonathan D. Glass
Daniel F. Hanley
Richard T. Johnson
Justin C. McArthur
Hans-Walter Pfister
David A. Ramsay
Karen L.Roos
Oren Sagher
Allan R. Tunkel
Brian Wispelwey
Eberhard Wilmes
G. Bryan Young

Acute Bacterial Meningitides

Common meningeal pathogens by age group

Neonates	Group B streptococci *Escherichia coli*
Children	*Haemophilus influenzae* type b *Neisseria meningitidis* *Streptococcus pneumoniae*
Adults	*S. pneumoniae* *Neisseria meningitidis*
Older adults (> 50 yrs)	*S. pneumoniae* Enteric gram-negative bacilli *Haemophilus influenzae* *Listeria monocytogenes*

Figure 3-1 Common meningeal pathogens by age group. The choice of empiric antimicrobial therapy for bacterial meningitis should be based on the most likely meningeal pathogen, which depends on the patient's age and associated conditions increasing the risk for bacterial infections.

Cerebrospinal fluid abnormalities in bacterial versus viral meningitis

	Bacterial	Viral
Opening pressure	200–500 mm H_2O	≤ 250 mm H_2O
White blood cells	10–10,000 mm^3 (predominance of PMNLs)	50–2000 mm^3 (predominance of lymphocytes)
Glucose concentration	< 40 mg/dL	> 45 mg/dL
CSF/serum glucose ratio	< 0.31	> 0.6
Protein concentration	> 50 mg/dL	< 200 mg/dL

Figure 3-2 CSF abnormalities in bacterial versus viral meningitis. A variety of CSF abnormalities help to distinguish bacterial from viral meningitis. The opening pressure, the degree and type of CSF pleocytosis, and the glucose concentration are particularly useful in making the distinction between these two types of meningitis. PMNLs–polymorphonuclear leukocytes.

Empiric antimicrobial therapy for bacterial meningitis

	Antimicrobial agent
Neonates	Ampicillin plus cefotaxime
Infants and children	Cefotaxime or ceftriaxone
Adults (15–50 yrs)	Third-generation cephalosporin or penicillin G
Older adults	Third-generation cephalosporin (ceftriaxone or ceftazidime) plus ampicillin
Neurosurgical procedure	Third-generation cephalosporin (ceftazidime) plus aminoglycoside plus vancomycin
Immunocompromised state	Ampicillin plus third-generation cephalosporin
Neutropenic state	Ceftazidime plus ampicillin

Figure 3-3 Empiric antimicrobial therapy for bacterial meningitis. The choice of an empiric agent for the treatment of bacterial meningitis should be based on the patient's age and any associated conditions (recent neurosurgical procedure, immunocompromised state, and so forth).

Recommended antibiotics for the treatment of bacterial meningitis by organism

Organism	Antibiotic
Haemophilus influenzae type b	Third-generation cephalosporin or ampicillin plus chloramphenicol
Neisseria meningitidis	Penicillin G or ampicillin
Streptococcus pneumoniae	Penicillin G or ampicillin
Pseudomonas aeruginosa	Ceftazidime (plus aminoglycoside)
Staphylococcus aureus (methicillin-sensitive)	Nafcillin or oxacillin
Staphylococcus aureus (methicillin-resistant)	Vancomycin
Coagulase-negative staphylococci	Vancomycin
Listeria monocytogenes	Ampicillin (plus aminoglycoside)
Enterobacteriaceae	Third-generation cephalosporin
Streptococcus agalactiae	Penicillin G or ampicillin (plus aminoglycoside)

Figure 3-4 Recommended antibiotics for treatment of bacterial meningitis by organism. Effective third-generation cephalosporins include cefotaxime or ceftriaxone. For meningitis due to coagulase-negative staphylococci, rifampin is added to vancomycin when there is no improvement after 48 hours of therapy. For that due to the Enterobacteriaceae, ceftazidime is used if *Pseudomonas aeruginosa* is suspected or proven. (*From* Roos *et al.* [1].)

Subacute and Chronic Meningitides

Common causes of chronic meningitis

Infectious	Noninfectious
Mycobacterium tuberculosis	Carcinoma
Cryptococcus neoformans	Sarcoid
Treponema pallidum	Granulomatous angiitis
Coccidioides immitis	Systemic lupus erythematosus
Histoplasma capsulatum	Behçet's disease
Borrelia burgdorferi	Vogt-Koyanagi-Harada syndrome

Figure 3-5 Common causes of chronic meningitis. (*From* Tucker and Ellner [2].)

Neurologic abnormalities in Lyme disease

Stage	CNS	PNS
I	Headache Neck stiffness without pleocytosis	
II	Lymphocytic meningitis Encephalitis Myelitis	Cranial neuritis Radiculitis Plexitis Mononeuritis Guillain-Barré syndrome
III	Progressive encephalomyelitis Late mental changes with MRI abnormalities Latent CNS borreliosis ? Amyotrophic lateral sclerosis ? Others	Distal axonopathy Neuropathy of ACA

Figure 3-6 Neurologic abnormalities in Lyme disease. ACA—acrodermatitis chronica atrophicans; PNS—peripheral nervous system. (*From* Reik [3].)

Antibiotic therapy for neurologic abnormalities of Lyme disease

Facial palsy alone

Adults

Amoxicillin, 500 mg orally qid × 2–4 wks (± probenecid, 500 mg orally qid)

Doxycycline, 100 mg orally bid × 2–4 wks

Children

Amoxicillin, 20–40 mg/kg/d orally qid × 2–4 wks

Erythromycin, 30 mg/kg/d orally qid × 2–4 wks

All other neurologic abnormalities

Adults

Ceftriaxone, 2 g/d iv × 2–4 wks

Penicillin G, 20–24 MU/d iv for 10–14 d

Doxycycline, 100 mg orally bid × 10–30 d *or* 200 mg iv × 2 d, then 100 mg/d iv × 8 d

Children

Ceftriaxone, 50–80 mg/kg/d iv × 2–4 wks

Penicillin G, 250,000 U/kg/d iv in divided doses

FIGURE 3-7 Antibiotic therapy for neurologic abnormalities of Lyme disease. The current recommendation is to treat most patients having Lyme meningitis with intravenous ceftriaxone at a dosage of 2 g/d for 2 to 4 weeks; the literature contains no agreement on the duration of therapy or on the minimal adequate dosage of antimicrobial. There is no evidence to support treatment durations longer than 4 weeks. No regimen has proven to be universally effective. (*Adapted from* Reik [4].)

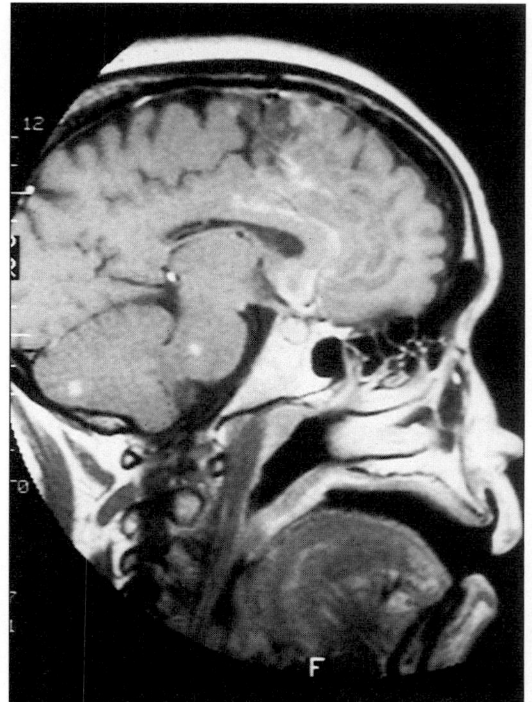

FIGURE 3-8 Sagittal view of cranial MRI in a patient with tuberculous meningitis revealing extensive leptomeningeal contrast enhancement. On this T1-weighted image with gadolinium, enhancement is particularly evident within the interhemispheric fissure; additional lesions are present in the pons and cerebellum. MRI may be superior to CT scanning in the identification of basilar meningeal inflammation and small tuberculoma formation.

Typical CSF findings in tuberculous meningitis

Opening pressure	180–300 mm H_2O
CSF WBC	50–300 cells/mm^3, usually lymphocytic
CSF glucose	< 45 mg/dL
CSF protein	50–200 mg/dL
Positive CSF smear	8%–29%
Positive CSF culture	25%–70%

FIGURE 3-9 Typical CSF findings in tuberculous meningitis. Because of the small population of tuberculous organisms in CSF, identification by specific stains is difficult; in many series, < 25% of specimens are smear-positive. One study found a rate of positive smears of 86% using multiple testing. False-negative CSF cultures are also common in patients with tuberculous meningitis, and even with as many as four CSF specimens, almost 20% of patients have persistently negative CSF cultures. WBC—white blood cell [5].

Clinical presentation of cryptococcal meningitis in non-AIDS and AIDS patients

	Non-AIDS, %	AIDS, %
Headache	87	81
Fever	60	88
Nausea, vomiting, malaise	53	38
Mental status changes	52	19
Meningeal signs	50	31
Visual changes, photophobia	33	19
Seizures	15	8
No symptoms or signs	10	12

FIGURE 3-10 Clinical presentation of cryptococcal meningitis. In non-AIDS patients, cryptococcal meningitis typically manifests as a subacute process after days to weeks of symptoms. In AIDS patients, the presentation of cryptococcal meningitis can be very subtle, with minimal, if any, symptoms. AIDS patients may present only with fever and headache. (*From* Tunkel and Scheld [6].)

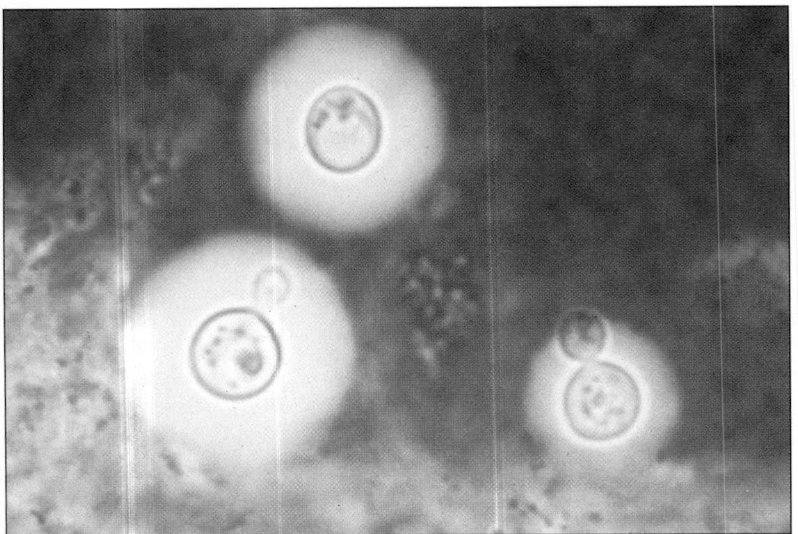

Figure 3-11 Cryptococcal meningitis. India ink preparation of CSF sediment demonstrates the prominent capsule of *Cryptococcus neoformans*. Note the highly refractile cell wall and internal structure of the yeast. The India ink test is positive in 50% to 75% of patients with cryptococcal meningitis; this yield increases up to 88% in patients with AIDS. (From Farrar *et al.* [7]; with permission. *Courtesy of* AE Prevost.)

Viral Encephalitis and Related Conditions

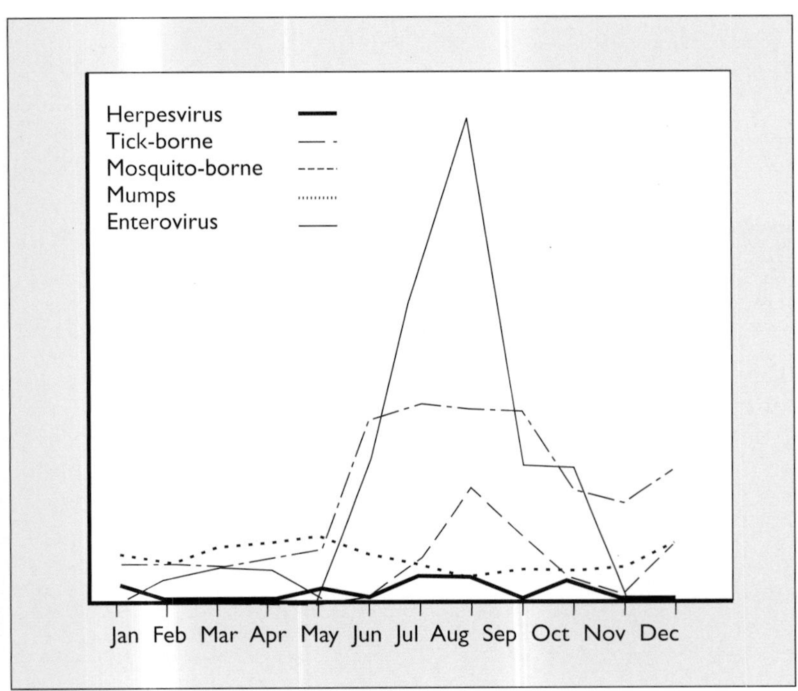

Figure 3-12 Seasonal variation of infections capable of causing viral encephalitis. In temperate climates of the northern hemisphere, the viral encephalitides have distinct seasonal occurrences that may be helpful in the differential diagnosis. Encephalitis caused by the mosquito-borne and tick-borne arboviruses peaks in the spring and summer, paralleling the periods of activity for their insect vectors. Others, such as the herpesvirus infections, may occur year-round. (*From* Griffin [8].)

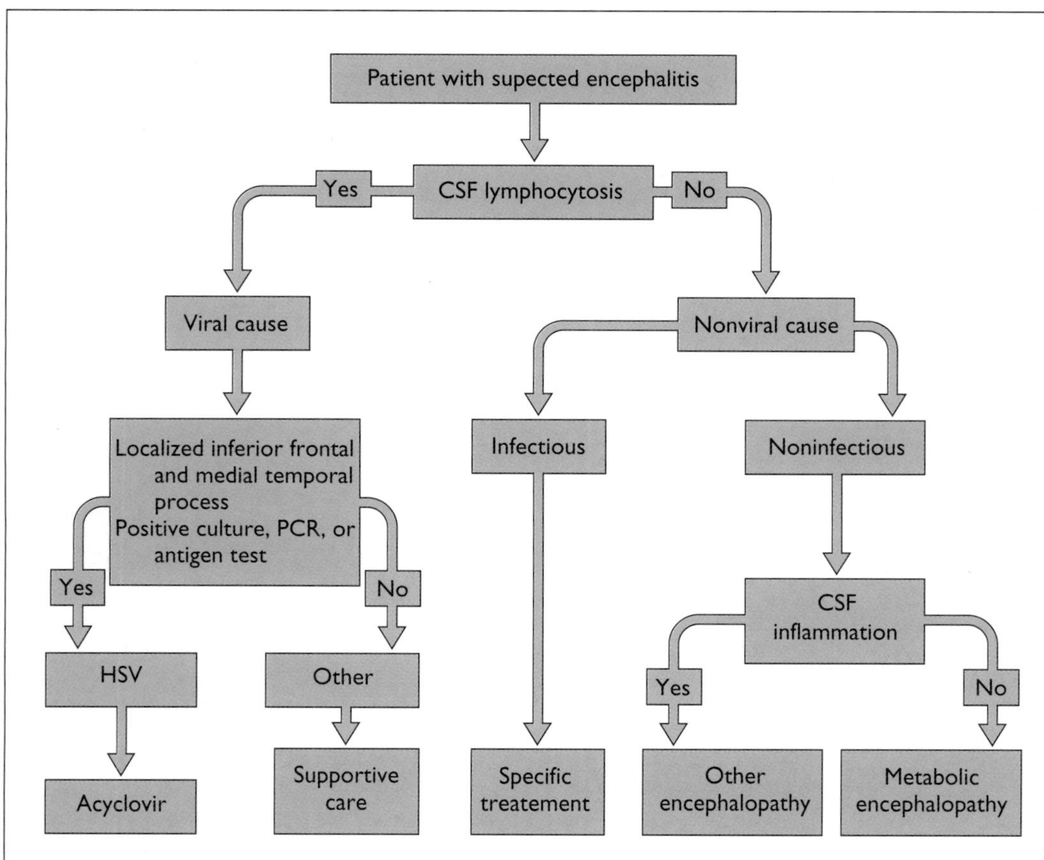

FIGURE 3-13 General approach to the patient with suspected encephalitis. In the febrile patient with depressed mental status, nonviral causes of encephalitis must first be considered and excluded, as treatment is available for many. Epidemiologic, clinical, and laboratory data are important in the differential diagnosis. If a viral encephalitis is suspected, a diagnosis of HSV encephalitis should next be considered. For HSV encephalitis, early treatment with acyclovir may be beneficial, whereas for most other viral encephalitides, treatment is supportive. CSF—cerebrospinal fluid; PCR—polymerase chain reaction.

Clinical and neurologic signs in herpes simplex encephalitis

Signs	%
Altered consciousness	97
CSF pleocytosis	93
Fever	85–87
Headache	79
Personality changes	70–80
Dysphasia	71
Autonomic dysfunction	58
Seizures (focal and generalized)	42–64
Vomiting	51
Ataxia	40
Hemiparesis	30–41
Cranial nerve defects	33
Memory loss	22
Visual field loss	13
Papilledema	13

FIGURE 3-14 Clinical and neurologic signs in herpes simplex encephalitis. A history of personality changes, bizarre behavior, hallucinations, focal seizures, or focal signs suggesting a temporal lobe lesion are common in HSV encephalitis, as this viral encephalitis usually is localized to the medial temporal and orbitofrontal areas and is often unilateral or asymmetrical. Signs do not differ significantly between patients with positive or negative cultures of brain biopsy material [9].

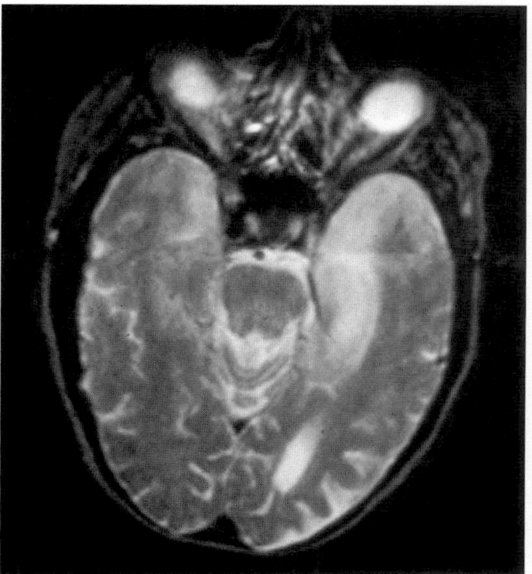

FIGURE 3-15 Brain edema in herpes simplex encephalitis. A rostral MRI section demonstrates contiguous medial and temporal extension of brain edema. The presence of medial and temporal findings suggests contiguous spread from the trigeminal ganglia, across the meningeal space to the inferior space of the temporal lobe, and then direct rostral extension.

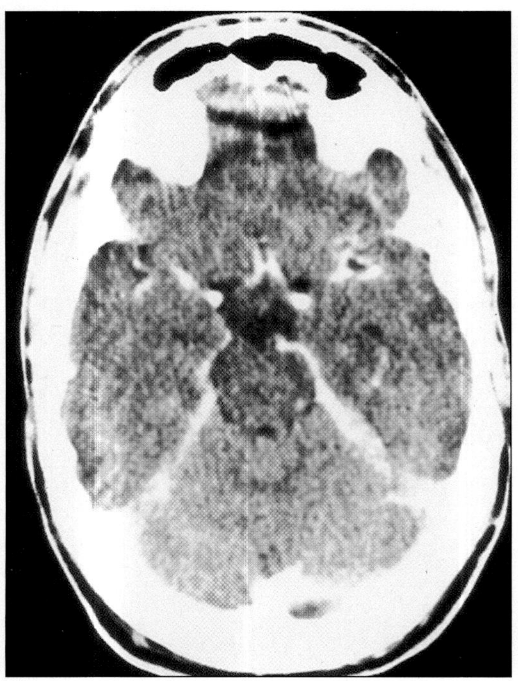

Figure 3-16 Temporal lucency and surface vessels on CT scan. A contrast-enhanced CT scan shows a medial temporal lucency and small linear enhancement suggestive of a cortical surface vessel. Dilation of surface vessels, increased number of surface vessels, and small areas of lucent tissue are early positive CT findings. However, the most common early CT picture in the first week of symptoms of HSV encephalitis is that of a normal CT.

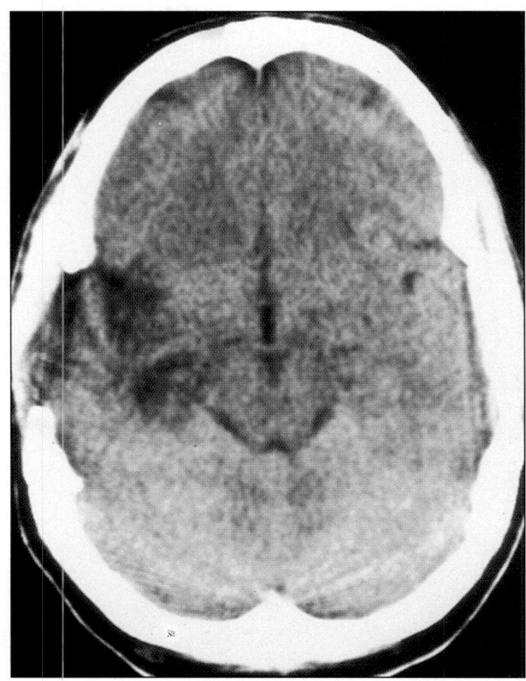

Figure 3-17 Temporal atrophy on CT scan. A post-biopsy CT scan demonstrates anterior and medial temporal atrophy. The absence of mass effect suggests that this CT was taken a month or more after the onset of HSV encephalitis and biopsy.

Differential diagnosis of common CNS complications of AIDS

	Clinical		Neuroimaging		
Disorder	**Onset**	**Alertness**	**Lesions, *n***	**Type of lesions**	**Location of lesions**
Cerebral toxoplasmosis	Days	Reduced	Multiple	Spherical, enhancing, mass effect	Cortex, basal ganglia
Primary CNS lymphoma	Days to weeks	Variable	One or few	Diffuse enhancement, mass effect	Periventricular, white matter
PML	Weeks	Preserved	Multiple	Nonenhancing, no mass effect	White matter, adjacent to cortex
AIDS dementia complex	Weeks to months	Preserved	None, multiple or diffuse	Increased T2 signal, no enhancement or mass effect	White matter, basal ganglia

Figure 3-18 Differential diagnosis of common CNS complications of AIDS. (*Adapted from* Price *et al.* [10]; with permission.)

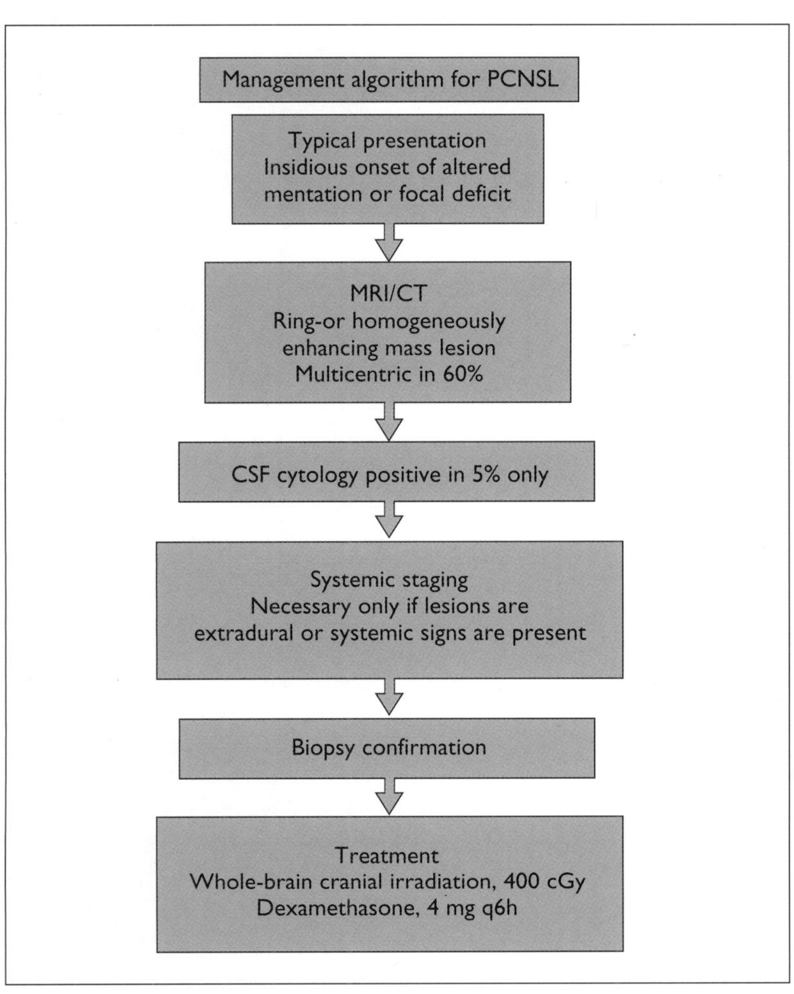

FIGURE 3-19 Management of primary CNS lymphoma. (*From* McArthur [11].)

BRAIN ABSCESSES

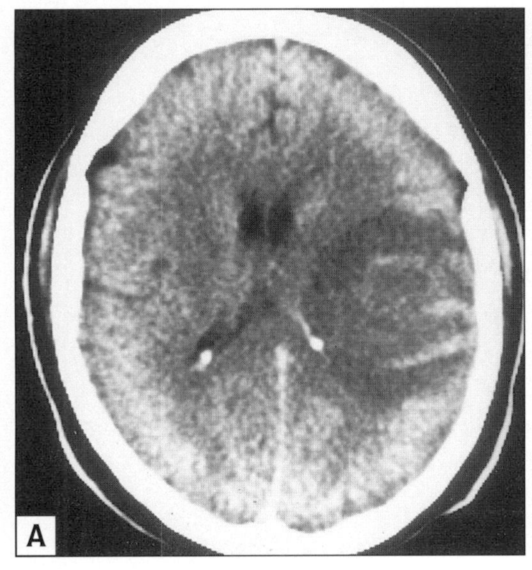

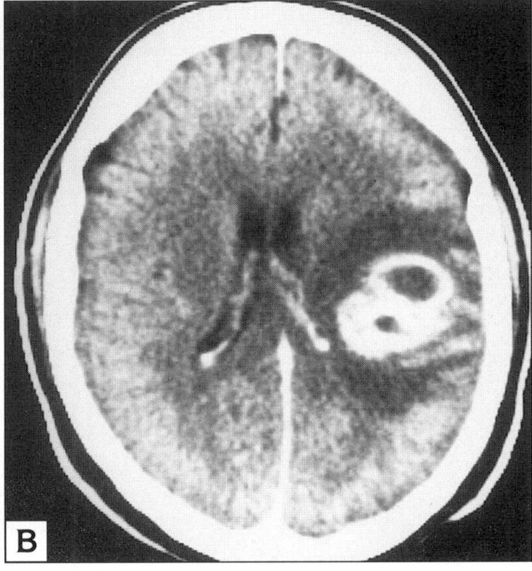

FIGURE 3-20 Unenhanced and enhanced axial CT scans. **A**, Unenhanced axial CT scan shows irregular areas of high and low attenuation producing effacement of the sylvian cistern and ipsilateral lateral ventricle on the left. **B**, After contrast enhancement, somewhat thick, irregular, ring-enhancing lesions with multiple loculi are seen to be surrounded by an area of decreased attenuation, indicating cerebral edema. (*From* Wispelwey *et al.* [12]; with permission.)

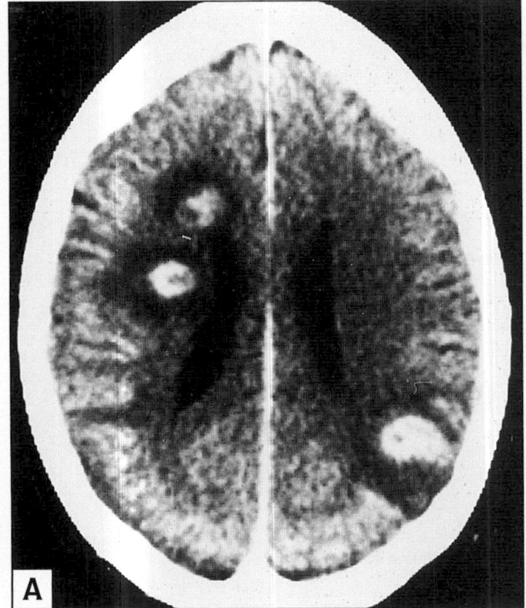

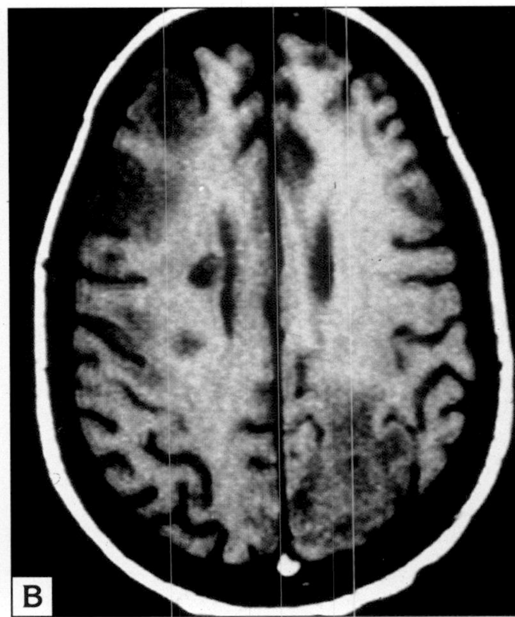

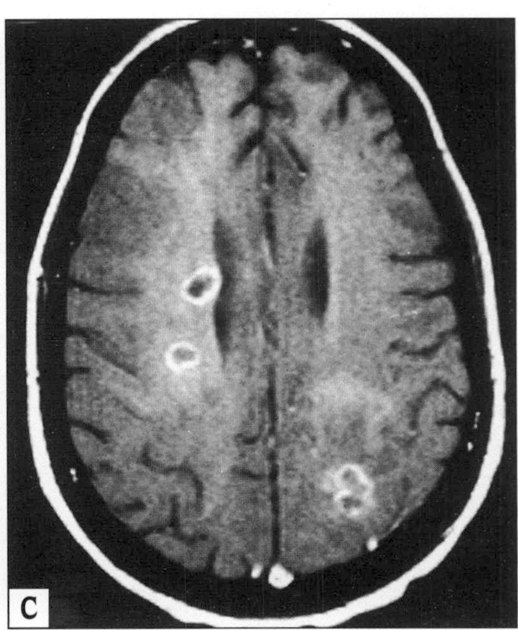

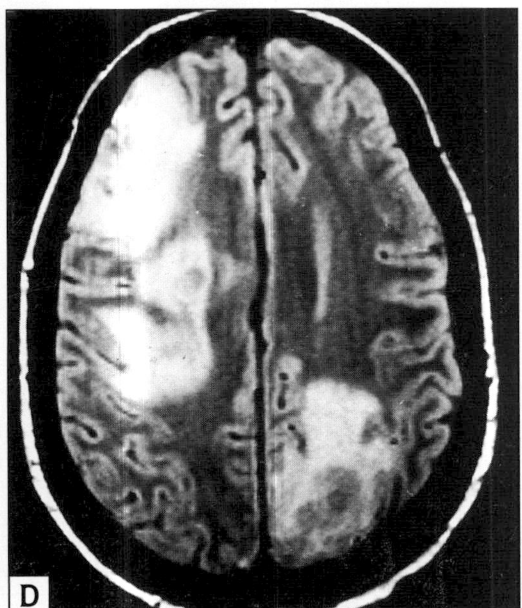

FIGURE 3-21 Cerebral toxoplasmosis in AIDS. **A**, An axial CT scan shows multiple areas of contrast enhancement in a patient with AIDS and cerebral toxoplasmosis. **B**, T1-weighted images show periventricular and gray-white junction lesions consistent with hematogenous dissemination. **C**, After gadolinium administration, contrast enhancement is seen on the T1-weighted image corresponding to that in *panel B*. **D**, Axial T2-weighted images show edema surrounding multiple cortical and subcortical lesions, further illustrating the increased information attainable by MRI relative to CT. (*From* Wispelwey *et al.* [12]; with permission.)

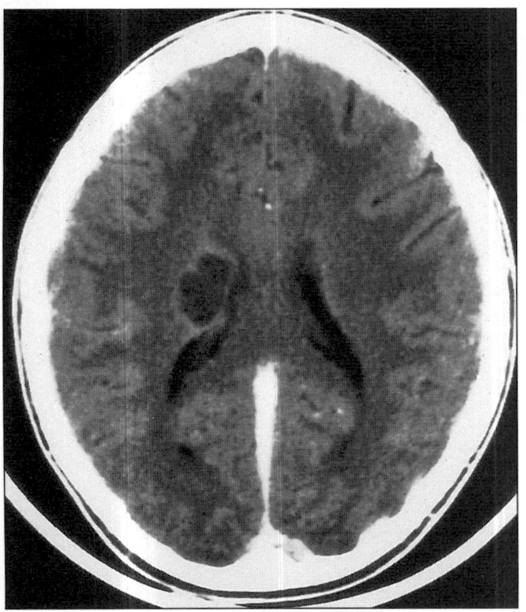

FIGURE 3-22 Cryptococcoma. A 15-year-old hemophiliac with AIDS and a fever of 2 weeks' duration developed a slowly progressive headache without focal findings. The enhanced CT scan revealed a large cystic-appearing periventricular mass with only minimal enhancement. Aspirate cultures revealed numerous budding yeast, and culture and antigen studies confirmed *Cryptococcus neoformans* as the etiologic agent. Cryptococcomas in the brain parenchyma are much less common than meningeal disease. Intraventricular cryptococcomas, as seen in this case, have been previously described and may originate in the choroid plexus. In AIDS patients, a ring-enhancing brain lesion, even in the setting of cryptococcal meningitis, could still represent a second etiologic agent such as toxoplasmosis.

Empiric antimicrobial therapy for brain abscess

Predisposing condition	Usual bacterial isolates	Antimicrobial regimen
Otitis media or mastoiditis	Streptococci (anaerobic or aerobic) *Bacteroides* spp. Enterobacteriaceae	Penicillin + metronidazole + third-generation cephalosporin
Sinusitis (frontoethmoidal or sphenoidal)	Streptococci *Bacteroides* spp. Enterobacteriaceae *Staphylococcus aureus* *Haemophilus* spp.	Vancomycin + metronidazole + third-generation cephalosporin
Dental sepsis	Mixed *Fusobacterium* *Bacteroides* spp. *Streptococcus* spp.	Penicillin + metronidazole
Penetrating trauma or postneurosurgical	*Staphylococcus aureus* Streptococci Enterobacteriaceae *Clostridium*	Vancomycin + third-generation cephalosporin
Congenital heart disease	Streptococci *Haemophilus* spp.	Penicillin + third-generation cephalosporin
Lung abscess, empyema, bronchiectasis	*Fusobacterium* *Actinomyces* *Bacteroides* spp. *Nocardia asteroides* Streptococci	Penicillin + metronidazole (+ trimethoprim-sulfamethoxazole)
Bacterial endocarditis	*Staphylococcus aureus* Streptococci	Vancomycin + gentamicin

FIGURE 3-23 Empiric antimicrobial therapy for brain abscess. When a diagnosis of brain abscess is made either presumptively by radiologic studies or by aspiration of the abscess, empiric antimicrobial therapy should be initiated based on knowledge of the likely etiologic agent associated with a given predisposing condition.

PARASITIC DISEASES OF THE NERVOUS SYSTEM

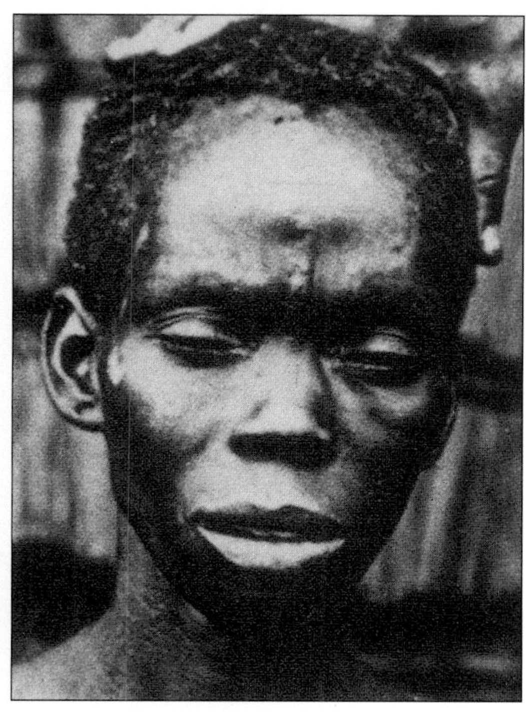

FIGURE 3-24 Characteristic facies of African trypanosomiasis. A stereotypic facial expression, characterized by somnolence and wasting, is seen with African trypanosomiasis in its advanced stages, which suggests the name sleeping sickness. (*From* Makerere Medical School Library; in Hutt and Wilks [13].)

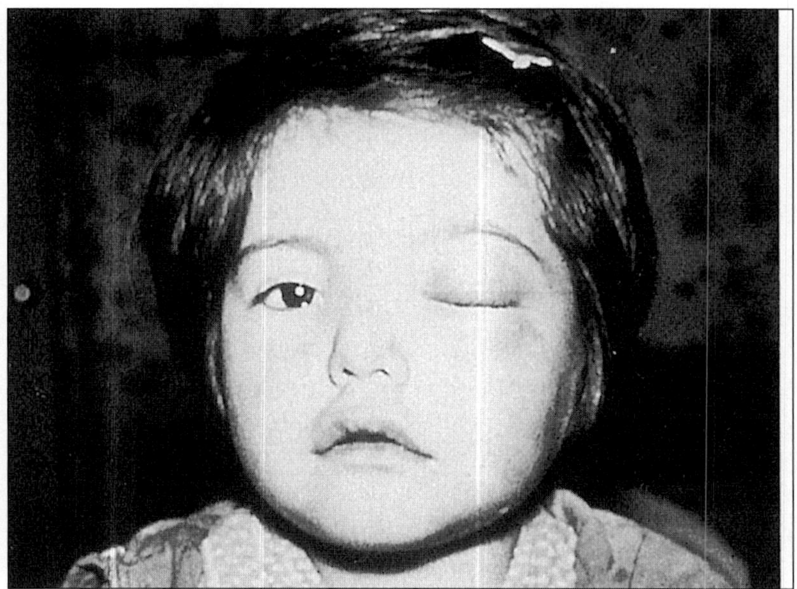

Figure 3-25 Romañna's sign in Chagas disease. Romañna's sign is a classic finding in acute Chagas disease and consists of unilateral painless edema of the palpebrae and periocular tissues that occurs when the conjunctiva is the portal of entry of the trypanosome. Malaise, fever, edema of face and lower extremities, generalized lymphadenopathy, and cardiac and gastrointestinal disorders subsequently appear. Meningoencephalitis is a rare complication. (*From* Moncayo [14]; with permission.)

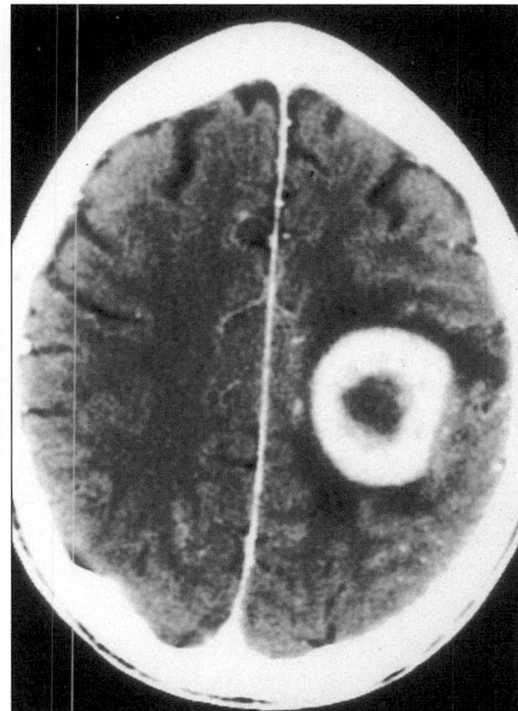

Figure 3-26 Computed tomographic (CT) scan of the brain in AIDS-related toxoplasmosis. The patient presented with right hemiparesis and a seizure disorder. CT scan with contrast shows the typical ring-enhancing lesion of toxoplasmosis. This ring enhancement, however, is not diagnostic and may be seen with tumors, abscesses, and vascular lesions.

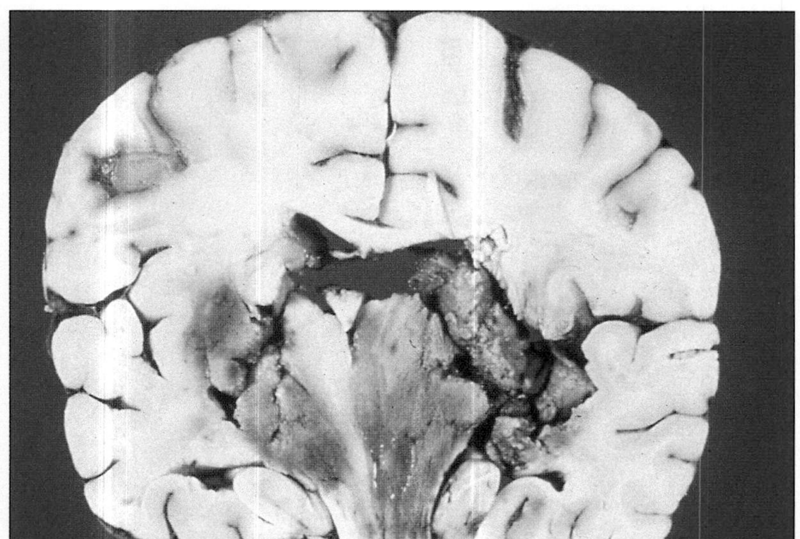

Figure 3-27 Gross brain specimen showing necrotic lesions of toxoplasma encephalitis. Lesions are present bilaterally in the basal ganglia and subcortically in the right frontal cortex.

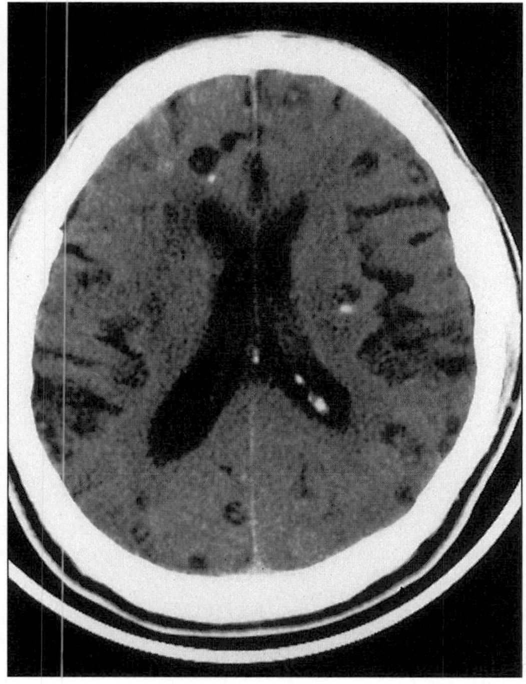

Figure 3-28 CT scan of the brain revealing multiple cysts within the parenchyma. The scolex of the cysticercus may be identified within many of these cysts, and calcification is observed as well. More than 50% of cases of neurocysticercosis are associated with calcification.

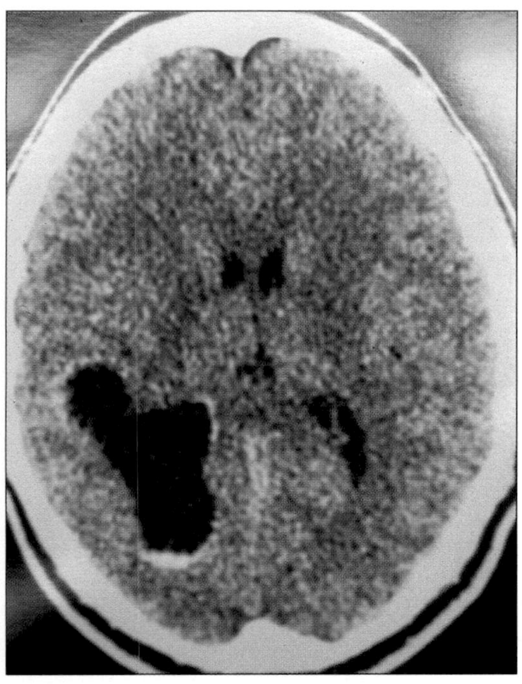

FIGURE 3-29 Intracranial hydatid cyst of echinococcosis. A CT scan of the brain shows a large cystic mass of the left temporoparietal region in a 40-year-old man from Honduras who presented with headache. At surgery, the cyst was inadvertently ruptured. Pathologic examination revealed hydatid disease. (*Courtesy of* Dr. Sara G. Austin, Houston, TX.)

EPIDURAL ABSCESS AND SUBDURAL EMPYEMA

Presenting signs and symptoms of intracranial subdural empyema and epidural abscess

Cranial subdural empyema	Cranial epidural abscess
Patient usually acutely ill at presentation:	Infection often an indolent course:
Fever	Headache
Headache	Fever
Depressed consciousness	Seizures
Hemiparesis	Focal neurologic signs
Seizures	Altered mental status
Malaise	
Gaze palsies/ataxia	
Nuchal rigidity	

FIGURE 3-30 Presenting signs and symptoms of intracranial subdural empyema and epidural abscess. Cranial subdural empyema and epidural abscess should be included in the differential diagnosis of any patient presenting with fever and focal neurologic deficits. Routine serologic testing rarely helps in diagnosing these disorders. Patients usually have a mild leukocytosis, but in some cases the total leukocyte count may be normal. Cerebrospinal fluid (CSF) may demonstrate signs of inflammation, including polymorphonuclear cells and elevated protein level. Particularly in cases of cranial epidural abscess, however, the CSF results may be normal. Blood and CSF cultures can assist in identifying the causative organism.

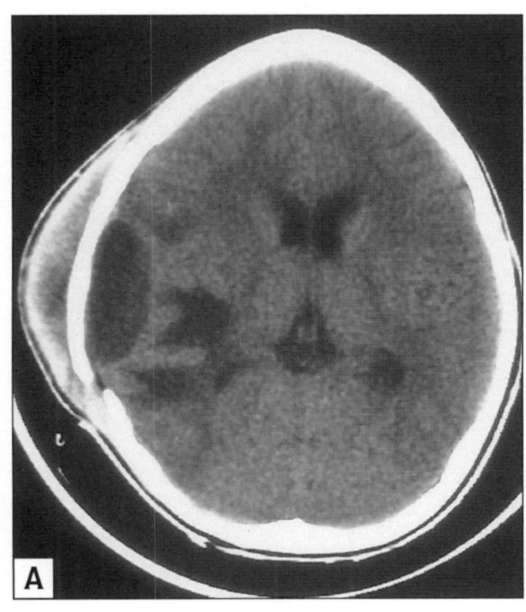

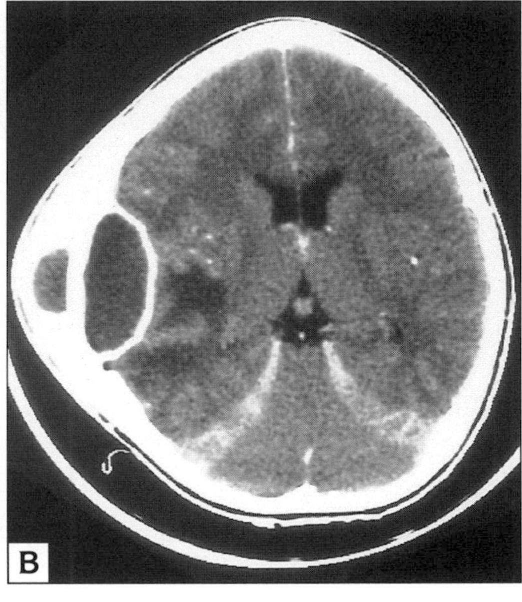

FIGURE 3-31 Typical computed tomographic (CT) appearance of an intracranial epidural abscess. This patient had an infected subgaleal hematoma which caused the epidural abscess. **A**, An uncontrasted CT scan shows a large, low-density mass with well-defined margins where the dura is being pulled away from the skull. There is prominent edema of the underlying cerebral hemisphere. **B**, The second CT with contrast demonstrates very intense contrast enhancement of the abscess rim. Note that the subgaleal abscess also enhances. Although CT scanning is usually adequate to diagnose an intracranial epidural abscess, some infections may be missed so magnetic resonance (MR) imaging should be considered if CT scanning is not diagnostic.

Clinical stages of spinal epidural abscess	
Stage I	Spinal ache usually at level of infection Possibly local edema, erythema, or percussion tenderness May last for weeks to months
Stage II	Radicular pain and paresthesias Progression over several days or < 1 day Headache, fever, and meningismus possible
Stage III	Impaired spinal cord function Urinary retention with progressive anesthesia and weakness May occur rapidly or over several days
Stage IV	Complete paralysis and anesthesia below the level of the abscess May develop within hours of the onset of Stage III

FIGURE 3-32 Clinical stages of spinal epidural abscess. The clinical features of spinal epidural abscess were first described in 1948 by Heusner and are still valid today. The rate of progression from stage I to stage IV varies dramatically between patients, and acute decompensation may occur over hours [15].

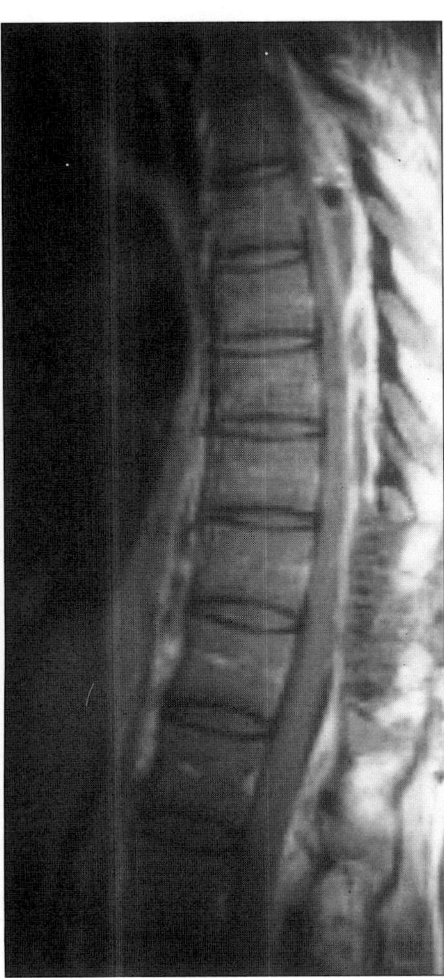

FIGURE 3-33 MR evaluation of spinal epidural abscess. A sagittal T1-weighted MR image after gadolinium-DTPA contrast administration demonstrates a large spinal epidural abscess in a patient who developed fever and back pain after a motor vehicle accident. There is an irregular enhancing septate lesion extending the length of the epidural space. The patient has already had a partial decompressive laminectomy from T9–11. MRI is becoming the preferred imaging study for spinal infections because of its high resolution, ability to image the entire length of the cord, ability to both localize infection and identify contiguous infections, and noninvasiveness [16].

Venous Sinus Infections

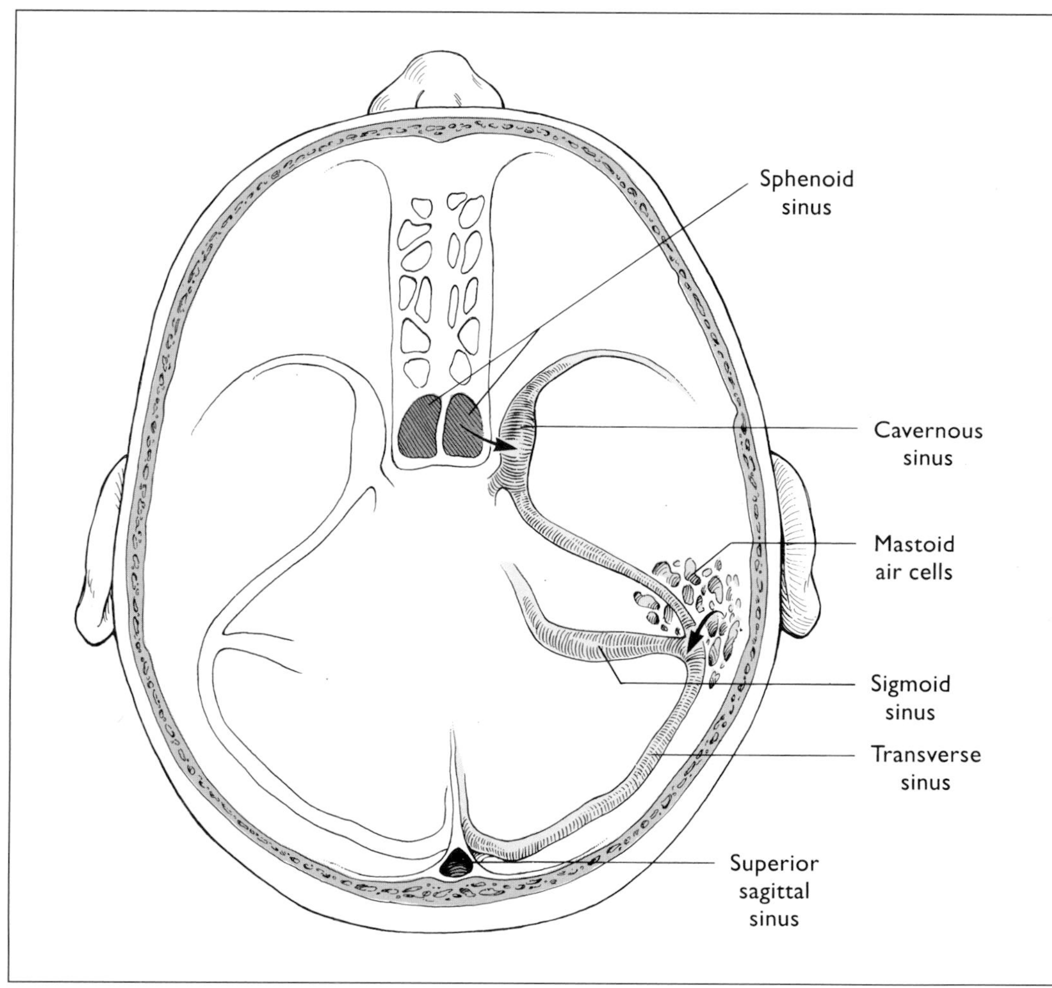

Figure 3-34 Dural venous sinuses. Septic thrombophlebitis may occur in any of the sinuses, but it is characteristically encountered in regions where the venous sinuses are in close proximity to air sinuses. Infectious processes within the air sinuses may extend to adjacent venous sinuses, either from direct involvement of the dura or by spread along emissary veins. As illustrated here, the cavernous sinus and sigmoid sinus are at risk for this type of direct extension.

Sigmoid sinus septic thrombosis: diagnosis

Risk factors	Signs
Otitis media	Infected middle ear
Mastoiditis	Postauricular swelling, tenderness
Symptoms	Obtundation
Headache	± Cranial nerve VI palsy
Ear pain	Papilledema
Ear drainage	Hemiparesis (rare)
Nausea/vomiting	
Fever	
Lethargy	

Figure 3-35 Sigmoid sinus septic thrombosis: diagnosis. Patients with sigmoid sinus septic thrombosis typically present with a history of partially treated ear infection and progressive headache, fever, and vomiting. Patients may be lethargic or obtunded due to elevated intracranial pressure. Focal neurologic findings (*eg*, hemiparesis) may also be present but raise the suspicion of a mass lesion, such as a brain abscess.

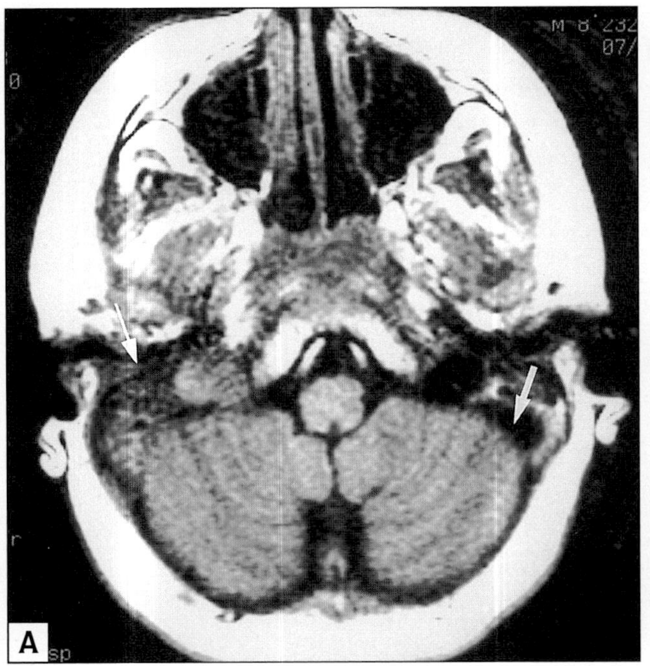

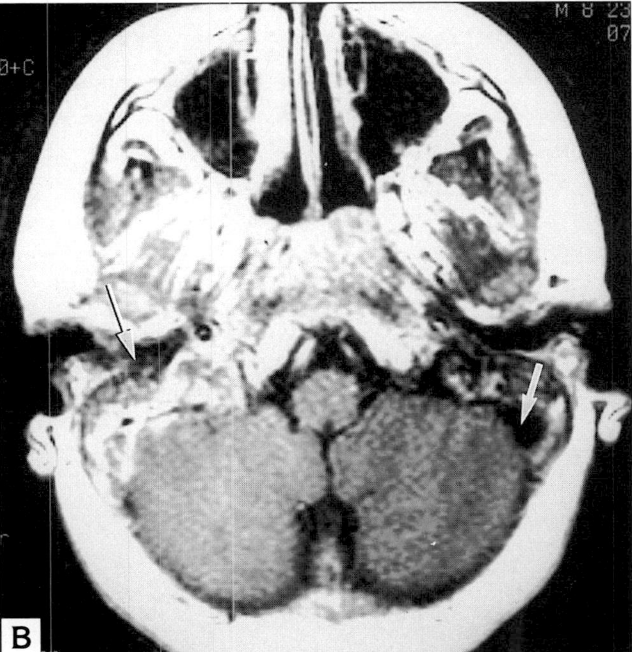

FIGURE 3-36 Mastoiditis and sigmoid sinus thrombosis in an 8-year-old boy with chronic otitis media. **A** and **B**, MRIs of the head before (*panel A*) and after (*panel B*) the administration of contrast. The inflammatory tissue within the right mastoid enhances brightly (*thin arrow*). The adjacent sigmoid sinus is occluded with inflammatory tissue and does not demonstrate the normal low signal seen in the sigmoid sinus on the other side (compare *thick arrow*).

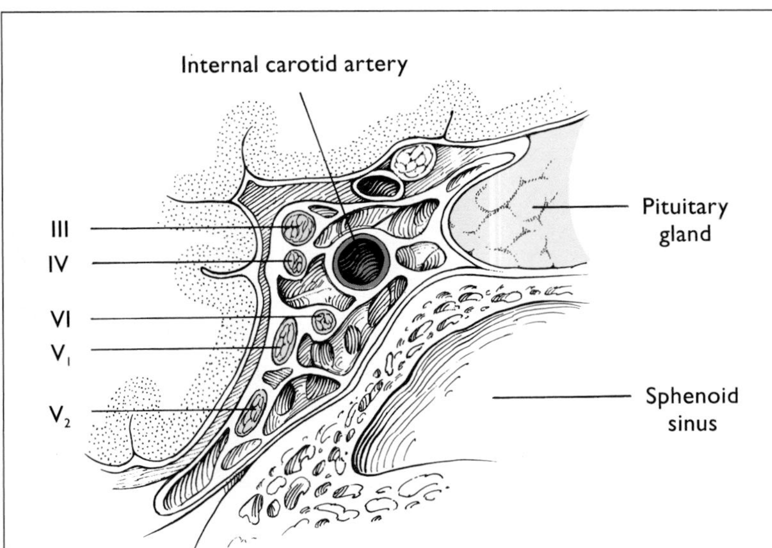

FIGURE 3-37 The cavernous sinus in cross-section. Infection and occlusion of this sinus may follow sphenoid sinusitis or septic thrombophlebitis of the orbital veins. The neurovascular structures within the cavernous sinus may be involved in the inflammatory process, resulting in a number of clinical signs and symptoms. Spread of the inflammation into the internal carotid artery may lead to narrowing or occlusion of the artery, an event which may result in a cerebral infarction. Cranial nerves III, IV, and VI are frequently involved in cavernous sinus thrombophlebitis, resulting in varying degrees of ocular motility deficits. Symptoms of involvement of cranial nerves V_1 and V_2 (*ie*, facial numbness or pain) are possible but are not frequently observed.

Cavernous sinus septic thrombosis: diagnosis

Risk factors	Signs
Paranasal sinusitis	Periorbital edema
Facial infection	Chemosis
Dental infection	Papillitis
	Oculomotor palsies
Symptoms	Proptosis
Headache	± Facial sensory changes
Facial pain	
Vision loss	
Fever	
Double vision	

FIGURE 3-38 Cavernous sinus septic thrombosis: diagnosis. Patients with cavernous sinus septic thrombosis typically present with headache, fever, and diplopia. A history of paranasal sinus infection may be obtained but is not necessary. Ophthalmoplegia and proptosis are often seen on examination.

Infections of the Skull and Bony Sinuses

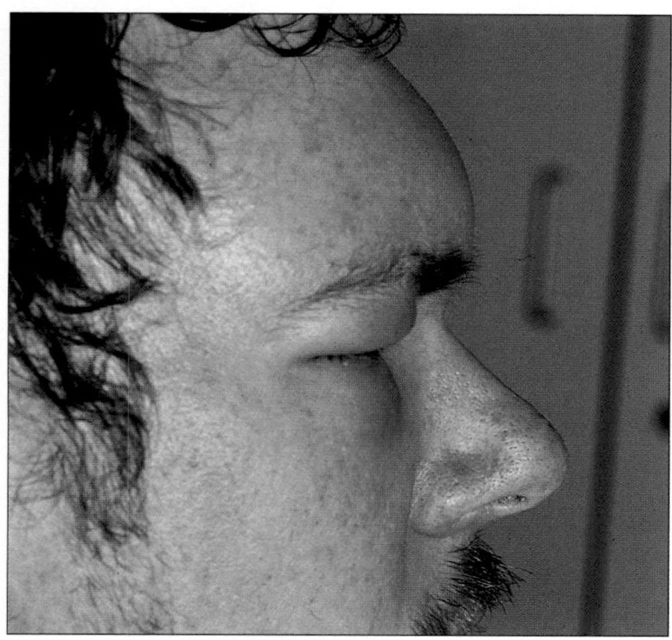

Figure 3-39 Osteomyelitis of the frontal bone. Side view of the patient shows marked edema of the periorbita and doughy swelling of the forehead.

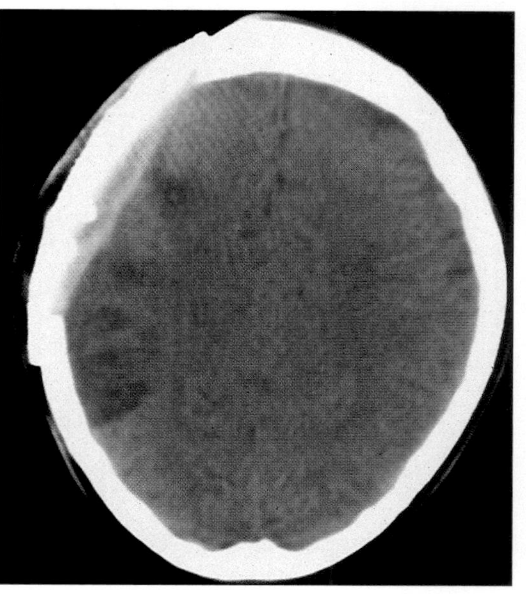

Figure 3-40 Cranial computed tomographic (CT) scan (axial section with bone window setting) revealing epidural empyema at the site of a previous cranioplasty with prosthetic material. Previous craniotomy was performed in this 23-year-old patient because of brain infarction with mass effect. (*Courtesy* of Dr. C. Hamburger.)

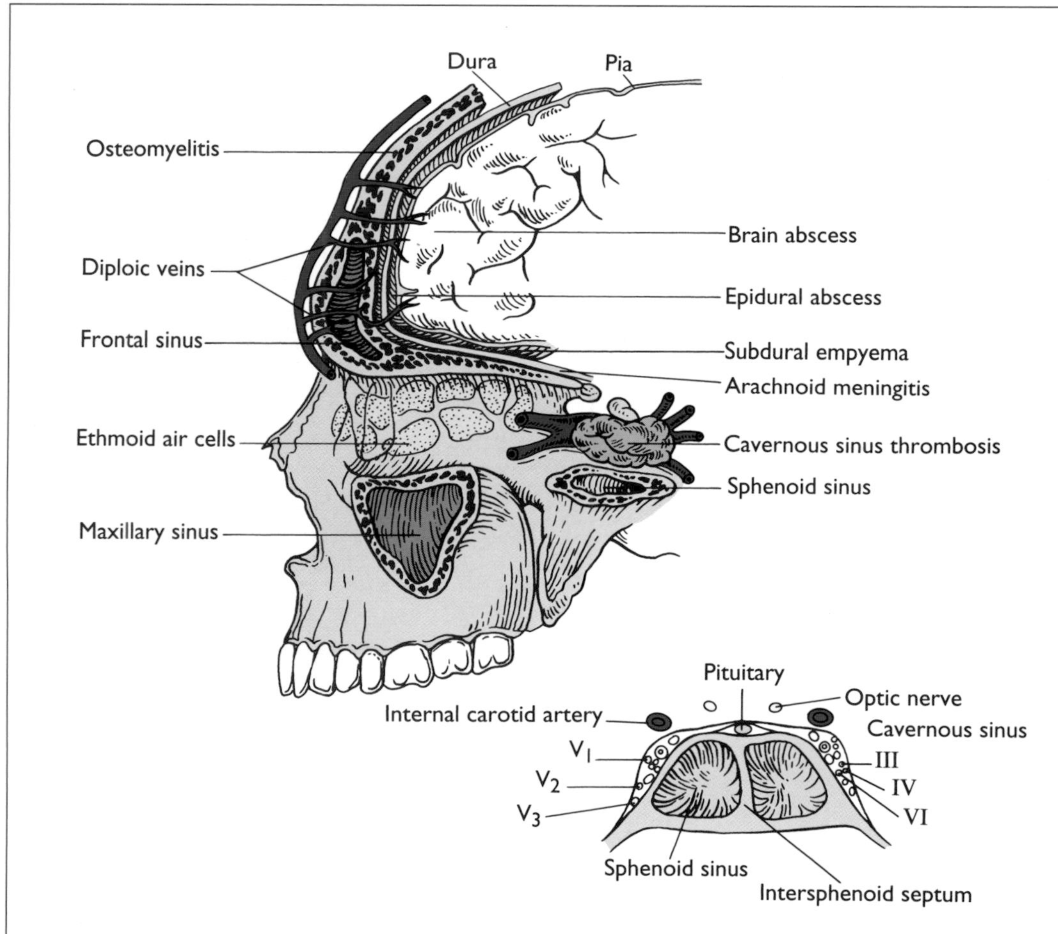

Figure 3-41 Intracranial complications of sinusitis. The sagittal section shows the major routes for intracranial extension of infection, either directly or via the vascular supply. Note the proximity of the diploic veins to the frontal sinus and of the cavernous sinuses to the sphenoid sinus. The coronal section (*inset*) demonstrates the structures adjoining the sphenoid sinus. (*From* Vortel and Chow [17].)

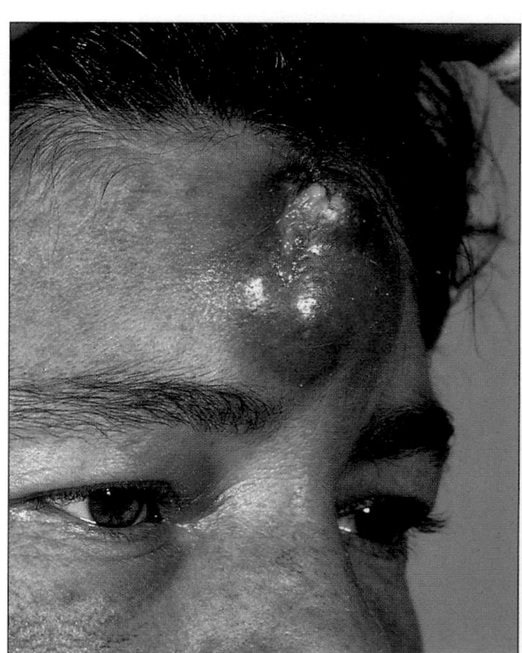

Figure 3-42 Mucopyocele of the frontal sinus with perforation. Preoperative view.

The Nervous System in Sepsis and Endocarditis

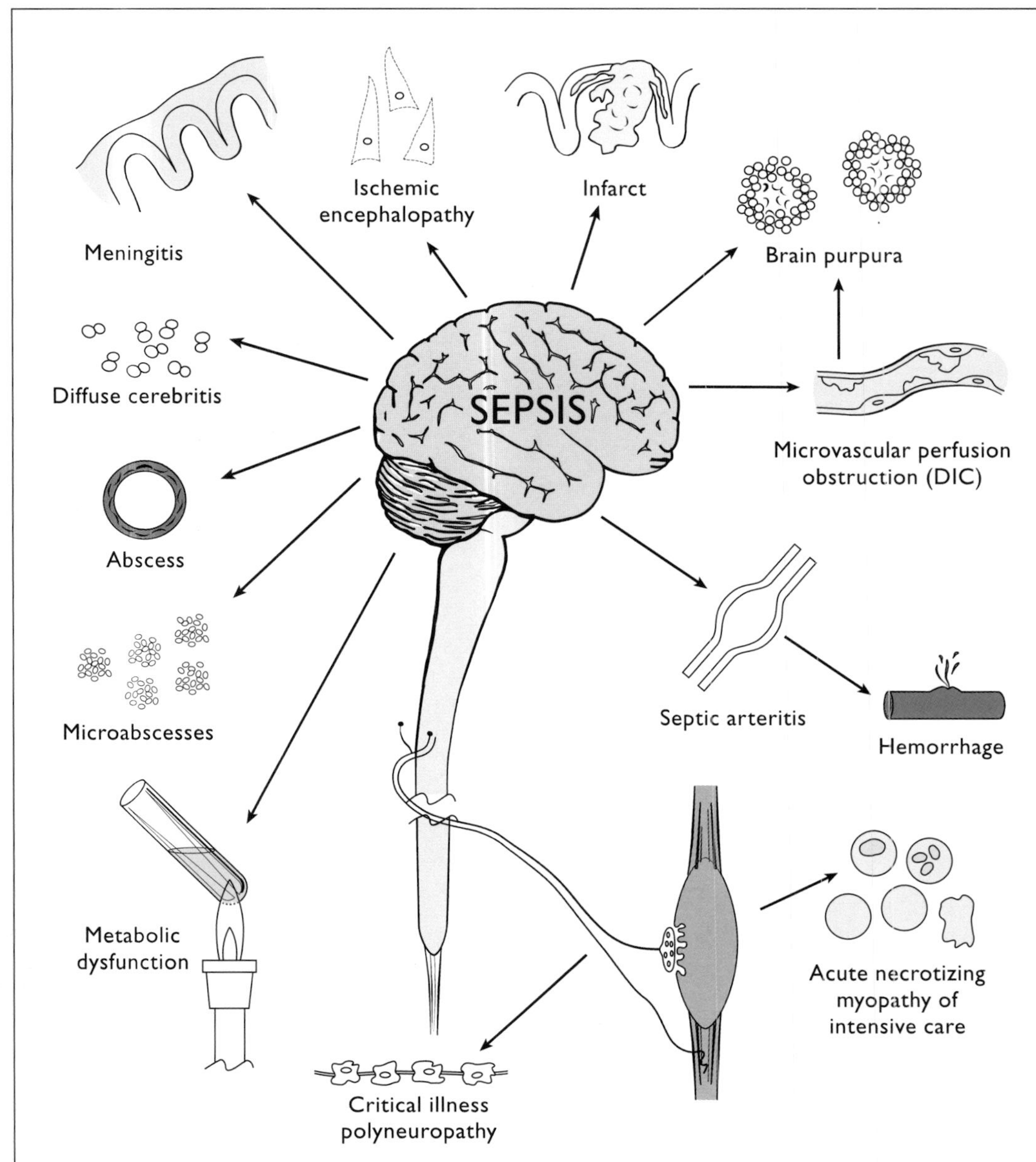

Figure 3-43 The effects of sepsis on the nervous system. *Sepsis* is a term that implies the presence of microorganisms or their toxins in the blood or tissues of the body *and* a systemic response or effect on at least one organ system. It must be emphasized that the otherwise helpful localizing signs and symptoms that characterize some of these disorders are masked in critically ill, often comatose, septic patients, who are, owing to their attachment to ventilators, monitors, and various lines, difficult to assess neurologically. Accordingly, extensive investigation, including electroencephalography, neuroimaging, and cerebrospinal fluid and blood analysis, is usually necessary to identify which of these often diffuse or multifocal complications of sepsis are present. DIC—disseminated intravascular coagulation [18–21].

Cerebrovascular complications of sepsis and their underlying causes

Process	Basis
Diffuse	
Vascular encephalopathy	Cardiorespiratory arrest (ischemic encephalomyelopathy)
	Microperfusion defects owing to DIC
	Microvasculitis (associated with cerebral microabscesses)
Focal	
Watershed region infarcts	Hypotension
Cerebral infarcts	Intravascular thrombosis on atheromatous plaque
	Embolus, atheromatous or fibrin-platelet
	Infective vasculitis with secondary arterial occlusion
Venous infarct	Venous sinus thrombosis
Intracerebral hemorrhage and microhemorrhage	Altered coagulation mechanisms, iatrogenic or secondary to sepsis
	Rupture of infected vessel

Figure 3-44 Cerebrovascular complications of sepsis and their underlying causes. The cerebrovascular complications of sepsis may be classified as diffuse or focal. Their bases or pathophysiologic mechanisms are noted.

Causes of impaired consciousness and fever

CNS infections
- Meningitis (bacterial, fungal, viral, or protozoal)
- Encephalitis
- Brain abscess (esp. multiple)
- Epidural or subdural empyema

Systemic inflammation
- Sepsis
- SIRS without infection (*eg*, following burns, trauma, or pancreatitis)
- Pneumonia
- Hepatitis
- Malaria

Drug related
- Aspirin poisoning
- Acute porphyria (esp. with seizures)
- Neuroleptic malignant syndrome
- Malignant hyperthermia
- Anticholinesterase toxicity
- Severe withdrawal syndromes (drugs or alcohol)
- Cocaine toxicity

Other intracranial events
- Severe head injury
- Infarction in hypothalamus or brainstem
- Status epilepticus (convulsive or, rarely, nonconvulsive)
- Sarcoid or tumor infiltration of hypothalamus

Endocrine and metabolic disturbances
- Thyroid storm
- Acute adrenal insufficiency (addisonian crisis)
- Acute porphyria
- Carcinoid syndrome

Other systemic illnesses (esp. if brain involved)
- Systemic malignancies (carcinoma of lung, pancreas, or liver or lymphomas)
- Hematologic disorders (sickle cell crisis)
- Autoimmune disorders (SLE, serum sickness)

Pulmonary embolism

Myocardial infarction (with failure)

Heatstroke or heat exhaustion

Figure 3-45 Causes of impaired consciousness and fever. A large number of conditions may cause impaired consciousness and fever; these should be excluded before making a diagnosis of sepsis-associated encephalopathy. SIRS—systemic inflammatory response syndrome; SLE—systemic lupus erythematosus.

Neurologic syndromes in patients with infective endocarditis

Syndrome (main clinical presentation)	Mechanisms
Stroke (hemiplegia, aphasia)	Emboli with bland or hemorrhagic infarction Intracranial hemorrhage due to mycotic aneurysm and necrotizing arteritis Brain abscess
Meningitis (meningitis ± focal signs)	Multiple causes: microabscesses Bacterial seeding of the meninges Brain abscess
"Toxic" encephalopathy (decreased level of consciousness)	Microemboli, microabscesses, cerebritis, CNS hypertension, drug toxicity, metabolic disturbances, vasculitis, other organic CNS complications
Psychiatric abnormalities (behavioral disorders, esp. in elderly patients)	Same as "toxic" encephalopathy Reactive to conditions surrounding the diagnosis of infective endocarditis
Seizures (focal or generalized)	Any of the underlying CNS lesions Drug toxicity, metabolic imbalance, hypoxia
Brain stem (nausea, vomiting, hiccup, dyskinesia, tremor)	Emboli in the vertebrobasillar territory
Cranial nerves (visual disturbances, disorders of eye movements, palsies, sensory impairment)	Emboli, space-occupying lesions
Spinal cord and peripheral disorders (para- or tetraplegia, mononeuropathy)	Emboli, metastatic abscesses, immune injury
Severe headache (severe, often localized)	Mycotic aneurysms or other CNS lesions
Subarachnoid hemorrhage (meningismus ± decreased consciousness)	Infectious arteritis with or without detectable mycotic aneurysm

Figure 3-46 Neurologic syndromes in patients with infective endocarditis. Several complications may occur simultaneously in a single patient, or complications may occur sequentially over the course of the illness. Also, there is often considerable variability and fluctuation in the severity of the illness. (*From* Francioli [22].)

Ocular and Orbital Infections

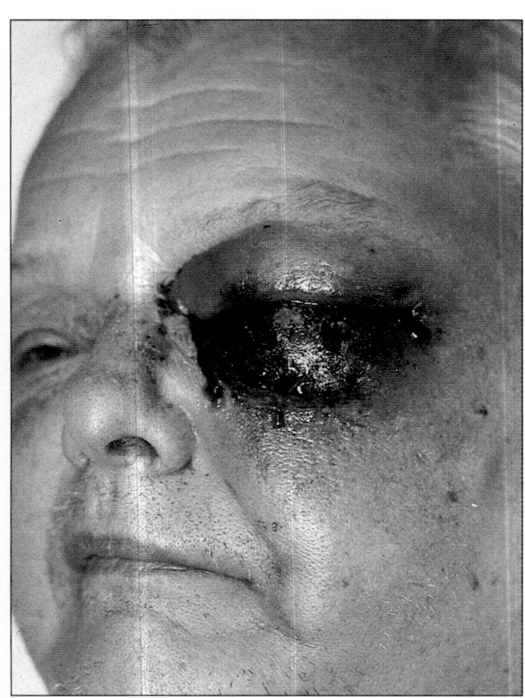

Figure 3-47 Preseptal cellulitis in an elderly man. This can be differentiated from orbital cellulitis by the intense preseptal inflammatory reaction, the cellulitis extending over the entire face, and extension onto the contralateral eyelids. In the presence of any recent skin injury, *Staphylococcus aureus* is a common causative organism. In the absence of any recent wound, the list of possible causative organisms is similar to that in acute sinusitis (*Haemophilus influenzae*, pneumococcus, *Streptococcus* spp., and *S. aureus*).

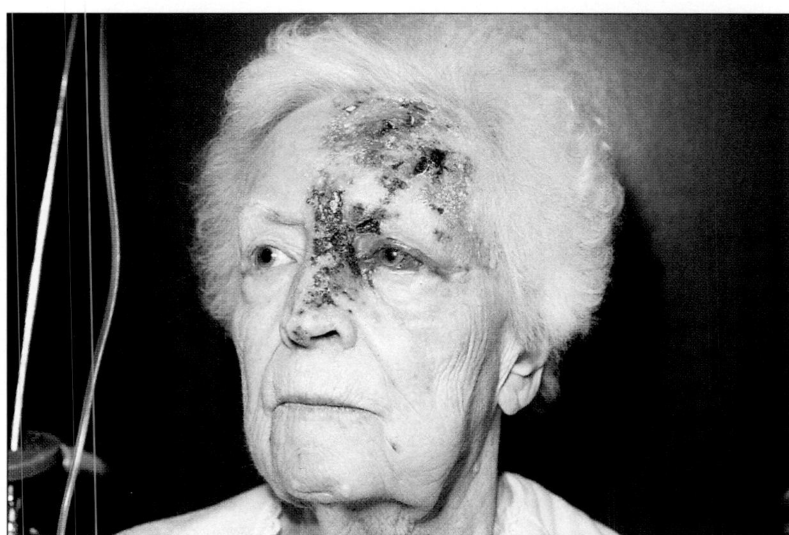

Figure 3-48 Acute herpes zoster ophthalmicus. An elderly woman presented with tingling and subsequent pain on the left side of her forehead. She developed vesicular lesions over the distribution of the ophthalmic branch of the trigeminal nerve. The involvement of the tip of her nose (Hutchinson's sign) suggests involvement of the nasociliary nerve, a nerve that also supplies the cornea. In this case, the cornea has become inflamed, the eye is red, and there is a danger that glaucoma will develop. Patients with acute herpes zoster ophthalmicus should be treated with acyclovir, 800 mg five times a day for 5 days, beginning within 72 hours of the onset of symptoms; this reduces the incidence of ocular involvement, but it does not alter the course of postherpetic neuralgia.

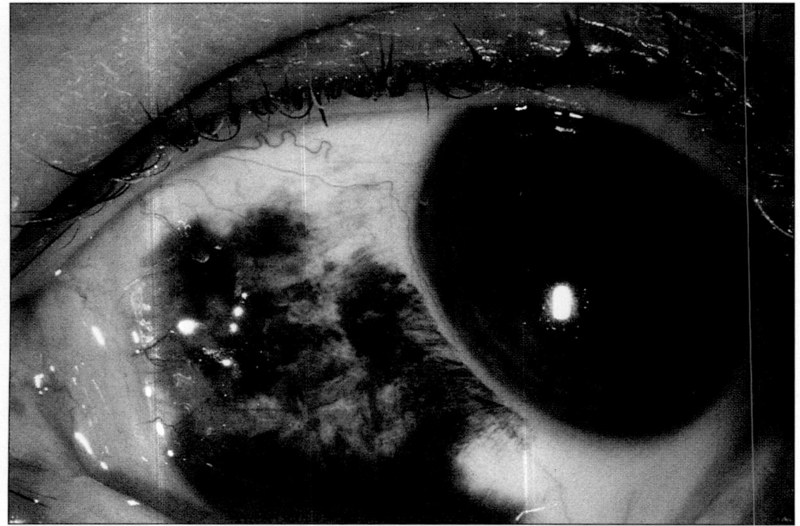

Figure 3-49 Subconjunctival hemorrhage. This focal area of redness contrasts with the diffuse erythema associated with conjunctivitis. This lesion is caused by a broken blood vessel, is self-limiting, and will resolve spontaneously within 10 days.

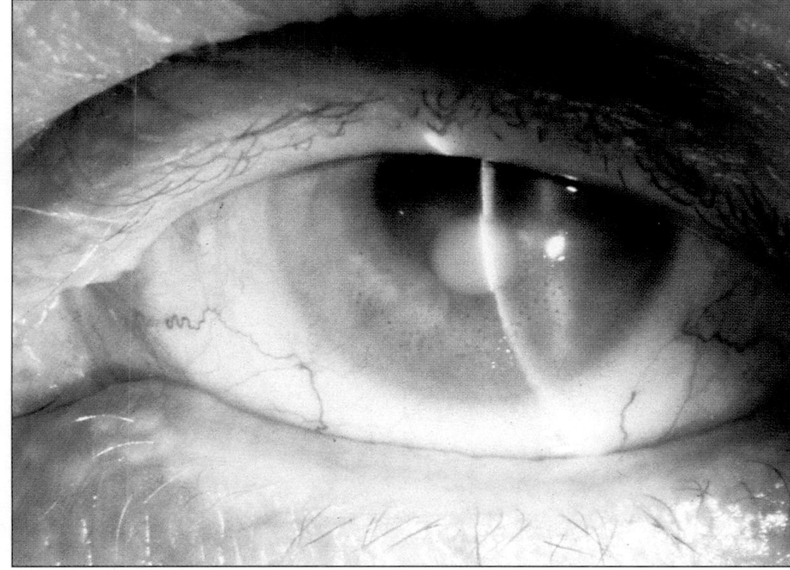

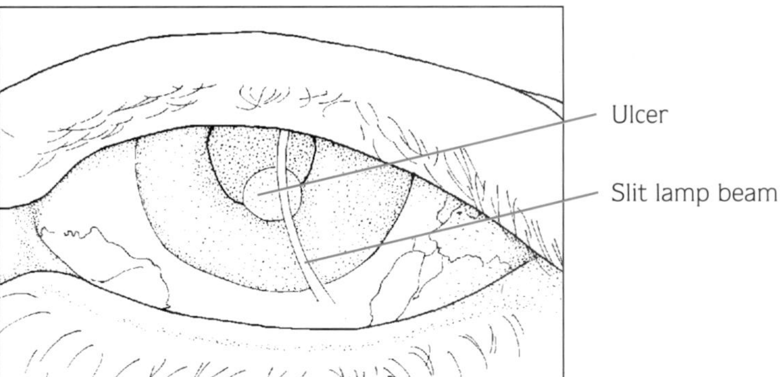

Figure 3-50 Bacterial corneal ulcer under a soft contact lens. The patient had been wearing extended-wear contact lenses for 2 weeks between cleanings. She developed an acute onset of irritation of this eye and was found to have a deep infiltrate of the cornea. The most common organism in this setting is *Pseudomonas* and, when present, can lead to rapid perforation of the cornea and permanent loss of vision.

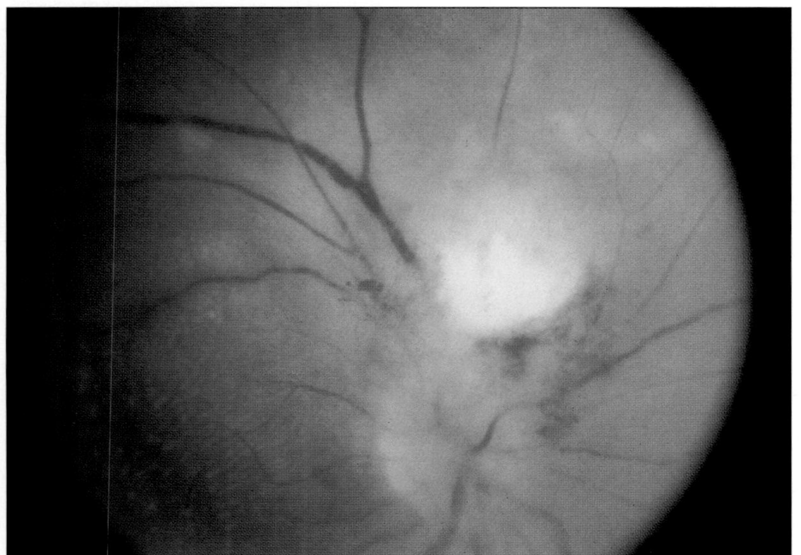

Figure 3-51 Acute acquired toxoplasmosis. A middle-aged woman developed acute toxoplasmic retinochoroiditis in the area of the optic nerve following a systemic toxoplasmosis infection. This finding is unusual in immunocompetent patients but has been seen increasingly in patients who are immunocompromised either iatrogenically or because of an underlying condition. Note the hemorrhagic and necrotic appearance of the retina, which is markedly edematous surrounding the area of infection.

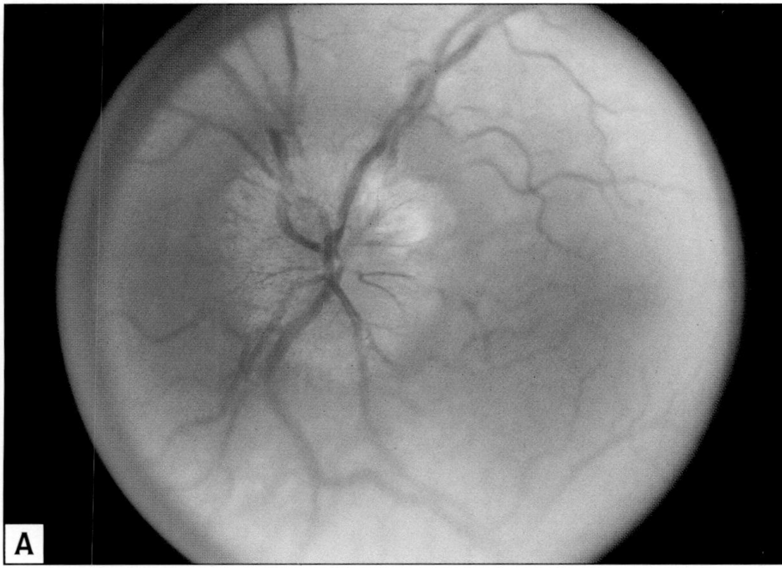

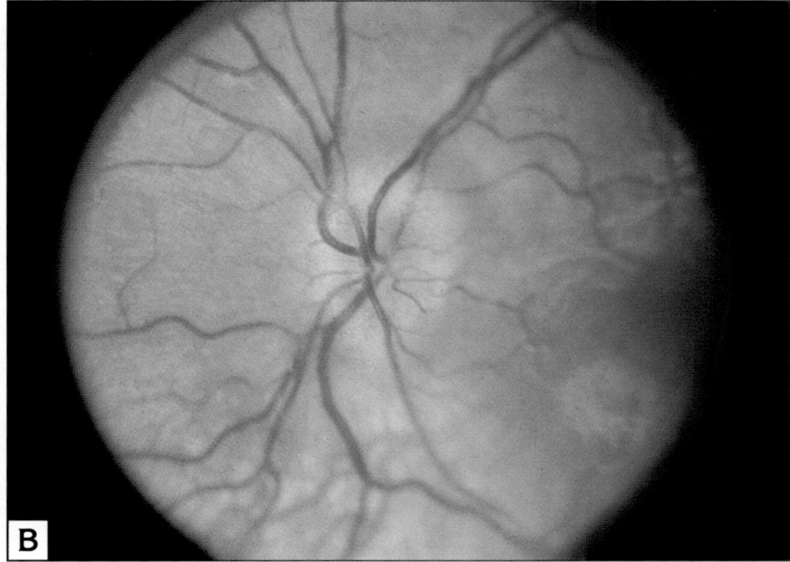

Figure 3-52 Papilledema. This patient had acute elevation of her intracranial pressure secondary to an abscess. **A**, Note that the margins of the optic nerve are blurred, there is hyperemia, and there is edema of the surrounding retina. Papilledema appears to result from pressure on the nerve axons with resultant back-up of axoplasmic flow. **B**, Three weeks following drainage of the abscess, the edema of the optic nerve has markedly abated. There remains some gliosis of surrounding tissue, but the peripapillary retina has flattened. The term *papilledema* is reserved for optic nerve swelling that is associated with elevated intracranial pressure.

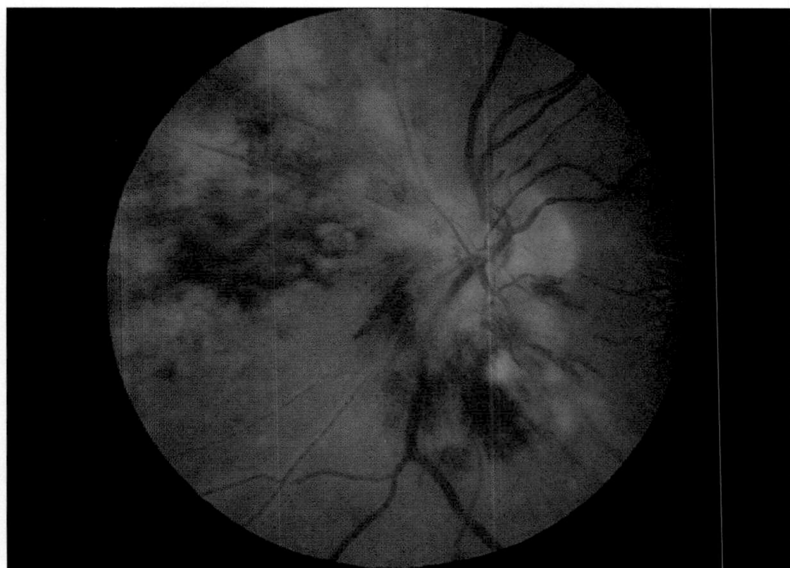

FIGURE 3-53 Cytomegalovirus (CMV) retinitis. This is the acute appearance of CMV retinitis affecting the posterior fundus. There is necrosis and hemorrhage of the retina and CMV optic neuritis. Following treatment with intravenous ganciclovir, the lesions lost their acute appearance and the edema subsided. However, the retinal tissue which was involved in the inflammation never recovered nor did the patient's central vision.

PRION DISEASES

Prion diseases

Disease	Host
Scrapie	Sheep, goats
Transmissible mink encephalopathy	Mink
Chronic wasting syndrome	Mule, deer, elk
Bovine spongiform encephalopathy	Cattle
Feline spongiform encephalopathy	Cats
Kuru	Humans
Jakob-Creutzfeldt disease	Humans
Gerstmann-Sträussler syndrome	Humans
Fatal familial insomnia	Humans

FIGURE 3-54 Prion diseases. In 1982, Prusiner proposed the name *prion*, *pro*teinaceous *in*fectious particle, to describe the agent responsible for a group of chronic, progressive, neurodegenerative disorders that share similar pathologic features and are caused by an inherited and transmissible agent with unconventional biologic properties. These rare disorders affect both humans and animals.

Characteristics of prion diseases

Diseases are mostly confined to the CNS
Prolonged incubation period of months to decades
Progressive clinical course of weeks to years leading to death
All diseases exhibit reactive astrocytosis with little inflammatory response and many show neuronal vacuolation
Infectious agents (prions) show properties distinguishing them from viruses, viroids, and other infectious agents

FIGURE 3-55 Characteristics of prion diseases. The prion diseases are heterogeneous human and animal diseases grouped together because they share certain features. The diseases have extended incubation times that can exceed 30 years before the onset of clinical disease. The central nervous system (CNS) receives the brunt of injury, with pathologic features of neuronal loss, reactive gliosis, and neuronal vacuolation (spongiform change). (*Adapted from* Prusiner and Hsaio [23].)

Clinical characteristics of Jakob-Creutzfeldt disease	
Transmission	Sporadic, familial, iatrogenic
Prevalence	Worldwide
Onset	57–62 yrs usually (range, 17–83)
Clinical features	Severe rapidly progressive dementia Myoclonus and movement disturbances Cerebellar dysfunction Visual disturbances
Course	Fatal in < 1 yr after onset
CSF findings	Typically normal
CT/MRI	Normal to generalized cortical atrophy
EEG	Periodic sharp wave complexes lasting 200–600 ms every 0.5–2.5 s (in 75%–95% of patients)

FIGURE 3-56 Clinical characteristics of Jakob-Creutzfeldt disease (JCD). JCD remains a rare disease, with a prevalence of approximately 1 case/million population worldwide, but it is the most commonly encountered of the human prion diseases. The overwhelming majority of cases (85%–95%) are sporadic. Familial transmission accounts for 5% to 15% of cases. Iatrogenic person-to-person spread is extremely rare and has followed transplantation of infected corneas or dural grafts, use of contaminated neurosurgical instruments, and use of contaminated growth hormone or pituitary gonadotropin. Dementia and myoclonus are the most prominent findings, but the clinical manifestations are highly variable, depending in part on the area of brain affected. One variant, the Heidenhain variant, has a predilection for the occipital and parietal lobes and may present with visual problems (hallucinations, hemianopia, and cortical blindness) before dementia becomes apparent.

Clinical characteristics of Gerstmann-Sträussler syndrome	
Transmission	Hereditary (autosomal diminant)
Onset	43–48 yrs (range, 24–66 yrs)
Clinical features	Progressive spinocerebellar degeneration Unsteadiness, clumsiness, incoordination, gait disturbances (early) Ataxia, dysarthrias, tremor, nystagmus (late) Dementia (late or minor) Myoclonus absent (or minor)
Course	Fatal in approx 5 yrs

FIGURE 3-57 Clinical characteristics of Gerstmann-Sträussler syndrome (GSS). GSS is an exceedingly rare disease, with an incidence of 1 to 10 cases/100 million population/year. Most cases are familial, with an autosomal dominant pattern of inheritance and virtually complete penetrance. Approximately two dozen independent kindreds have been identified worldwide. The onset typically is in midlife, with prominent cerebellar features and absent or late dementia.

REFERENCES

1. Roos KL, Tunkel AR, Scheld WM: Acute bacterial meningitis in children and adults. *In* Scheld WM, Whitley RJ, Durack DT (eds.): *Infections of the Central Nervous System*. New York: Raven Press; 1991:335–410.
2. Tucker T, Ellner JJ: Chronic meningitis. *In* Scheld WM, Whitely RJ, Durack DT (eds.): *Infections of the Central Nervous System*. New York: Raven Press; 1991:704.
3. Reik L Jr: Lyme disease. *In* Scheld WM, Whitely RJ, Durack DT (eds.): *Infections of the Central Nervous System*. New York: Raven Press; 1991:668.
4. Reik L Jr: Lyme disease. *In* Scheld WM, Whitley RS, Durack DT (eds.): *Infections of the Central Nervous System*. New York: Raven Press; 1991:681.
5. Zuger A, Lowy FD: Tuberculosis of the central nervous system. *In* Scheld WM, Whitely RJ, Durack DT (eds.): *Infections of the Central Nervous System*. New York: Raven Press; 1991:424–455.
6. Tunkel AR, Scheld WM: Central nervous system infections in the compromised host. *In* Rubin RH, Young LS (eds.): *Clinical Approach to Infection in the Compromised Host*, 3rd ed. New York: Plenum; 1994:187.
7. *Infectious Diseases: Text and Color Atlas*, 2nd ed. by WE Farrar, MJ Wood, JA Innes, H Tubbs. Gower Medical Publishing: an imprint of Times Mirror International Publishers Ltd., London, UK, 1992.
8. Griffin DE: Encephalitis, myelitis, and neuritis. *In* Mandell GL, Bennett JE, Dolin R (eds.): *Principles and Practice of Infectious Diseases*, 4th ed. New York: Churchill Livingstone; 1995:877.
9. Whitley RJ, *et al.*: Herpes simplex encephalitis: clinical assessment. *JAMA* 1982, 247:317–320.
10. Price RW, Brew BJ, Roke M: Central and peripheral nervous system complications of HIV-1 infections and AIDS. *In* DeVita VT Jr, Hellman S, Rosenberg SA, *et al.* (eds.): *AIDS: Etiology, Diagnosis, Treatment, and Prevention*. Philadelphia: J.B. Lippincott; 1992:237–254.
11. McArthur JC: Neurologic complications of human immunodeficiency virus infection. *In* Gorbach SL, Bartlett JG, Blacklow NR (eds.): *Infectious Diseases*. Philadelphia: W.B. Saunders; 1992:956–972.
12. Wispelwey B, Dacey R Jr, Scheld WM: Brain abscess. *In* Scheld WM, Durack D, Whitley R (eds.): *Infections of the Central Nervous System*. New York: Raven Press; 1991.
13. Hutt MRS, Wilks NE: African trypanosomiasis (sleeping sickness). *In* Macial-Rojas RA (ed.): *Pathology of Protozoal and Helminthic Diseases*. Huntington, NY: Robert E. Kreiger; 1975:57–68.
14. Moncayo A: Chagas disease. In *Tropical Disease Research: Progress 1991–1992 [11th Programme Report of the UNDP/World Bank/WHO Special Programme for Research and Training in Tropical Diseases]*. Geneva: World Health Organization; 1993:67.

15. Heusner AP: Nontuberculous spinal epidural infections. *N Engl J Med* 1948, 239:845–854.
16. Post MJD, Sze G, Quencer RM, *et al.*: Gadolinium-enhanced MR in spinal infection. *J Comput Assist Tomogr* 1990, 14:721–725.
17. Vortel JJ, Chow AW: Infections of the sinuses and parameningeal structures. *In* Gorbach SL, Bartlett JG, Blacklow NR (eds.): *Infectious Diseaes.* Philadelphia: W.B. Saunders; 1992:432.
18. Barton R, Cerra FB: The hypermetabolism–multiple organ failure syndrome. *Chest* 1989, 115:136–140.
19. Bone RC: Sepsis syndrome: New insights into its pathogenesis and treatment. *Intensive Care World* 1992, 4:50–59.
20. Nava E, Palmer RMF, Moncada S: Inhibition of nitric oxide synthesis in septic shock: How much is beneficial? *Lancet* 1991, 338:1557–1558.
21. Sprung C, Cerra FB, Freund HR, *et al.*: Plasma amino acids as predictors of the severity and outcome of sepsis. *Crit Care Med* 1991, 19:753–757.
22. Francioli P: Central nervous system complications of infective endocarditis. *In* Scheld WM, Whitley RJ, Durack DT (eds.): *Infections of the Central Nervous System.* New York: Raven Press; 1991:529.
23. Prusiner SB, Hsaio KK: Prions causing transmissible neurodegenerative diseases. *In* Schlossberg D (ed.): *Infections of the Nervous System.* New York: Springer-Verlag; 1990:153–168.

Chapter 4

Upper Respiratory and Head and Neck Infections

Editor
Itzhak Brook

Contributors

Stephen G. Baum
James N. Endicott
Theodore W. Fetter
Marlin E. Gher, Jr
Kenneth M. Grundfast
Rande H. Lazar
Andrew M. Margileth
Moses Nussbaum
George Quintero
Janet Seper
Harris R. Stutman
Debra A. Tristram
Ellen R. Wald
Ayal Willner

EYE AND ORBIT INFECTIONS

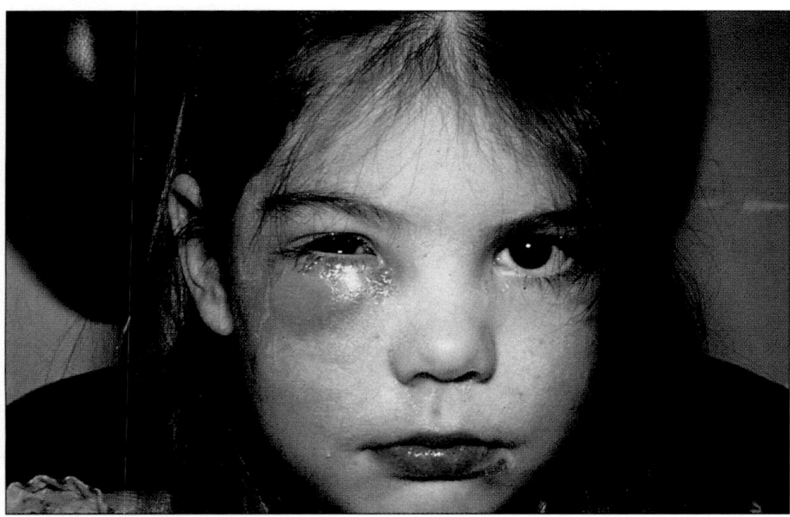

FIGURE 4-1 Dacryocystitis. This child had an upper respiratory tract infection for 3–4 days and then developed fever and an erythematous area beneath the medial canthus. This area is indurated, warm to touch, and exquisitely tender. This is an example of dacryocystitis, a bacterial infection of the lacrimal sac and duct. These infections are rare, although they can occur at any age as a complication of a viral upper respiratory tract infection.

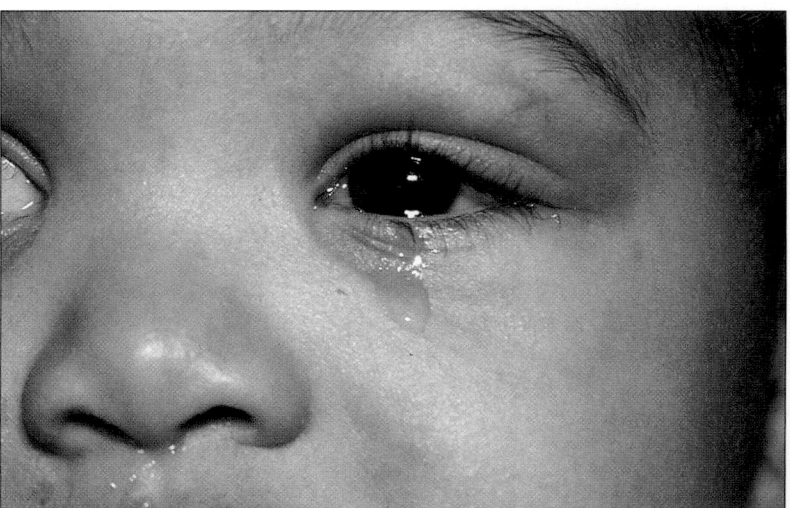

FIGURE 4-2 Dacryoadenitis. A 2-year-old girl, who had a viral upper respiratory tract infection for the preceding 5 days, developed swelling and erythema above the lateral portion of her upper lid. The swelling was painless and occurred during the fourth day of amoxicillin therapy, which was prescribed for the treatment of a right-sided otitis media. No additional treatment was instituted. The swelling resolved spontaneously over the next 2 days. This child had dacryoadenitis, or inflammation of the lacrimal gland. The location of the swelling, above the lateral portion of the upper lid, is the key to the diagnosis.

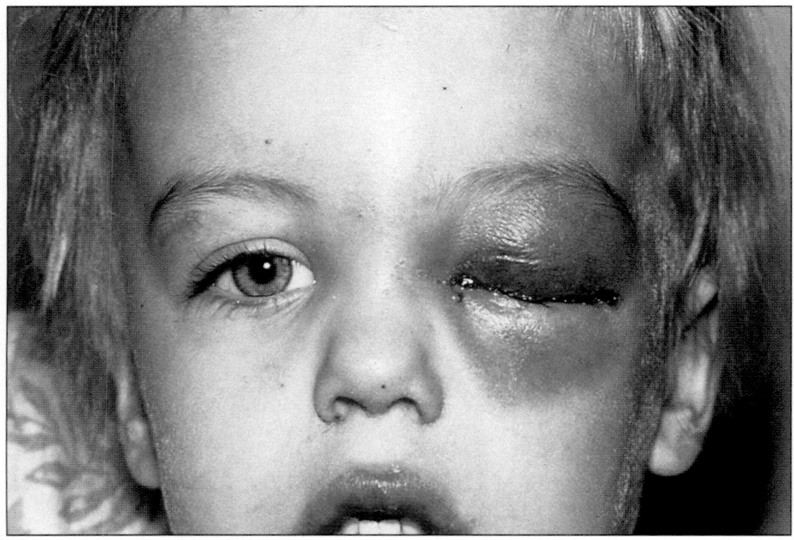

FIGURE 4-3 Streptococcal bacterial cellulitis secondary to orbital trauma. A 2-year-old boy had nasal discharge, nasal congestion, and low-grade fever for about 10 days. The morning before presentation, he fell and sustained a 7-mm laceration just lateral to his left eye. Despite careful cleansing of the area, he developed dramatic periorbital swelling and erythema over the next 24–36 hours. His 9-year-old brother had had a "strep" throat the preceding week. Group A streptococcus was recovered from the culture of the wound. Bacterial cellulitis secondary to trauma is usually due to *Staphylococcus aureus* or *Streptococcus pyogenes* (group A streptococcus). Parenteral therapy was initiated with good response.

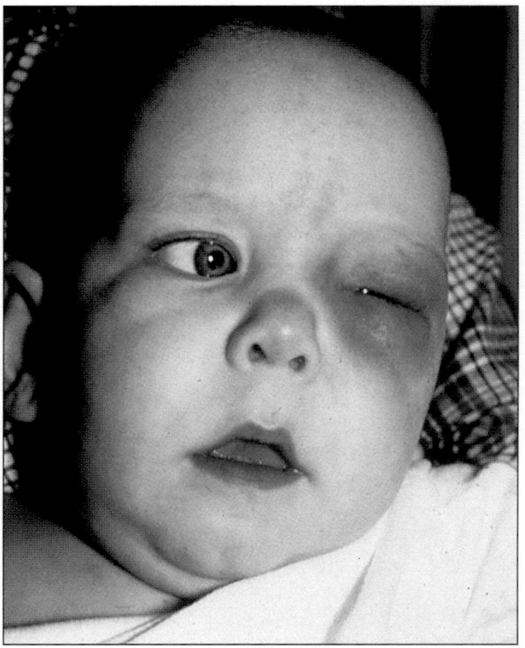

FIGURE 4-4 *Haemophilus influenzae* type b bacteremic cellulitis. A 9-month-old boy had an upper respiratory tract infection for 3 days. On the morning of admission, he had a temperature of 40° C (104° F) and a small erythematous area under the medial portion of the lower lid. Within 6 hours, the erythema and swelling progressed to involve both upper and lower lids. The area was nontender. Eversion of the lids showed the globe to be normally placed with intact extraocular movements. The blood culture was positive for *H. influenzae* type b. Parenteral antibiotics were initiated and resolution was prompt. Within 24 hours, the erythema had receded partially, and the eye was approximately 25% open. In 48 hours, the eye was nearly completely open, and the cutaneous findings had resolved.

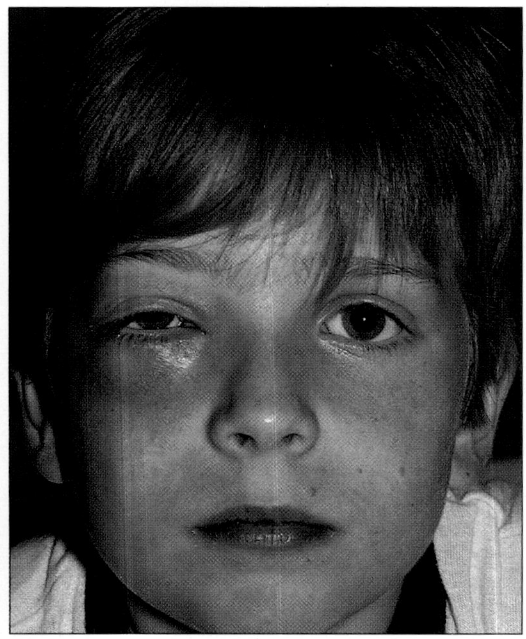

FIGURE 4-5 Inflammatory edema. A 10-year-old boy had an upper respiratory tract infection for several days with clear nasal discharge and daytime cough. The onset of eye swelling prompted a visit to his pediatrician. The globe was normally placed, and extraocular eye movements were within normal limits. The periorbital area was puffy but neither tender nor indurated. A computed tomography (CT) scan showed that the primary site of infection was the ethmoid sinus. Within the bony orbit, the muscle and globe of the eye were normal. All the swelling was in the eyelid. Accordingly, this is a case of preseptal cellulitis.

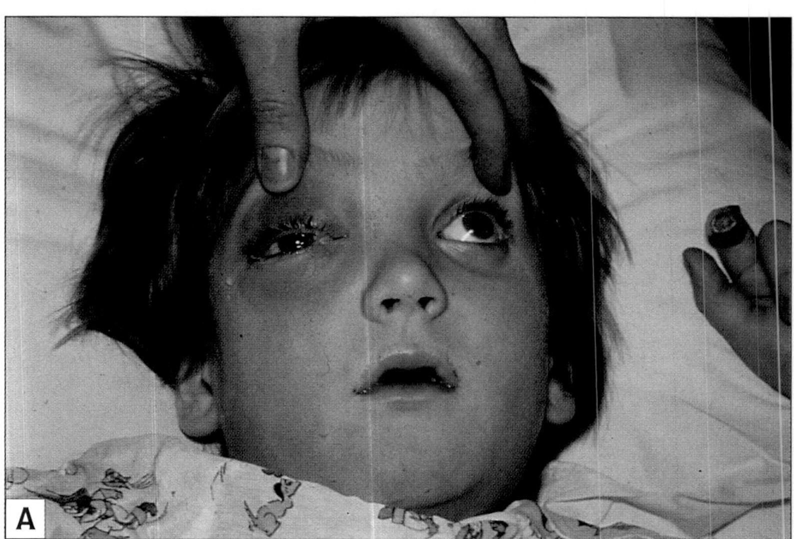

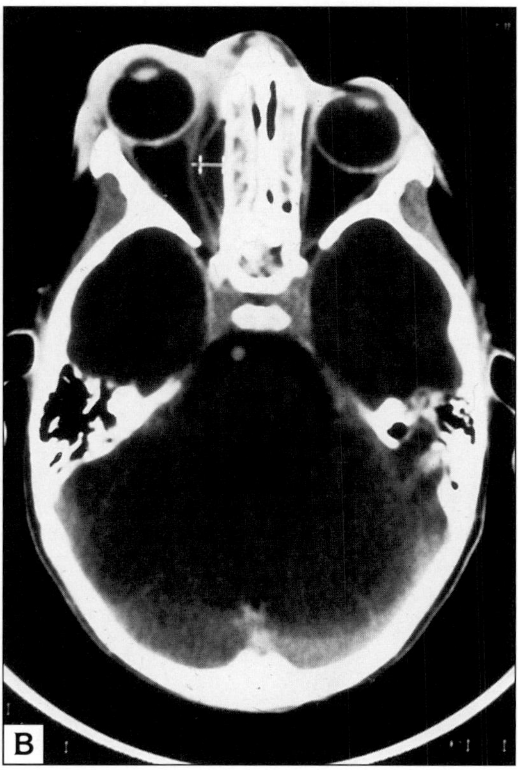

FIGURE 4-6 Subperiosteal abscess. A 6-year-old boy had an upper respiratory tract infection for 5 days. He had been complaining of eye discomfort and headache behind his eye for 12 hours. On physical examination, he was afebrile. His eyelid was swollen and could not be opened spontaneously. When his lids were everted manually, the globe of his right eye was anteriorly displaced (proptotic). **A.** When he is moving his eyes up, there is an impairment of upward gaze. The remaining extraocular eye movements were within normal limits. The hallmark of a true orbital infection is 1) displacement of the globe, 2) impairment of extraocular eye movements, or 3) loss of visual acuity. **B**, Computed tomography (CT) scan shows that the ethmoid sinus is completely opacified. There is a subperiosteal abscess consequent to osteitis of the lateral wall of the ethmoid sinus (lamina papyracea), as evident in the coronal planes (*panel B*). This finding mandates surgical exploration and drainage of the abscess and the sinuses as well. In the axial view (not shown) there was a bilateral maxillary involvement: complete opacification on the right and mucosal thickening on the left. High-dose parenteral antibiotics are indicated. Culture of the subperiosteal abscess grew *Streptococcus pneumoniae*. (Panel B *from* Wald [1]; with permission.)

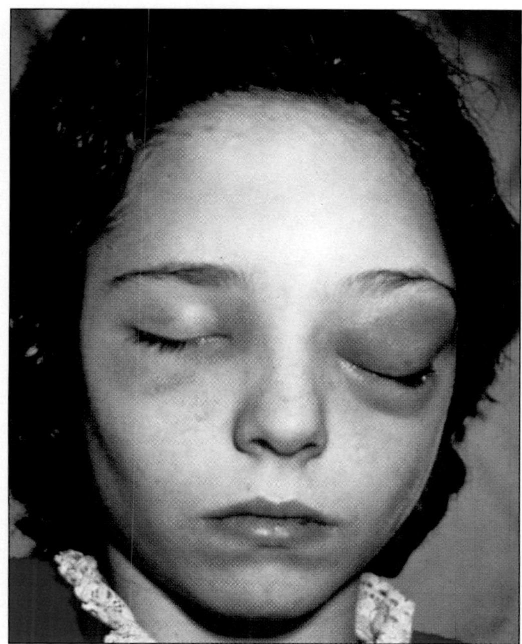

FIGURE 4-7 Subperiosteal abscess. A 14-year-old girl had a 1-week history of nasal congestion, cough, and low-grade fever. She developed a frontal headache, bilateral eye pain, and erythema first around the left eye and then around the right for 2 days before visiting her physician. Her left eye appeared to be bulging. On physical examination, there was modest proptosis of her left globe with limitation of upward gaze of her left eye. A computed tomography scan showed a possible accumulation of pus between the left medial rectus and the left ethmoid sinus. Because the abscess was not well defined, high-dose parenteral therapy was initiated. She did very well, and surgery was not required. (*Courtesy of* R. Moriarity, MD.)

OTITIS MEDIA AND INFECTIONS OF THE INNER EAR

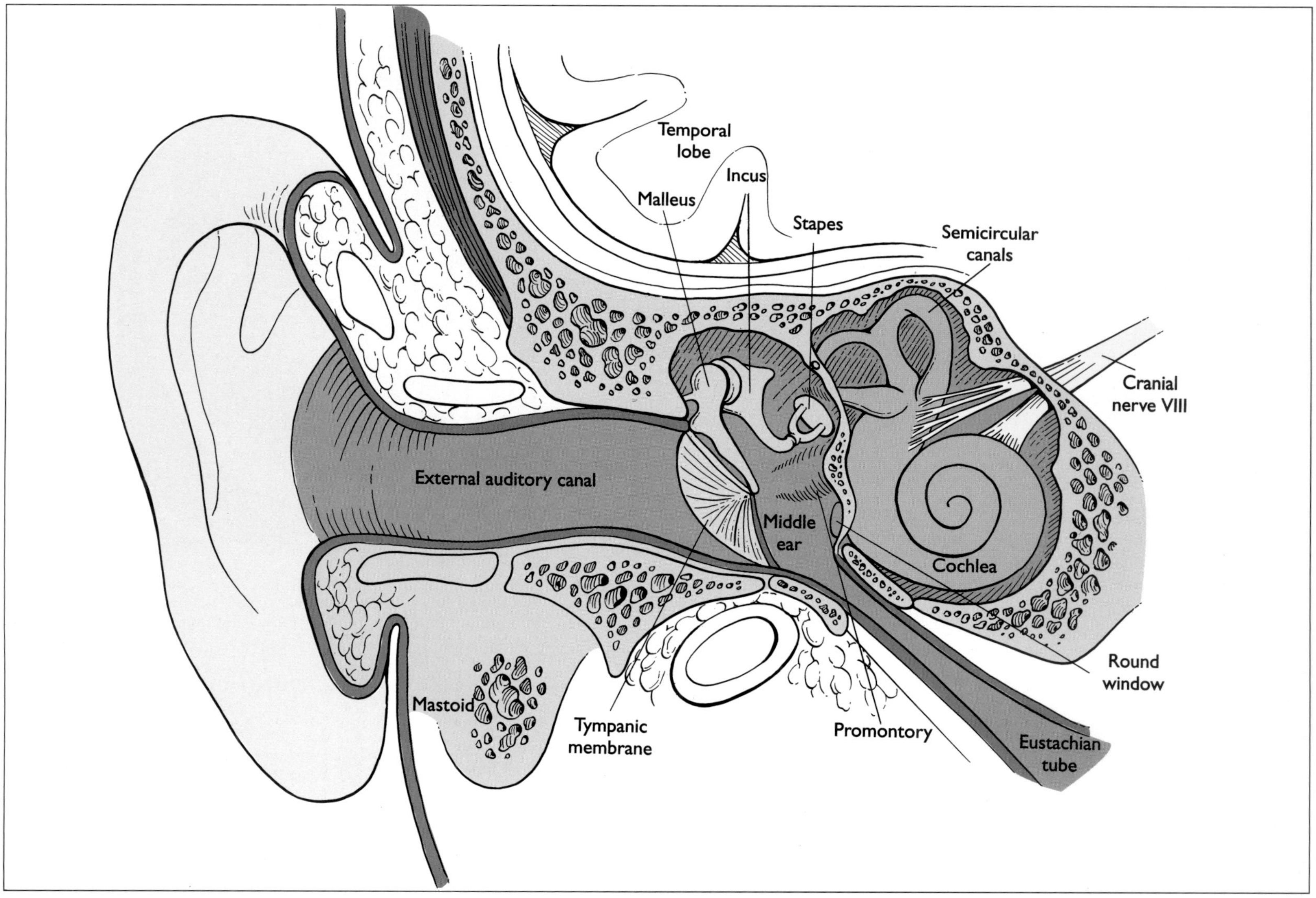

FIGURE 4-8 Normal cross-sectional anatomy of the ear. The external, middle, and inner ear comprise a compact group of components situated in the temporal bone. Sound is funneled by the pinna into the external auditory canal, where it causes vibration of the tympanic membrane. Attached to the tympanic membrane is the malleus, which, with the incus, increases sound pressure by 30%. The stapes articulates with the long process of the incus, and the stapes footplate acts as a piston to transfer the sound vibrations to the cochlea, where the vibratory stimuli are transformed to nerve impulses. The inner ear also houses the semicircular canals, which, via a portion of the eighth cranial nerve, give dynamic and static information on the motion and position of the head.

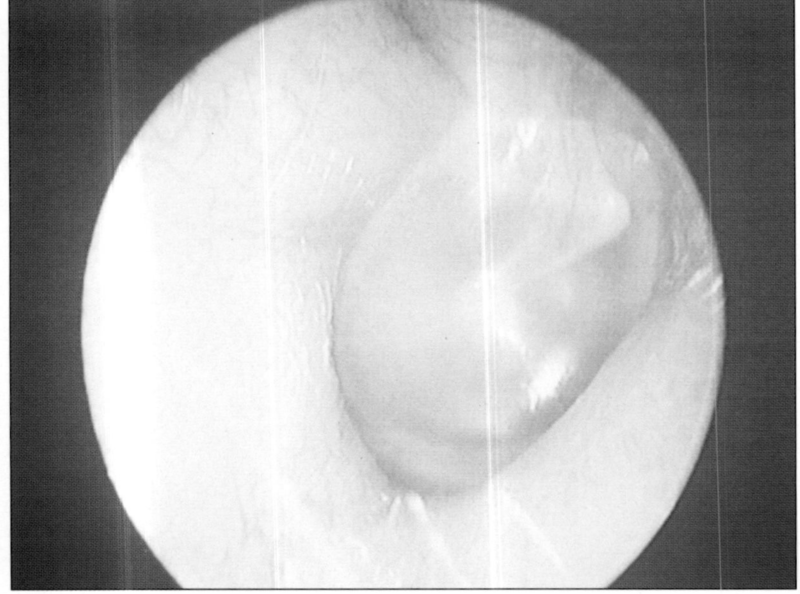

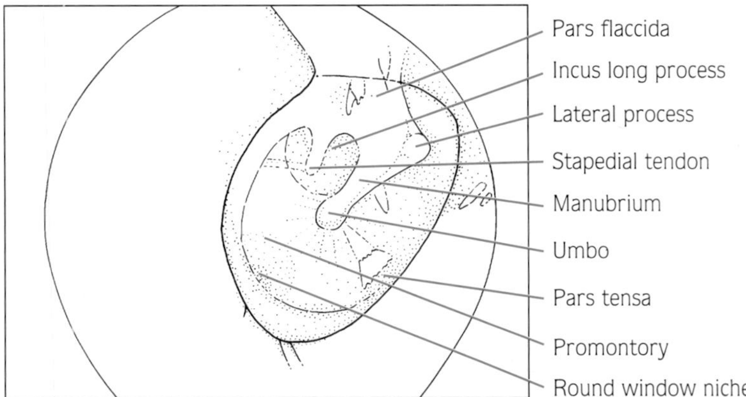

FIGURE 4-9 Normal eardrum (tympanic membrane). The normal eardrum, as viewed with an otoscope, is a translucent gray structure. During physical examination, two parts of the drum normally can be seen: the pars tensa, which encompasses the area of the drum inferior to the lateral process, and the pars flaccida, above the level of the lateral process. Several bony landmarks can be identified: the lateral process, manubrium of the malleus, umbo, incus, stapedial tendon, promontory, and round window niche.

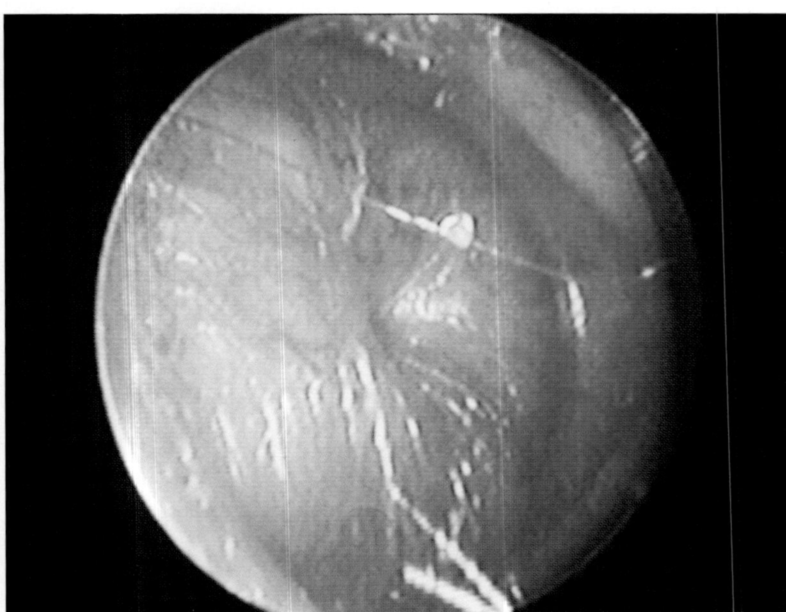

FIGURE 4-10 Acute otitis media with bulging drum. An operative photograph of acute otitis media shows the drum to be inflamed with thickening and erythema, and the landmarks have been obliterated by the bulging drum. This acute process usually, though not invariably, is accompanied by fever and otalgia. Of note, bulging of the tympanic membrane may be seen in any acute inflammatory process of the ear, including acute mastoiditis, coalescent mastoiditis, and complicated mastoiditis. (*From* Bull [2]; with permission.)

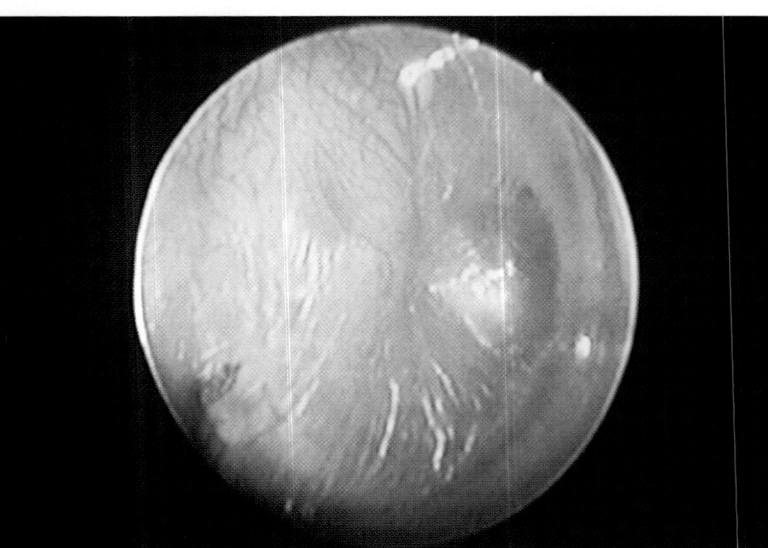

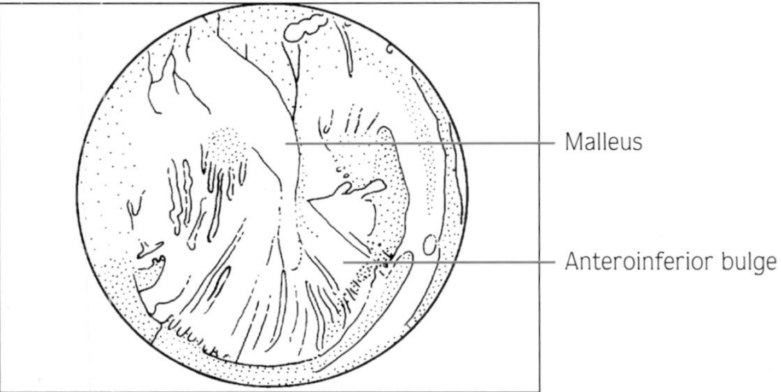

FIGURE 4-11 Otoscopic view of otitis media with effusion, showing bulging drum. As early inflammation progresses, there is an increase in the amount of fluid produced by the cells lining the middle ear cleft and mastoid air cell system. In such cases, the drum may be seen to bulge. Generally, otitis media effusion is painless. However, as the amount of fluid increases and the drum bulges, pain may develop. In this photograph, the bulging of the drum is most prominent at the anteroinferior quadrant. This area may have been the site of a previous perforation or ventilation tube. The fluid seen at this stage of otitis media with effusion is usually clear or may give a bluish hue to the drum, because purulent material has not yet developed.

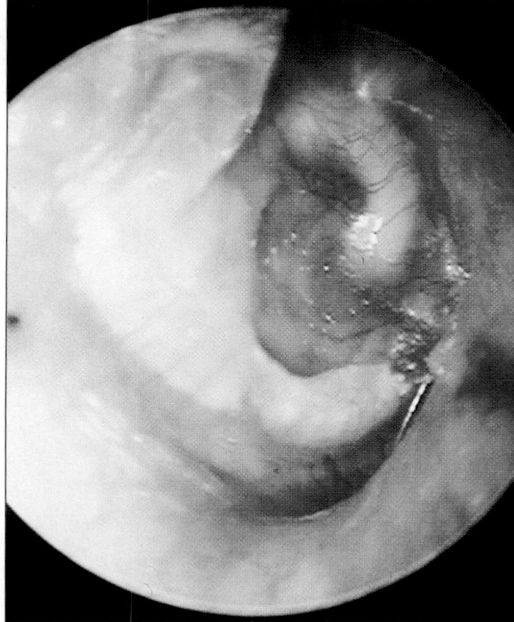

Figure 4-12 Tympanosclerosis. Tympanosclerosis is the deposition of hyaline material within the middle layer of the tympanic membrane. This condition results from recurrent infection and sometimes as a consequence of ventilation tube placement. Usually, this phenomenon is of no importance, but when severe, it can progress to involve the entire drum and ossicular chain, resulting in a conductive hearing loss.

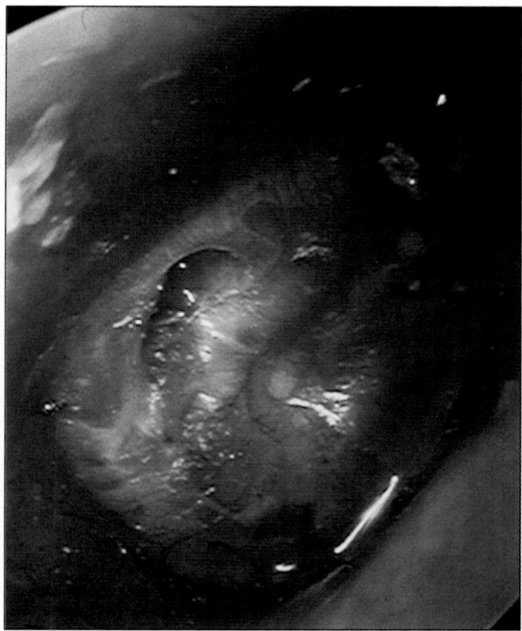

Figure 4-13 Tympanic membrane changes associated with cholesteatoma. A slitlike opening can be seen. Over a long period of time, negative pressure within the middle ear, along with recurrent and chronic infection, can lead to flaccidity of the drum and creation of a retraction pocket. As keratinaceous debris and desquamated cells build up within this pocket, it enlarges to form a sac. With further buildup of debris, the advancing surface of this sac will fill the interstices of the epitympanum and erode the middle and inner ear structures. In addition, chronic otorrhea results from infection arising from both the underlying chronic ear disease and the inspissated debris within the sac itself.

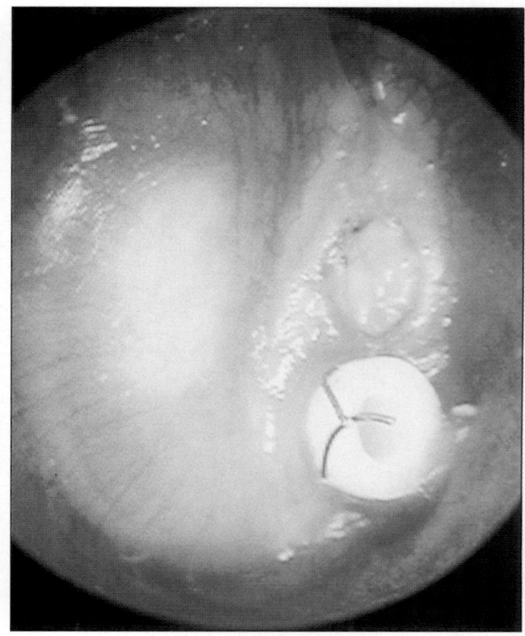

Figure 4-14 Cholesteatoma behind the tympanic membrane. An otoscopic view shows a white sac behind an anterosuperior perforation. A ventilation tube is seen in the antero-inferior quadrant. In this case, insertion of a tube did not prevent the formation of cholesteatoma. It may be that the process of cholesteatoma development had started before insertion of the tube or that this case represents a congenital cholesteatoma that developed in the mesotympanum but which has eroded through the tympanic membrane.

Infections of the External Ear

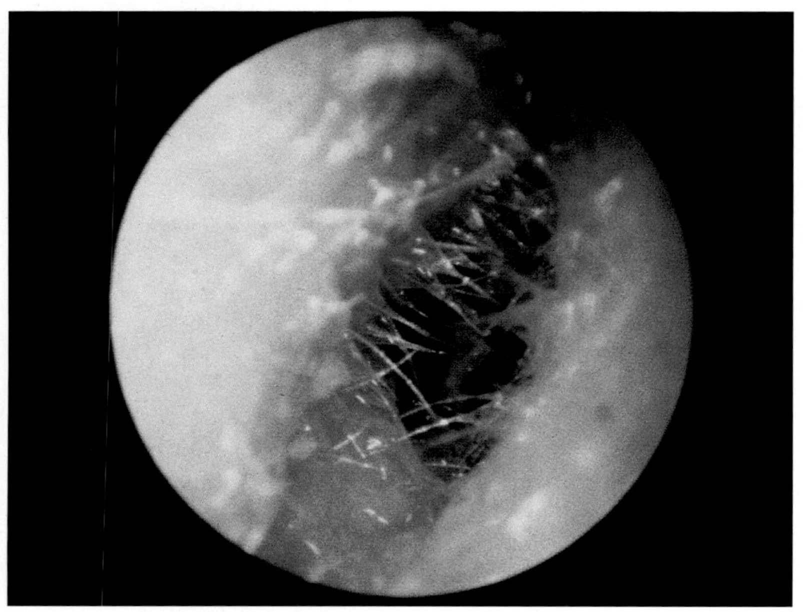

Figure 4-15 Otoscopic view of early acute diffuse otitis externa. Acute diffuse otitis externa (swimmer's ear) is a nonlocalized inflammation of the external auditory canal and is the most commonly seen type of otitis externa. It is commonly associated with swimming and hot, humid climates. The patient presents with complaints of itching, pain (which may be severe), a blocked feeling or sense of pressure in the ear, and possible aural discharge. On otoscopy, the skin of the cartilaginous external canal is edematous and tender and has a shiny, red appearance. The lumen is narrowed, and a yellow mucopurulent exudate may be seen. Gram-negative bacteria, particularly *Pseudomonas aeruginosa*, are the usual pathogens, but *Staphylococcus aureus* also is isolated frequently. (*From* Hawke *et al* [3]; with permission.)

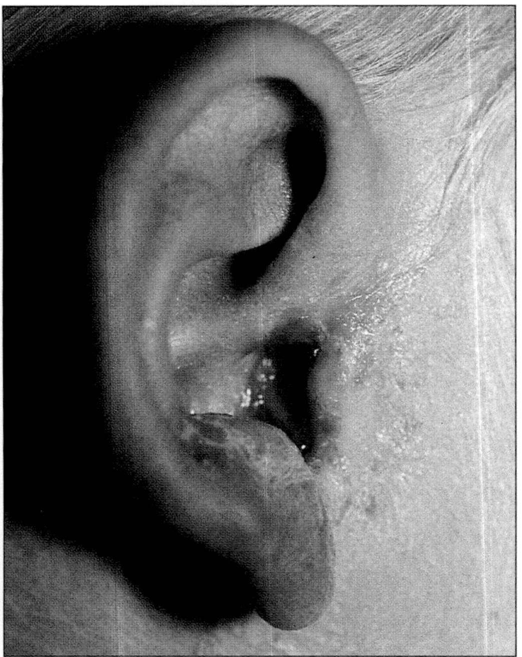

Figure 4-16 Lateral view of the ear in acute diffuse otitis externa. External examination shows swelling of the ear canal and lymphadenopathy anterior to the tragus. A yellow, mucopurulent discharge may ooze from the ear opening, especially as the condition progresses. Movement of the tragus or auricle is extremely painful, which may limit or prevent otoscopic examination. (*Courtesy of* A. Willner, MD.)

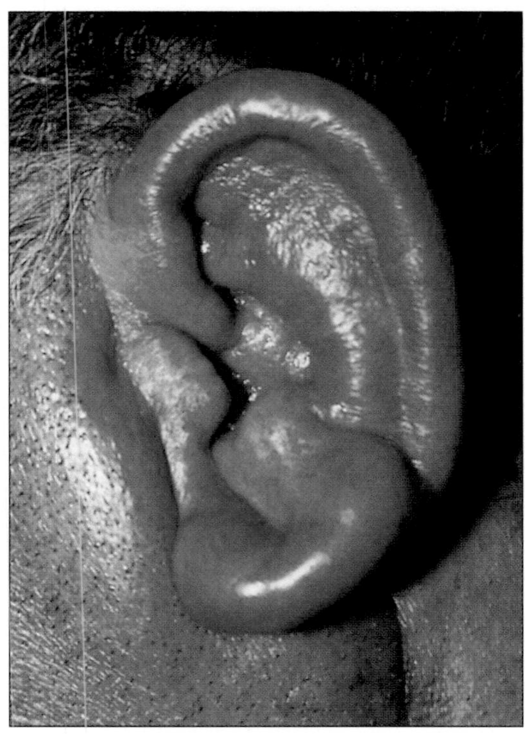

Figure 4-17 Auricular erysipelas. Erysipelas is an acute, localized but spreading form of superficial cellulitis. It usually involves only the pinna in the ear and can spread to adjacent facial areas. It is caused mainly by group A β-hemolytic streptococci. The lesions are characteristically bright red, well demarcated, and tender, with an elevated and distinct advancing peripheral margin. Penicillin therapy brings a rapid response. (*Courtesy of* B. Benjamin, MD.)

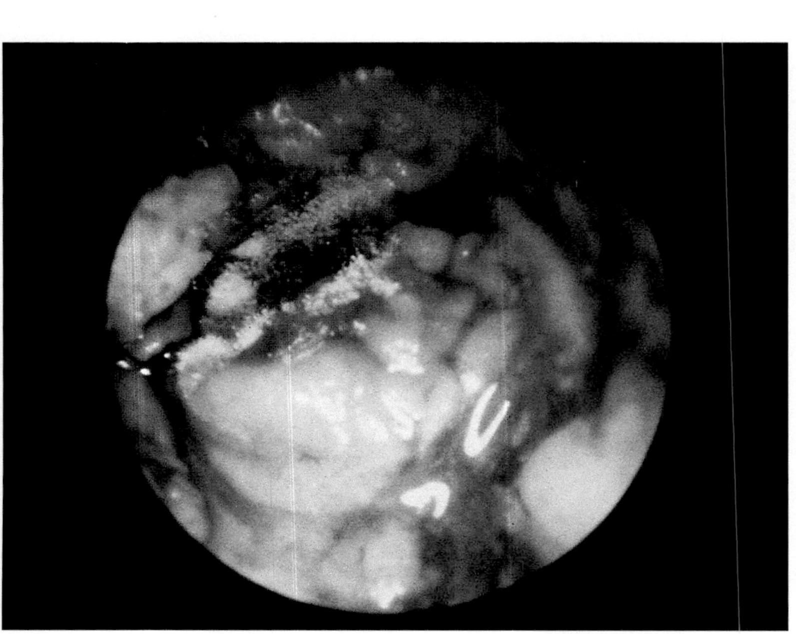

Figure 4-18 *Aspergillus niger* otomycosis. *Aspergillus* is responsible for up to 90% of cases of otomycosis. Otomycosis due to *A. niger* can usually be diagnosed by the presence of white, fluffy, cottonlike material, which represents the fungal hyphae. A creamy white mucopurulent exudate may fill the ear canal. Numerous mycelia (shown here) with grayish-black or brown fruiting heads (conidiophores) can be seen in *Aspergillus* infection. A brownish-yellow mucopurulent exudate is present behind, and often the underlying canal skin is inflamed and granular due to invasion by the fungal mycelia. (*From* Hawke *et al* [4]; with permission.)

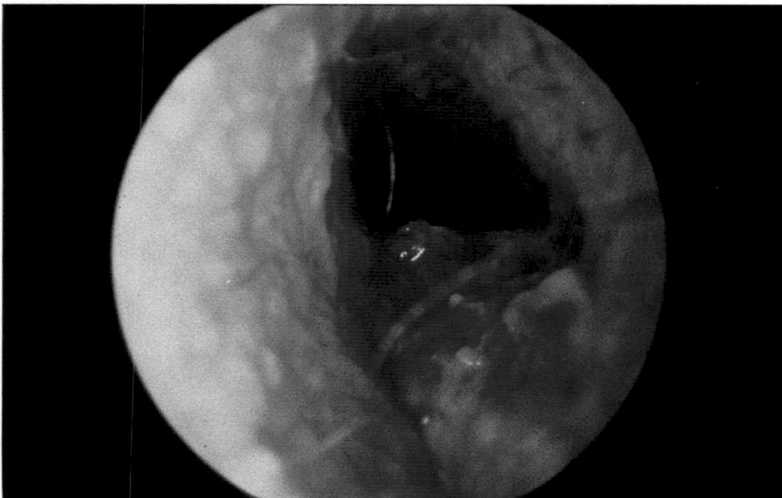

Figure 4-19 Otoscopic view of necrotizing (malignant) otitis externa. Necrotizing otitis externa is a severe, invasive, locally aggressive infection that occurs primarily in elderly diabetics and immunocompromised patients. The condition almost always is caused by *Pseudomonas aeruginosa* infection. Classically, necrotizing otitis externa presents as severe otalgia associated with the presence of exuberant granulation tissue arising from the floor of the external auditory canal at the junction of the bony and cartilaginous portions with persistent purulent otorrhea. Despite the misleading nomenclature, this is a bacterial infection, not a neoplastic condition. (*From* Hawke *et al* [5]; with permission.)

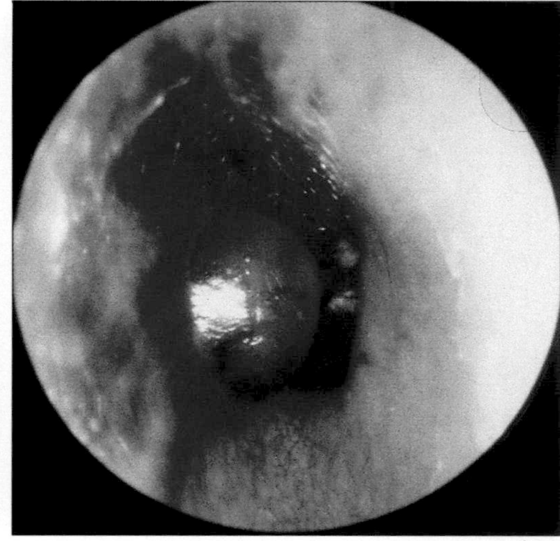

Figure 4-20 Otoscopic view of bullous myringitis. Bullous myringitis is an acute inflammation of the tympanic membrane and surrounding meatal skin that is characterized by severe pain and the presence of hemorrhagic blebs. The condition is thought to be due to an influenza-like virus, but in some cases, *Mycoplasma pneumoniae* has been cultured. A large hemorrhagic bleb is present on the posterior bony canal wall and adjacent tympanic membrane. The bleb contains a serous effusion with a collection of blood in the inferior portion. After rupture and aspiration of the bleb, extensive subcutaneous and intracutaneous hemorrhage could be seen. There was extensive hemorrhage along the handle of the malleus. (*From* Hawke *et al* [6]; with permission.)

Sinusitis

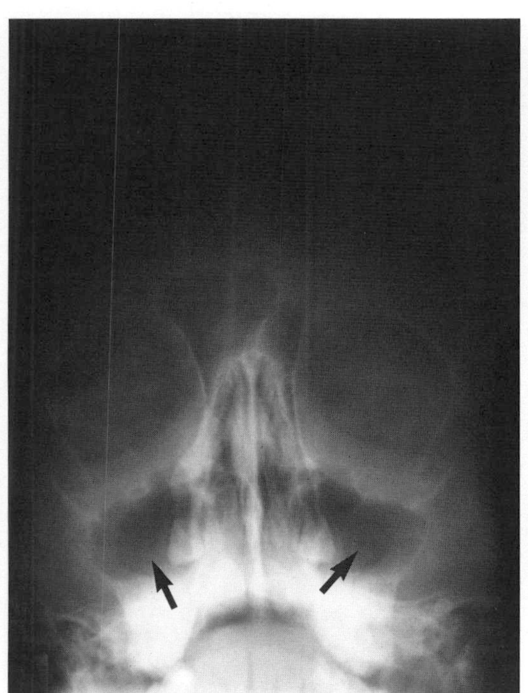

Figure 4-21 Radiographic evaluation. Radiographs can be used to confirm the clinical suspicion of acute sinusitis. Three radiographic views should be obtained as follows: Anteroposterior, to visualize the ethmoid air cells; lateral, to visualize the frontal and sphenoid sinuses; occipitomental, to visualize the maxillary sinuses. This radiograph shows an occipitomental view.

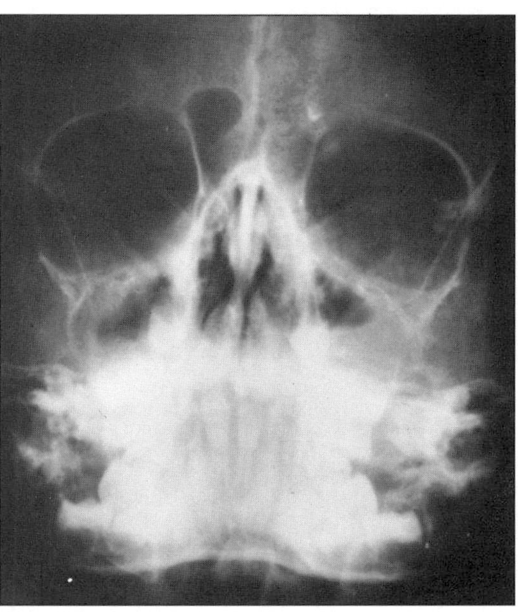

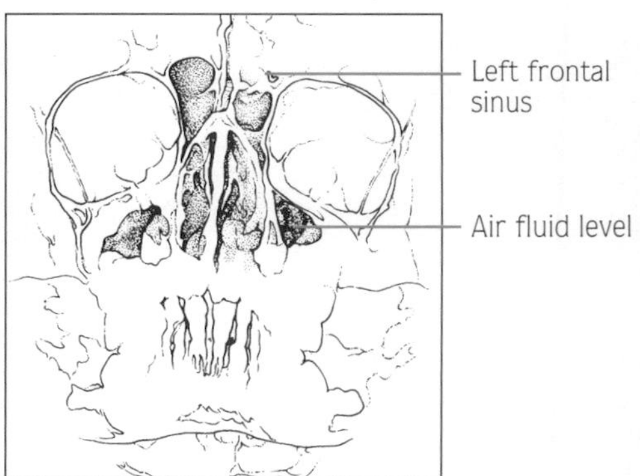

Figure 4-22 Diagnostic radiographic findings. An occipitomental view demonstrates significant mucosal thickening in the right maxillary sinus. There is an air-fluid level in the left maxillary sinus, an unusual finding in children with acute sinusitis. The left frontal sinus, although rudimentary, is opacified.

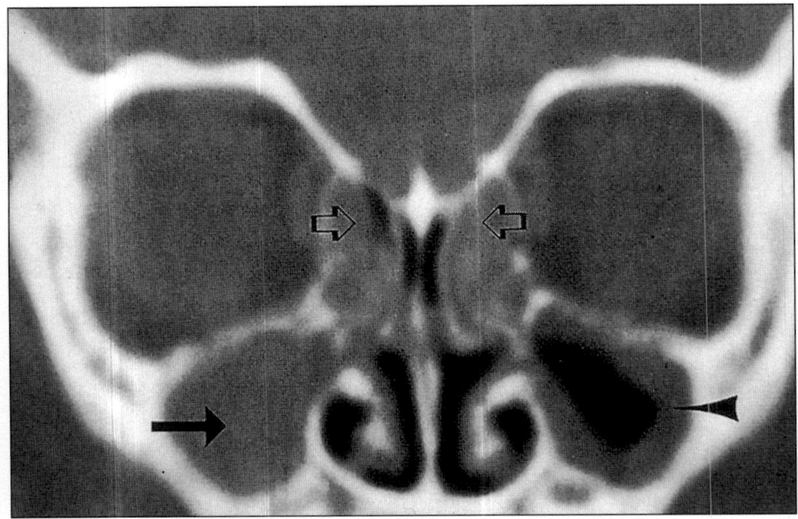

FIGURE 4-23 Other imaging modalities used to confirm a diagnosis of sinusitis include Computed tomographic (CT) and magnetic resonance (MR) imaging. These studies are usually reserved for patients with very protracted symptoms or patients in whom complications of sinusitis have developed. This coronal CT evaluation shows a completely opacified right maxillary sinus (*arrow*), significant mucosal thickening in the left maxillary sinus (*arrowhead*), and opacification of the ethmoids bilaterally (*open arrows*). (*Courtesy of* M. Casselbrant, MD.)

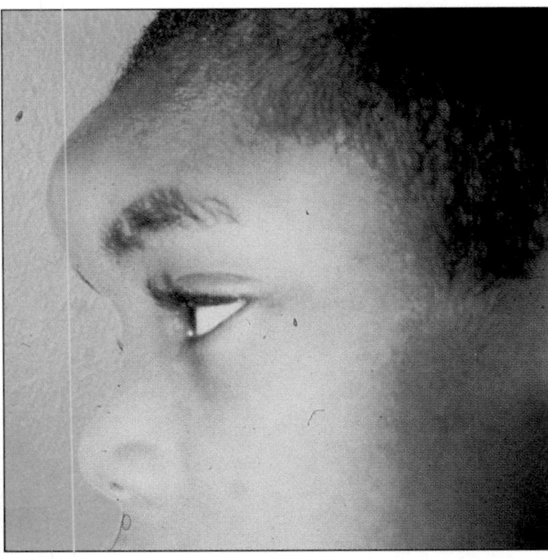

FIGURE 4-24 Pott's puffy tumor. A 13-year-old boy presented with a 10-day history of respiratory symptoms and headache. His fever had been low-grade. The headache was not relieved by acetaminophen. During the last 3 days, his forehead had become tender to touch. On physical examination, the middle of his forehead was swollen, tender, and fluctuant. This is an example of Pott's puffy tumor—subperiosteal abscess of the frontal bone, secondary to frontal sinusitis.

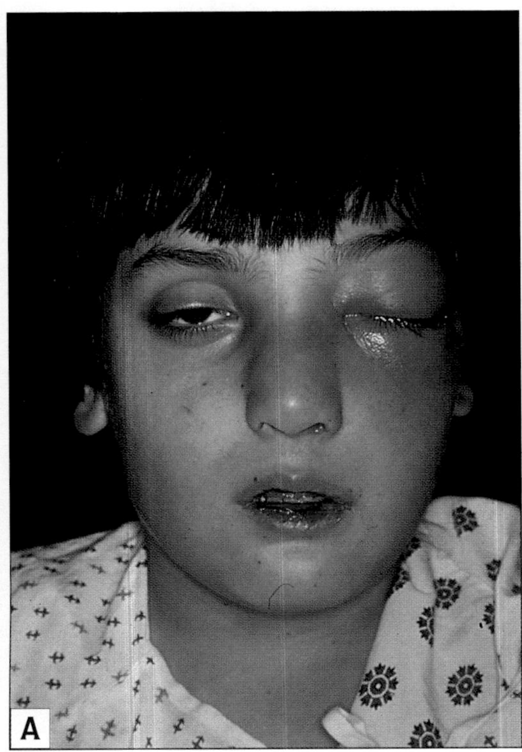

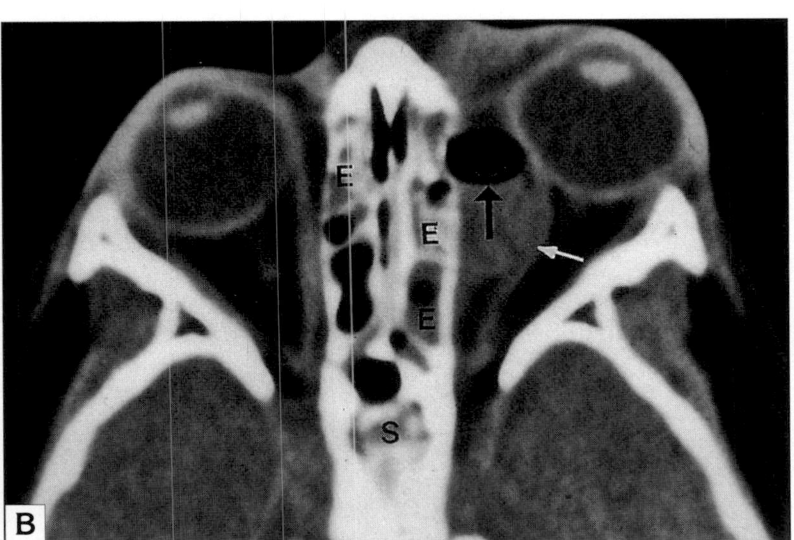

FIGURE 4-25 Intra- and extraorbital suppurative complications of sinusitis. **A**, A 10-year-old boy had long-standing allergic symptoms, including chronic nasal discharge and congestion. For 3 days, he had left-sided facial pain and headache, with progressive swelling of his left eye. On physical examination, he was febrile to 38.4° C (101.2° F). When his lids were mechanically everted, his left globe was frozen and there was intense chemosis of the conjunctiva. **B**, An axial computed tomography (CT) scan shows anterior and lateral displacement of his left eye. There is an air-fluid level (*black arrow*) in the area between the lateral border of the left ethmoid and the medial rectus of his left eye (*white arrow*). (E—ethmoid air cells; S—sphenoid sinus.)

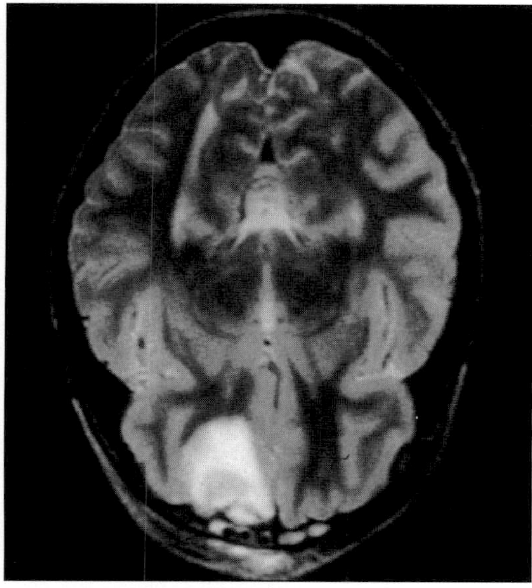

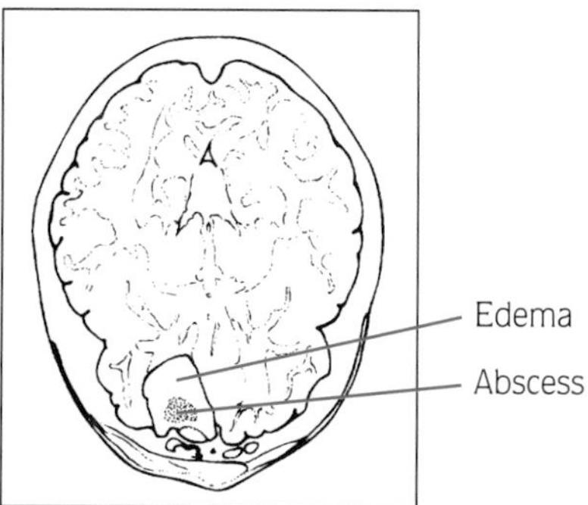

FIGURE 4-26 Epidural abscess. A 30-year-old man had nasal congestion and headache for 1 month. During the last 3 days, the headache became extremely intense; he was vomiting daily and developed a low-grade fever. On physical examination, he appeared very uncomfortable. His face was tender to touch, especially over his brow. Computed tomography (CT) scan and magnetic resonance (MR) imaging were done. The MR scan demonstrates the abscess and a large area of edema posterior to it in the right frontal area.

INFECTIOUS DISEASES OF THE ORAL CAVITY

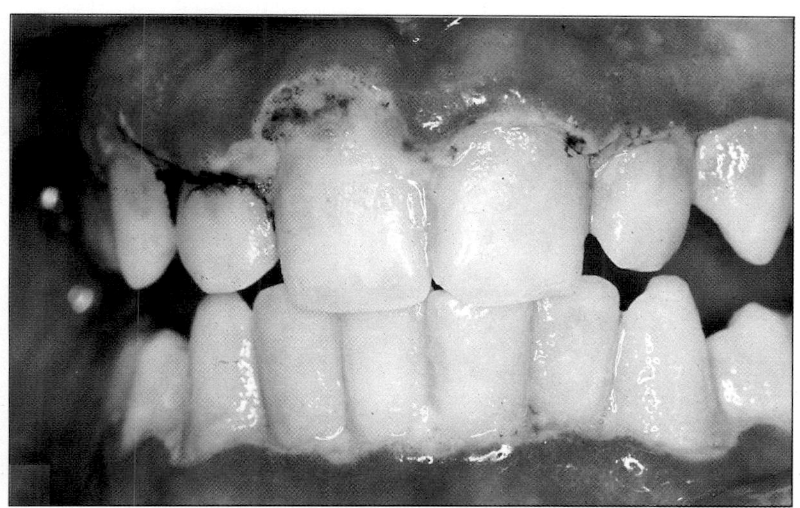

FIGURE 4-27 Acute necrotizing ulcerative gingivitis (ANUG). Generalized severe view. Also termed *Vincent's infection* and *trench mouth*, ANUG is a severe form of gingivitis associated with infection by spirochetes, fusiform bacteria, and *Prevotella intermedia*. This rapidly progressing infection is characterized by acute fiery-red gingivitis, soft-tissue necrosis with formation of a necrotic surface layer (referred to as a pseudomembrane), severe pain, fetid odor, and, at times, malaise, lymphadenopathy, and low-grade fever. The hallmark sign of ANUG is necrosis and cratering of the interproximal papillae, referred to as "punched-out papillae." ANUG may be localized, generalized, or generalized severe (shown here) in its presentation.

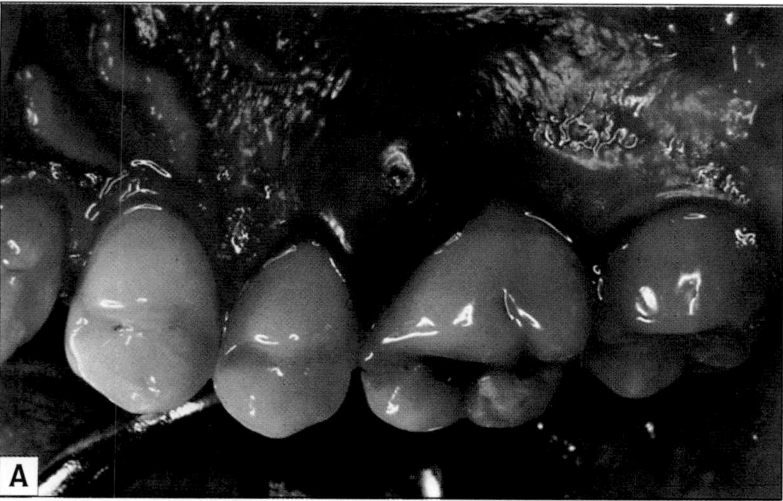

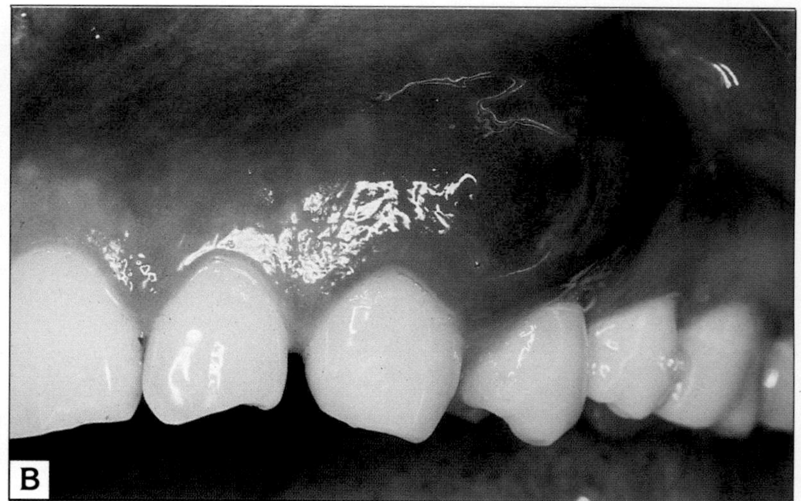

FIGURE 4-28 Periodontal abscess. A periodontal abscess is a localized purulent inflammatory process, which is initiated by the pathogenic organisms associated with periodontitis and involves the subgingival periodontal structures. Comprehensive evaluation of the patient usually shows generalized periodontal disease in conjunction with the periodontal abscess. Often, the abscess is associated with root surface accretions and deep tortuous periodontal pockets. Clinically, patients present with pain and percussion sensitivity, mobility, and slight elevation of the involved tooth, or with a feeling of "pressure in the gums." The periodontal abscess may present interproximally (*panel A*) or buccally (*panelB*) or in the furcation areas (not shown). The periodontal abscess must be differentiated from abscesses resulting from necrosis of the dental pulp to ensure proper treatment. Clinical and radiographic evaluation combined with tests to determine the pulp vitality of the affected tooth help differentiate these lesions. Debridement of the affected root surface aborts the acute symptoms and leads to healing if the area is maintained plaque-free. The use of systemic antibiotics is rarely indicated.

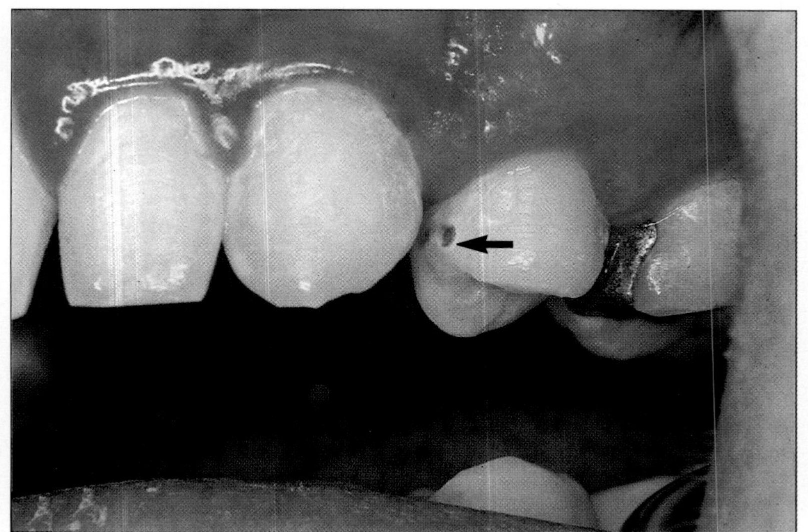

FIGURE 4-29 Dental caries. One of the most common bacterial infections in humans, dental caries is the process of decalcification of the inorganic portion of the tooth, followed by disintegration of the organic portion leading to cavitation. This disease is caused by the *Lactobacillus* and *Streptococcus mutans* class of acid-producing bacteria, which metabolize carbohydrates that have been ingested into the mouth and produce lactic acid, which in turn dissolves the mineralized portion of the tooth. Though this is considered a life-long disease, there are varying degrees of susceptibility within population groups. Some individuals remain at low risk for this disease whereas others are chronically affected. The use of systemic and topical fluorides, restricting the frequency of sucrose intake, and the removal of bacterial plaque are the major preventive measures used to control dental caries. Dental caries is subclassified principally by location, recurrence, and severity as coronal (smooth surface shown [dental caries, *arrow*] and fissure), cervical and root, recurrent (at the margins of dental restorations), and rampant caries. Root caries increases in prevalence with age due to gingival recession, which exposes the root surface and makes it susceptible to colonization by caries-producing organisms. The etiology of root caries is similar to coronal caries, with the addition of *Actinomyces* sp. as causative organisms. Rampant caries is seen principally in young individuals with high sucrose intake and high lactobacillus counts and in xerostomic individuals.

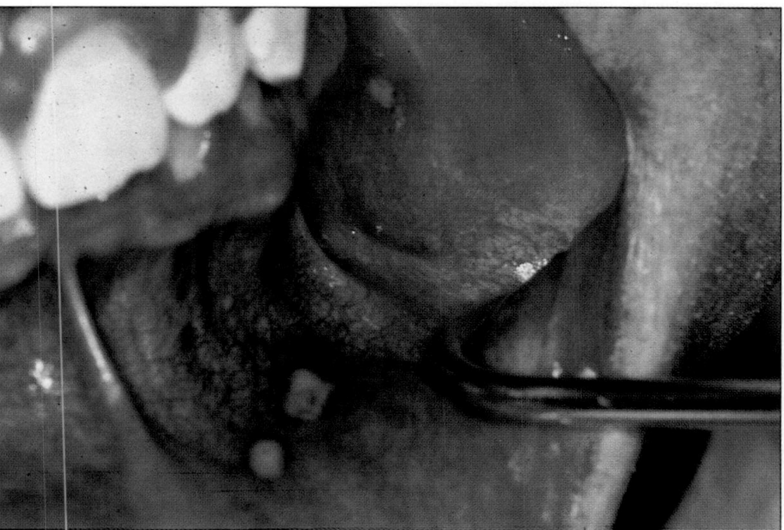

FIGURE 4-30 Primary herpetic gingivostomatitis. Primary herpetic gingivostomatitis is a contagious disease caused by the herpes simplex virus type 1 and, less frequently, type 2. It may be subclinical or acute, affecting all of the soft tissues of the mouth including the gingiva, mucosa, tongue, lips, pharynx, and palate. Clinical signs include fiery red, swollen, and bleeding gingiva and formation of clusters of small vesicles that burst to form yellowish ulcers with a circumscribing red halo (*shown here*). The small ulcers may coalesce to form large ulcers. Symptoms include fever, malaise, and localized pain associated with ulceration. This phase of the infection usually regresses spontaneously in 10–14 days. Supportive treatment includes the use of a liquid diet, topical anesthetics, and acyclovir in severe cases. Following the primary infection, the patient continues to harbor the virus, which can later reactivate causing recurrent herpes simplex lesions. Primary herpetic gingivostomatitis should be clinically differentiated from erythema multiforme, which can produce similar appearing oral lesions.

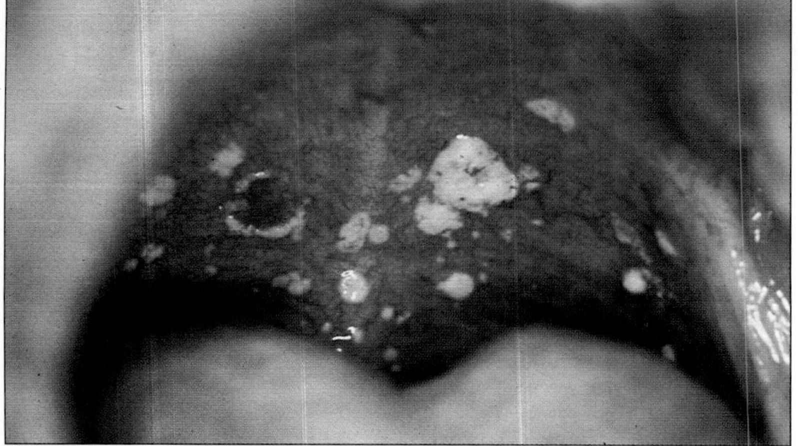

FIGURE 4-31 Pseudomembranous candidiasis (thrush). Thrush presents clinically as white patches on the oral mucosa, which wipe off to reveal a red or ulcerated area. Diagnosis is made by clinical appearance and demonstration of the organism on a stained smear from the lesion.

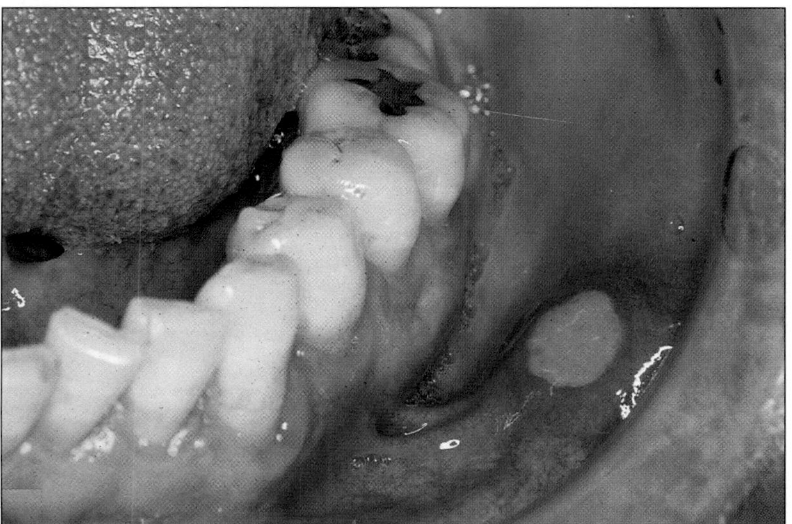

Figure 4-32 Recurrent aphthous stomatitis. Recurrent aphthous stomatitis clinically presents as single or multiple painful ulcerations of the buccal and labial mucosa. It is considered to be an immune reaction to oral bacteria, particularly *Streptococcus sanguis* 2A. Up to six recurrences per year are common. Minor lesions (seen here) are 0.3–1.0 cm in diameter and heal within 10–14 days of onset. Major aphthae range in size from 1.0–5.0 cm (Sutton's disease, periadenitis mucosa necrotica recurrens) and can be disabling due to their frequent recurrences, severe pain, and prolonged duration of months. This disease may actually represent a spectrum of diseases that ranges from minor aphthae to major aphthae to Behçet's disease, which presents as ulcerative lesions of the oral cavity, eyes, and genitals. Treatment includes analgesics and topical corticosteroids for minor aphthae and topical tetracycline and steroid mouthrinse or lozenges in refractory cases of major aphthae.

Pharyngotonsillitis

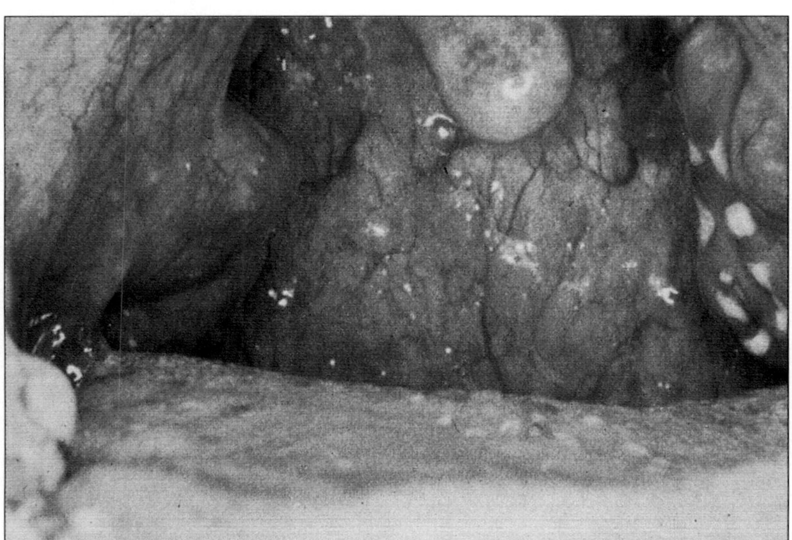

Figure 4-33 Marked pharyngeal erythema with edema. Marked pharyngeal erythema with edema and bilaterally enlarged and boggy tonsils with whitish or whitish-yellow exudate are the most characteristic features of pharyngitis due to GABHS. Although these features are occasionally seen in infectious mononucleosis, other pathogens producing this picture (diphtheria, tularemia, and candidiasis) are much less common. Uvulitis is also typical for streptococcal etiologies. Because *Haemophilus influenzae* type b may also rarely be a cause, coincident epiglottitis should be considered in cases in which uvulitis is seen without pharyngitis.

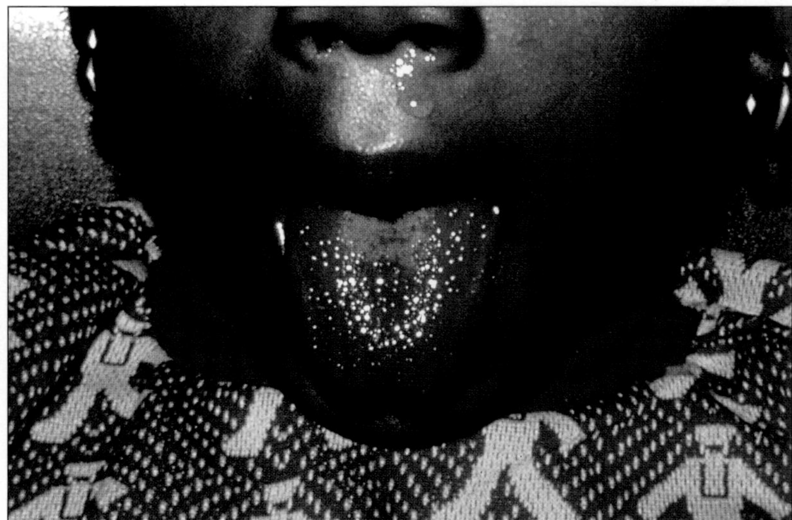

Figure 4-34 Circumoral pallor and strawberry tongue in scarlet fever. Patients with streptococcal pharyngitis often have circumoral pallor and a strawberry tongue. The circumoral pallor is relative to the facial flushing and labial erythema often seen in this infection. The tongue is often erythematous with prominent papillation, giving a strawberry-like appearance. These features are often more noteworthy in patients with scarlet fever than those without.

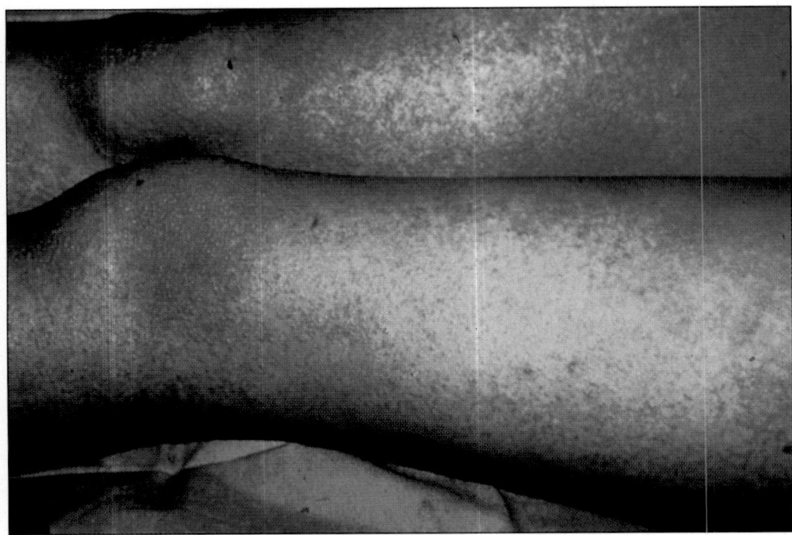

FIGURE 4-35 Scarlatiniform rash in scarlet fever. The scarlatiniform rash of scarlet fever is due to an erythrogenic toxin produced by some strains of GABHS that results in a macular or maculopapular rash that is dry and sandpapery. This rash usually begins within 2 days of disease onset, is most prominent on the trunk and proximal extremities, and is accentuated in the flexor creases (Pastia's lines). Macular rash is evident on the patient's legs.

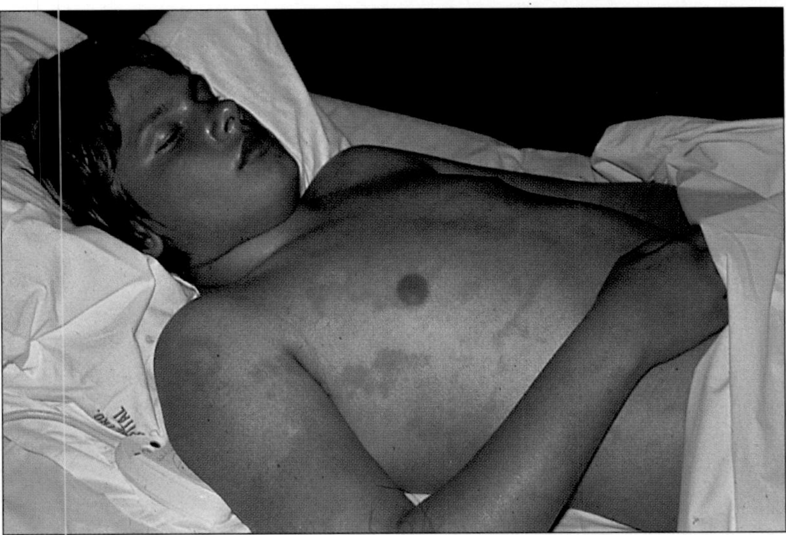

FIGURE 4-36 Erythema margination in rheumatic fever. Of all the major criteria for acute rheumatic fever, erythema marginatum is the most clearly pathognomonic. This serpentine, raised rash occurs in 3% to 13% of patients with rheumatic fever. Carditis and arthritis are more common features, each occurring in 30% to 50% of affected patients, but are not specific for the diagnosis.

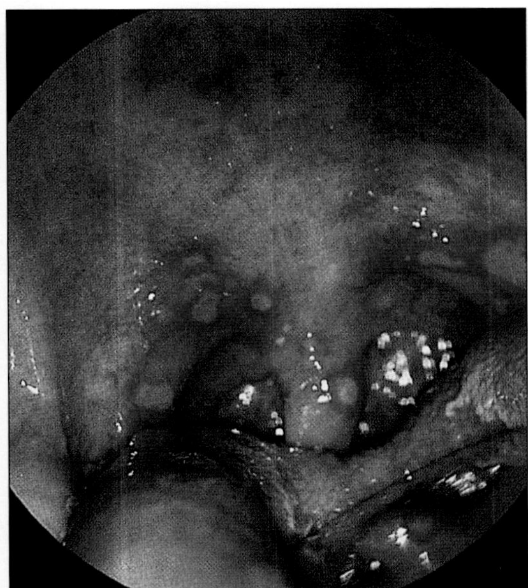

FIGURE 4-37 Hand-foot-mouth syndrome (coxsackie A virus infection). A papulovesicular rash on the palms and soles is a rare clinical finding. When seen in association with pharyngitis, or pharyngostomatitis, especially in the summer or fall, the diagnosis of hand-foot-mouth syndrome, typically due to coxsackie A viruses, is strongly suggested. Oral lesions of hand-foot-mouth syndrome on the uvula and palate.

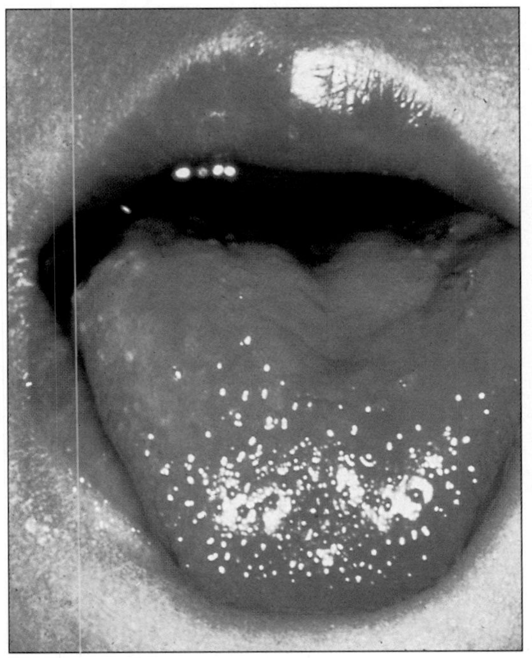

FIGURE 4-38 Kawasaki syndrome. Kawasaki syndrome is a condition of unknown etiology associated with fever, mucosal and cutaneous manifestations, swollen hands and feet, lymphadenopathy, and periungual desquamation. Prolonged fever and extreme irritability are characteristic. The oral manifestations include nonexudative pharyngitis, strawberry tongue, and swollen, red, cracked lips. This is a generalized vasculitis, and other features may include hepatitis, hydrops of the gallbladder, sterile pyuria, aseptic meningitis, and pleuritis. The most ominous feature is coronary arteritis with aneurysm formation. In some recent studies, Kawasaki disease has been a more common form of acquired heart disease in children than acute rheumatic fever. When diagnosed early, high-dose immunoglobulin therapy (2 g/kg) has proven useful in speeding resolution of acute symptoms and significantly decreasing the incidence of coronary aneurysms. [7,8]

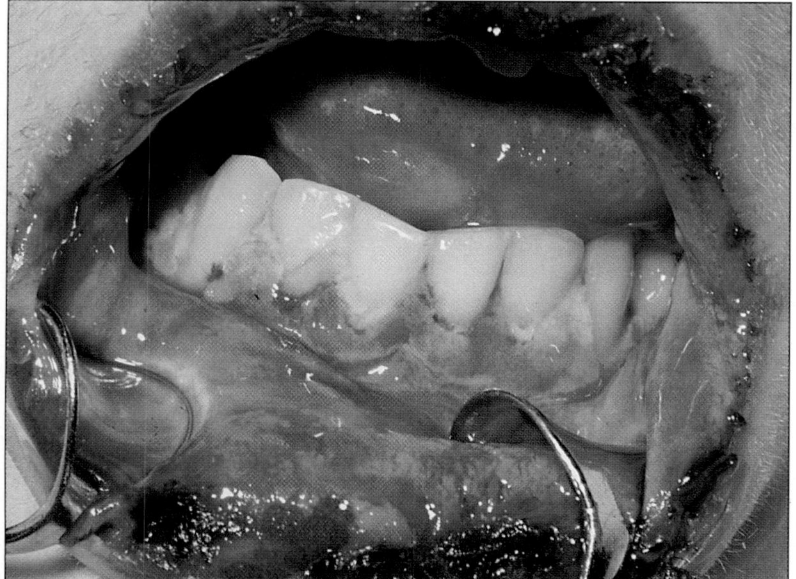

FIGURE 4-39 Stevens-Johnson syndrome. Patients with erythema multiforme major (Stevens-Johnson syndrome) have both cutaneous and mucosal findings. The mucosal inflammation may include the oral and conjunctival mucosa, pharynx, and genitourinary and perineal mucosa. The pharyngitis is nonexudative, and tonsillar involvement is unusual. The syndrome is immunologically mediated, although some infectious agents, particularly *Mycoplasma pneumoniae* and herpes simplex virus, have been associated with recurrent cases. Therapy is largely supportive, although those with large areas of involved skin may be treated in a fashion similar to burned patients.

EPIGLOTTITIS, CROUP, LARYNGITIS, AND TRACHEITIS

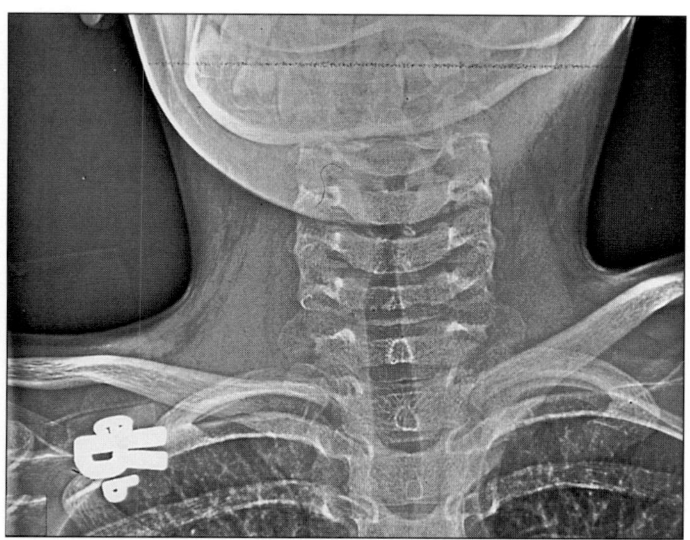

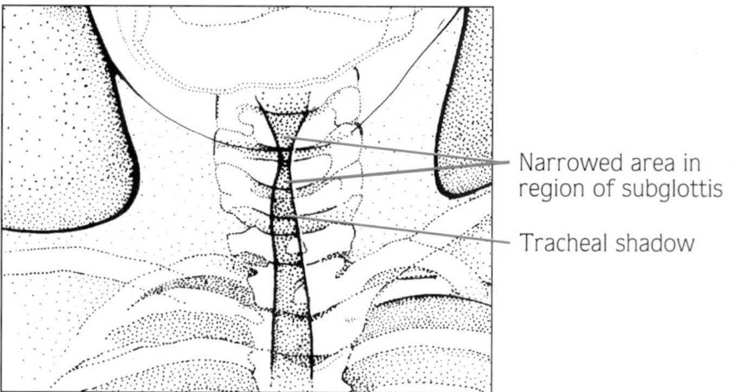

FIGURE 4-40 Epiglottitis, as seen by xeroradiography. Anteroposterior view of the neck of a child with documented epiglottitis shows narrowing in the diameter of the trachea, which can be confused with acute viral croup. The lateral neck view is preferable because it can demonstrate the enlarged epiglottis, or "thumb sign."

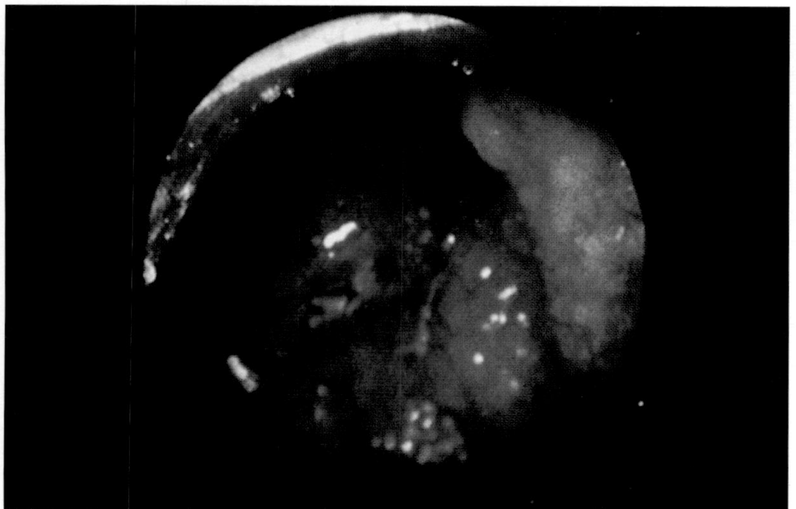

FIGURE 4-41 Epiglottitis, as seen by laryngoscopy. On direct laryngoscopy, a beefy red appearance of the epiglottis is characteristic of acute epiglottitis in children. In addition, the epiglottis may be infolded during severe swelling. This child was intubated to protect his airway during the initial 3–4 days of acute epiglottic swelling. Cultures were taken at the time of intubation and grew *Haemophilus influenzae* type B. In adults, the epiglottis may be swollen but is often pale in color. (*From* Riley [9]; with permission.)

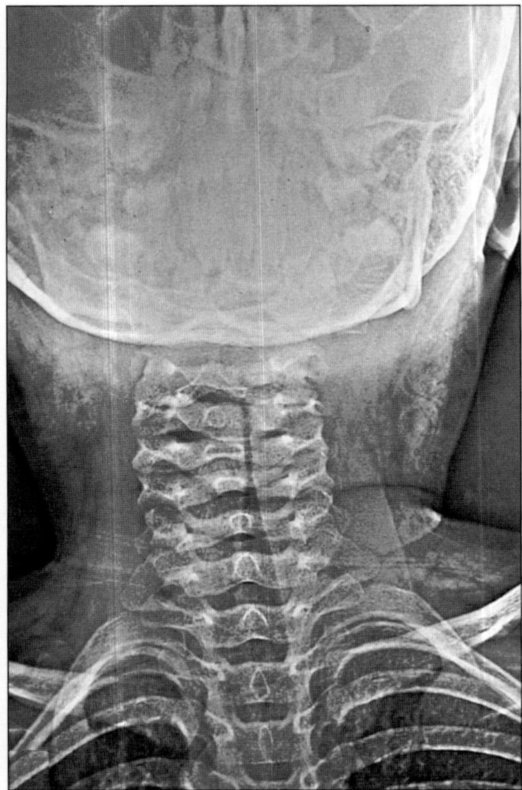

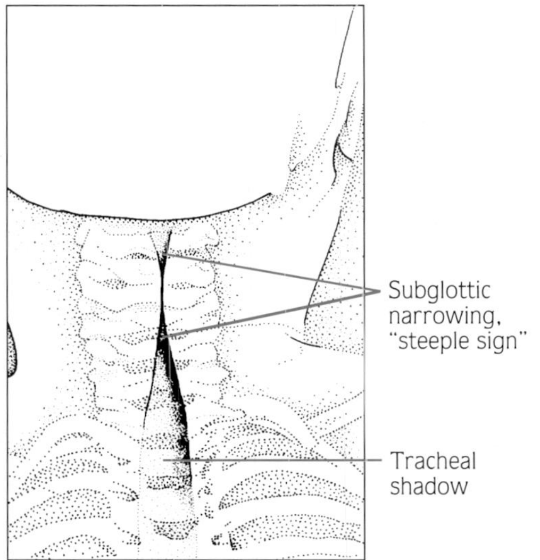

FIGURE 4-42 Croup, radiographic views. A xeroradiograph of the neck demonstrates a long area of narrowing extending well below the normal anatomic narrowing seen at the level of the larynx. This finding is called the *steeple sign* and is characteristic of children with croup. However, this finding is occasionally seen in cases of epiglottitis as well.

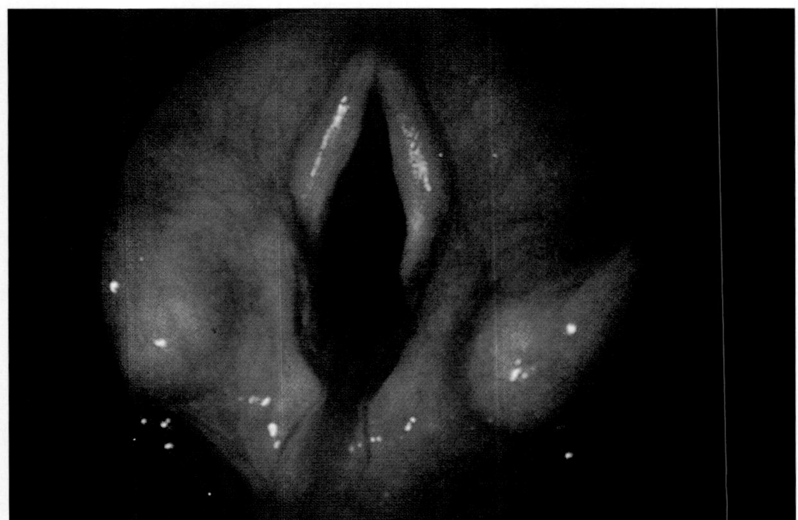

FIGURE 4-43 Examination of the larynx. Chronic laryngitis with substantial edema (*From* Benjamin [10]; with permission.)

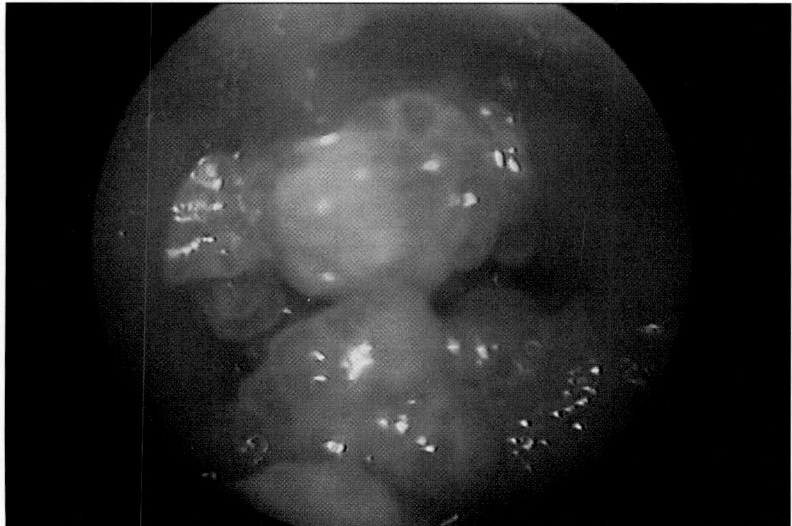

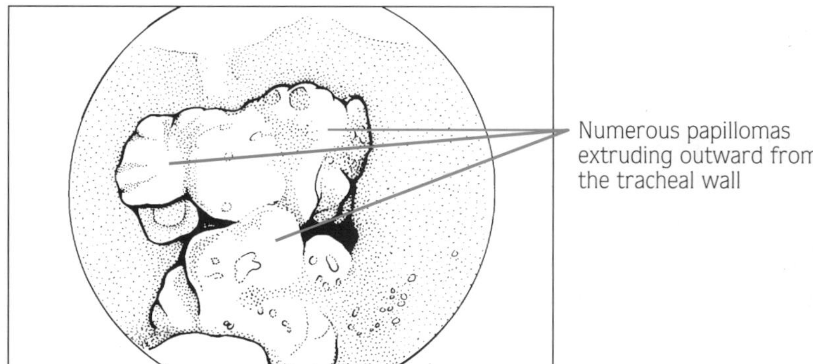

FIGURE 4-44 Laryngeal and tracheal papillomatosis. Laryngeal papillomatosis is a rare cause of laryngitis. Bronchoscopy of the larynx of a child who presented with increasing larygitis and shortness of breath showed fleshy growths on the vocal cords. More severe narrowing of the trachea was seen on lower-level bronchoscopy (seen here). Such lesions commonly occur on the vocal cords, but other sites in the respiratory tract have been documented as well (nose, trachea, lungs, oral cavity). The majority of such papillomas are caused by human papillomaviruses type 6 and 11. These are the most common isolates from exophytic genital condylomata and are thought to be acquired at the time of vaginal delivery in patients with juvenile onset of papillomas. Most cases are seen in children < 10 years of age, but papillomas can occur in adulthood as well. Although these growths can be removed surgically, they often recur. Viral genome is present in normal epithelium adjacent to the papillomas and is believed to account for latency and recurrence of such lesions [11].

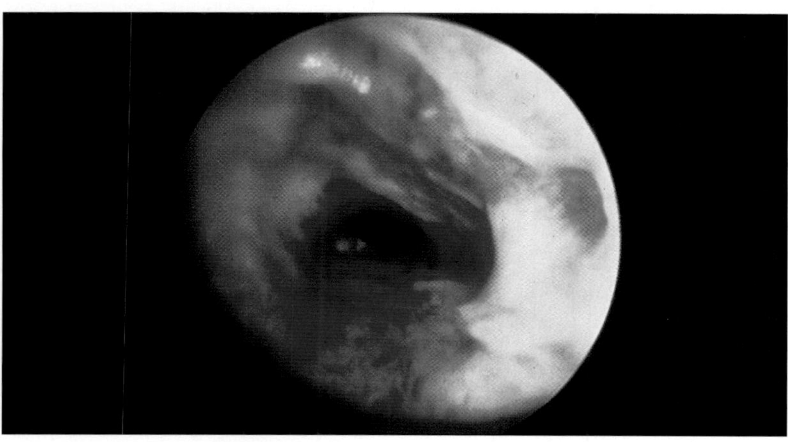

FIGURE 4-45 Acute bacterial tracheitis. Bronchoscopy of a patient with worsening airway compromise reveals marked narrowing, erythema, and edema of the trachea. Pus is easily removed from the walls of the trachea. (*Courtesy of* L. Brodsky, MD.)

Cervical Lymphadenopathy

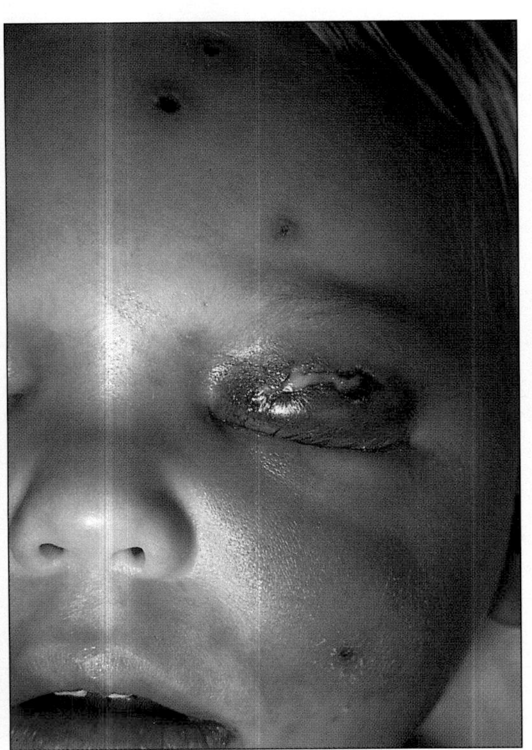

Figure 4-46 Cellulitis. Orbital and facial cellulitis developed in a 2-year-old child 3 days after the onset of chickenpox. The patient presented with fever (41.1° C, 106° F), grand mal seizures, and a generalized pruritic vesiculopustular exanthem, with cultures of blood and skin pustules positive for group A β-hemolytic streptococcus. Penicillin therapy was effective.

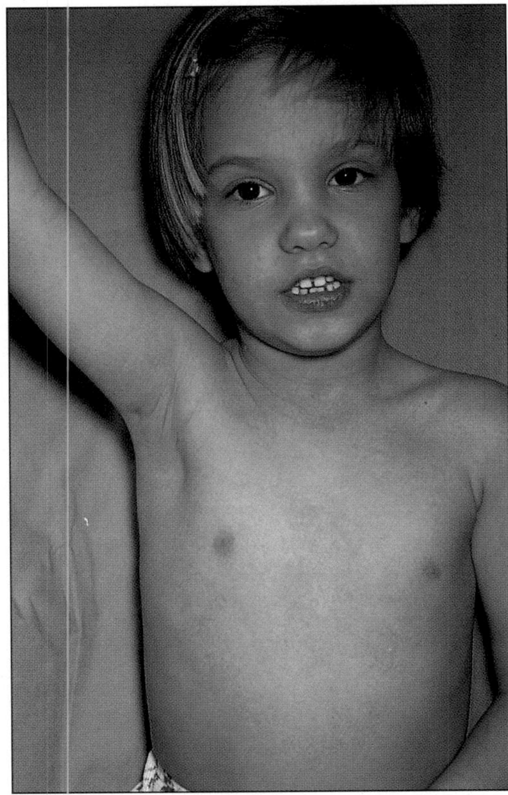

Figure 4-47 Staphylococcal scarlet fever. A 5 year-old girl, the sister of the girl with staphylococcal scalded skin disease in Fig.8-15, simultaneously had staphylococal scarlet fever due to the same phage type iiB *Staphylococcus aureus* strain. Her symptoms included fever, tonsillopharyngitis, cervical adenitis, and a fine papular scarlatinform exanthem for 3 days, as well as characteristic Pastia's lines in the right axilla and anterior neck (also seen in streptococcal scarlet fever. Oxacillin therapy was effective for both siblings

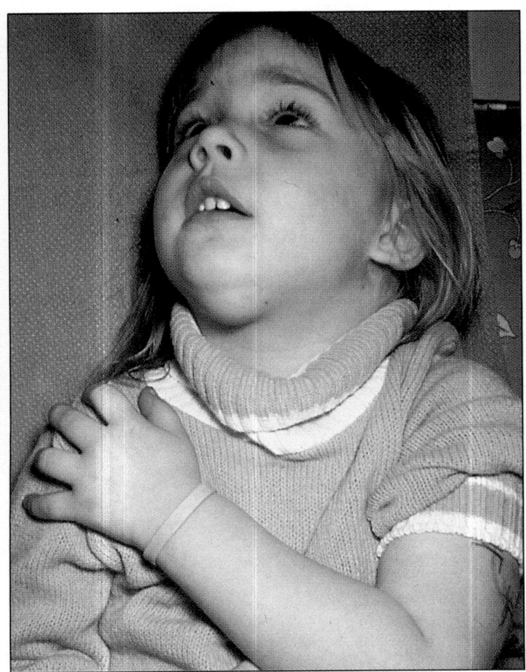

Figure 4-48 Submental node cat scratch disease (CSD). A healthy asymptomatic 3-year-old girl had a primary inoculation papule in the center of her chin for 3 weeks. Note the positive 28-mm CSD skin test on the left arm. The father had concurrent CSD of the inguinal nodes with cat scratches and a primary papule on his knee. Resolution occurred in 6 weeks, after application of local warm saline compresses.

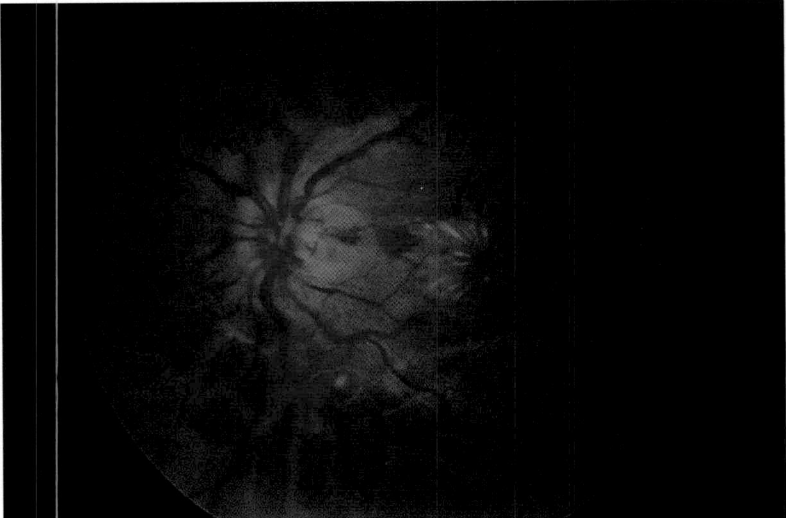

Figure 4-49 Cat scratch disease (CSD) neuroretinitis. A healthy 31-year-old man had flulike symptoms for 4 weeks, fever for 1 week, decreased vision in his right eye for 20 days, a papular rash on his abdomen and arms for 4 weeks secondary to flea bites and cat scratches, and submental adenopathy. The right fundus, (here shown) revealed optic edema with a macular star; visual acuity was 20/50. His left eye showed normal fundus and visual acuity. A CSD skin test was 35 mm. Spontaneous resolution of adenopathy and return of normal vision occurred in 3 months, and the maculopapular rash resolved in 6 months. (*From* Margileth and Hatfield [12]; with permission.)

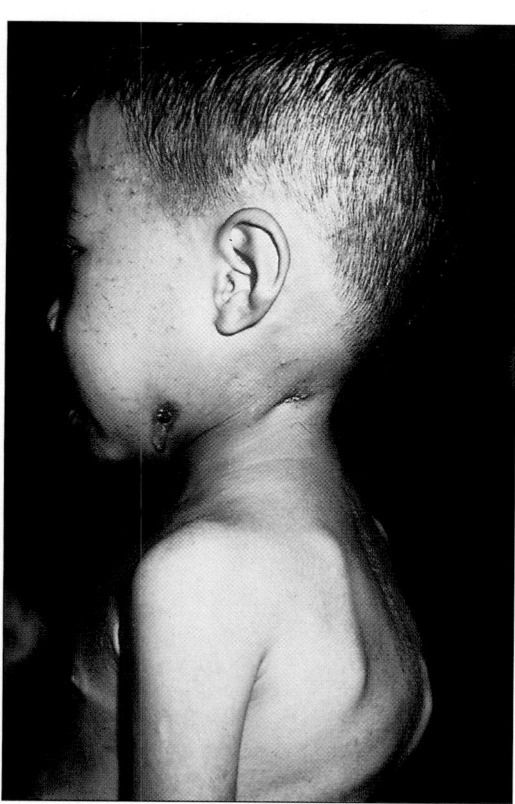

FIGURE 4-50 *Mycobacterium tuberculosis* scrofula with draining sinus tracts. Pulmonary infiltrates and Pott's disease of the spine of unknown duration were also seen in a Haitian child. Note the severe gibbus deformity of the thoracic spine, which usually occurs in the thoracolumbar region in children.

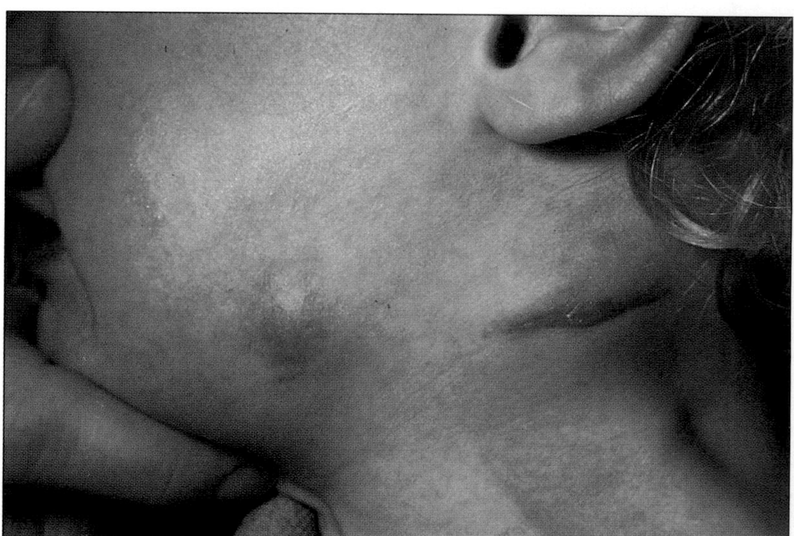

FIGURE 4-51 Nontuberculous mycobacterial lymphadenitis. A 3-year-old, healthy, asymptomatic child had lymphadenitis for several weeks. Incision and drainage produced a thick pus that grew *Mycobacterium avium-intracellulare*. PPD-T was 16 mm; PPD-Battey was 52 mm. Spontaneous drainage of caseous material from a mandibular node occurred several weeks later. Spontaneous healing of both lesions occurred over 24 months [13]. (*From* Margileth and Zawadsky [14]; with permission.)

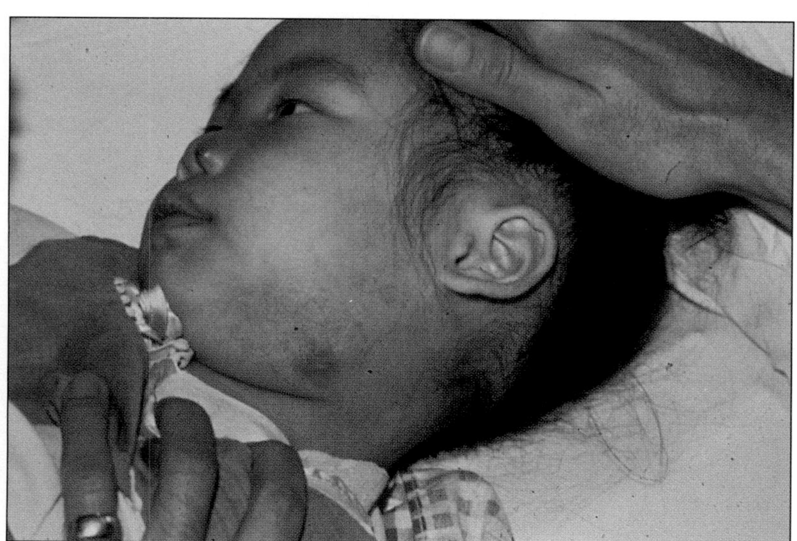

FIGURE 4-52 Cervicofacial nocardiosis. A 3-year-old child with cervicofacial nocardiosis for 7 days' duration presented with submandibular adenopathy and a draining left naris pustule that grew *Nocardia caviae* on culture. Trimethoprim-sulfamethoxazole therapy for 3 months was effective [15].

Parotitis and Thyroiditis

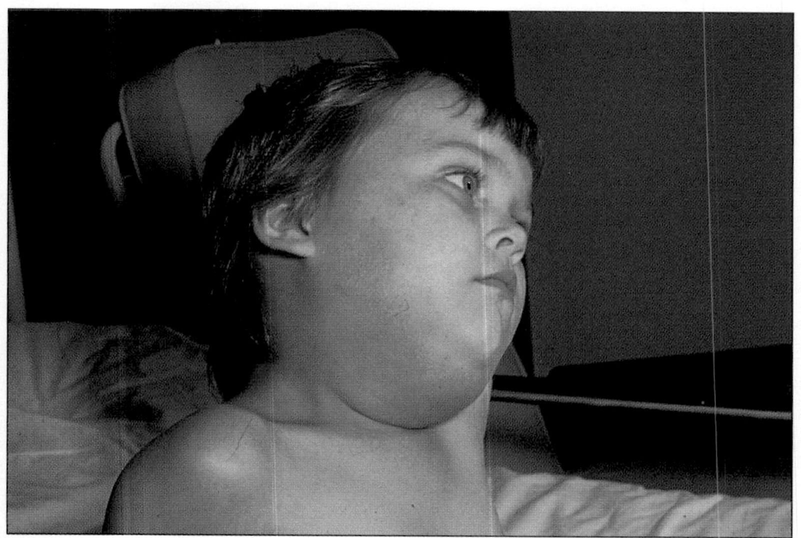

Figure 4-53 Unilateral parotitis due to mumps virus infection in a 4-year-old girl. The angle of the jaw is obliterated, and the earlobe is tilted forward, hallmark findings of parotitis. (*Courtesy of* the Centers for Disease Control and Prevention.)

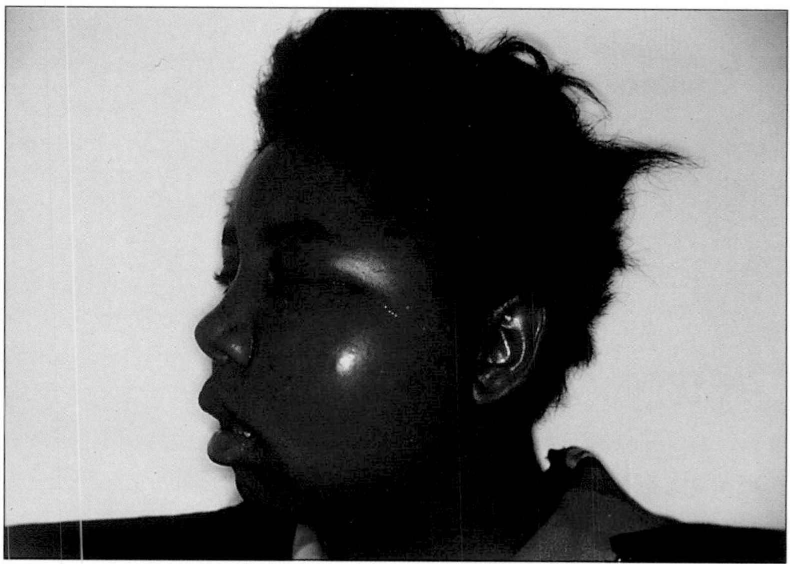

Figure 4-54 Suppurative parotitis. A female patient had become dehydrated and developed suppurative parotitis. The area around the angle of the jaw and extending up to the ear was red, swollen, rock hard, and exquisitely tender. Inspissated secretions had produced inflammation in Stensen's duct. *Staphylococcus aureus* was isolated from the pus in Stensen's duct. (*Courtesy of* A.M. Schwimmer, DDS.)

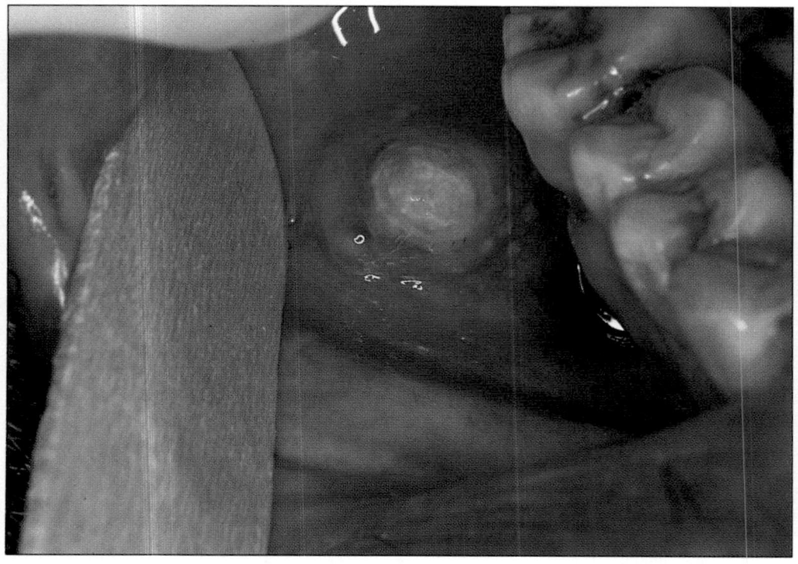

Figure 4-55 Stensen's duct showing inflammation and purulent discharge. (*Courtesy of* C.E. Barr, DDS.)

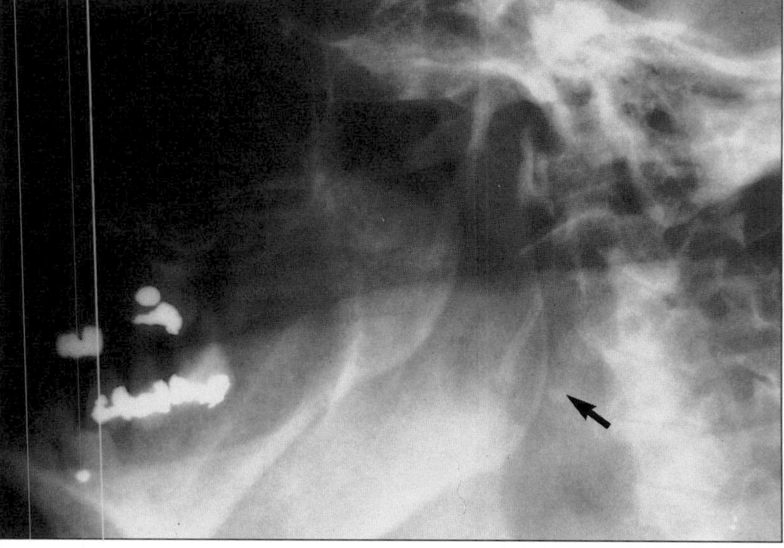

Figure 4-56 Sialogram showing a stone in Stensen's duct (*arrow*)..(*Courtesy of* B.A. Zeifer, MD.)

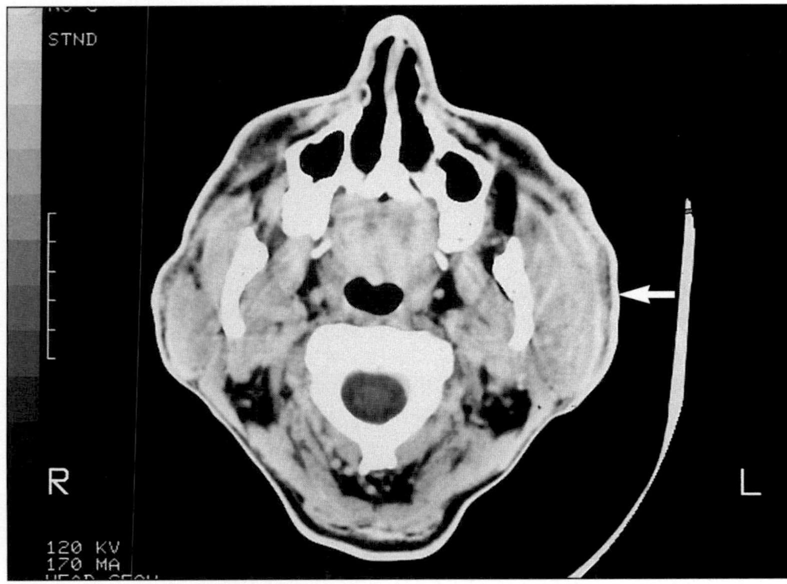

Figure 4-57 Computed tomographic scan of the parotid showing a well-circumscribed mass on the left (*arrow*). This mass, in the patient shown in Figure 9-12, underwent biopsy and yielded primarily red blood cells. The skin over the parotid underwent biopsy. (*Courtesy of* S.R. Yancovitz, MD, and L.M. Laya, MD.)

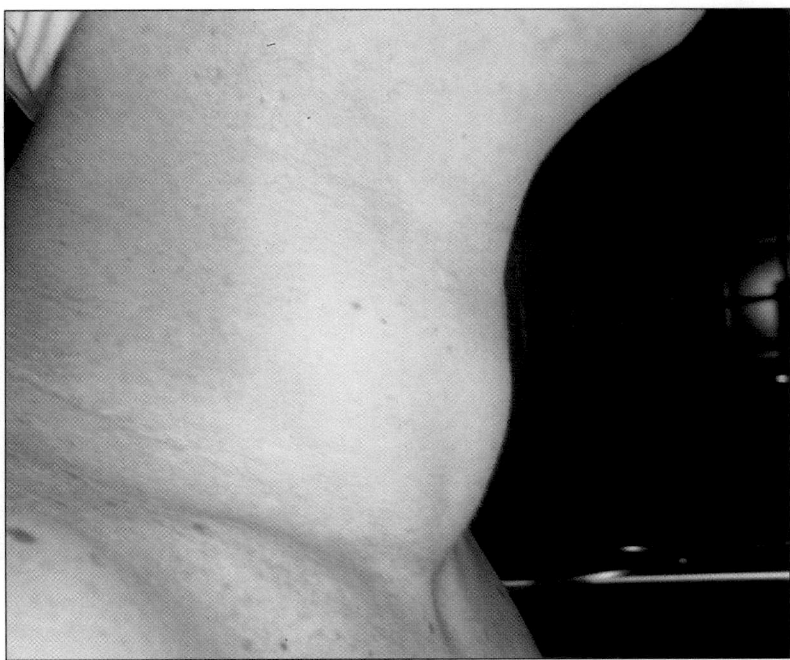

Figure 4-58 Subacute thyroiditis in a 40-year-old woman. This episode was the second bout of thyroiditis in this patient, and it was thought that the swelling was a thyroid tumor until biopsy revealed Hashimoto's thyroiditis.

Deep Neck Infections and Postoperative Infections

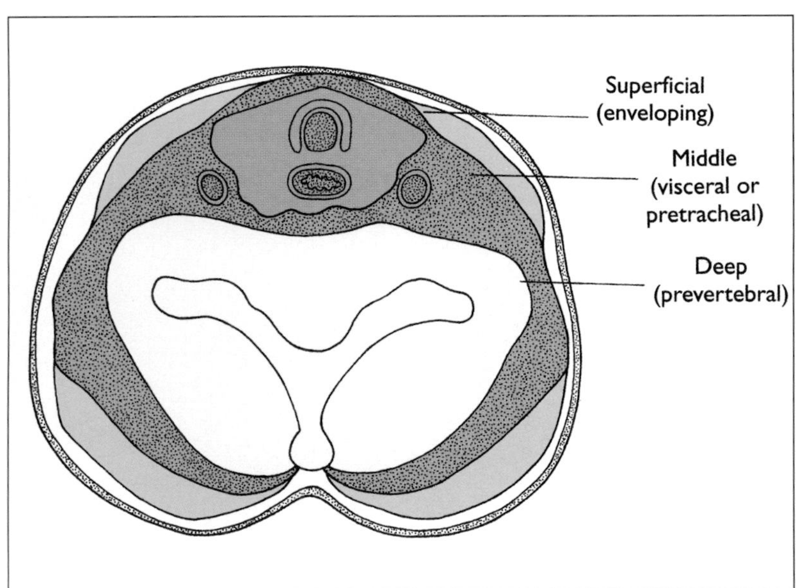

Figure 4-59 Anatomy of the neck. Deep neck infections, although uncommon, may have life-threatening sequelae despite antibiotic therapy. An understanding of the anatomic relationships of the fascial planes and potential spaces of the neck is essential for the surgical management required for most deep neck infections. The "tube within the tube" concept helps one to visualize the three layers of the deep cervical fascia.

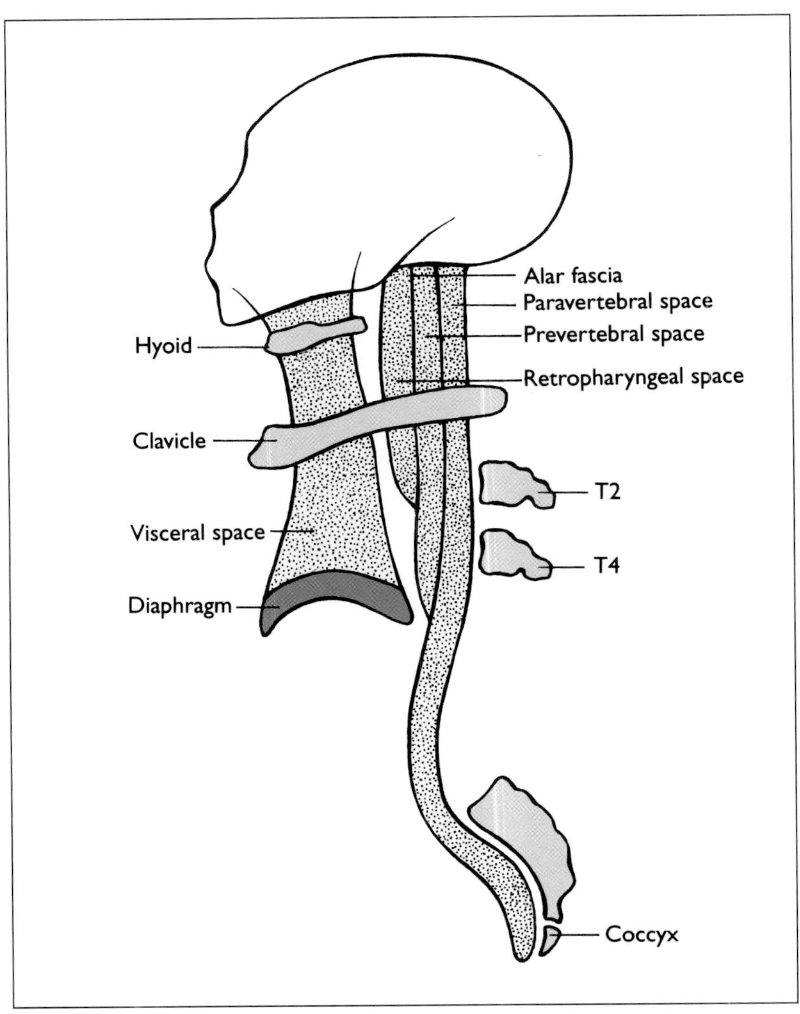

Figure 4-60 The fascial layers of the neck (sagittal view). A fascial plane represents a condensation of connective tissue lying between adjacent structures. Fascial spaces are the potential spaces between these connective tissue planes. When an abscess forms in a space, spread to other spaces occurs along planes of least resistance because of the interrelationship and continuity of all the deep cervical fascia and potential spaces. The fascial layers and space relationships through the length of the neck are shown. The alar fascia is a portion of the deep layer, extending inferiorly from the skull base and attaching to the transverse processes of the vertebrae as it descends to the level of the tracheal bifurcation at T2. This fascial layer separates the retropharyngeal space from the prevertebral space. (*From* Endicott [16].)

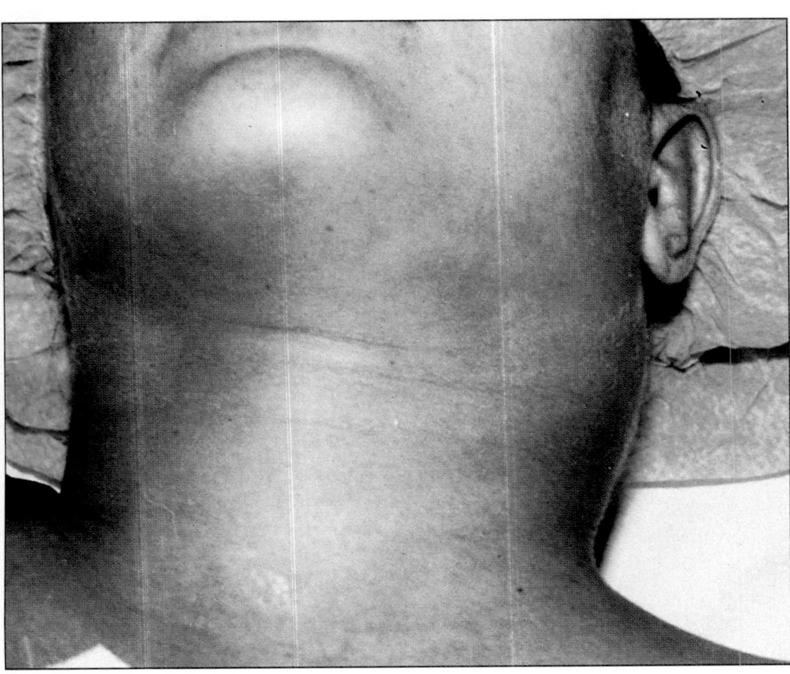

Figure 4-61 Parapharyngeal space abscess. The infection in this patient presented as a rapidly growing unilateral tender neck mass obliterating the angle of the mandible. Such a patient with a deep neck abscess may have an elevated temperature. Sepsis may be present. The most common organisms are *Staphylococcus aureus, Streptococcus* sp., and anaerobic bacteria. The patient should be treated with maximum therapeutic doses of intravenous antibiotics after blood is drawn for culture. High-dose aqueous penicillin G plus clindamycin is the recommended antibiotic treatment for a deep neck abscess. However, β-lactamase–producing aerobic and anaerobic organisms were found in almost one half of head and neck abscesses in children, suggesting that penicillin may no longer be the drug of choice. Clindamycin, chloramphenicol, metronidazole, cefoxitin, imipenem, and the combination of a penicillin (*ie,* amoxicillin or ticarcillin) plus a β-lactamase inhibitor (clavulanic acid) are more appropriate antibiotics for these infections. Surgical drainage is an important adjuvant treatment to antibiotic coverage [17].

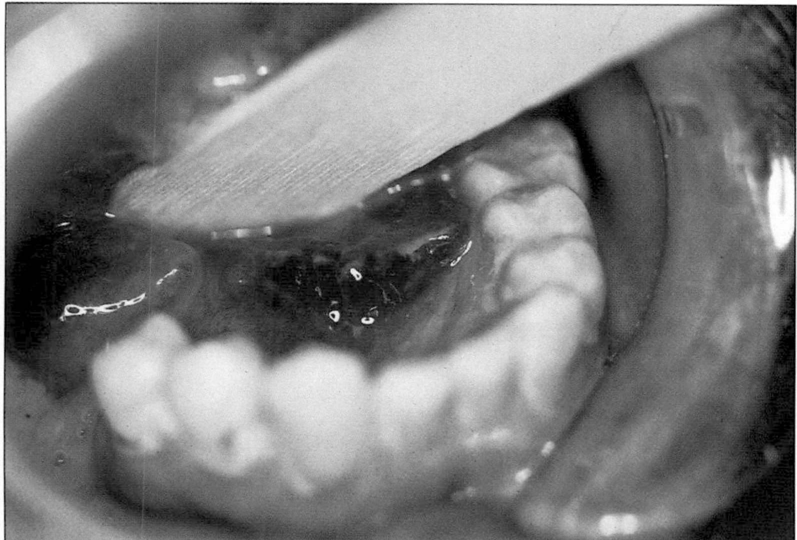

Figure 4-62 Ludwig's angina with bilateral sublingual space infection. A sublingual space abscess responds to intraoral drainage, but when it progresses to the submandibular space followed by a crossover to the opposite side and involvement of similar compartments, Ludwig's angina has developed. This highly virulent infection is a cellulitis and not a true abscess and can cause rapid death from upper airway obstruction or mediastinitis if it descends past the hyoid. Most abscesses in these spaces are of dental origin. A computed tomography scan for this abscess is not helpful in management decisions.

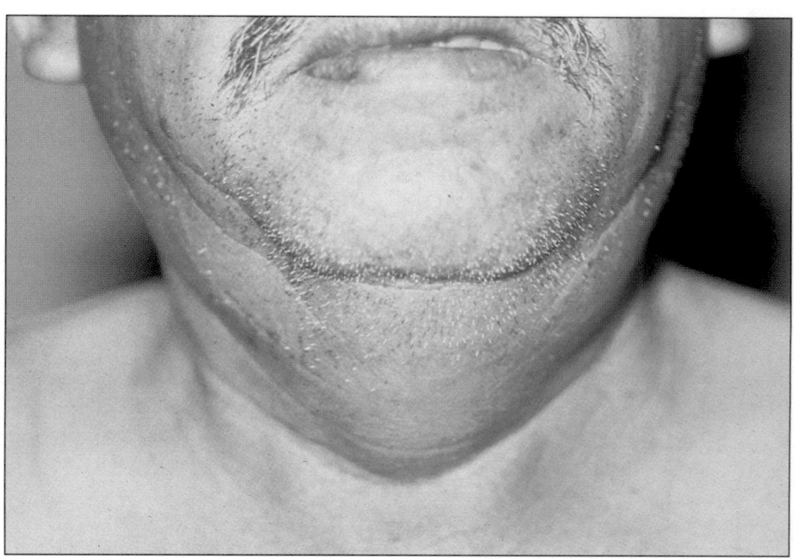

Figure 4-63 Tender bilateral suprahyoid swelling in Ludwig's angina. Originally described by Ludwig in 1836, Ludwig's angina is characterized by a patient in acute distress with the following findings: 1) all the tissues of the floor of the mouth are greatly swollen and extremely inflamed, 2) displacement of the tongue upward and backward toward the palatal vault, 3) woodenlike induration at first confined to the submandibular compartment, 4) trismus, and 5) hoarseness and dyspnea. (*From* Endicott [16]; with permission.)

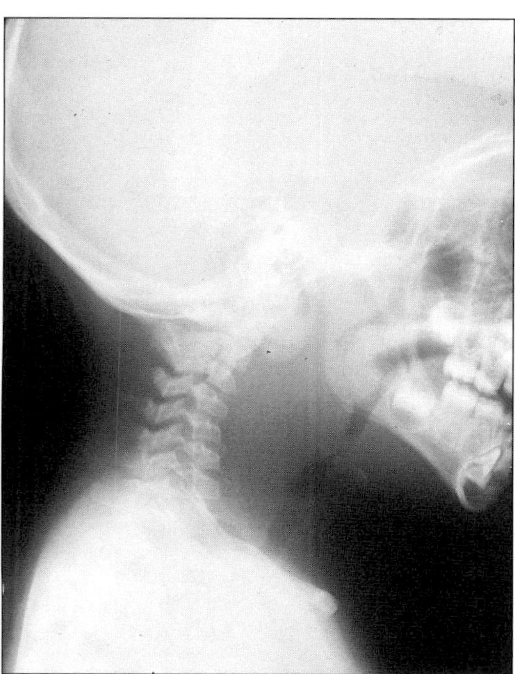

Figure 4-64 Retropharyngeal abscess. Retropharyngeal tissue on this lateral plain film is equal to the width of the body of C_2 in this small child. Normally, it should be no more than one third the width of C_2. Air in the retropharyngeal soft tissues or widening of the prevertebral retropharyngeal soft tissues may also be noted. Although no mass is palpable, this abscess may threaten the airway. Abscesses localized above the hyoid are more common in children under age 4 years secondary to suppurative retropharyngeal nodes, which drain the posterior two thirds of the nose, paranasal sinuses, pharynx, and eustachian tube. A midline fascia divides the retropharyngeal space, restricting abscesses to a position lateral to the midline. The classical appearance of the retropharyngeal abscess is a unilateral swelling of the posterior pharyngeal wall, which may push the palate forward.

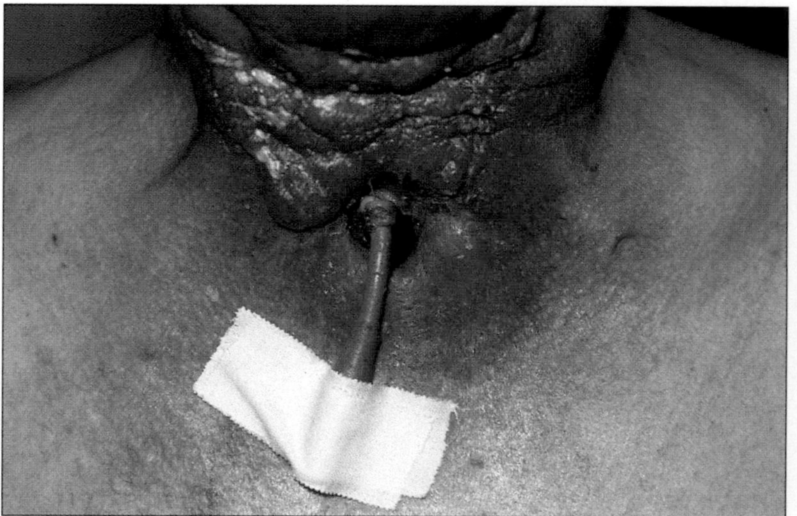

Figure 4-65 Cellulitis after tracheoesophageal puncture. Tracheoesophageal puncture is a major advance in the vocal rehabilitation of laryngectomy patients. The procedure involves the creation of a tracheal-esophageal fistula for placement of a one-way valve prosthesis. Though the procedure is not complex, significant infectious complications are possible. Cellulitis around the puncture site, as illustrated, may occur, requiring postoperative antibiotic coverage for gram-positive organisms and anaerobes. Mediastinitis may occur secondary to puncture of the posterior wall of the esophagus. Pneumonia may result from aspiration of saliva into the trachea secondary to leakage around the prosthesis.

REFERENCES

1. Wald ER:Rhinitis and acute and chronic sinusitis. *In* Bluestone CB, Stool SE (eds.): *Pediatric Otolaryngology*, 2nd ed. Philadelphia: W.B. Saunders; 1990:736.
2. Bull TR: *A Color Atlas of E.N.T. Diagnosis*, 2nd ed. London: Wolfe Medical Publications; 1987:96.
3. Hawke M, Keene M, Alberti PW: *Clinical Otoscopy: A Text and Color Atlas.* Edinburgh: Churchill Livingstone; 1990:59.
4. Hawke M, Keene M, Alberti PW: *Clinical Otoscopy: An Introduction to Ear Diseases*, 2nd ed. Edinburgh: Churchill Livingstone; 1990:79–80.
5. Hawke M, Keene M, Alberti PW: *Clinical Otoscopy: A Text and Color Atlas.* Edinburgh: Churchill Livingstone; 1984:65.
6. Hawke M, Keene M, Alberti PW: *Clinical Otoscopy: A Text and Color Atlas*, Edinburgh: Churchill Livingstone; 1984:76.
7. Taubert KA, Rowley AH, Shulman ST: Nationwide survey of Kawasaki disease and acute rheumatic fever. *J Pediatr* 1991, 119:279–282.
8. Newburger JW, Takahashi M, Beiser AS, *et al.*: A single intravenous infusion of gamma globulin as compared with four infusions in the treatment of acute Kawasaki syndrome. *N Engl J Med* 1991, 324:1663–1639.
9. Riley J, Davis H: Pediatric Otolaryngology. *In* Zitelli B, Davis H (eds.): *The Atlas of Pediatric Diagnosis.* St. Louis: C.V. Mosby; 1987.
10. Benjamin BNP: *Diagnostic Laryngology: Adults and Children.* Philadelphia: W.B. Saunders; 1990.
11. Shah KV, Howley PM: Papillomaviruses. *In* Fields BN, Knipe DM, *et al.* (eds.): *Virology.* New York: Raven Press; 1990:1651–1676.
12. Margileth AM, Hatfield T: A new look at old cat scratch. *Contemp Pediatr* 1990, 7:27.
13. Margileth AM: Nontuberculous [atypical] mycobacterial disease. *Semin Pediatr Infect Dis* 1993, 4:307–315.
14. Margileth AM, Zawadsky P: Chronic adenopathy in children and adolescents. *Am Fam Physician* 1985, 31:178.
15. Lampe RL, *et al.*: Cervicofacial nocardiosis in children. *J Pediatr* 1981, 99:563–565.
16. Endicott J: Infections of the deep fascial spaces of the head and neck: Update of diagnosis and management. *In* Johnson JT, *et al.* (eds.): *AAO-HNS Instructional Courses*, vol 3. St. Louis: Mosby Year-Book; 1990.
17. Brook I: Microbiology of abscesses of the head and neck in children. *Ann Otol Rhinol Laryngol* 1987, 96:429–433.

CHAPTER 5

Sexually Transmitted Diseases

Editor
Michael F. Rein

Contributors
Lawrence Corey
Nicholas J. Fiumara
Laura T. Gutman
Sharon L. Hillier
Robert B. Jones
John N. Krieger
Sandra A. Larsen
Per-Anders Mårdh
Birger Möller
Daniel M. Musher
Jorma Paavonen
Richard Reid
Michael F. Rein
Allan Ronald
Navjeet K. Sidhu-Malik
Jack D. Sobel
Lars Weström
Barbara B. Wilson
Jonathan M. Zenilman

Gonorrhea

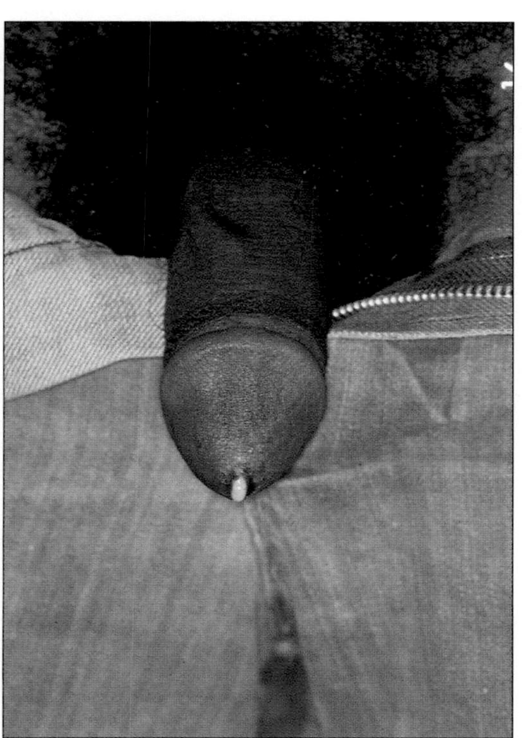

Figure 5-1 Gonococcal urethritis with urethral discharge. On physical examination, a urethral discharge, which is usually purulent, is seen in 90% to 95% of men. The purulent discharge may appear spontaneously at the urethra, without urethral manipulation (stripping). Such appearance of discharge prior to stripping is more common in gonococcal than in nongonococcal urethritis. (*Courtesy of* M.F. Rein, MD.)

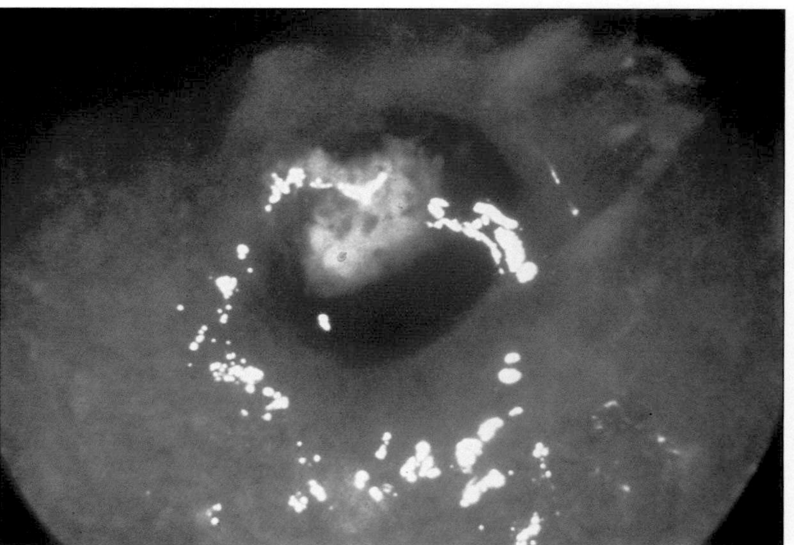

Figure 5-2 Mucopurulent gonococcal cervicitis. On physical examination, the typical appearance of gonococcal infection in women includes cervical edema, erythema, and mucopurulent discharge, yielding mucopurulent cervicitis. The differential diagnosis of mucopurulent cervicitis includes gonococcal cervicitis, chlamydial cervicitis, herpetic cervicitis, chronic dysplastic changes due to human papillomavirus disease, and cervical inflammation due to chronic vaginitis.

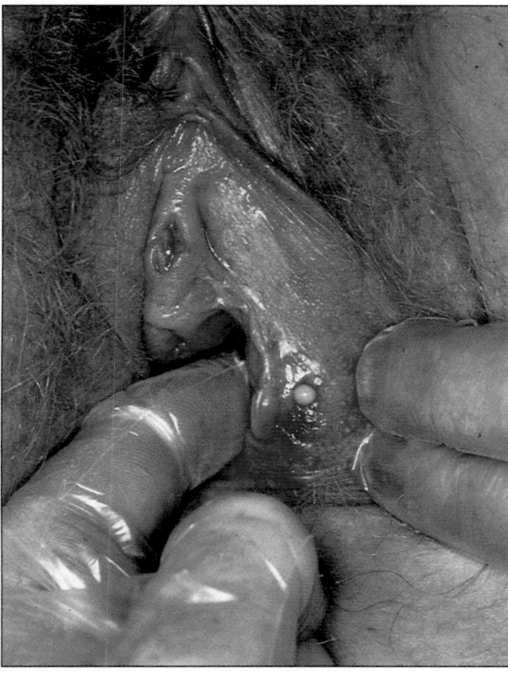

Figure 5-3 Bartholinitis. Bartholinitis and inflammation of the labial glandular structures are occasionally seen in women with gonococcal infection. These conditions manifest as acute, painful swelling of the labial folds, and often, a discrete mass can be visualized on physical examination. In bartholinitis, purulent discharge can be expressed from the duct by applying pressure to the gland. The swollen gland itself is visible in this image, but normally Bartholin's glands are neither palpable nor visible.

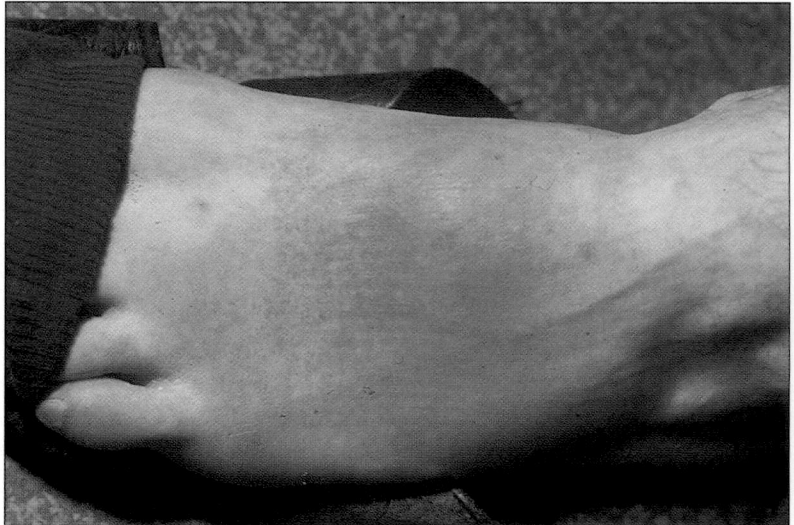

Figure 5-4 Gonococcal tenosynovitis. The arthritis of disseminated gonococcal infection is often accompanied by inflammation of the overlying tendons. This finding helps differentiate gonococcal arthritis from other infections. The tenosynovitis is sometimes visible as erythema overlying the tendons. (*Courtesy of* the Centers for Disease Control and Prevention.)

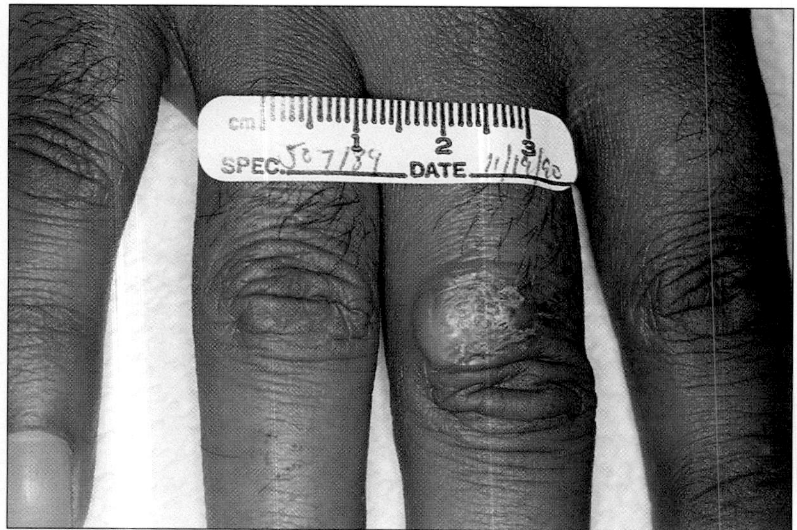

FIGURE 5-5 Rash of disseminated gonococcal infection. The rash of disseminated gonococcal infection manifests as a sparse distribution of papular, vesicular, or pustular lesions, usually on the extensor surfaces of the extremities. Pustular lesion of disseminated gonococcal infection on the right middle finger. Disseminated gonococcal infection is easily treated with appropriate antibiotics, such as quinolones or third-generation cephalosporins. Current recommendations call for a full week of antibiotic treatment.

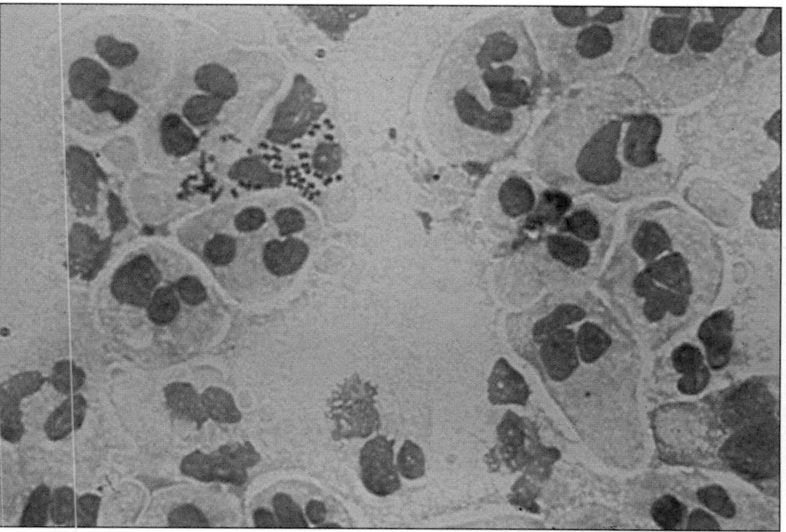

FIGURE 5-6 Positive Gram stain of urethral smear. In the clinic setting, the Gram stain usually is used for presumptive diagnosis of gonococcal infection. Urethral Gram stain in symptomatic men has a sensitivity and specificity of > 95%. Gonococcal urethritis is demonstrated by the presence of > 5 leukocytes/oil-immersion field and observation of gram-negative intracellular diplococci. Some men, particularly those who have recently urinated, have smaller numbers of leukocytes.

CHLAMYDIAL INFECTIONS

Laboratory diagnosis of uncomplicated *Chlamydia trachomatis* infection

	Sensitivity, %	Specificity, %
Culture	52–92	99–100
Antigen detection or nucleic acid hybridization	50–70	95–99
Rapid tests	48–75	95–98
PCR	65–95	> 99
LCR	85–95	> 99
Serology	85–100	< 65

LCR—ligase chain reaction; PCR—polymerase chain reaction.

FIGURE 5-7 Laboratory diagnosis of uncomplicated *Chlamydia trachomatis* infection. Although culture remains the gold standard for diagnosis of chlamydia infection, antigen detection or nucleic acid hybridization techniques have been developed that may be used instead. These include enzyme-linked immunosorbent assays, direct fluorescent antibody tests, and nucleic acid hybridization. Rapid tests refer to kits designed for office use and are based on an immunosorbent or nucleic acid hybridization assay. Both the polymerase chain reaction and the ligase chain reaction appear to be more sensitive than culture by 30% or more. However, both have problems with inhibitors causing falsely negative results at some body sites (particularly the endocervix) and cross-contamination in inexperienced laboratories. Both tests have been used successfully to detect genital infection using urine as a primary specimen and may offer a means for noninvasive screening in the future. Serologic evaluation, including complement fixation and microimmunofluorescence tests, is useful in population-based studies but, because of its low specificity, is not useful in the diagnosis of current (as opposed to past) infection in individuals [1].

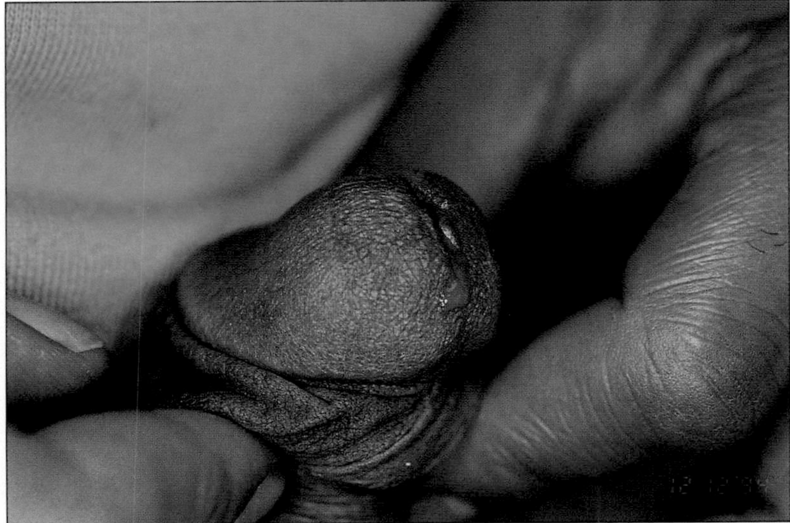

Figure 5-8 Urethral discharge from a man with chlamydial urethritis. There is considerable overlap between signs and symptoms of gonococcal and chlamydial urethritis. However, in newly acquired chlamydial urethritis, the discharge tends to be scant, thin, and watery, whereas in gonococcal urethritis, it is usually more copious and purulent. The incubation period usually is longer in chlamydial urethritis (7–10 days) than in gonococcal urethritis (3–5 days).

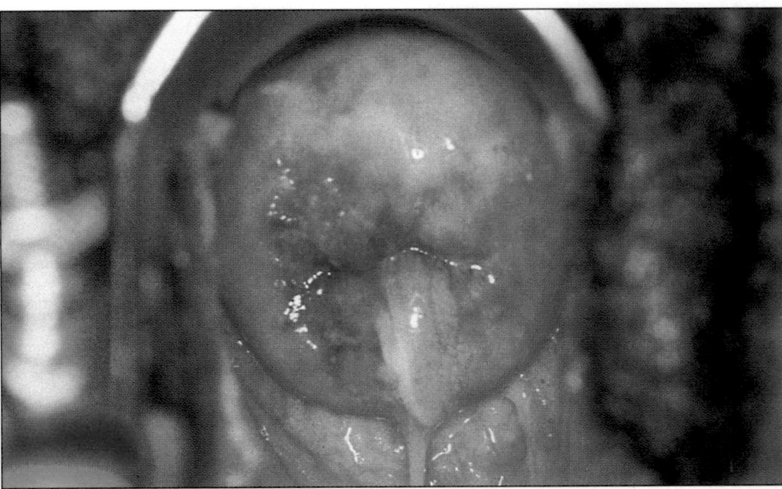

Figure 5-9 Mucopurulent cervicitis photographed at colposcopy. Mucopurulent cervicitis is a clinical diagnosis made during a speculum examination of the cervix. The diagnosis depends on the presence of yellow-green discharge in the endocervical os (although the color is better assessed against the white background of a swab). Mucopurulent cervicitis is highly associated with infection with *Neisseria gonorrhoeae* and *Chlamydia trachomatis*, but especially with the latter. Recovery of *C. trachomatis* also is associated in a linear fashion with the number of polymorphonuclear leukocytes detected per high-power field in a Gram stain of the endocervical exudate. (*Courtesy of* D. Soper, MD.)

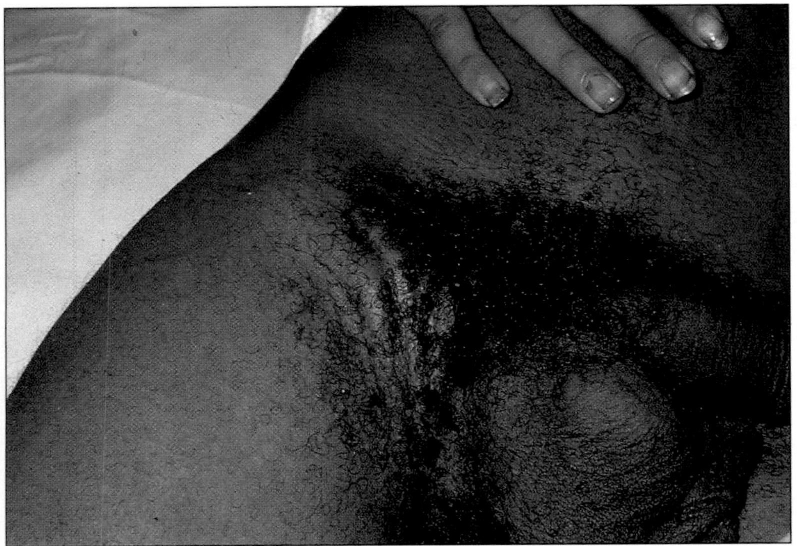

Figure 5-10 Unilateral inguinal and femoral lymphadenopathy in a man with lymphogranuloma venereum. The inguinal and femoral nodes on the patient's right are enlarged with overlying erythema, and they are divided by the inguinal ligament (groove sign). A vesicular primary lesion is evident near the base of the penile shaft. Untreated, the involved nodes would continue to enlarge with periadenitis to form a firm mass or bubo. Over time, the buboes may become fluctuant and drain spontaneously or involute. (*Courtesy of* A. Hood, MD.)

Bacterial Vaginosis

Diagnostic criteria for bacterial vaginosis
1. Homogeneous discharge
2. Distinct fishy odor released immediately after mixing vaginal secretions with 10% KOH (amine whiff test)
3. Vaginal pH > 4.5
4. Clue cells and characteristic alterations of vaginal microflora on microscopy

KOH—potassium hydroxide.

Figure 5-11 Diagnostic criteria for bacterial vaginosis. Patients complaining of vaginal discharge and odor and having a grayish-white, thin, adherent, homogeneous discharge on speculum examination can be diagnosed with bacterial vaginosis with reasonable certainty if they meet three of the four criteria outlined in the table. Wet mount microscopy demonstrating many "clue" cells and Gram stain showing altered vaginal flora are the most specific criteria for establishing the diagnosis [2].

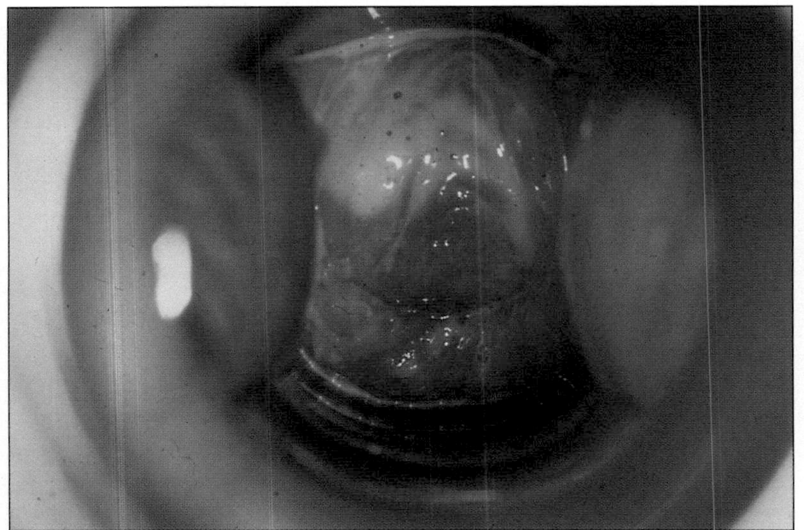

FIGURE 5-12 Speculum examination of a women with bacterial vaginosis showing adherent homogeneous discharge. Whereas the normal vaginal discharge is finely floccular, the discharge in bacterial vaginosis is homogeneous and often manifests small bubbles. The discharge is relatively thin, but, as here, it adheres to vaginal structures. An inflammatory response with erythema of the vaginal walls is usually absent. (*Courtesy of* H.L. Gardner, MD.)

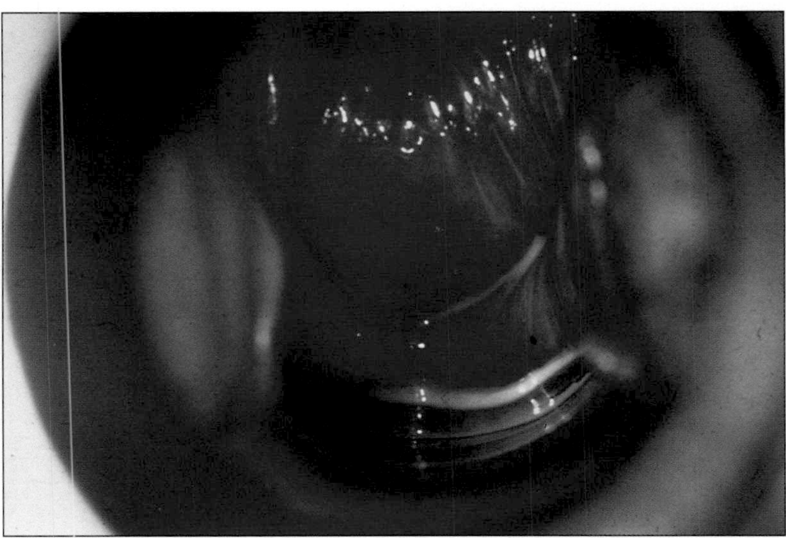

FIGURE 5-13 Speculum examination of a women with bacterial vaginosis showing little discharge. In many women, little discharge is present. Here, a very small amount of discharge has pooled in the posterior fornix. A characteristic bubble can be seen. Women with limited discharge may note vaginal odor as the only symptom of disease. The examiner should recognize that because of the adherent nature of the discharge, the discharge may be observed only as an increased light reflex returned from the vagina walls. (*Courtesy of* H.L. Gardner, MD.)

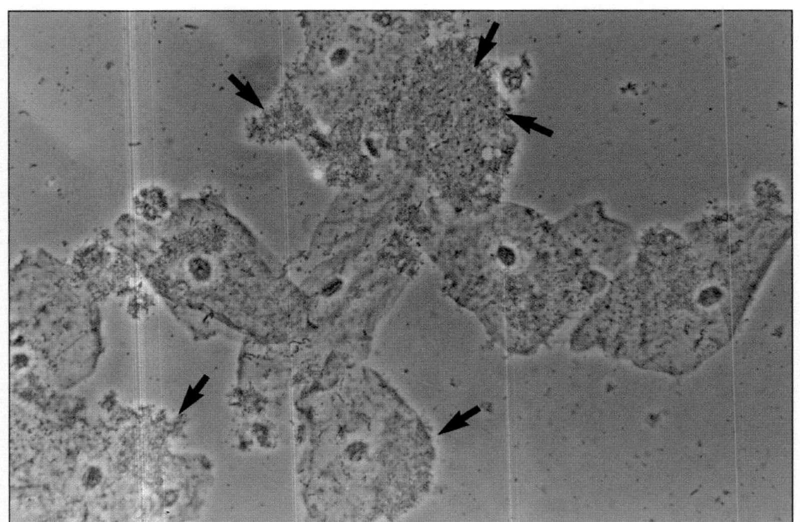

FIGURE 5-14 Microscopic examination for clue cells in vaginal fluid from a woman with bacterial vaginosis. A second wet mount preparation of vaginal fluid is examined under high-power (× 400) microscopy for clue cells (*arrows*). Clue cells are squamous epithelial cells having a granular appearance and indistinct cell borders obscured by adherent microorganisms. Clue cells are the single best clinical indicator of bacterial vaginosis and result from the attachment of *Gardnerella vaginalis*, anaerobic gram-negative rods, and gram-positive cocci to the cells. If at least one in five epithelial cells in the vaginal fluid is a clue cell, the specimen is categorized as clue cell positive. A few clue cells may be present in the vaginal fluid of women without bacterial vaginosis, caused by lactobacilli that bind to vaginal epithelial cells.

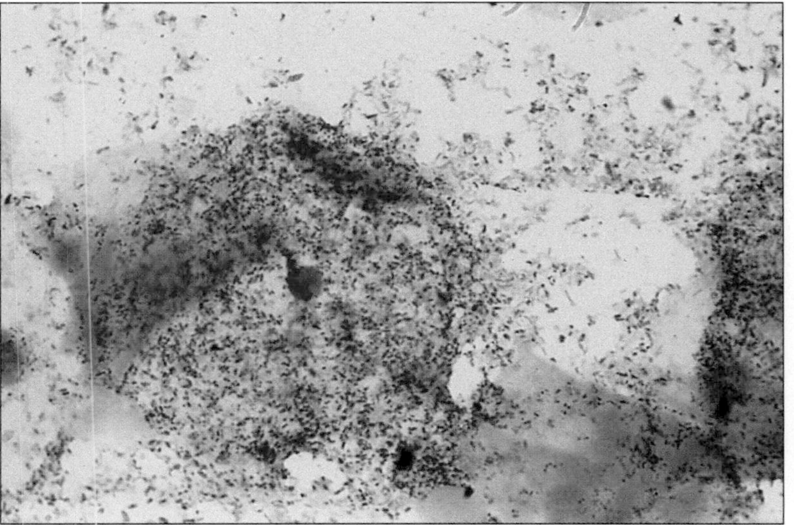

FIGURE 5-15 Gram-stained vaginal smear from a women with bacterial vaginosis. A large clue cell with edges covered by bacteria is visible in the center of the field. The *Lactobacillus* morphotypes have been replaced by small gram-negative anaerobic rods (*Prevotella*, *Porphyromonas*, *Bacteroides*) and small gram-variable rods (*Gardnerella vaginalis*). Mycoplasmas lack cell walls and therefore are not visible by Gram stain. The epithelial cell at the bottom of the field is a squamous epithelial cell without attached bacteria.

Pelvic Inflammatory Disease

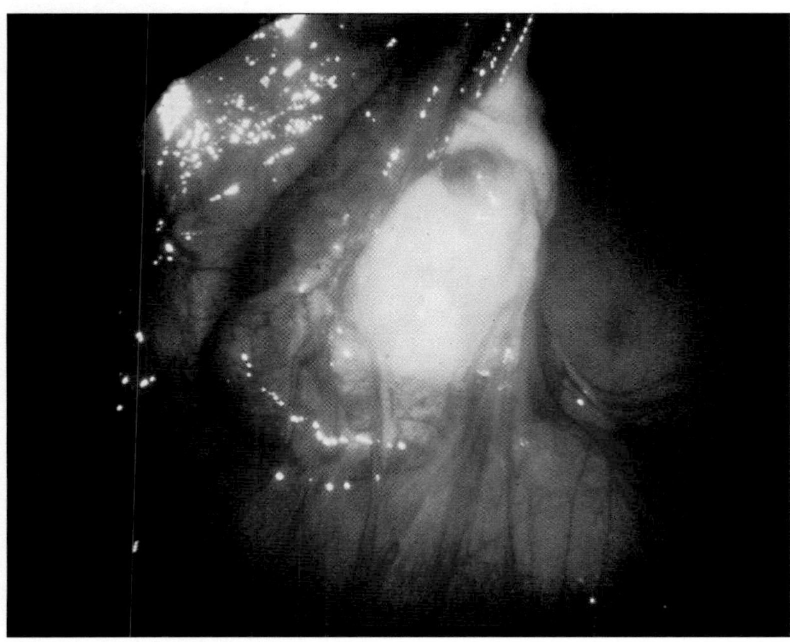

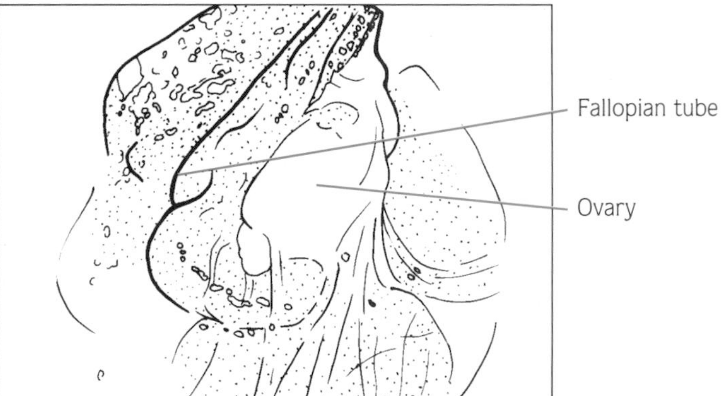

Figure 5-16 Laparoscopic view of moderately severe PID, showing distended, inflamed fallopian tube and ovary. The fallopian tube is slightly distended and hyperemic. Purulent exudate, exiting the fimbriated end of the tube, covers the ovary. Laparoscopy provides the opportunity to examine the fallopian tubes, appendix, liver, and other intra-abdominal organs, as well as to grade the severity of salpingitis. Intra-abdominal spread may occur in up to one fourth of chlamydial PID cases.

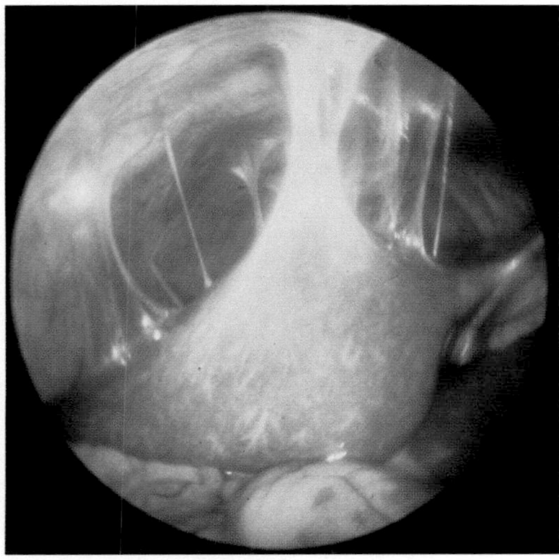

Figure 5-17 Violin-string adhesions in chlamydial PID and perihepatitis. The role of the violin-string adhesions in the pathogenesis of chronic abdominal pain is uncertain. Some gynecologists recommend resolving the adhesions to improve mobility of structures in the abdominal cavity. Before chlamydiae were known to be genital tract pathogens, these adhesions were considered typical for intra-abdominal gonococcal infection.

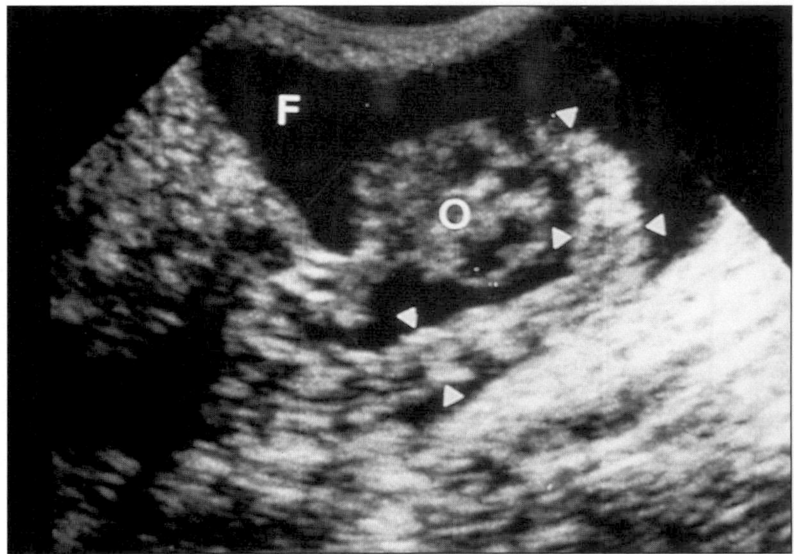

Figure 5-18 Vaginal ultrasound in PID, showing free pelvic fluid (*F*) and enlarged ovary (*O*). The fallopian tube (*arrowheads*) is thickened, the ovary is enlarged, and free fluid is seen in the peritoneum. Although not a diagnostic test, ultrasound is useful in distinguishing among the complications of PID, such as tuboovarian abscess, and other pelvic masses, such as ectopic pregnancy or ovarian cysts.

Trichomoniasis

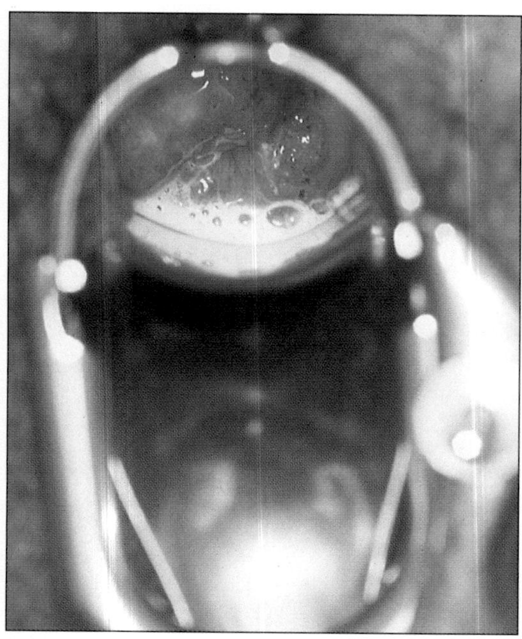

Figure 5-19 Frothy vaginal discharge in trichomoniasis. Speculum examination of woman with trichomoniasis reveals a profuse, foul-smelling discharge containing bubbles. The discharge is loose and pools in the posterior fornix. Redness of the exocervix is also appreciated. Some workers claim that the bubbles in trichomoniasis appear larger than those frequently accompanying bacterial vaginosis. The cervical discharge is seen to be mucoid; *Trichomonas vaginalis* causes vaginitis and exocervicitis but not endocervicitis; thus, a mucopurulent cervical discharge should raise suspicion of coincident gonococcal or chlamydial infection. (*From* Rein [3]; with permission.)

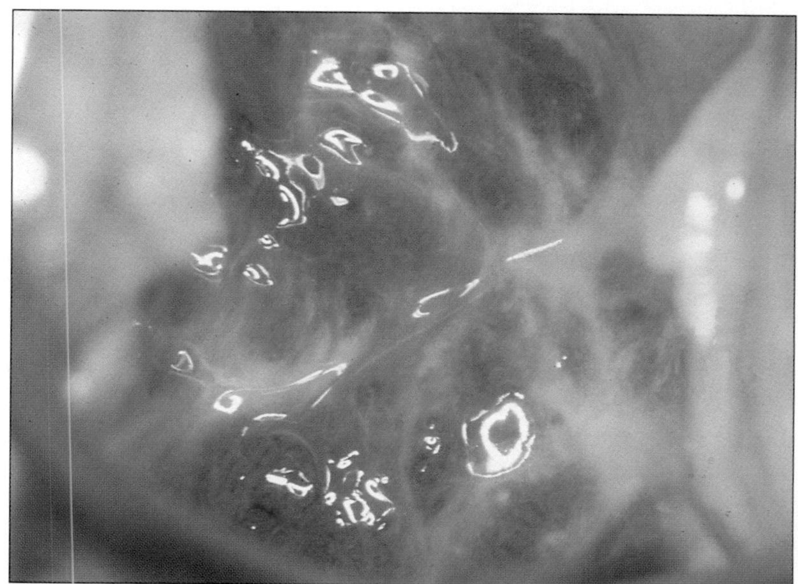

Figure 5-20 Speculum examination demonstrating florid granular vaginitis in a woman with chronic trichomoniasis. With the naked eye, the vaginal walls are recognized as erythematous in one to two thirds of women with trichomoniasis. In severe infection, the vaginal walls are characterized by dilation of blood vessels and capillary proliferation, yielding the granular appearance. When viewed through the colposcope, such inflamed vaginal walls reveal a characteristic double cresting of capillaries [4]. (*From* Rein [5]; with permission.)

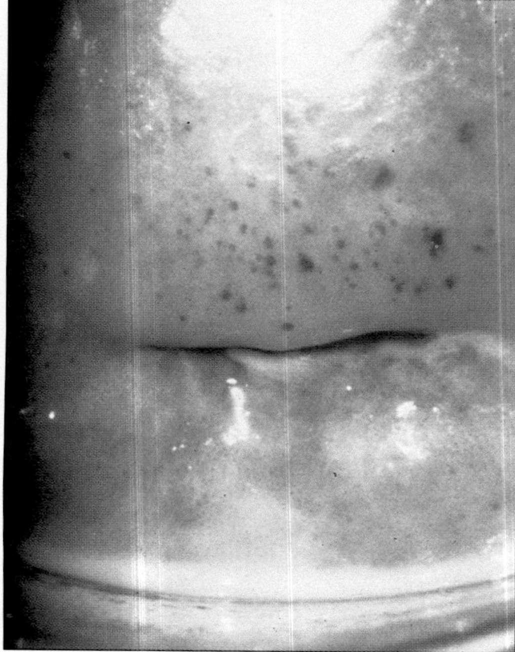

Figure 5-21 Colposcopic view of colpitis macularis in trichomoniasis showing small hemorrhages. Such hemorrhages are quite specific for trichomoniasis. Microscopic examination of biopsy specimens reveals superficial ulcerations and infiltration with polymorphonuclear neutrophils [6].

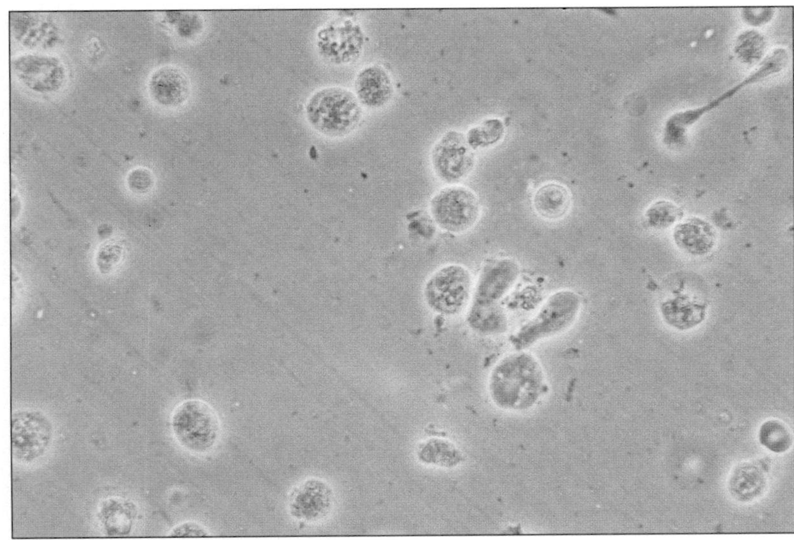

Figure 5-22 Phase photomicrograph of vaginal wet mount in trichomoniasis. Wet mount shows four trichomonads, numerous, polymorphonuclear neutrophils (which are close in size to trichomonads), and occasional red blood cells. The wet mount will identify trichomonads in about two-thirds of infected women. (Original magnification, × 400.) [7]

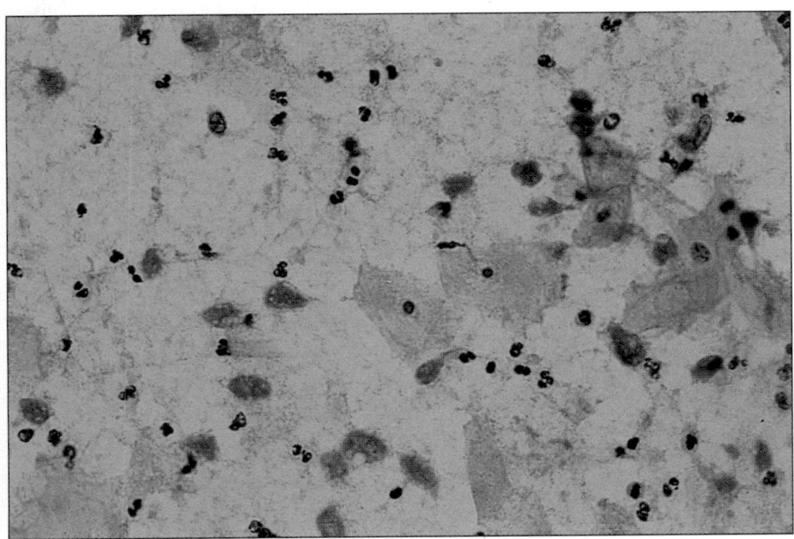

Figure 5-23 Papanicolaou-stained specimen containing *Trichomonas vaginalis*. The Papanicolaou smear, which stains the trichomonads green, has a sensitivity of about 60%. False-positive smears are also reported, even by experienced cytologists. Thus, cytologic diagnosis should be confirmed using another method [8].

Vulvovaginal Candidiasis

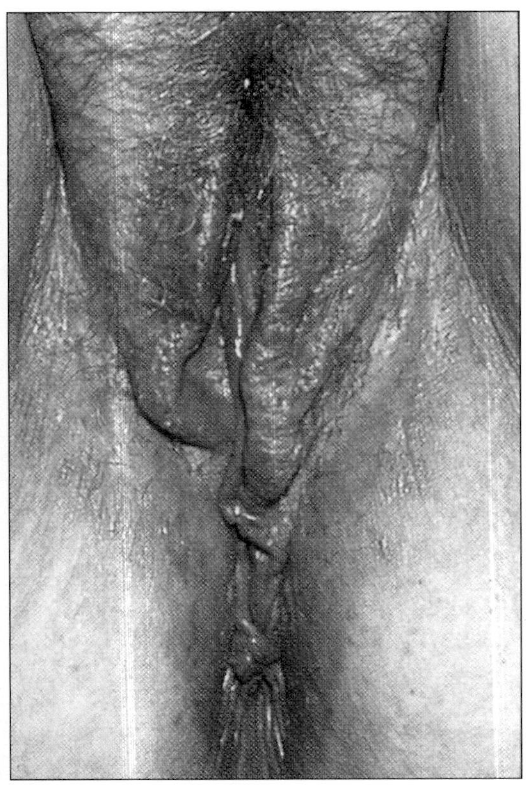

Figure 5-24 Vulvar edema and erythema. Characteristic findings in vulvovaginal candidiasis include edema, erythema, and fissures, with prominent vulvar manifestations.

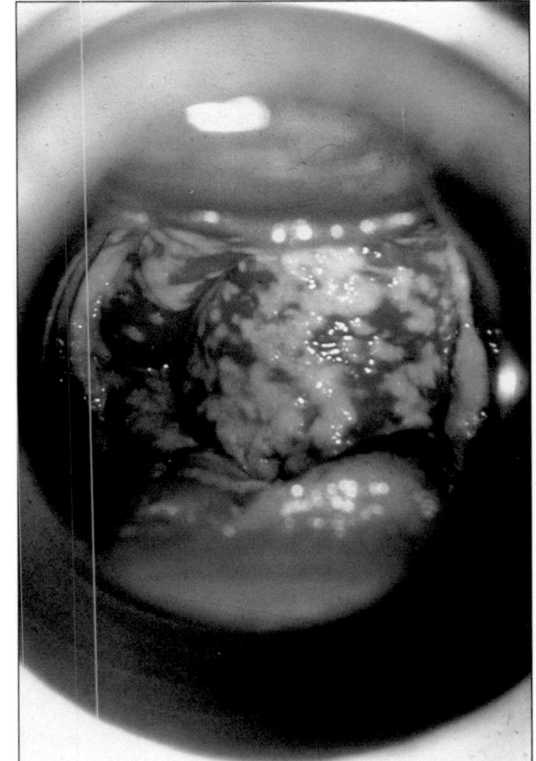

Figure 5-25 Typical cottage cheese–like discharge in vaginal candidiasis. The typical "cottage cheese," white discharge seen on speculum examination is found in only a minority of patients with *Candida* vaginitis. Most women manifest a thinner discharge that is less etiologically specific.

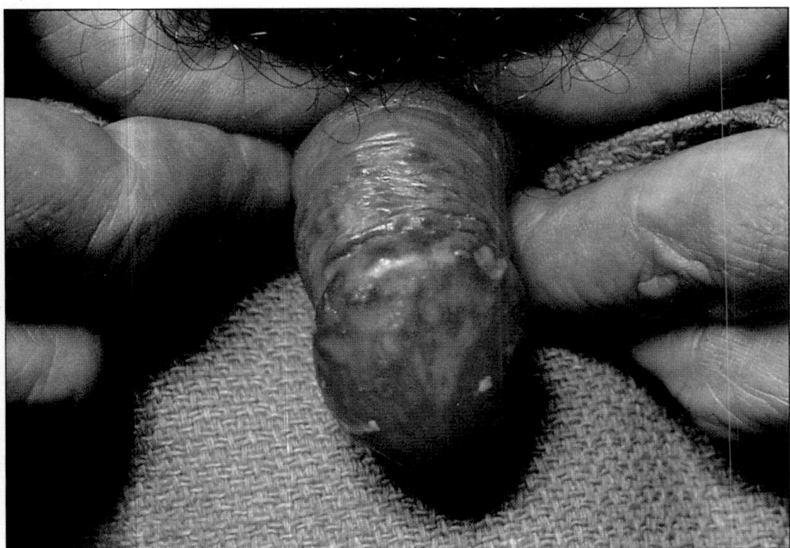

Figure 5-26 *Candida* balanoposthitis. Candida balanoposthitis presents with penile itching, irritation, and soreness, accompanied by edema, erythema, and excoriation. It is seen in the male partners of women with a vaginal culture positive for *Candida albicans*. Only a small fraction of the male partners of women with vulvovaginal candidiasis will develop superficial genital candidiasis.

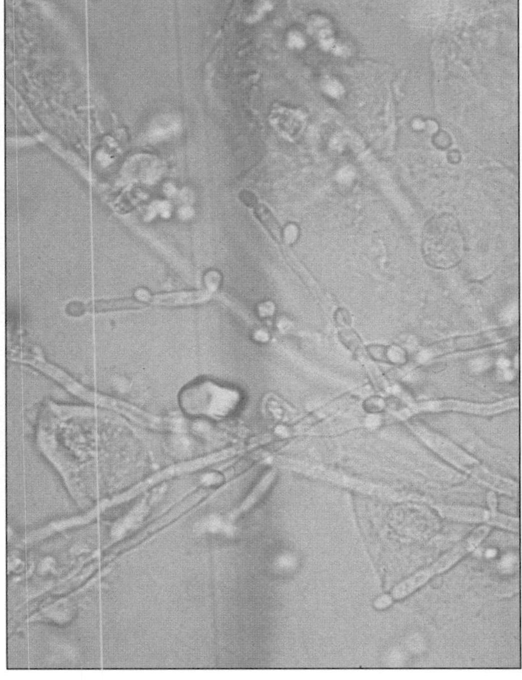

Figure 5-27 Saline microscopy. Although a number of techniques are used, most frequently a swab obtained from the middle third of the vagina is immediately placed in 0.5 mL of saline in a test tube. Then, a single drop of the resultant solution is placed on a clean dry slide and a coverslip applied. Initially under low power, the presence of motile trichomonads, polymorphonuclear neutrophils (PMNs), and hyphae can be detected. Under high-power magnification, a search is made for clue cells, trichomonads, PMNs, yeast blastospores and pseudohyphae, and epithelial cell maturation (squamous versus basal and parabasal cells). Finally, the bacterial flora is assessed (rods versus cocci).

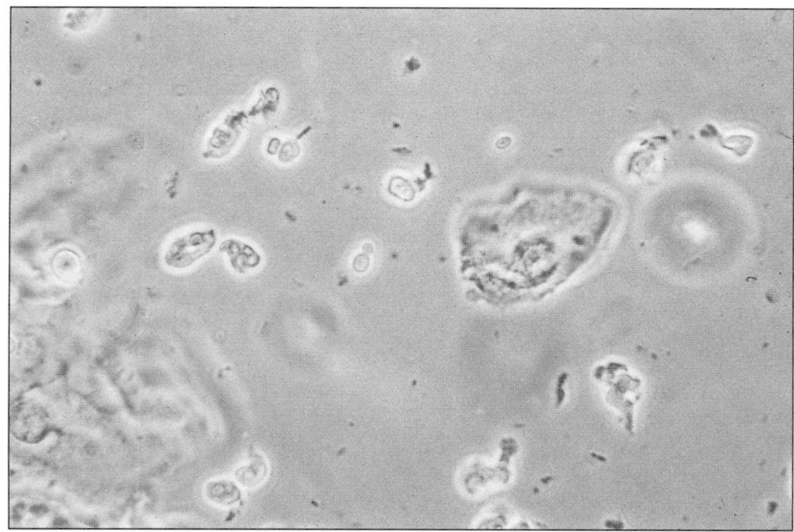

FIGURE 5-28 Phase microscopic examination (wet mount) of vaginal discharge in vulvovaginal candidiasis (VVC). Many patients with symptomatic VVC have small numbers of yeasts in the vaginal pool. The overall sensitivity of wet mount in the diagnosis of VVC may be as low as 50%, and thus, a negative wet mount does not rule out the diagnosis. This figure shows a single budding yeast and, above it and to the right, a single yeast cell. There are several epithelial cells, alone or in clumps. Polymorphonuclear neutrophils are present, as are bacilli, which presumably represent normal lactobacillary flora. (*Courtesy of* M.F. Rein, MD.)

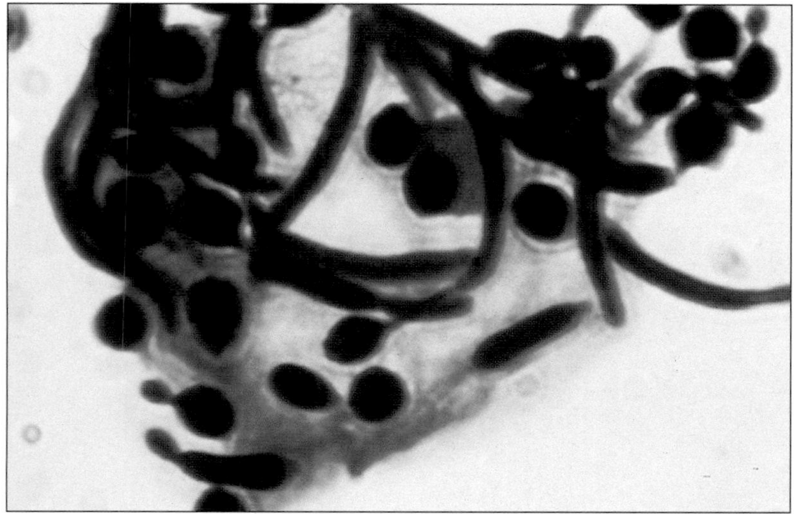

FIGURE 5-29 Gram stain of vaginal squamous epithelial cell with adherent blastospores, budding yeast, and pseudohyphae. The pseudohyphae often have a beaded appearance on Gram stain.

SYPHILIS: EPIDEMIOLOGY AND LABORATORY TESTING

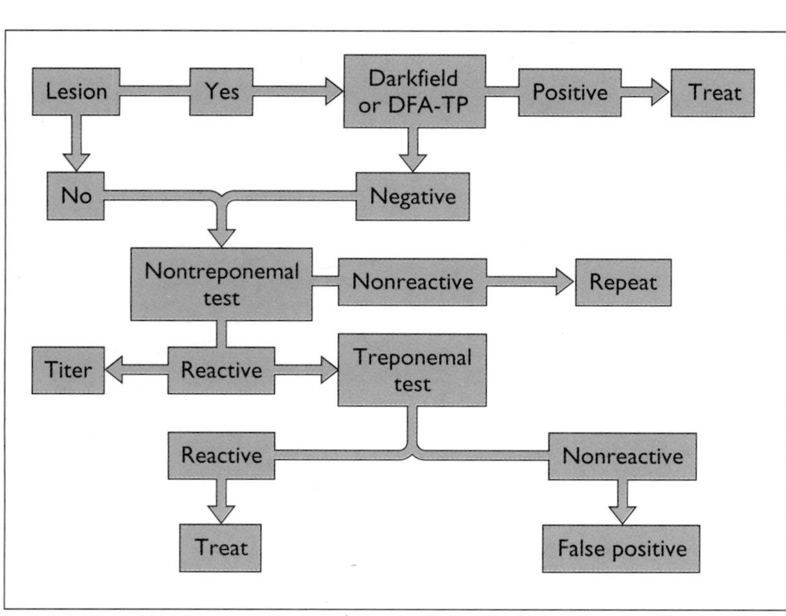

FIGURE 5-30 Routine testing scheme for syphilis. If lesions are present, routine testing consists of direct microscopic examination, either by darkfield microscopy or direct fluorescent antibody for *Treponema pallidum* (DFA-TP). If lesions are not present or are healing, then first a nontreponemal test is used to screen for syphilis, with a reactive result confirmed by a treponemal test. The nontreponemal tests can be quantitated to determine an endpoint titer. A fourfold decrease in titer after treatment indicates a successful response to treatment, whereas a fourfold increase in titer usually indicates relapse or reinfection. The routine testing scheme does not need to be altered for HIV-positive individuals, but direct microscopic examination is even more important in these individuals because a delay in antibody response may occur in immunosuppressed individuals [9].

Primary and Secondary Syphilis

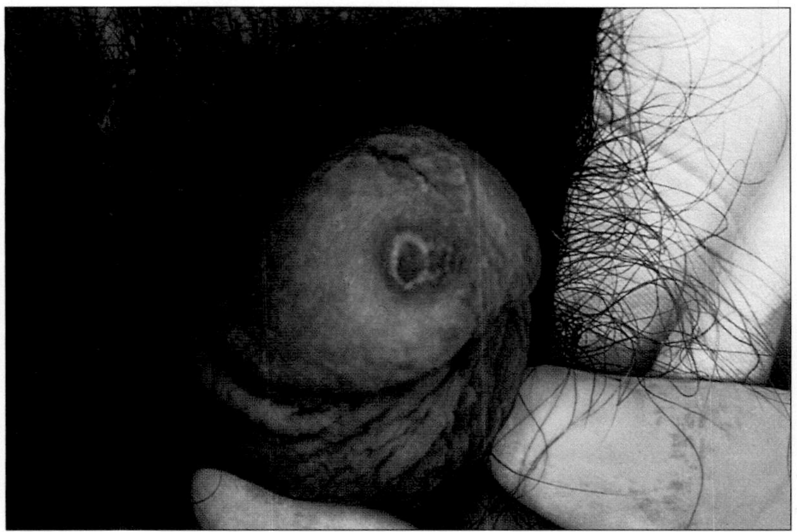

Figure 5-31 Typical chancre of primary syphilis on glans penis. The typical appearance of the chancre is shown. Such lesions are usually indurated, indolent, and nontender. The ulcerations may be large or small but are always indurated and sharply demarcated. The chancre appears after an average of 3 weeks after infection, but the incubation period can range from 9 to 90 days. Intercurrent antibiotics can delay or dramatically modify the appearance of the chancre. Regional lymphadenopathy accompanies the chancre. Classically referred to as satellite bubo, involved nodes are moderately enlarged, discrete, and nontender. The inguinal nodes regularly enlarge because syphilis first spreads throughout the lymphatic vessels. The chancre heals spontaneously within about 3 to 6 weeks but may persist for up to 3 months and overlap the manifestations of secondary syphilis.

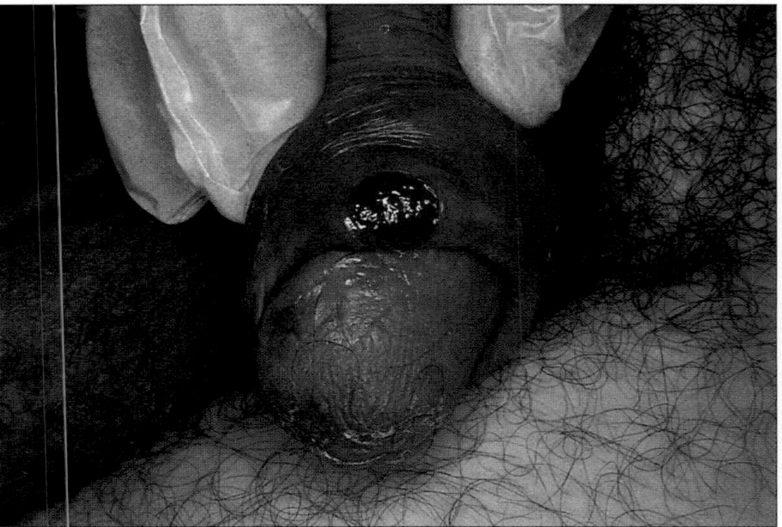

Figure 5-32 Chancre on the prepuce in primary syphilis. Chancres of the prepuce, like those of the glans, are indurated and nontender. Several studies have suggested an increased incidence of sexually transmitted diseases among uncircumcised men; the mechanism is unknown, but theories include delays in diagnosis of hidden lesions, increased proliferation of organisms beneath the foreskin, or even increased susceptibility of the foreskin itself.

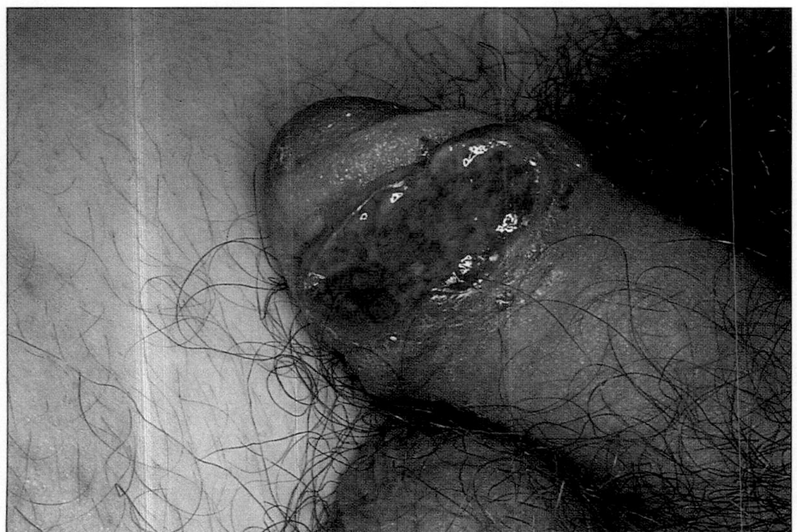

Figure 5-33 Multiple penile chancres in primary syphilis. Multiple chancres have merged together, forming a large ulceration at the corona of the penis, which is the most common site for penile chancres. Multiple chancres are seen in approximately 40% of cases. The rapid plasma reagin blood test is universally reactive when the chancre is 7 days old.

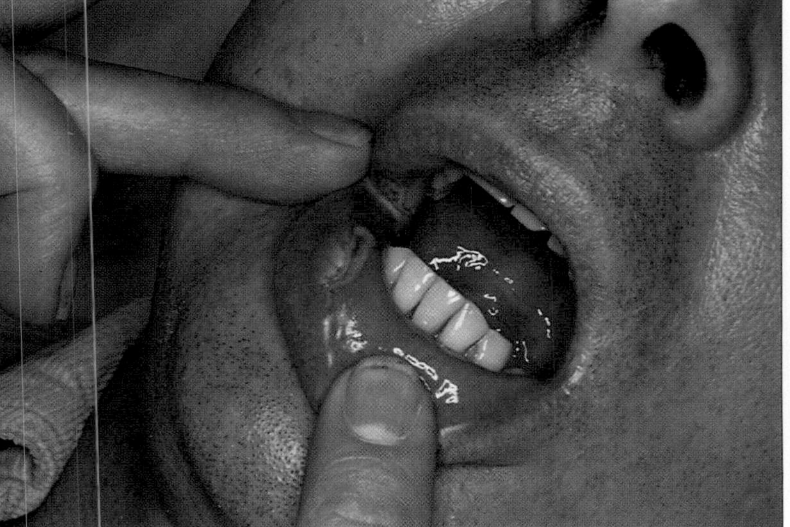

Figure 5-34 Oral chancres in primary syphilis. A chancre developed on the lower lip of a man, caused by performing fellatio. Most chancres of the lip result from open-mouth or "wet" kisses and tend to occur on the upper lip in the man and the lower lip in the woman (due to the mechanics of kissing in our culture). The infecting partner is usually in the secondary stage of syphilis, with mucous patches in the mouth. Chancres resulting from fellatio are usually on the lower lip or at the commissure of the mouth. During preliminary sex play, whether kissing or fellatio, microscopic tears occur that become the portal of entry for the spirochete of syphilis. (*From* Fiumara [10]; with permission.)

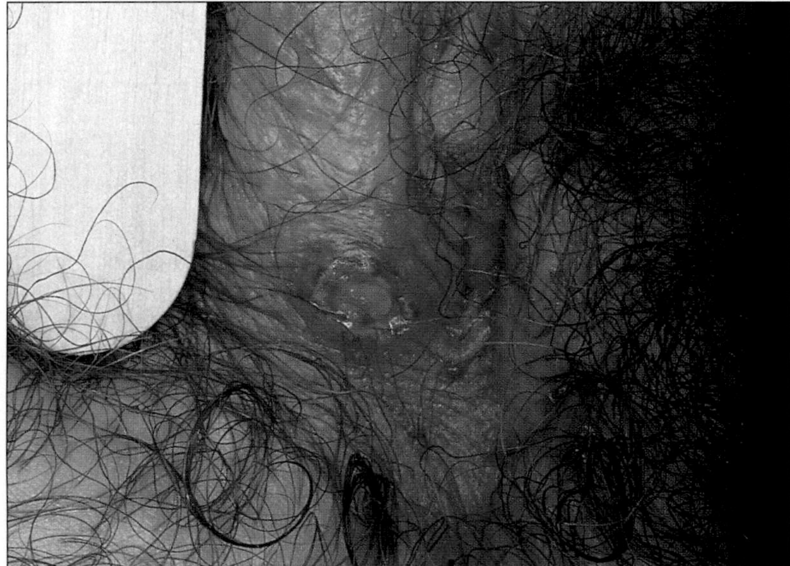

Figure 5-35 Vaginal chancre in primary syphilis. A typical indurated, nontender chancre is seen on the lower pole of the right labium. The right inguinal node is discretely enlarged and also nontender. Most chancres in women appear in the lower portions of the labia. Whereas the external genitalia and distal two thirds of the vagina drain to the inguinofemoral nodes, the cervix and proximal third of the vagina drain to the deep iliac nodes. Thus, chancres at these latter locations may not be accompanied by palpable lymphadenopathy.

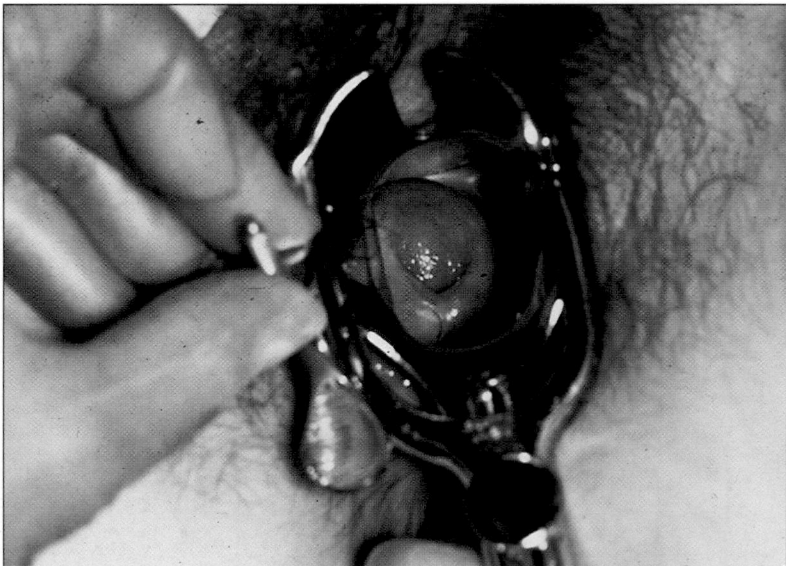

Figure 5-36 Cervical chancre in primary syphilis. A sharply circumscribed ulceration is seen on the cervix. Chancres are often not noticed in women, and primary syphilis is usually not detected unless the woman is identified as a contact of an individual with infectious syphilis.

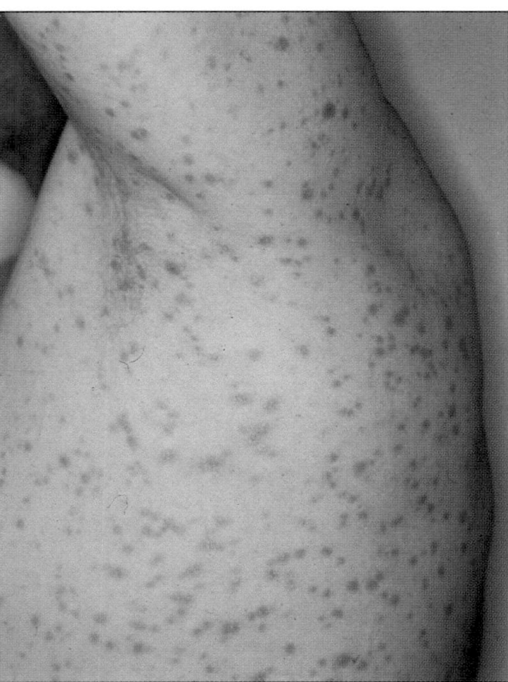

Figure 5-37 Maculopapular rash of secondary syphilis on the trunk. The symptoms of secondary syphilis appear about a month after the onset of primary syphilis or about 8 weeks after the infectious exposure. This patient had flulike symptoms, rash, and generalized adenopathy. The rash may be macular, maculopapular, papular, or pustular. In this patient, the maculopapular rash also involved the midface, with mucous patches in the mouth, oval lesions in the lines of cleavage of the skin, which superficially resembled pityriasis rosea, and lesions on the palms and soles.

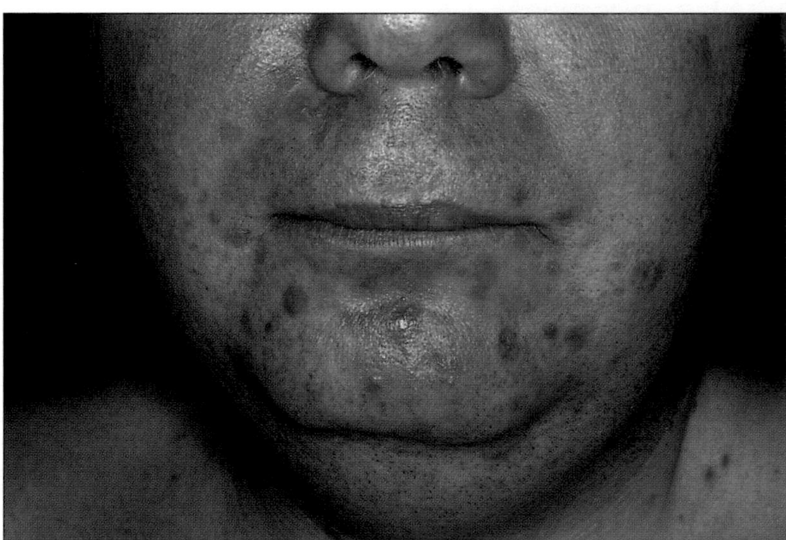

Figure 5-38 Papular lesions of secondary syphilis on the face and chin. Papular lesions are seen on the middle of the face and the chin in this patient who also has AIDS. A few case reports suggest an increased frequency of malignant syphilis, with rapidly progressive and destructive lesions, in patients with advanced HIV disease. These lesions may also occur on the upper trunk.

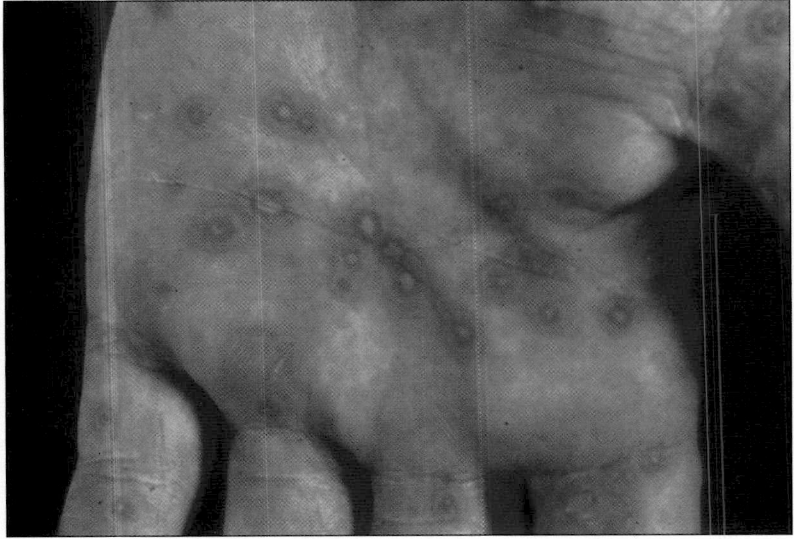

FIGURE 5-39 Palmar lesions of secondary syphilis. Papular lesions of the palms are seen crossing the creases. If lesions of secondary syphilis are present on the palms, they should also be looked for elsewhere on the skin and mucous membranes.

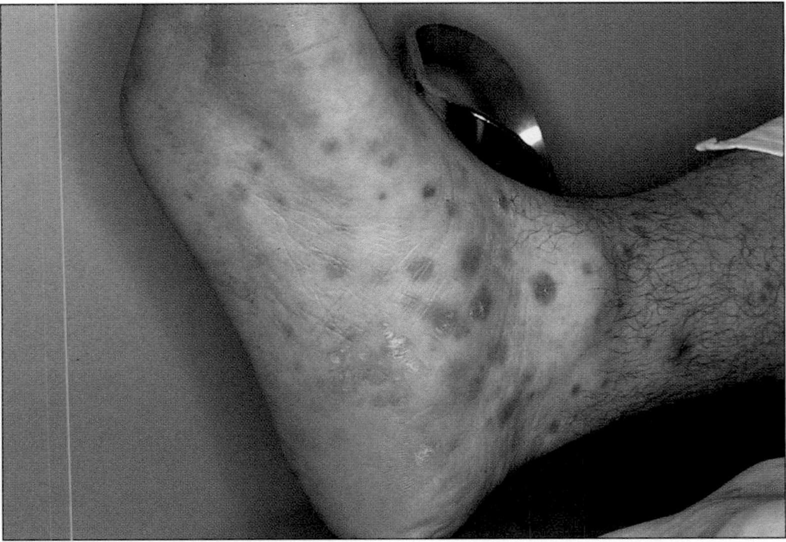

FIGURE 5-40 Papular lesions of secondary syphilis on the soles and ankles. These lesions are hard, nontender, and nonpruritic. One half to two thirds of patients will have lesions on the palms and soles.

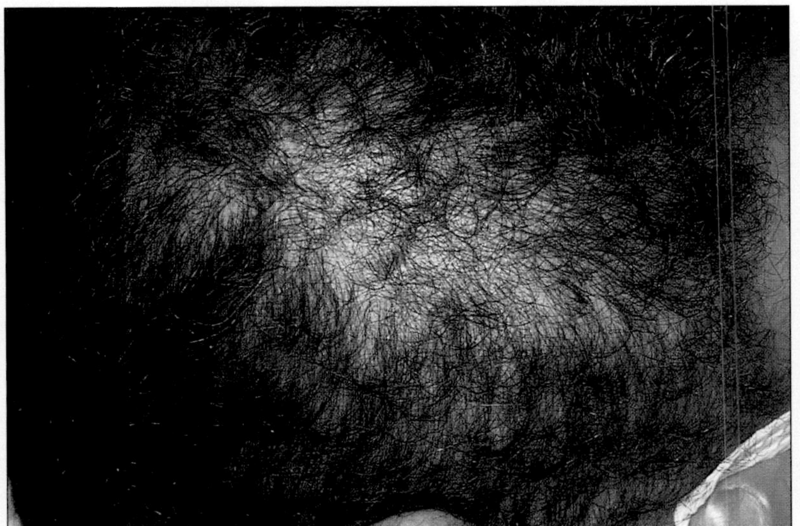

FIGURE 5-41 Papular lesions of the scalp in secondary syphilis. Involvement of hair follicles will produce papular lesions of the scalp, leading to patchy, moth-eaten, nonerythematous, nonscarring alopecia. The hair regrows after treatment. The differential diagnosis may initially include superficial fungal infection, but in syphilis, broken hair shafts are not observed.

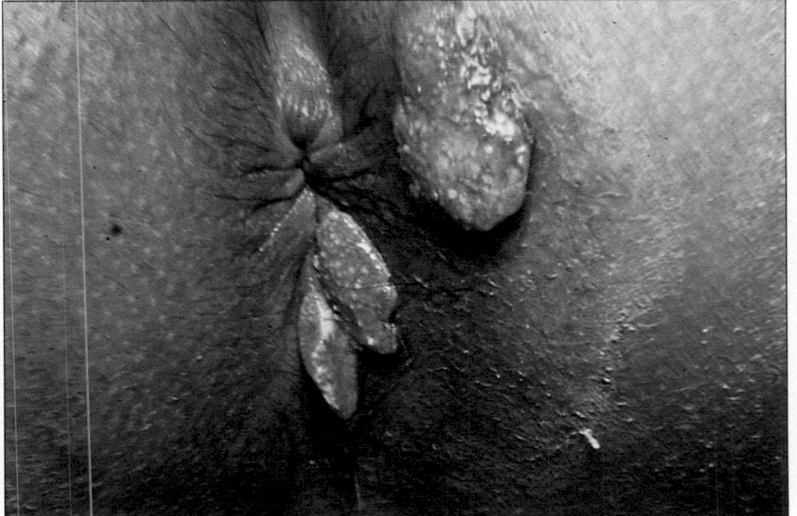

FIGURE 5-42 Condyloma lata in the perianal region. Papular lesions on moist, intertriginous areas may coalesce to form broad, moist, highly infectious plaques called *condyloma lata*. These flat, wartlike lesions develop at sites to which *Treponema pallidum* has disseminated and are frequently seen around the anus, as in this image. They may also occur on the vulva or scrotum and are less commonly found in the axillae, under the breasts, or between the toes. Condyloma lata must be differentiated from condyloma acuminata, caused by human papillomavirus, which are generally more verrucous and exuberant.

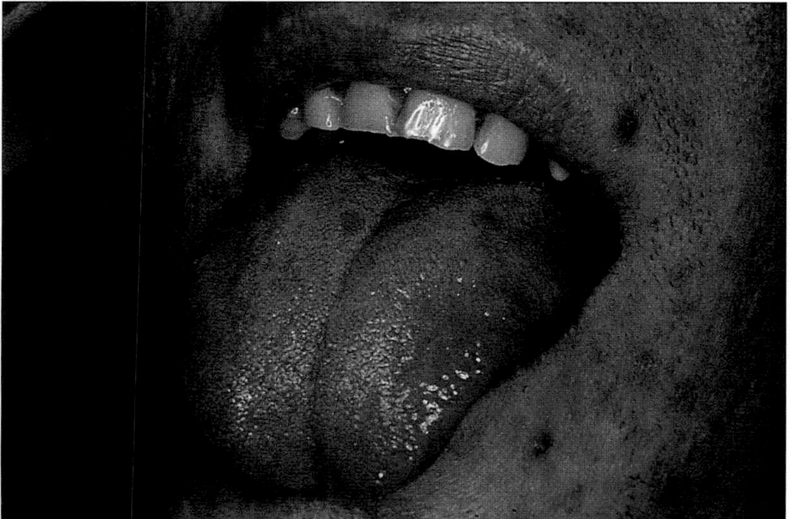

Figure 5-43 Mucous patches on the tongue in secondary syphilis. Secondary syphilis results from systemic dissemination of the spirochetes. Lesions on the skin contain small numbers of organisms and are not contagious. Mucous membrane lesions, on the other hand, contain large numbers of organisms and can easily result in disease transmission. Mucous patches are painless ulcerations, often displaying a dirty, yellowish base.

Late Syphilis

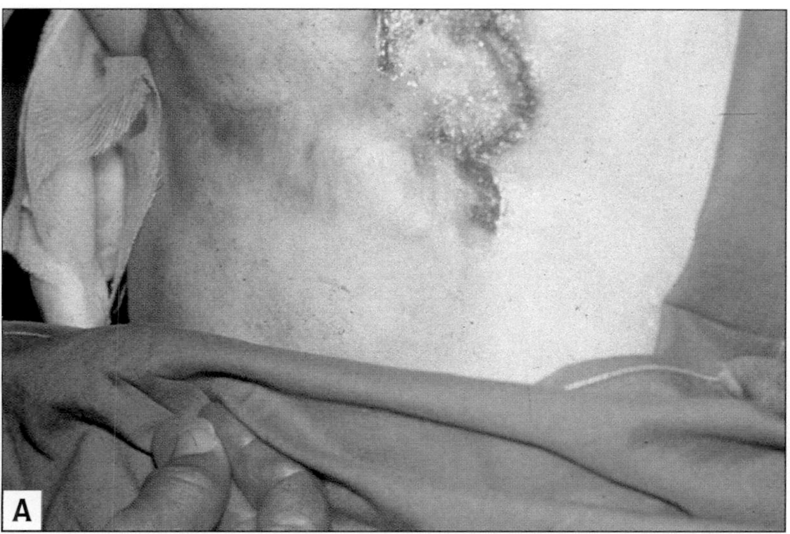

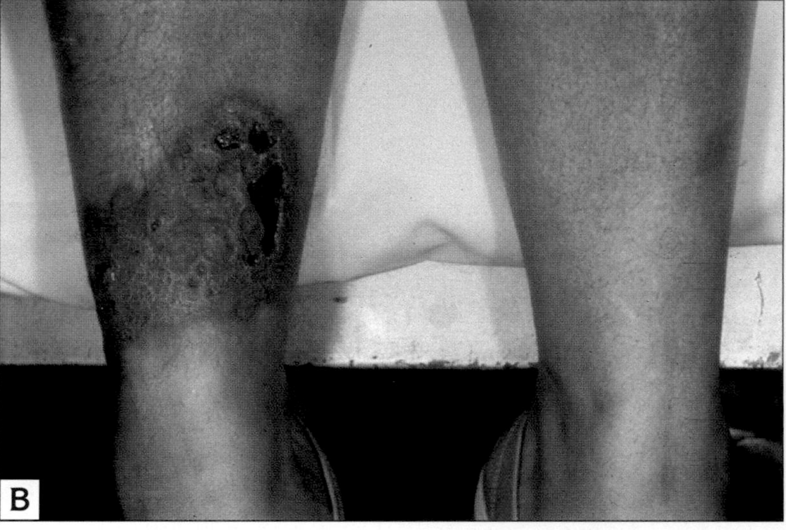

Figure 5-44 Cutaneous gummas in late syphilis. Gummas may affect virtually any part of the body and range from small nodules to deep, necrotizing, ulcerative lesions. They are typically indolent and painless and develop from 2 to 35 years after initial infection. **A**, Cutaneous gumma on the lower back. **B**, Cutaneous gumma on the lower leg. These two lesions show nearly all of the typical characteristics of late cutaneous syphilis, as described by Stokes: 1) solitary character; 2) asymmetry; 3) induration; 4) indolence; 5) arciform (circinate) configuration; 6) sharp margination of the lesion, with a punched-out appearance of ulcers; 7) tissue destruction and replacement; 8) tendency to one-sided healing with extension; 9) scar formation that is atrophic and noncontractile, retaining the arciform configuration of the original lesion; 10) peripheral hyperpigmentation that persists [11]. (*Courtesy of* J.F. Mullins, MD.)

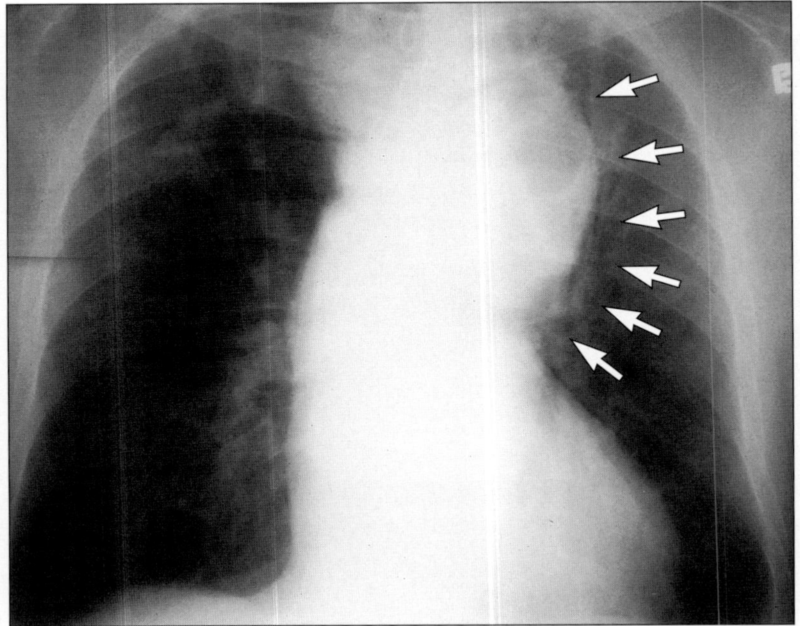

FIGURE 5-45 Admission chest radiograph showing a large aneurysm of the ascending aorta. A 54-year-old man presented with substernal chest pain on exertion that radiated down his left arm. His rapid plasma reagin titer was 1:8, and his fluorescent treponemal antibody absorbed test was reactive. He gave a history of a generalized rash some 30 years previously but denied having genital lesions. He had a grade II/VI diastolic decrescendo murmur at the left sternal border, and the electrocardiogram suggested ischemia. The chest radiograph revealed a large aneurysm of the ascending aorta (*arrows*).

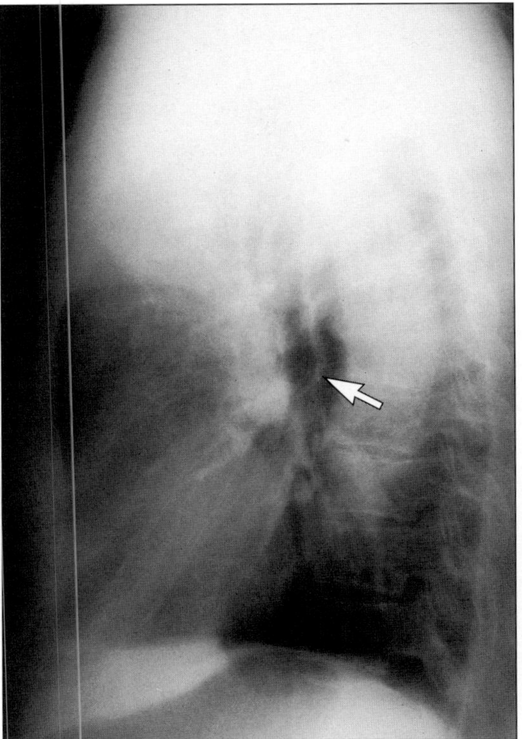

FIGURE 5-46 Lateral chest radiograph showing the ascending aortic aneurysm as an upper lobe density. In the same patient as seen in Fig. 5-45, some fine, "eggshell" calcification is seen within the descending aorta (*arrow*); this finding is observed in 20% of cases of syphilitic aortitis as well as in atherosclerotic disease. Observing linear calcification in the *ascending* aorta should raise the question of syphilitic aortitis, because in the absence of syphilis, such calcifications are rare in that location (although they may be seen in severe atherosclerotic disease) [12,13].

CONGENITAL SYPHILIS

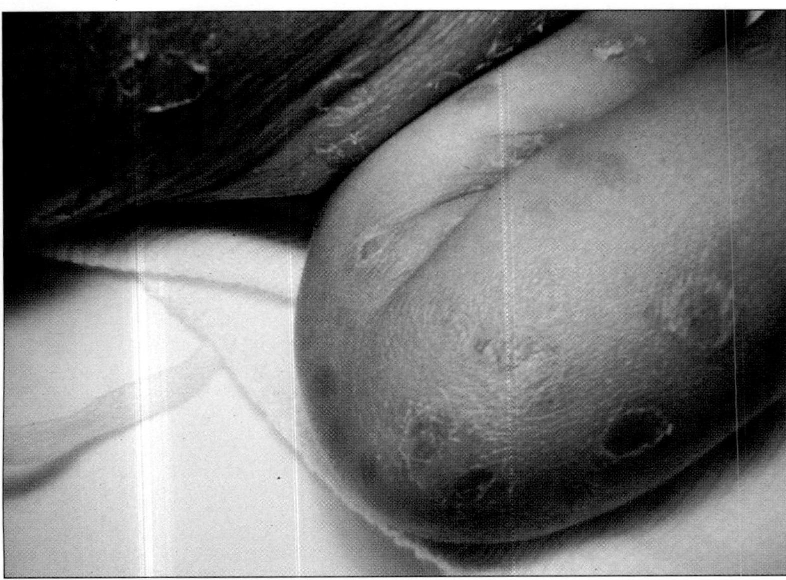

FIGURE 5-47 Plaquelike dermal lesions of congenital syphilis. This child developed signs of congenital syphilis at 5 weeks of age. Plaquelike lesions, which were scaly, rough, pigmented, and round, appeared on all external skin surfaces.

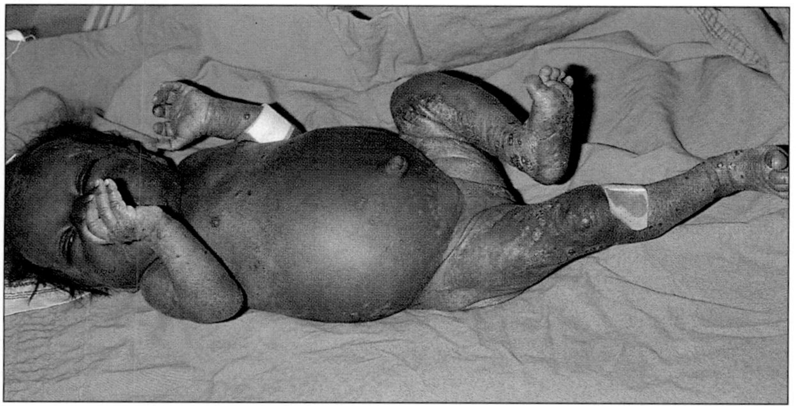

Figure 5-48 Dermal lesions and ascites in congenital syphilis. Ascites associated with a chronic hemolytic process is apparent. The hemolytic process seen with congenital syphilis is not fully understood and has been the subject of relatively little research. At least one aspect of the disorder is the production of Forssman antibodies. Forssman hapten is a naturally occurring glycolipid coupled to a ceramide lipid and is widely distributed on mammalian membranes, including circulating erythrocytes and precursors. Following damage by treponemal infection, antibody to Forssman may be produced and directed toward the host tissues. Children with hemolytic processes of congenital syphilis characteristically continue to exhibit chronic hemolysis for an extended period (months) after treatment of syphilis has been completed.

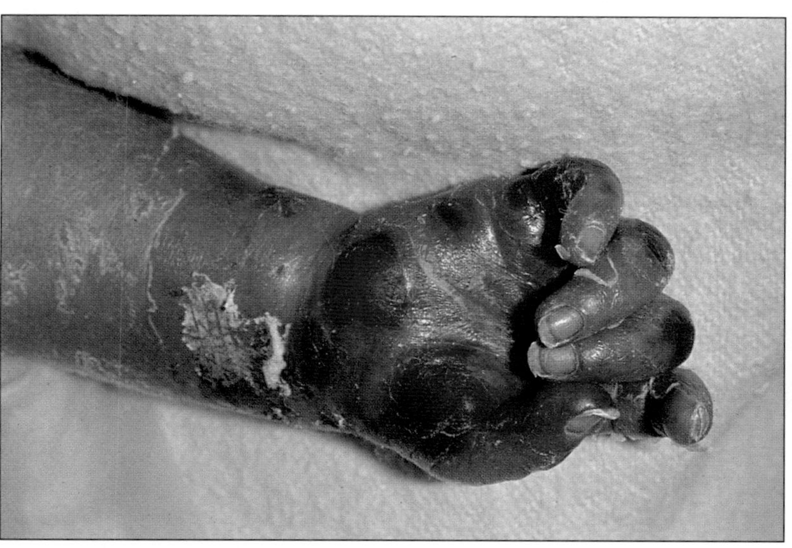

Figure 5-49 Hemorrhagic bullous lesions of the hand. Congenital syphilis is one of the few conditions in which there occur vesicular, bullous, and hemorrhagic lesions of the hands and feet, especially involving the palms and soles.

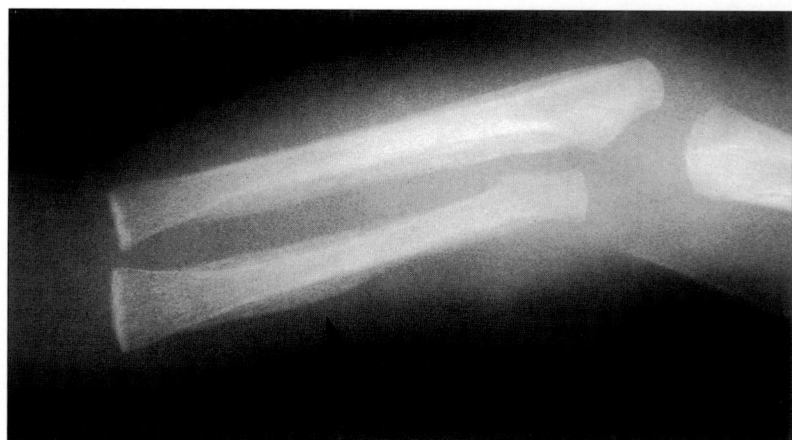

Figure 5-50 Bony lesions in early congenital syphilis. Periosteal new bone formation (*arrow*) is seen at the metaphyseal region. Epiphysitis is seen at the ends of both humerus and ulna. Irregular demineralization of the metaphyses and focal areas of cortical atrophy have occurred. These lesions are painful and cause the child to avoid motion, leading to the appearance of paralysis (pseudoparalysis).

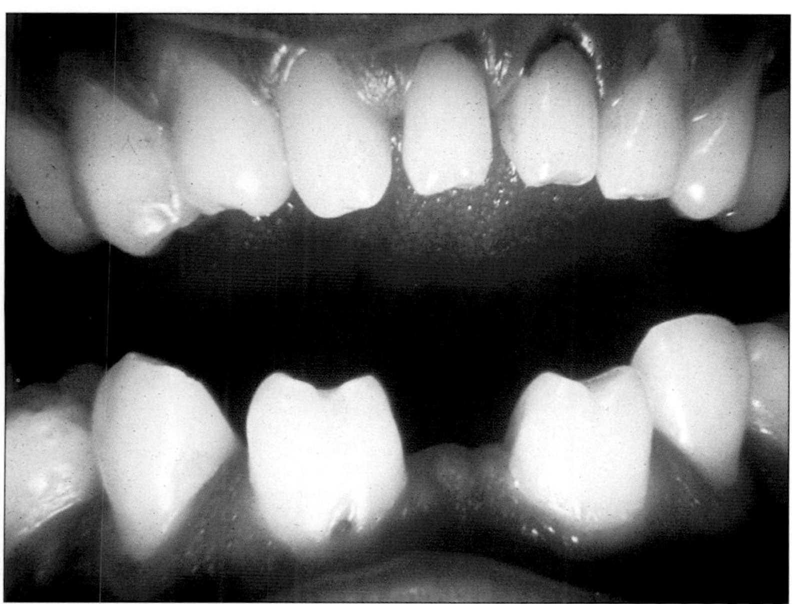

Figure 5-51 Hutchinson's teeth. Congenital syphilis causes abnormalities of the teeth, which are manifested by the small size of affected teeth, defective enamelization, and apical notching of incisors. The incisors of this child aged 6 years demonstrate notching.

Human Papillomavirus–Associated Diseases

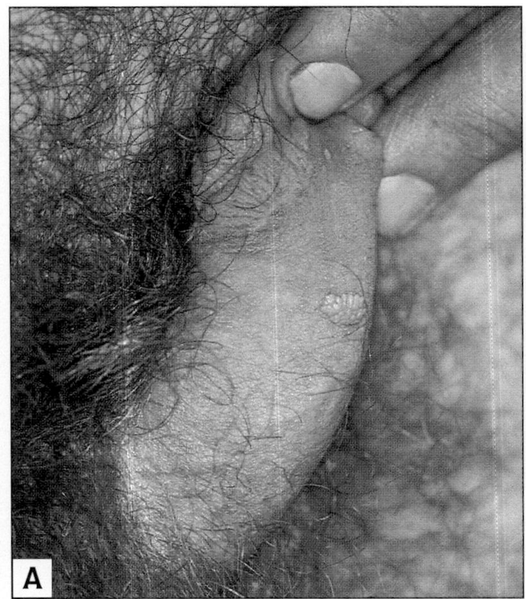

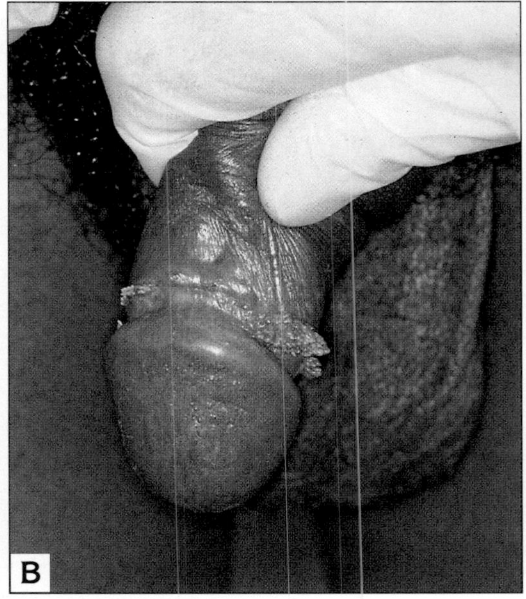

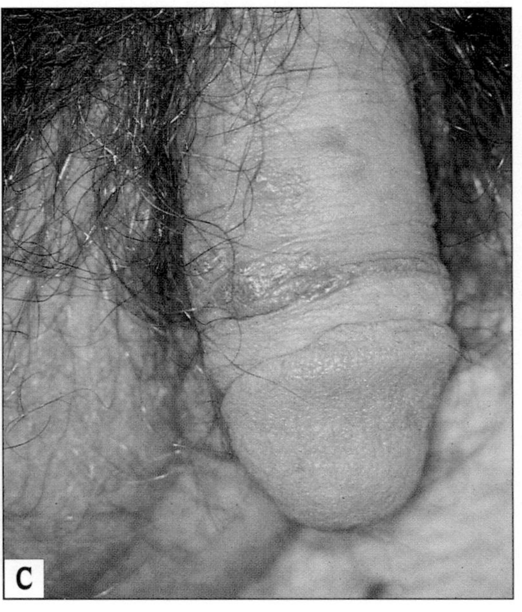

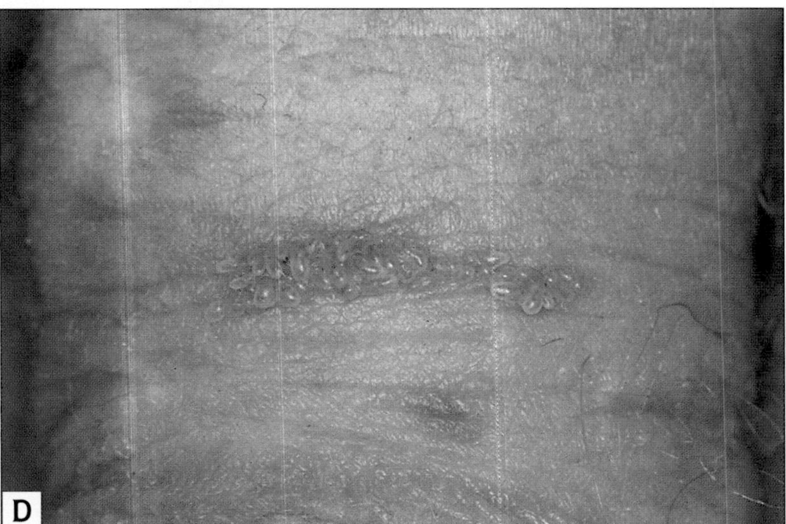

Figure 5-52 Penile warts. **A**, Typical papilliferous wart of the penis in a healthy man. These exophytic lesions are initially soft and fleshy. They occur most frequently on the shaft and coronal sulcus and are commonly found under the prepuce. When lesions have the typical verrucous appearance seen here, a clinical diagnosis is made easily. The lesions may spread linearly or circumferentially. A smaller lesion is seen distally, just beneath the patient's fingers. **B**, Papilliferous warts of the penis involving the coronal sulcus. The coronal sulcus is a common site for condyloma acuminata in men, perhaps because of the susceptibility of this site to subclinical trauma during intercourse. Here, the warts have spread circumferentially, with the initial lesions to the patient's left. These older lesions have become hyperpigmented. **C**, Flatter, more chronic warts on the penis. These lesions were an incidental finding on a man who presented as an asymptomatic contact to a woman with chlamydial cervicitis. Chronic warts are likely to become keratinized. **D**, Recurrent warts on the penile shaft. This patient had been treated 3 months previously, with complete resolution of visible lesions, but returned with recurrent, tiny lesions. A blush may be seen at the base of some of the individual lesions, which are highly vascular. The appearance of a tiny blood vessel running along the side of a lesion may assist in identifying it as a wart (as opposed to molluscum contagiosum) [14]. (*Courtesy of* M.F. Rein, MD.)

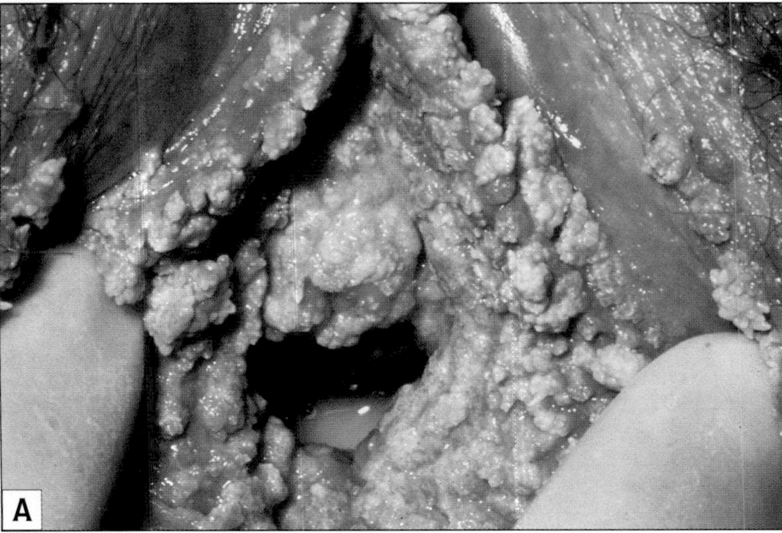

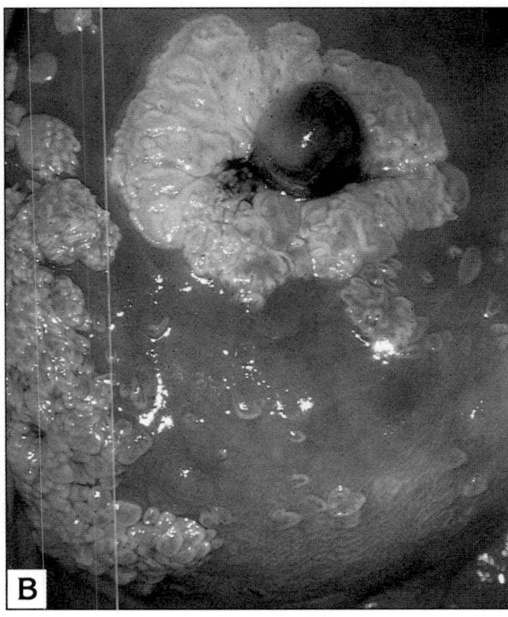

Figure 5-53 **A** and **B**, Typical papilliferous warts (condyloma acuminata) affecting the vulva and vagina (*panel A*) and cervix (*panel B*) of an immunologically healthy young woman. (*Courtesy of* E. Pixley, MD.)

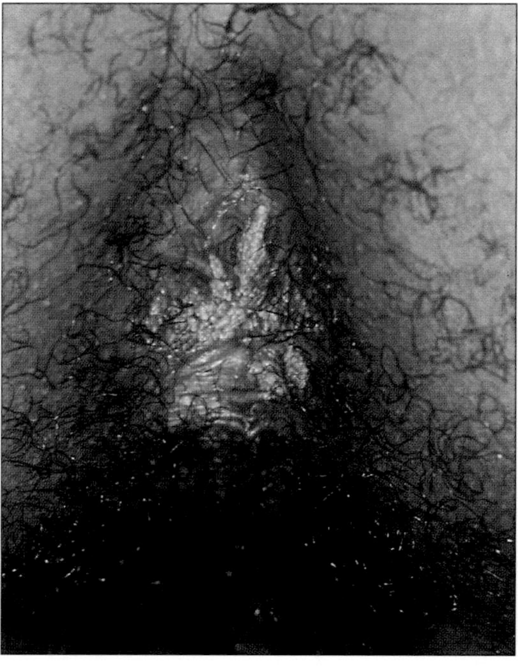

Figure 5-54 Perianal warts. This patient was seen in 1977, before the identification of HIV, and was presumably immunologically intact. The presence of such perianal lesions in a man is possible evidence that the patient has engaged in receptive anal intercourse. Such patients should undergo anoscopy to look for internal lesions and should be evaluated for other anorectal sexually transmitted diseases, such as gonorrhea or chlamydial infection. They also should be strongly encouraged to undergo testing for HIV antibody. (*Courtesy of* M.F. Rein, MD.)

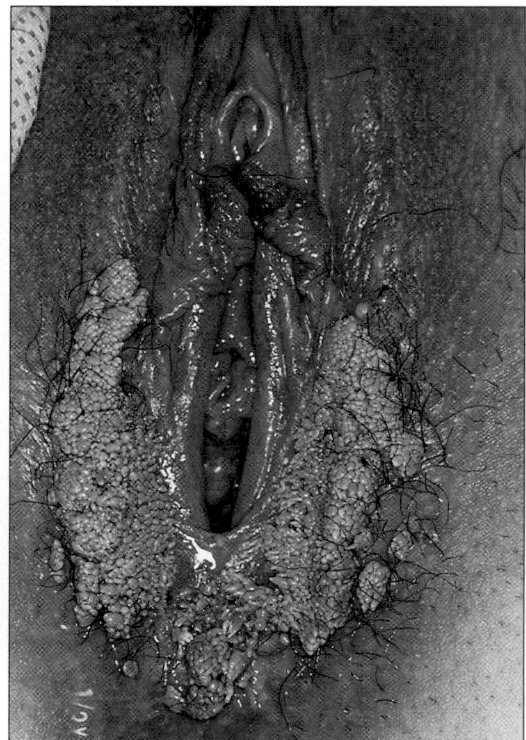

Figure 5-55 Condylomas of nonglabrous skin. Classic appearance of recent-onset condylomas within the nonglabrous skin. There is sufficient surface keratosis to make these lesions flesh-colored prior to the application of acetic acid. With vinegar soaking, the lesions are highlighted by prominent acetowhitening, sufficient to mask the underlying vascularity.

Ectoparasitic Infestations

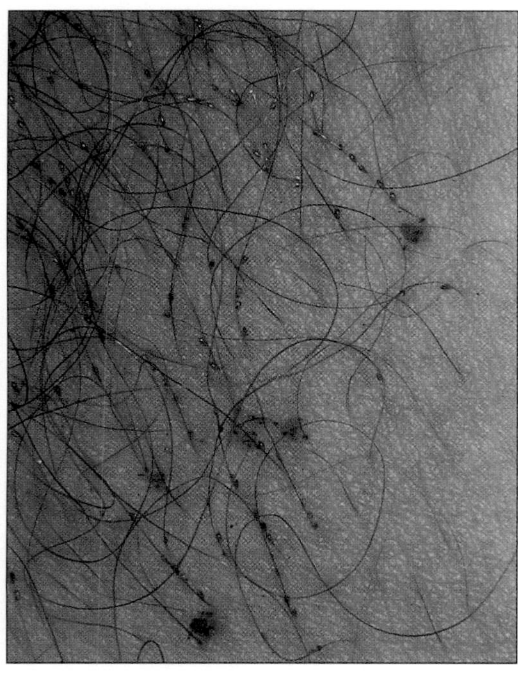

Figure 5-56 Infestation of the pubic hair by crab lice. The crab lice can be seen attached between the hairs, and a large number of nits are attached to the hair shafts. The diagnosis is made by clinical examination of affected areas to detect the adult lice and nits. The crab lice are often found at the base of hairs, with the terminal claws of their legs grabbing the hairs and their heads embedded in the skin. The nits appear as small dots of firm material along the hair shaft.

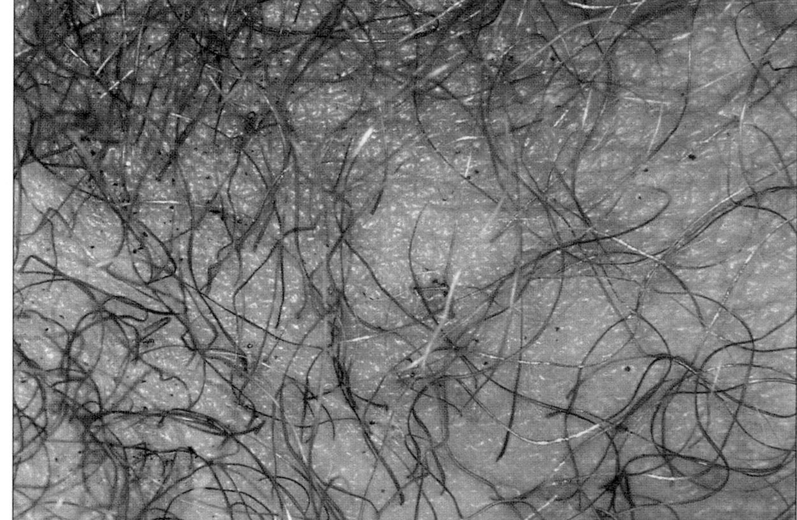

Figure 5-57 Louse feces on skin. The feces are deposited after a blood meal and appear as reddish-brown dots on the affected skin. They may also be found in the underwear by the patient or examiner.

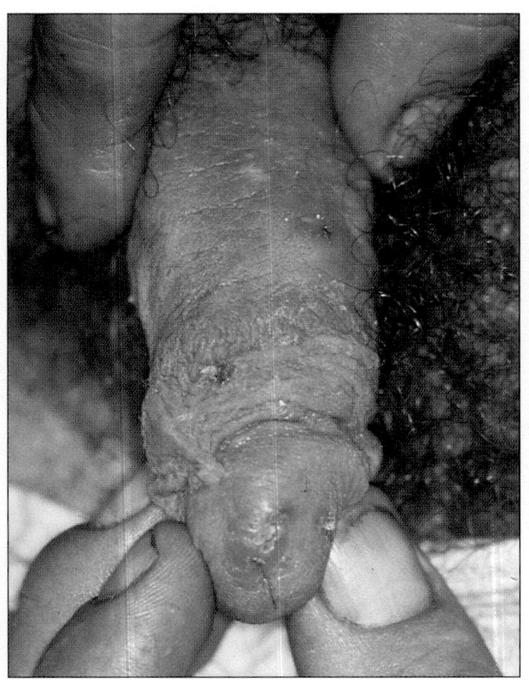

Figure 5-58 Penile scabies with weeping lesions. Typically penile lesions are often weepy and crusted. Herpetic lesions also often heal with crusts but are far less pruritic at that stage; in addition, herpetic lesions are often clustered rather than scattered over the penis.

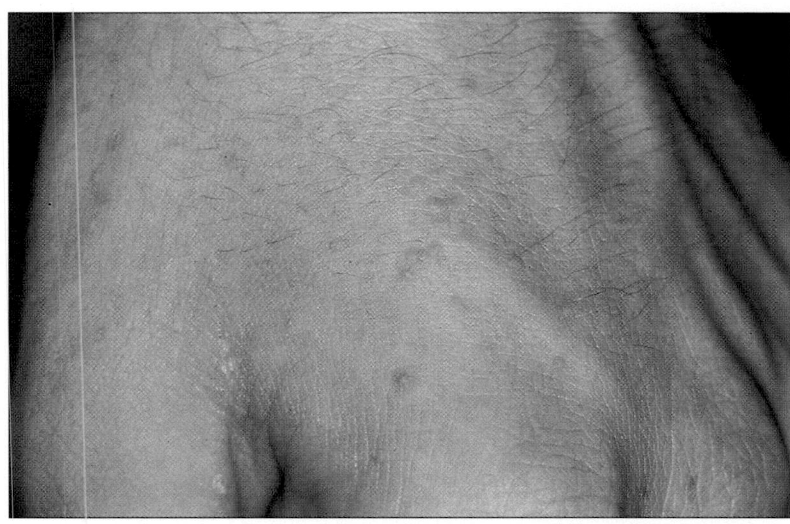

Figure 5-59 Scabies of the hand, showing typical moist papules. The hands are commonly involved in venereal scabies and may be the first site of symptoms. The typical moist papules of scabies are seen in this patient [15].

Molluscum Contagiosum

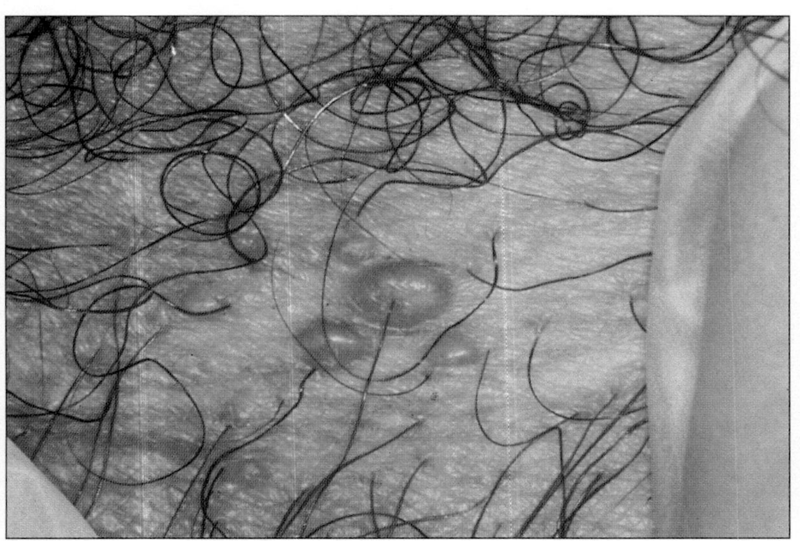

Figure 5-60 Molluscum contagiosum lesions in the pubic hair of a 32-year-old woman. Umbilications on the lesions are barely visible. Additional lesions were present on the thighs. (*Courtesy of* M.F. Rein, MD.)

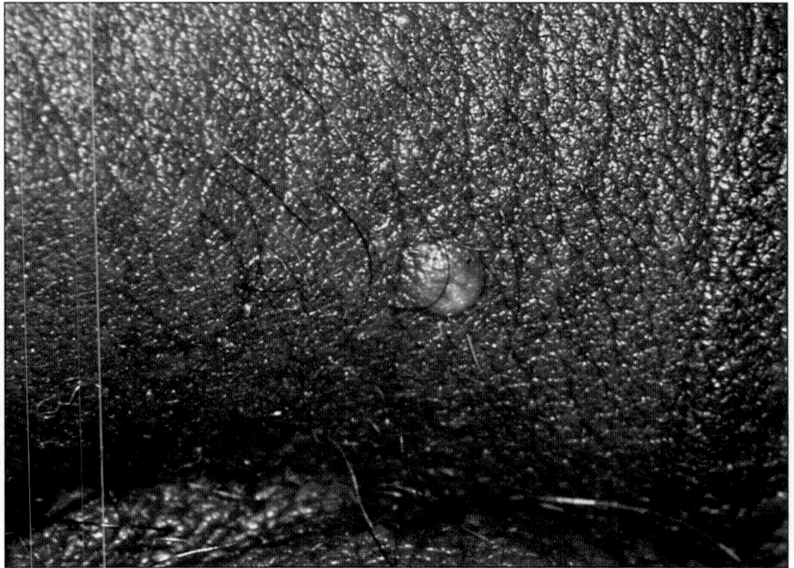

Figure 5-61 Solitary lesion of molluscum contagiosum on the penile shaft. A 28-year-old man presented with urethral discharge and dysuria, and the lesion was an incidental finding. (*Courtesy of* M.F. Rein, MD.)

Herpes Simplex Virus Infections

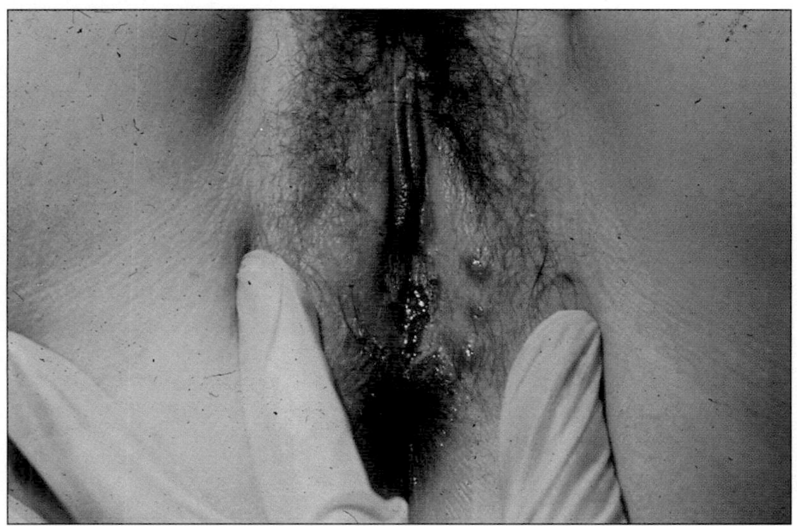

Figure 5-62 Primary genital herpes of the vulva. A woman with classic primary genital herpes shows the bilaterally distributed lesions. She complained of headache, malaise, and myalgias and had a low-grade fever. Primary HSV infection also involved the urethra and cervix in this woman, and HSV-2 was isolated from urethral swabs and urine. Clinically, one cannot distinguish primary genital herpes due to HSV-1 from that due to HSV-2; only laboratory assays can distinguish between the two viral subtypes.

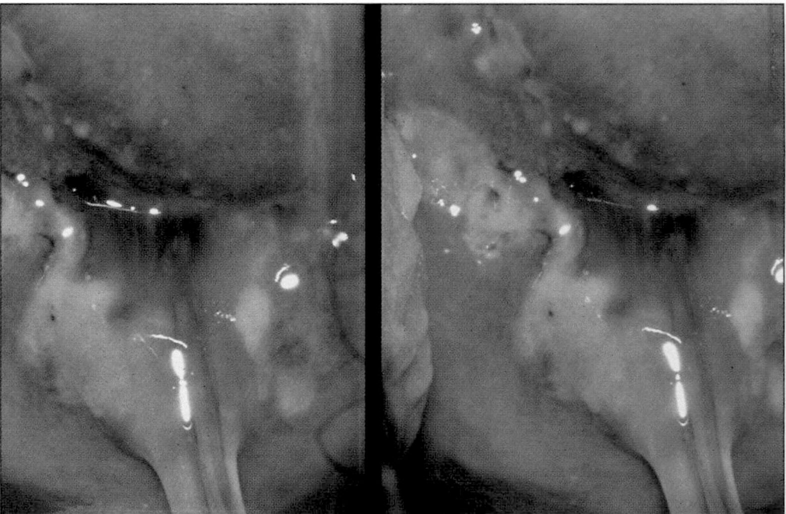

Figure 5-63 Colposcopic view of purulent HSV cervicitis. A colposcopic view of the cervix from the patient in Fig. 5-62 shows a characteristic purulent HSV cervicitis. Note the purulent exudates and characteristic erosive lesions on the exocervix. She responded well to treatment with oral acyclovir, 400 mg three times daily (or 200 mg five times daily) for 10 days.

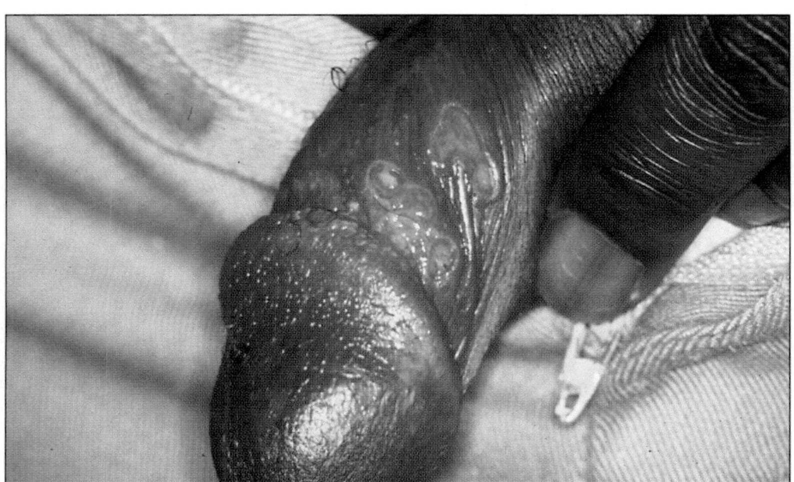

Figure 5-64 Primary genital HSV infection in a man. Two clusters of large ulcers are seen on the left side of the penile shaft. Although these appear to be single lesions, each actually is formed from the coalescence of multiple ulcers. Such lesions are tender and nonindurated. Herpetic lesions tend all to be similar in size, whereas lesions of chancroid may vary in size. This patient also had bilateral tender lymphadenopathy of the inguinal nodes and was slightly febrile. He improved on oral acyclovir therapy. (*Courtesy of* M.F. Rein, MD.)

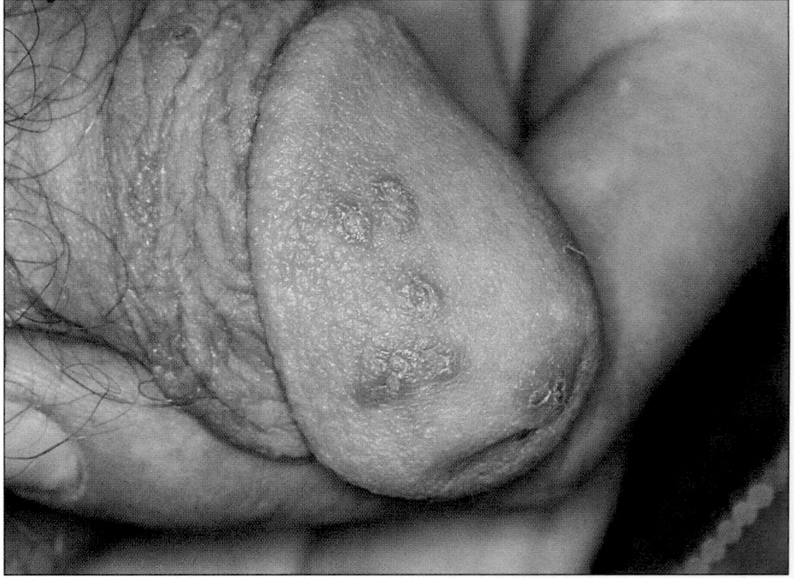

Figure 5-65 Healing HSV lesions on the penis. Herpetic lesions tend to heal by crusting over, as seen on the glans and coronal sulcus in this patient. Culture of material from crusted lesions has a sensitivity of only 27% for the virus. The pattern of crusts seen on the glans in this patient suggests the clustering of initial lesions, which is characteristic in genital HSV infections. The differential diagnosis of crusted lesions includes scabies, which tend to be scattered rather than clustered, are markedly pruritic, and usually do not involve inguinal adenopathy [16]. (*Courtesy of* M.F. Rein, MD.)

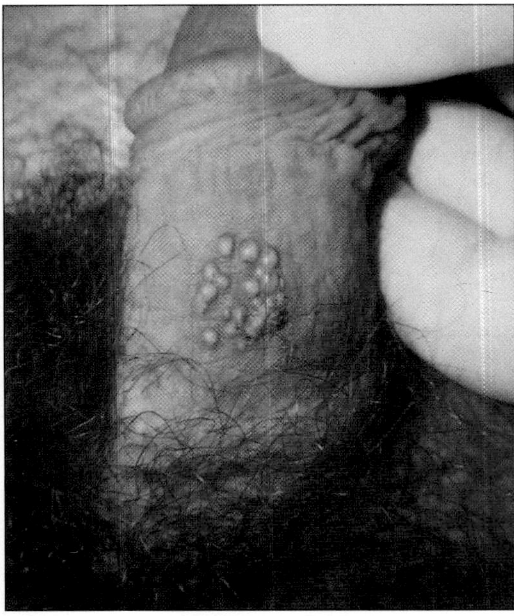

Figure 5-66 Recurrent genital HSV lesions on the penile shaft. In men, genital herpes recurs as clusters of vesicular lesions on an erythematous base, usually on the penile shaft or glans. This patient reported episodes of exacerbations every other month. He was both HSV-1– and HSV-2–seropositive by Western blot analysis, with HSV-2 being isolated from the genital lesions. He elected to initiate suppressive acyclovir therapy, 400 mg orally twice daily, and did not have any recurrences during the initial year of therapy.

Chancroid

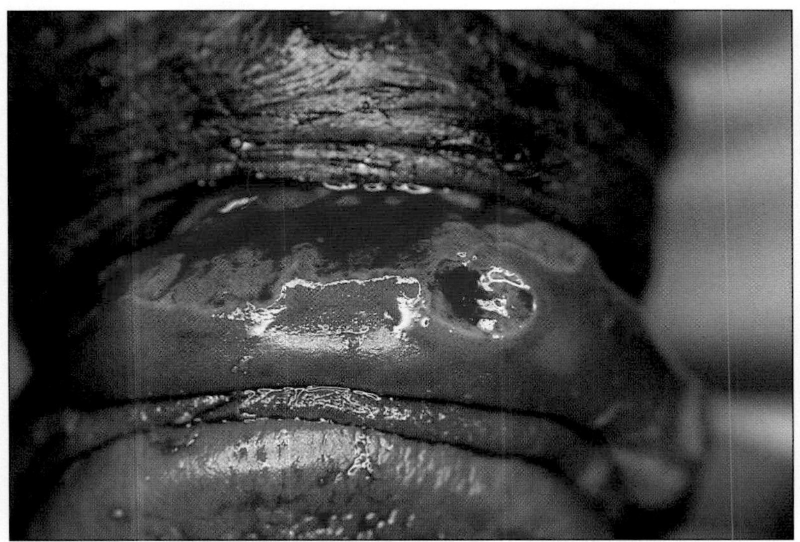

Figure 5-67 Classic, purulent chancroid lesion on the distal penis. A purulent, bleeding lesion 2 cm in diameter is seen on the prepuce. This patient had two other smaller lesions on the shaft of the penis. The most common sites of involvement in men are the distal prepuce, the mucosal surface of the prepuce on the frenulum, and the coronal sulcus.

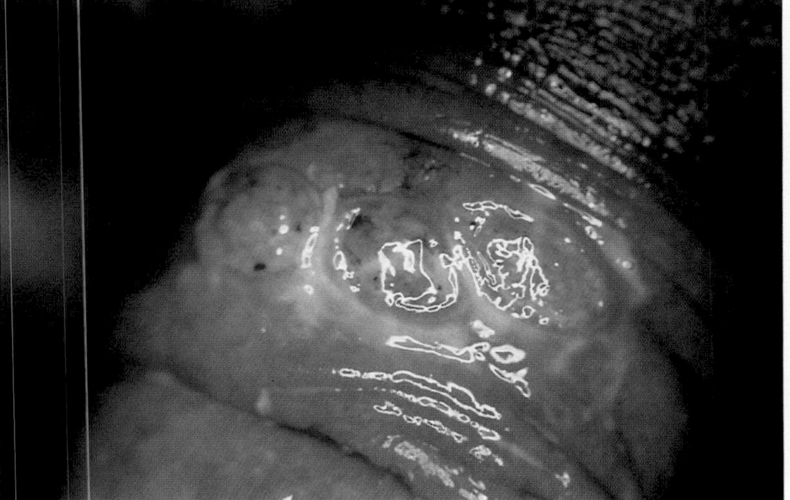

Figure 5-68 Multiple chancroid lesions on the coronal sulcus. The coronal sulcus is a very common site for chancroid, particularly in uncircumcised patients, and often the lesions merge to form an entire ring around the circumference of the penis.

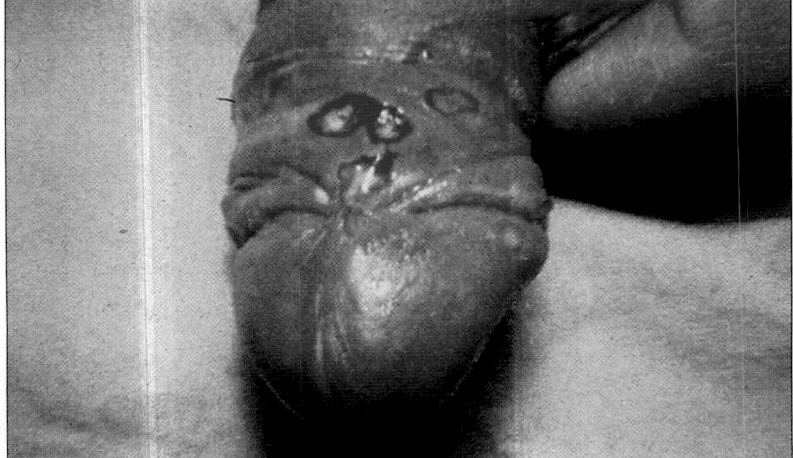

Figure 5-69 Four dwarf chancroid lesions on the underside of the penis. These lesions were never vesiculated. Although these small lesions appear initially to be herpetiform, about 10% of chancroid cases present in this way. Many would resolve without treatment over the course of 1 to 3 weeks.

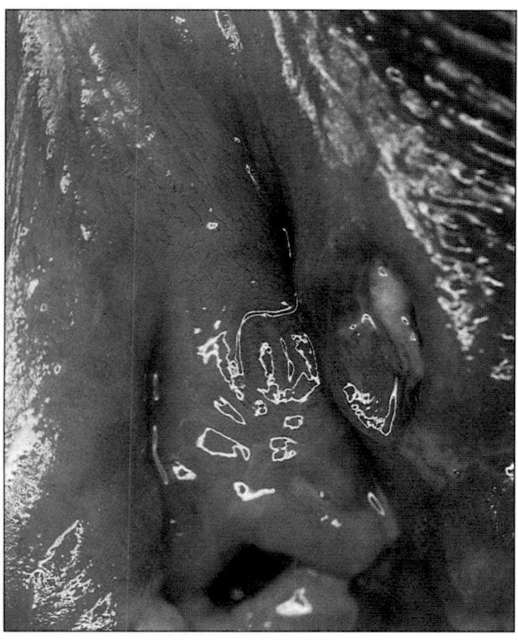

Figure 5-70 Chancroid lesion on the inner aspect of the labium majorum. Again, this 6-mm lesion was minimally symptomatic and was not recognized until the patient was examined.

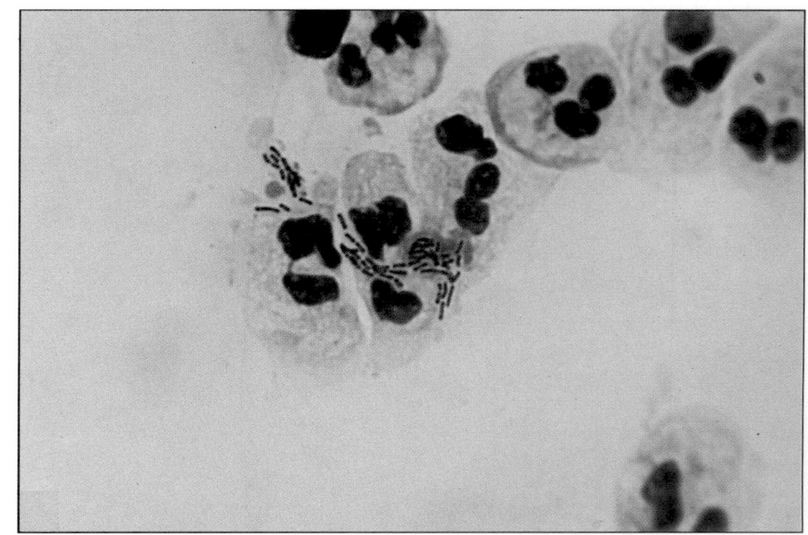

Figure 5-71 Classically, Gram stains of chancroid lesions are described as showing the organisms in "school-of-fish" patterns. These patterns are seen in only one third to one half of patients, and the finding is not specific for chancroid because other gram-negative rods can have similar arrangements. However, intracellular *H. ducreyi* is usually seen only in patients with chancroid, and Gram stain showing this finding can be a more specific, if insensitive, result from the chancroidal lesion. (*Courtesy of* E.J. Bottone, MD.)

References

1. Schachter J: Diagnosis of *Chlamydia trachomatis* infection. *In* Orfila J, Byrne GI, Chernesky MA, *et al.* (eds.): *Chlamydial Infections: Proceedings of the Eighth International Symposium on Human Chlamydial Infections*. Bologna, Italy: Società Editrice Esculapio; 1994:293–302.
2. Holmes KK, Handsfield HH: Sexually transmitted diseases. *In* Isselbacher KJ, *et al.* (eds.): *Harrison's Principles of Internal Medicine*, 13th ed. New York: McGraw-Hill; 1994:538–539.
3. Rein MF: *In* Holmes KK, *et al.* (eds.): *Sexually Transmitted Diseases*. New York: McGraw-Hill; 1984.
4. Kolstad P: The colposcopic picture of *Trichomonas vaginalis. Acta Obstet Gynecol Scand* 1965, 43:388–398.
5. Rein MF: Clinical manifestations of urogenital trichomoniasis in women. *In* Honigberg BM (ed.): *Trichomonads Parasitic in Humans*. New York: Springer-Verlag: 1989:228.
6. Gupta PK, Frost JK: Cytopathology and histopathology of the female genital tract in *Trichomonas vaginalis* infection. *In* Honigberg BM (ed.): *Trichomonads Parasitic in Humans*. New York: Springer-Verlag; 1989:274–290.
7. Rein MF, Sullivan JA, Mandell GL: Trichomonacidal activity of human polymorphonuclear neutrophils: Killing by disruption and fragmentation. *J Infect Dis* 1980, 142:575–585.
8. Krieger JN, Tam MR, Stevens CE, *et al.*: Diagnosis of trichomoniasis: Comparison of conventional wet-mount examination with cytologic studies, cultures and monoclonal antibody staining of direct specimens. *JAMA* 1988, 259:1223–1227.
9. Larsen SA, Steiner BM, Rudolph AH: Laboratory diagnosis and interpretation of tests for syphilis. *Clin Microbiol Rev* 1995, 8:1–21.
10. Fiumara NJ: *Pictorial Guide to Sexually Transmitted Diseases*. New York: Cahners Publ.; 1989:42.
11. Stokes JH: *Modern Clinical Syphilology: Diagnosis-Treatment-Case Study*. Philadelphia: W.B. Saunders; 1934.
12. MacFarlane WV, Swan WGA, Irvine RE: Cardiovascular disease in syphilis: A review of 1330 patients. *BMJ* 1956, 1:827–832.
13. Higgins CB, Reinke RT: Nonsyphilitic etiology of linear calcification of the ascending aorta. *Radiology* 1974, 113:609–613.
14. Oriel D: Genital human papillomavirus infection. *In* Holmes KK, Mårdh P-A, Sparling PF, *et al.* (eds.): *Sexually Transmitted Diseases*, 2nd ed. New York: McGraw Hill; 1990:435.
15. Orkin M, Maibach HI: Scabies. *In* Holmes KK, Mårdh P-A, Sparling PF, Wiesner PJ (eds.): *Sexually Transmitted Diseases*, 2nd ed. New York: McGraw-Hill; 1990:473–479.
16. Moseley RC, Corey L, Benjamin D, *et al.*: Comparison of viral isolation, direct immunofluorescence, and indirect immunoperoxidase techniques for detection of genital herpes simplex virus infection. *J Clin Microbiol* 1981, 13:913–918.

CHAPTER 6

Pleuropulmonary and Bronchial Infections

Editor
Michael S. Simberkoff

Contributors

Donald Armstrong
Robert F. Betts
Roger C. Bone
Richard E. Bryant
Scott F. Davies
Ann R. Falsey
Jay A. Fishman
John Froude
Caroline B. Hall
James J. Herdegen
Jaishree Jagirdar
Howard L. Leaf
Melanie J. Maslow
Herbert Y. Reynolds
Richard B. Roberts
Robert H. Rubin
Christopher J. Salmon
George A. Sarosi
Michael S. Simberkoff
John J. Treanor

Gram-Positive Bacterial Infections of the Lungs

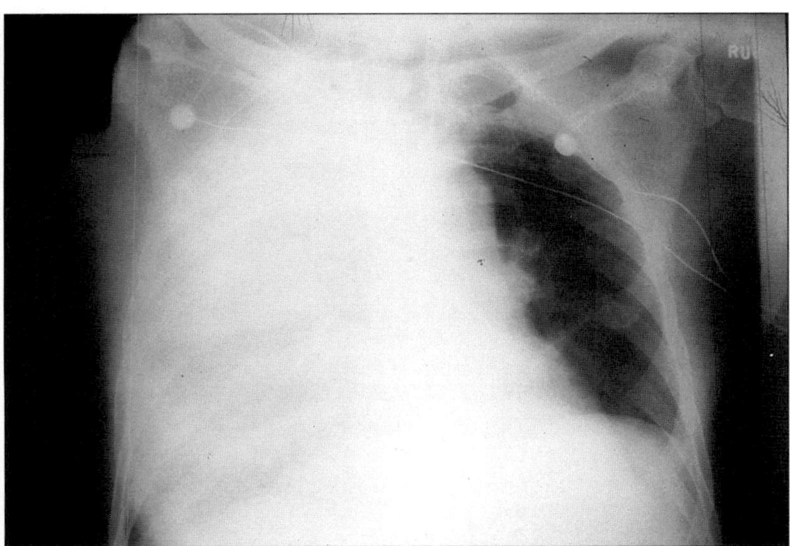

Figure 6-1 Chest radiograph showing multilobar consolidation in pneumococcal pneumonia. A 64-year-old man presented with a 6-day history of fever, shaking chills, chest pain, and cough productive of rust-cultured sputum. One day before admission, he developed dyspnea and confusion. His past medical history was remarkable for mild hypertension and a 150-pack-year smoking history. The patient had not received pneumococcal vaccination. An admission chest film revealed consolidation of the right upper, middle, and lower lobes.

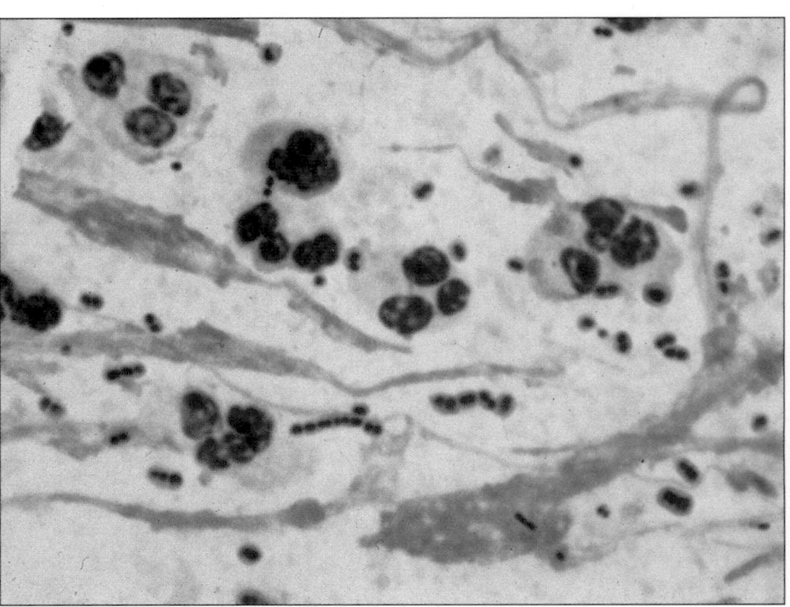

Figure 6-2 Microbiologic studies in pneumococcal pneumonia. Sputum Gram stain from the patient in Figure 6-1. Many polymorphonuclear leukocytes with lancet-shaped, gram-positive cocci in pairs and chains can be seen, indicative of *Streptococcus pneumoniae*. To be adequate for evaluation, a sputum sample must have ≥ 25 leukocytes per low-power field.

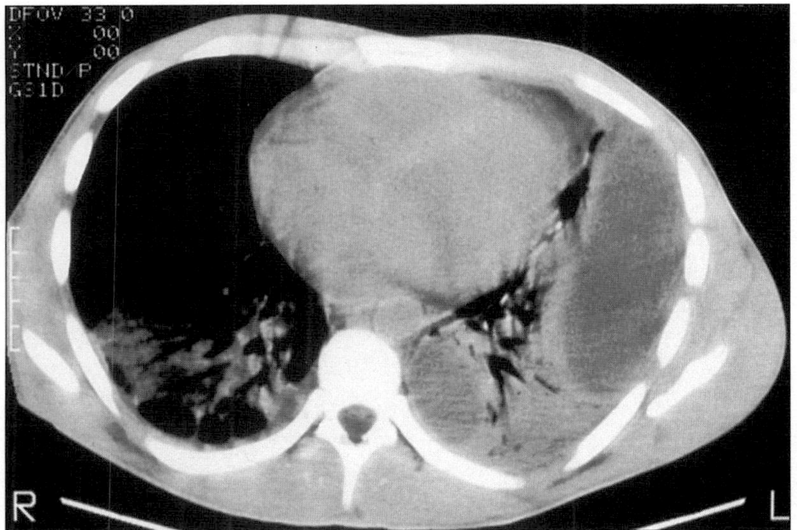

Figure 6-3 Pneumococcal pneumonia with empyema. A previously healthy 25-year-old man, presumably HIV positive with a CD+ count of 21/mm^3, was hospitalized with a 4-day history of fever, productive cough, dyspnea, and pleuritic chest pain. Admission chest film revealed left lower, right lower, and right middle lobar consolidation with a left pleural effusion. Blood cultures were positive for type-14 *Streptococcus pneumoniae*. Six days after admission, computed tomography of the chest (shown here) revealed bibasilar infiltrates and a large loculated left pleural effusion. Radiographic-guided thoracentesis yielded 280 mL of cloudy fluid with a leukocyte count of 39,000/mm^3 with 99% polymorphonuclear leukocytes, protein of 4.0 mg/dL, and glucose of 5 mg/dL, which are consistent with empyema.

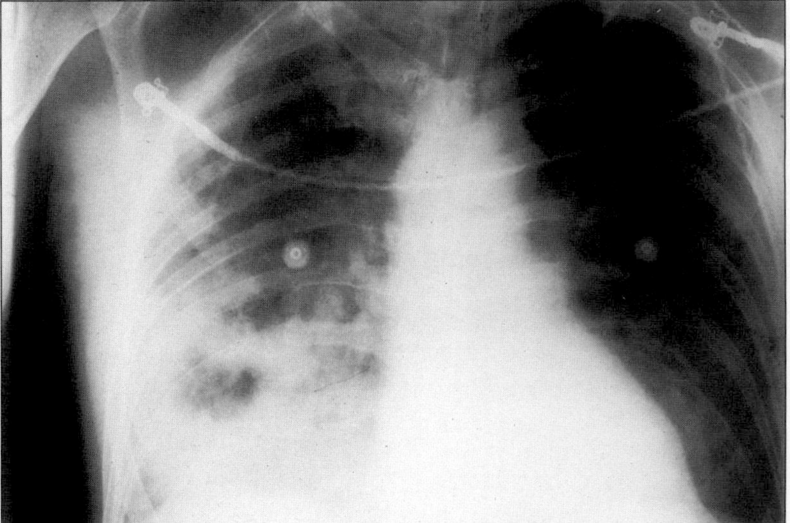

Figure 6-4 Progression of chest radiographic abnormalities in streptococcal toxic shock syndrome. A 53-year-old man walked into the emergency department with dyspnea and palpitations for 12 hours. He had been well until 3 days before admission when he noted an influenza-like syndrome, followed by blood-tinged sputum, drenching sweats, and dyspnea on the day of admission. Repeat chest film revealed progression of the infiltrates and two radiolucencies in the right lower lung field. By 12 hours after admission, he had had two spontaneous pneumothoraces, and chest films revealed bilateral infiltrates consistent with adult respiratory distress syndrome. He developed disseminated intravascular coagulation (platelets, 32,000/mm^3; prothrombin time, 18.3 $_s$; partial thromboplastin time, 87.7; fibrinogen, 300 mg/dL). He died 8 hours later.

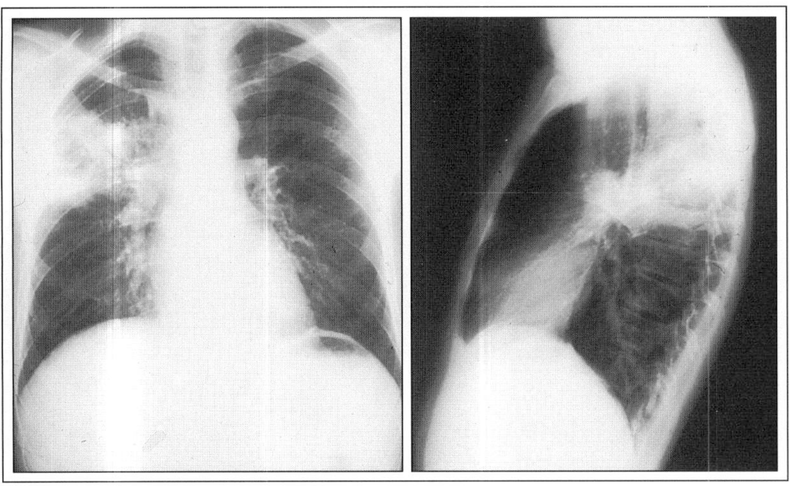

Figure 6-5 Posteroanterior and lateral chest films demonstrating staphylococcal aspiration pneumonia. A 27-year-old man developed fever, cough productive of blood-tinged sputum, and pleuritic chest pain 2 days following an episode of acute emesis. Admission chest film revealed consolidation of the posterior segment of the right upper lobe with cavitation. Sputum cultures grew *Staphylococcus aureus*. His hospital course was complicated by desquamation of the palms and severe hemoptysis. Patients with primary staphylococcal pneumonia are usually very toxic and may respond more slowly to appropriate antimicrobial therapy than patients with other bacterial pneumonias.

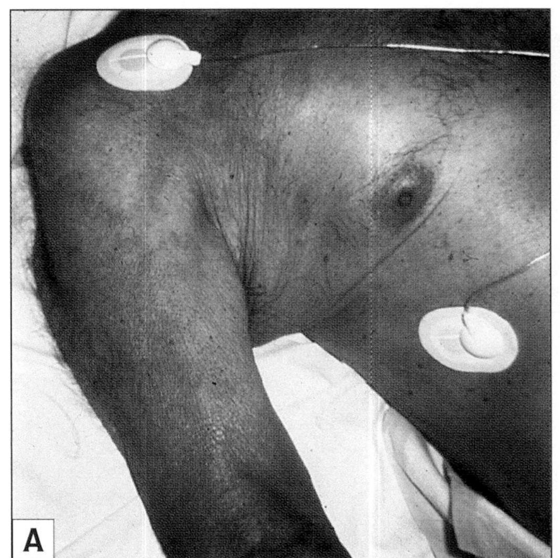

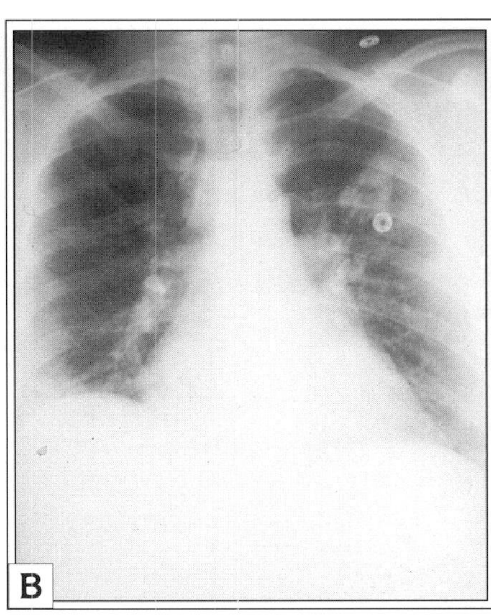

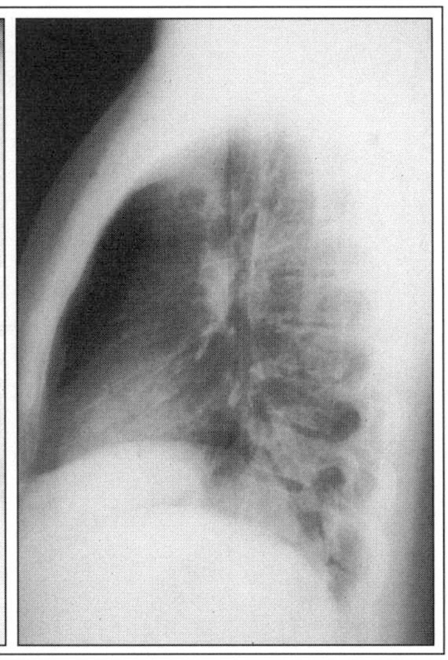

Figure 6-6 Suppurative phlebitis, metastatic pneumonia, and endocarditis due to intravenous catheter-related staphylococcal bacteremia. A 78-year-old man was transferred to the intensive care unit because of hypotension and obtundation several hours following a transurethral prostatic resection. An intravenous catheter was placed in the right cephalic vein to monitor central venous pressure. Fever subsequently developed, and blood cultures repeated over a 48-hour period grew *Staphylococcus aureus*. **A**, Phlebitis and surrounding cellulitis that extended to the anterior chest wall were noted. The intravenous catheter was removed, and 4 mL of purulent material was expressed from the puncture site. **B**, As seen on chest radiographs, multiple pulmonary infiltrates developed secondary to prolonged staphylococcal bacteremia. The entire cephalic vein was resected, which upon incising open revealed suppurative phlebitis. Gram stain of the purulent material demonstrated gram-positive cocci in clusters, and cultures grew *S. aureus*. Postoperatively, the patient deteriorated clinically and died 5 weeks later.

Gram-Negative Bacterial Infections of the Lungs

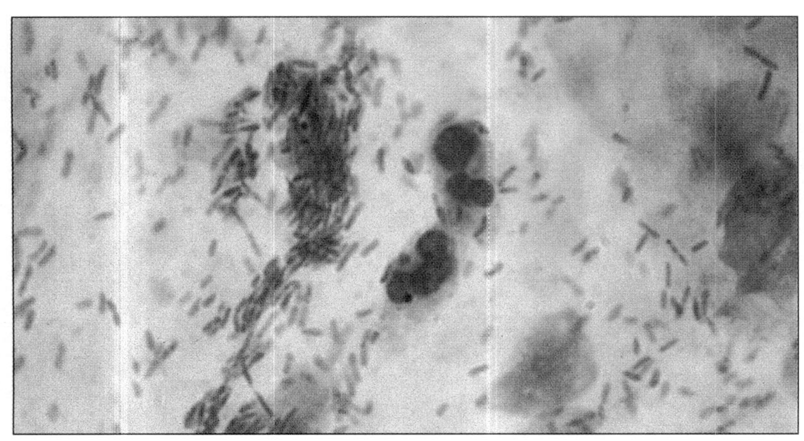

Figure 6-7 Sputum Gram stain showing polymorphonuclear leukocytes and numerous gram-negative bacilli. Gram-negative aerobic bacteria account for approximately 60% of cases of nosocomial pneumonia and are estimated to cause between 6% and 20% of community-acquired bacterial pneumonia. The mortality rate from gram-negative pneumonia ranges from 30% to 50%. This high rate is a function of both underlying host factors and the special virulence factors associated with these organisms [1].

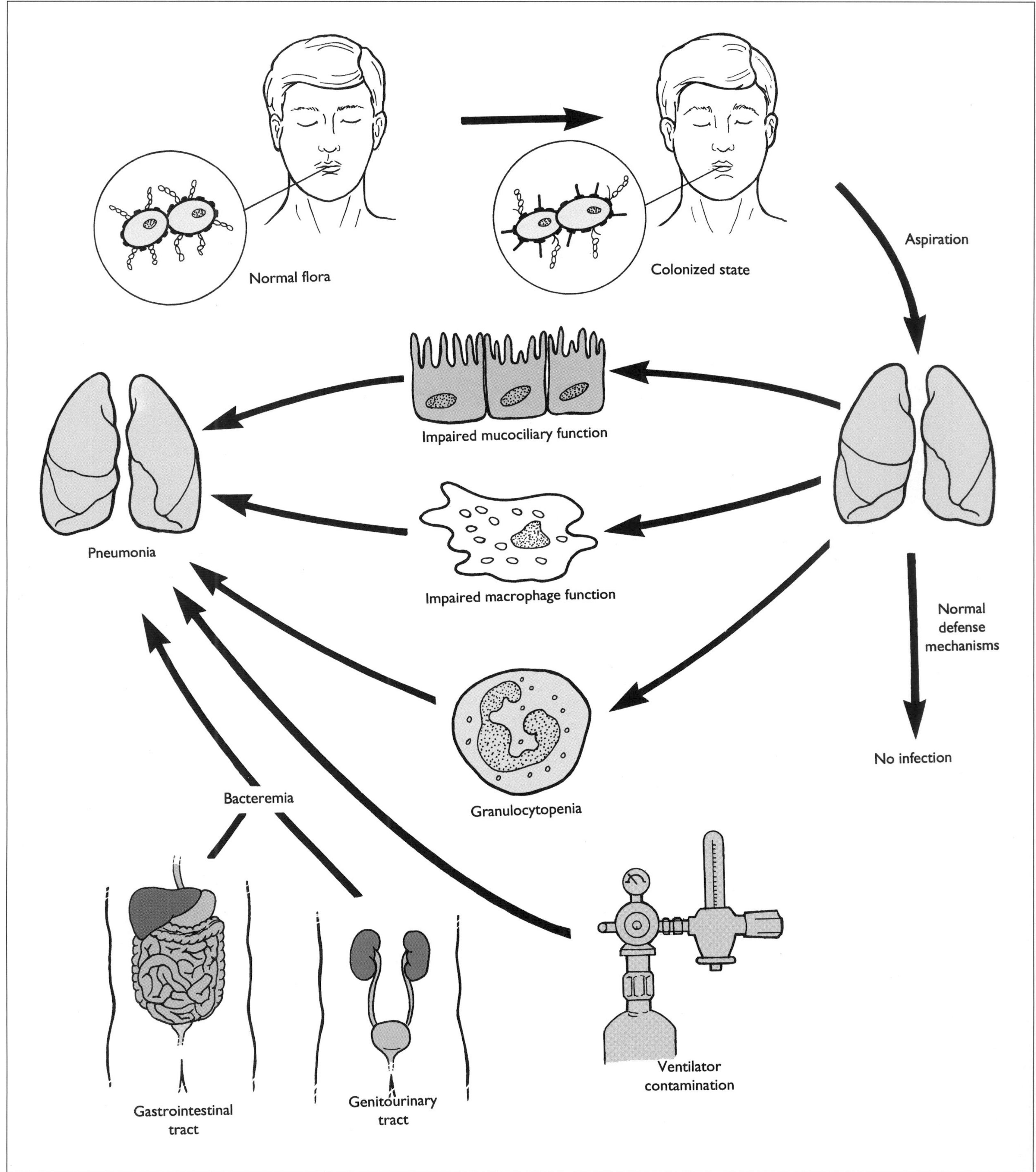

Figure 6-8 Pathogenesis of gram-negative pneumonia. Once gram-negative bacilli have established colonization, multiplication results in high bacterial concentrations in oral secretions. Secretions are then aspirated in small liquid boluses into the lungs. Pneumonia results if the pulmonary defense mechanisms are impaired by various mechanisms, including alveolar hypoxia, decreased mucociliary clearance, decreased phagocyte migration associated with alcoholism, and neutropenia. Other less frequent routes of infection are bacteremic spread to the lung from other foci of infection and aerosol contamination through respiratory equipment.

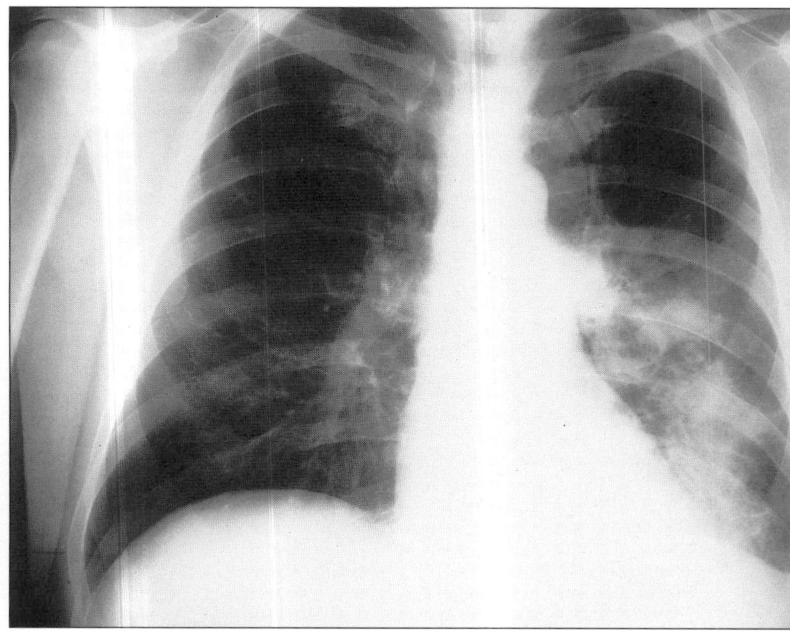

FIGURE 6-9 Chest radiograph from an alcoholic man with left lower lobe pneumonia due to *Haemophilus influenzae*. Predisposing factors to *H. influenzae* pneumonia in adults include chronic lung disease, diabetes, neoplasm, alcoholism, and immunodeficiency states. Adults with chronic bronchitis are at increased risk of both community-acquired and nosocomial *H. influenzae* pneumonia. The clinical presentation of pneumonia is similar to that of *Streptococcus pneumoniae* except that *Haemophilus* infection may have a slower clinical onset. The spectrum of radiologic findings includes segmental, lobar, bronchopneumonic, and interstitial infiltrates. Pleural effusion occurs in one half of cases.

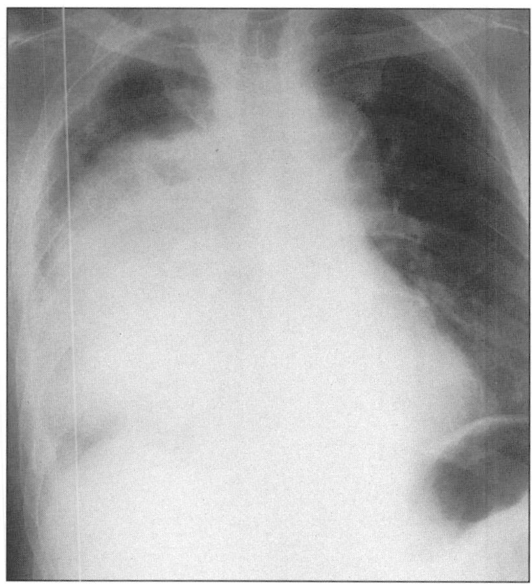

FIGURE 6-10 Chest radiographs of cavitary pneumonia due to *Pseudomonas aeruginosa*. A 75-year-old black man admitted with cavitary pneumonia involving the right upper, right middle, and right lower lobes. A follow-up chest radiograph 3 days later shows progression of infection with cavitary lesions and air-fluid levels in the right middle and right upper lobes. The abscesses slowly contracted and healed with scarring over 6 months.

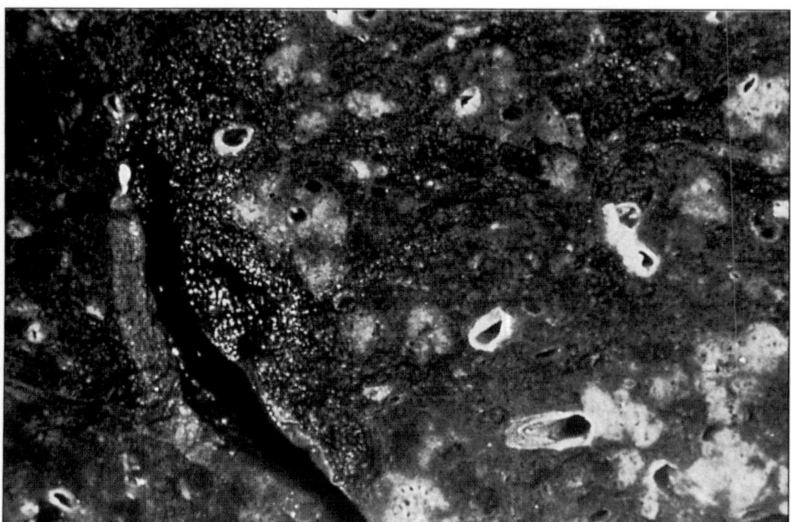

FIGURE 6-11 Autopsy sample of lung parenchyma from a patient with *Pseudomonas aeruginosa* pneumonia. A close-up photograph shows areas of hemorrhage with multiple yellow-white abscesses. Diffuse *Pseudomonas* bronchopneumonia may be associated with microabscess or macroabscess formation, necrosis of alveolar septa, and focal hemorrhage.

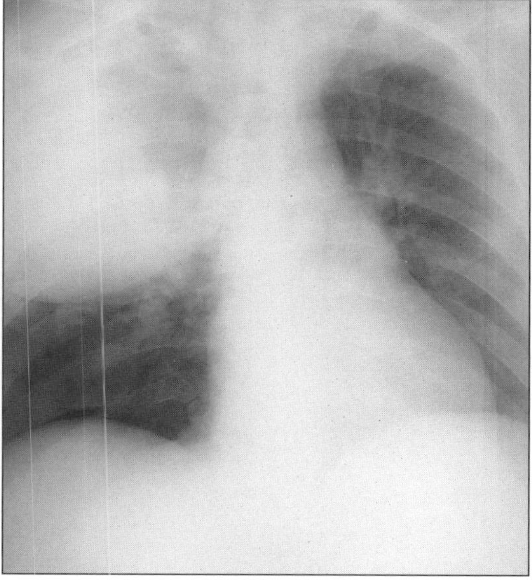

FIGURE 6-12 Chest radiograph of right upper lobe pneumonia due to *Klebsiella pneumoniae*, demonstrating the classic picture of infiltration with a bulging fissure. This radiologic finding occurs secondary to underlying necrotic inflammation and hemorrhage. Extensive scarring, necrosis, and abscess formation are characteristic of *Klebsiella* pneumonia. Microscopically, acute *Klebsiella* pneumonia is characterized by a diffuse intra-alveolar inflammatory exudate that contains a large number of foamy macrophages in addition to neutrophils. Grossly, the lung is red to gray in color, and the cut surface may have a mucoid appearance. Posteroanterior view.

Atypical Pneumonia and Pneumonia Due to Higher Bacteria

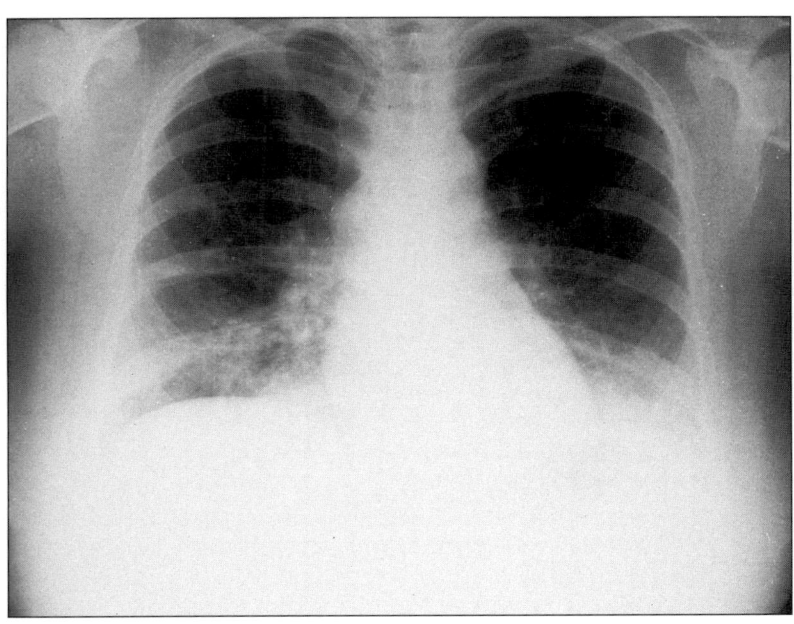

Figure 6-13 Chest radiograph of a young woman with *Mycoplasma pneumoniae* pneumonia showing bilateral patchy alveolar opacities of the lower lobes. There is a wide spectrum of radiographic presentations in *M. pneumoniae* pneumonia, including alveolar disease, interstitial disease, or combined interstitial/alveolar disease. Infiltrates are characteristically unilateral patchy areas of bronchopneumonia, usually involving the lower lobes; multilobar involvement, pleural effusion, and hilar adenopathy have been described. *M. pneumoniae* infection often begins insidiously with gradual onset of constitutional and pneumonic symptoms. As the disease progresses, fever and a hacking cough productive of mucoid or mucopurulent sputum develop. (*From* Marrie [2]; with permission.)

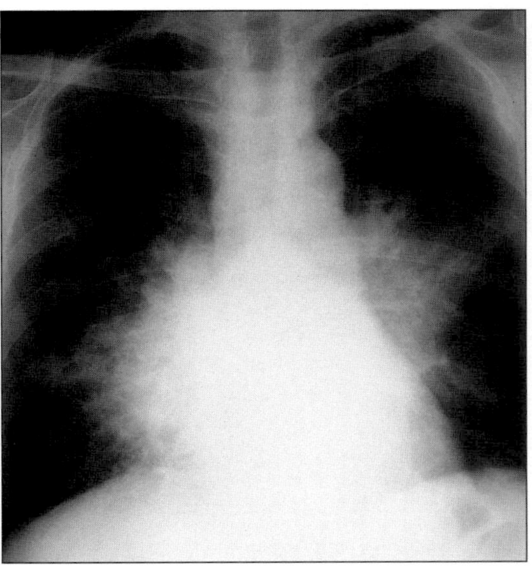

Figure 6-14 Chest radiograph of a patient with chronic lymphocytic leukemia demonstrating confluent right middle lobe and lingular infiltrates secondary to *Legionella pneumophila* pneumonia. Risk factors for *Legionella* infection include cigarette smoking, chronic obstructive pulmonary disease, steroid therapy, transplantation, and old age. *Legionella* species rank among the top three microbial agents of community-acquired pneumonia in several studies. (*Courtesy of* N. Ettinger, MD.)

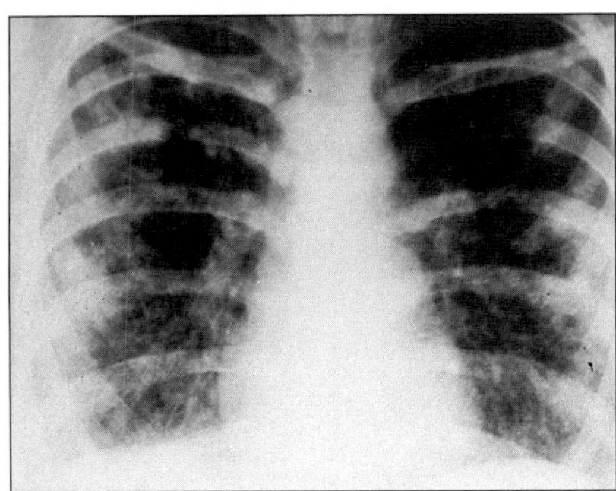

Figure 6-15 Chest radiograph of psittacosis demonstrating a patchy symmetrical interstitial infiltrate, especially involving the lower lobes. After the organism is inhaled, *Chlamydia psittaci* is taken up by the reticuloendothelial cells of the liver and spleen, where it replicates and spreads hematogenously to the lungs. Radiographic findings are varied. The most common presentation is as a patchy infiltrate radiating outward from the hilum; but miliary patterns, consolidation, and pleural effusion may be seen. (*From* Schaffner [3]; with permission.)

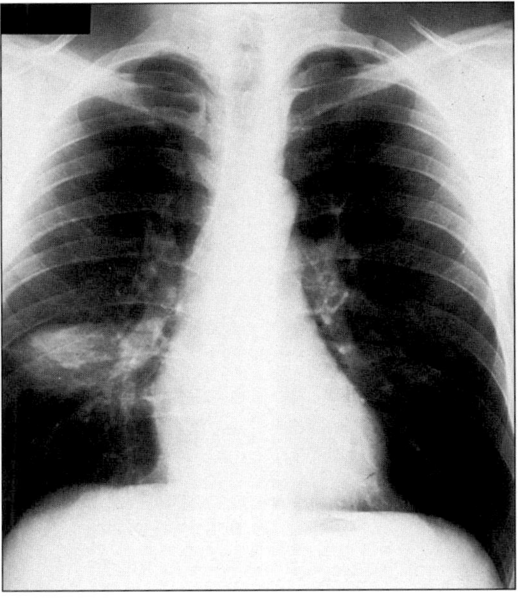

Figure 6-16 Chest radiograph of a right upper lobe segmental infiltrate secondary to *Coxiella burnetii* infection. Chest radiograph abnormalities in Q fever most resemble those seen with viral and *Mycoplasma pneumoniae* infection. There are usually single or multiple rounded segmental densities in the lower lobes; lobar consolidation, coin lesions, hilar adenopathy, atelectasis, and pleural effusions have been reported. The presence of a severe headache may be a clue to the diagnosis, which is confirmed serologically because isolation is difficult and hazardous to laboratory personnel. The treatment of choice for *C. burnetii* pneumonia is tetracycline. (*Courtesy of* T.J. Marrie, MD.)

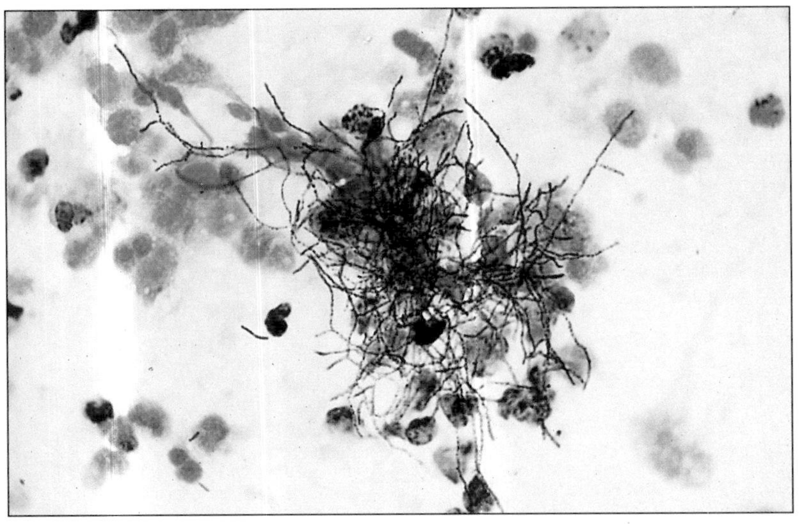

Figure 6-17 Sputum Gram stain from a patient with *Nocardia asteroides* pneumonia. The organism appears as thin, weakly gram positive, branching, often beaded filaments. *Nocardia* is a member of the order Actinomycetales, along with *Actinomyces* and *Streptomyces*, and was first described by Nocard in 1889 during an outbreak of bovine farcy. Although *Nocardia* exhibits the fungal characteristic of aerial hyphae, it is considered a higher bacterium because the cell wall consists of peptidoglycans and lacks chitin and cellulose. *Nocardia* is ubiquitous and is found primarily in soil and organic matter.

Tuberculosis and Other Mycobacterial Infections of the Lungs

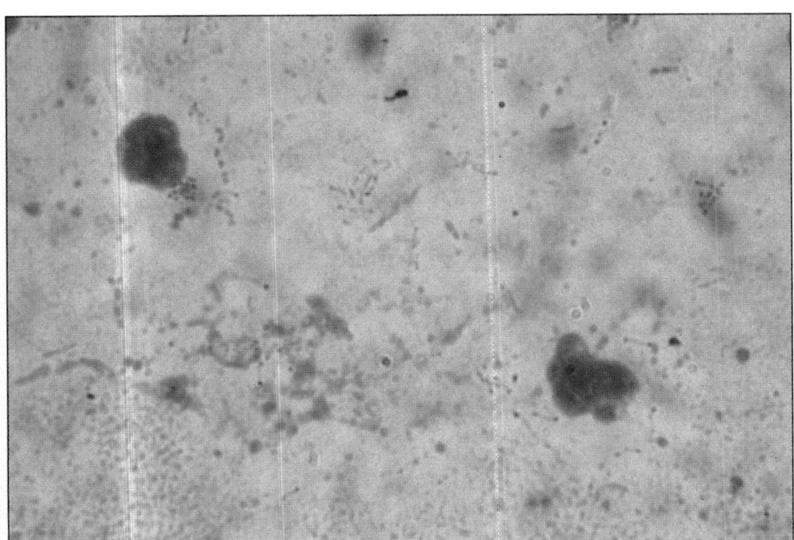

Figure 6-18 Kinyoun stain of sputum demonstrating numerous acid-fast bacilli. Approximately 10,000 acid-fast bacilli are needed per milliliter of sputum to be detected microscopically. Sputum for culture must first be treated by decontamination and digestion to reduce bacterial overgrowth and release trapped mycobacterial cells from liquefied mucus. The specimen then undergoes high-speed centrifugation to concentrate the organisms in the sediment.

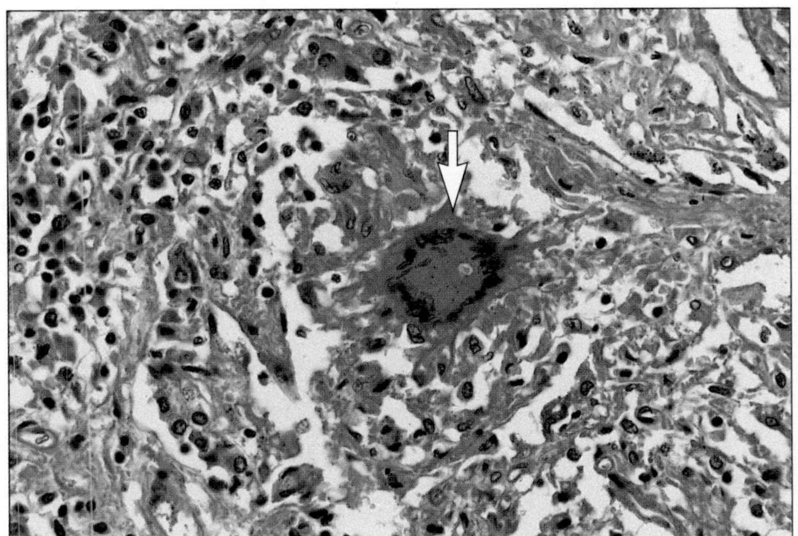

Figure 6-19 Epithelioid cell granuloma containing Langhans' giant cells. Epithelioid cells are highly stimulated macrophages. The Langhans' giant cell (*arrow*) represents fused macrophages oriented around tuberculous antigen, with the multiple nuclei in a peripheral position. Activated macrophages secrete a fibroblast-stimulating substance that leads to collagen production and eventual fibrosis. This hard tubercle is able to contain infection and heals with fibrosis, encapsulation, and scar formation (*Courtesy of* G. Sidhu, MD.)

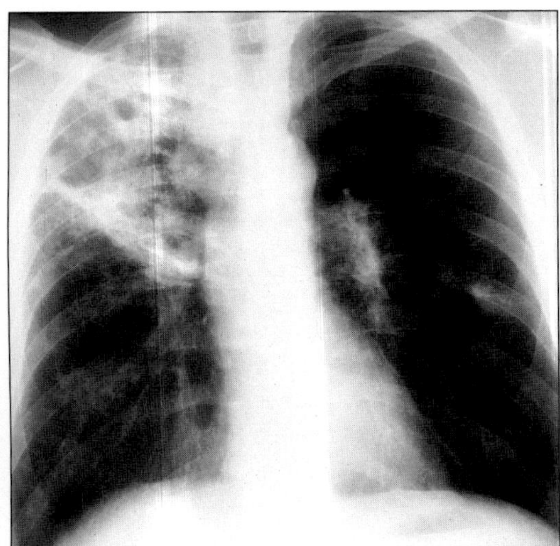

Figure 6-20 Chest radiograph of a 39-year-old man with acute upper lobe tuberculosis demonstrating typical cavitary infiltrates. Apical localization of pulmonary tuberculosis is characteristic of adult infection. This localization has been attributed to the hyperoxic environment of the apices, but another theory proposes that lymph production is deficient at the apices, favoring retention of antigens at this location [4]. (*Courtesy of* N. Ettinger, MD.)

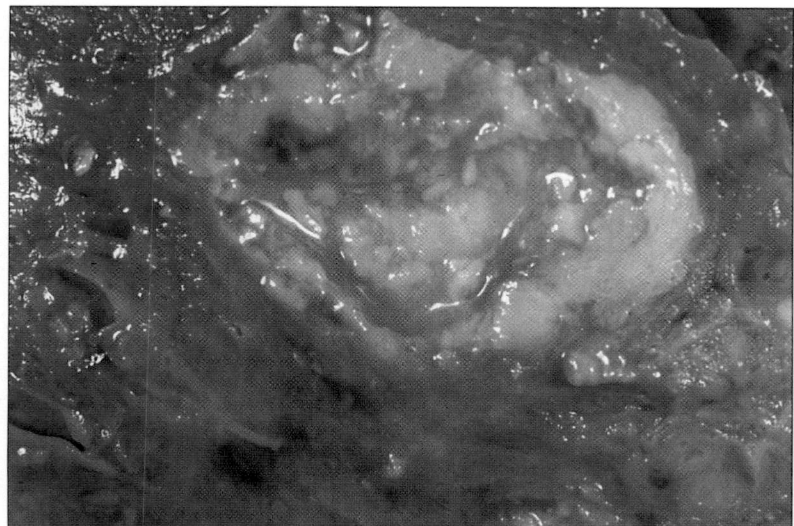

Figure 6-21 Gross photograph of a tuberculous cavity with caseous content. An active, freshly opened cavity exemplifies the many pathologic reactions that occur with tuberculous infection. Microscopically, the cavity contains a central core of many bacilli lined by a layer of caseous material with fewer organisms; a more peripheral layer of macrophages and lymphocytes with still fewer organisms; a layer of epithelioid cells and Langhans' giant cells; and finally a layer of encapsulating fibrosis. (*Courtesy of* G. Sidhu, MD.)

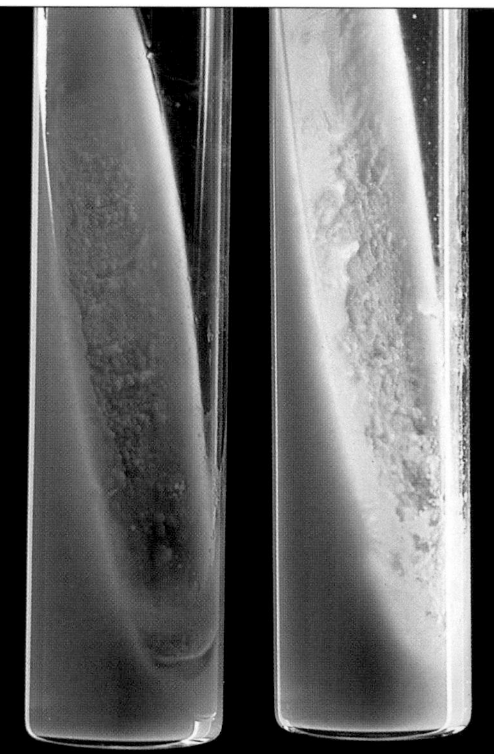

Figure 6-22 *Mycobacterium kansasii* colonies on Löwenstein-Jensen media. The distinctive feature of this photochromogenic species is dependence on light exposure for production of yellow pigment. Both tubes are shielded from light during incubation; the tube on the right was exposed to light for several hours and developed pigmented colonies. Typical strains grow at about the same rate or slightly faster than *Mycobacterium tuberculosis*. Colonies are intermediate between fully rough and fully smooth.

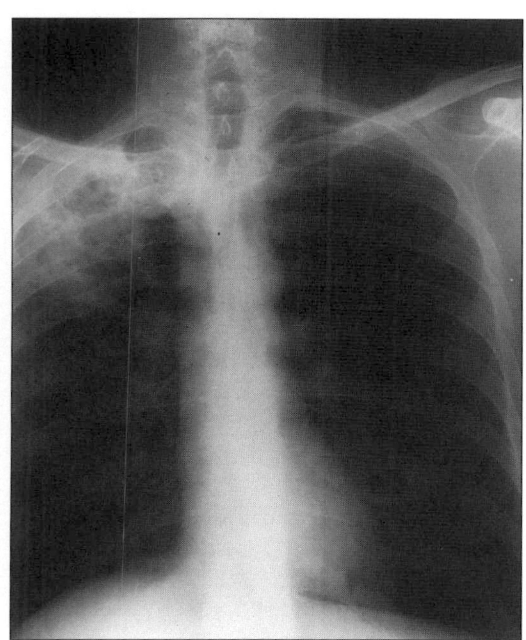

Figure 6-23 Chest radiograph from a 50-year-old man with chronic *Mycobacterium avium-intracellulare* pulmonary infection. This radiograph, taken after 2 years of therapy with a five-drug antibiotic regimen, shows persistence of a right upper lobe infiltrate with areas of cavitation. In most immunocompetent patients, infection follows an indolent course and is similar to tuberculosis radiographically. Treatment is complicated by the wide resistance of strains to the first-line agents. Treatment regimens include ethambutol, a macrolide antibiotic (clarithromycin or azithromycin), ciprofloxacin, rifabutin, clofazamine, and amikacin. In non-AIDS patients, resectional surgery may be used in conjunction with chemotherapy [5]. (*Courtesy of* N. Ettinger, MD.)

Fungal Infections

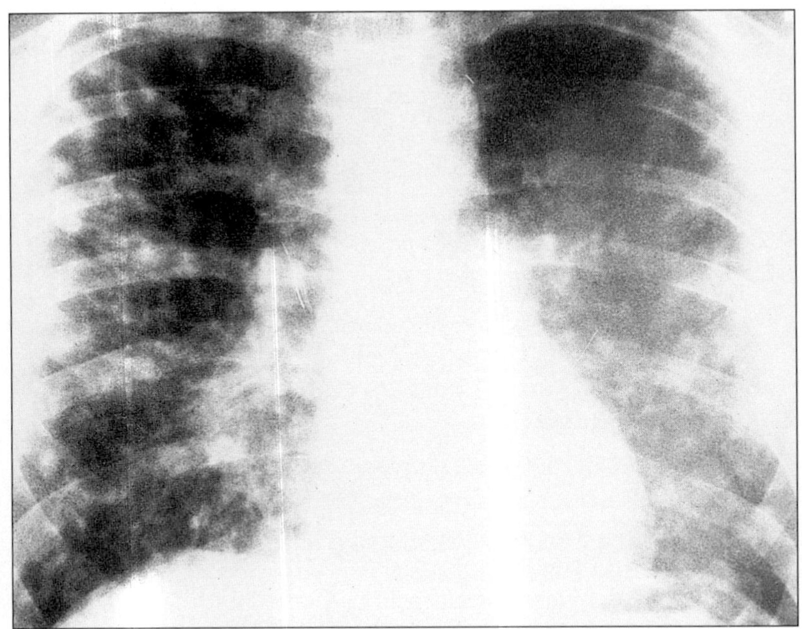

Figure 6-24 Chest radiograph showing diffuse, bilateral micronodular infiltrates in inhalational histoplasmosis. A 32-year-old man was exposed to large concentrations of *Histoplasma capsulatum* spores in a closed space while cleaning an attic contaminated by large amounts of bat droppings. Exactly 2 weeks later, he presented with headache, cough, and fever. His chest radiograph showed diffuse micronodular infiltrates throughout both lung fields. Serologic tests were positive. An immunodiffusion test was positive for H and M bands, and the competent fixation test was positive at a titer of 1:64. The patient was febrile for almost 2 weeks but eventually made a complete recovery without any specific antifungal therapy.

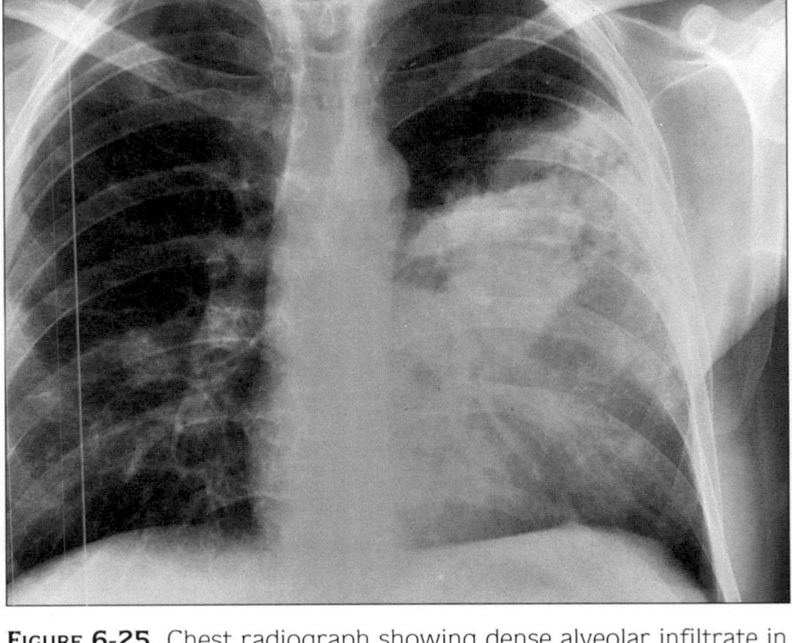

Figure 6-25 Chest radiograph showing dense alveolar infiltrate in blastomycosis. A posteroanterior chest radiograph shows a large, dense alveolar infiltrate involving the left midlung in a 33-year-old intravenous drug user. Direct smears of sputum after potassium hydroxide digestion were positive for *Blastomyces dermatitidis*. Sputum cultures were also positive. The dense alveolar infiltrates can resemble infiltrates of pneumococcal or other bacterial pneumonia. This patient was initially started on oral ketoconazole therapy, but while receiving that therapy, he developed multiple skin lesions and blastomycotic meningitis. Therapy was switched to intravenous amphotericin B, and he fully recovered. (*From* Bone *et al.* [6]; with permission.)

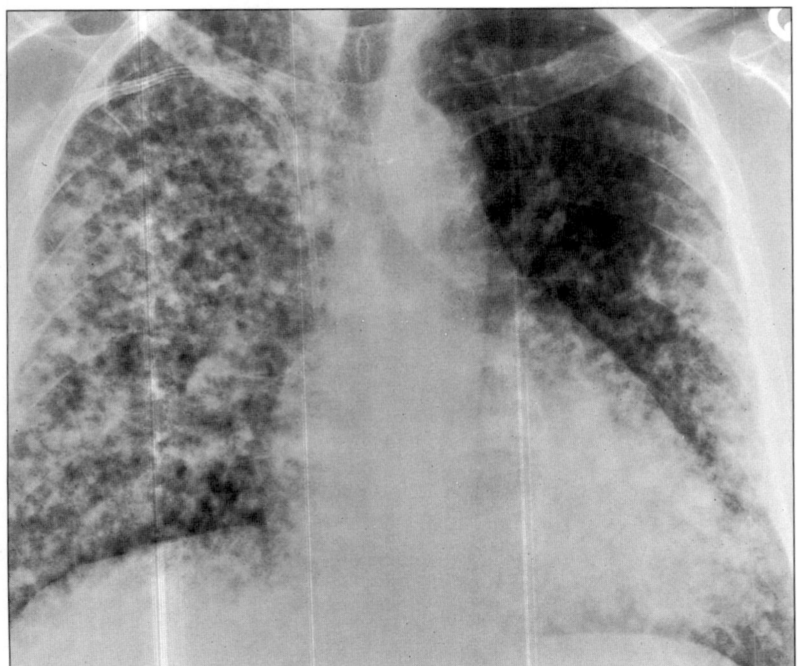

Figure 6-26 Chest radiograph showing diffuse nodular infiltrates in blastomycosis. A 50-year-old dialysis patient presented with fever and chills and progressive respiratory failure. The initial suspicion was tuberculosis, but an open-lung biopsy showed *Blastomyces dermatitidis* on histopathologic sections and on cultures. The patient recovered after treatment with intravenous amphotericin B. Diffuse infiltrates in blastomycosis can range from fine interstitial infiltrates to diffuse nodular infiltrates or even to diffuse alveolar infiltrates with prominent air bronchograms typical for noncardiac pulmonary edema. (*From* Bone *et al.* [6]; with permission.)

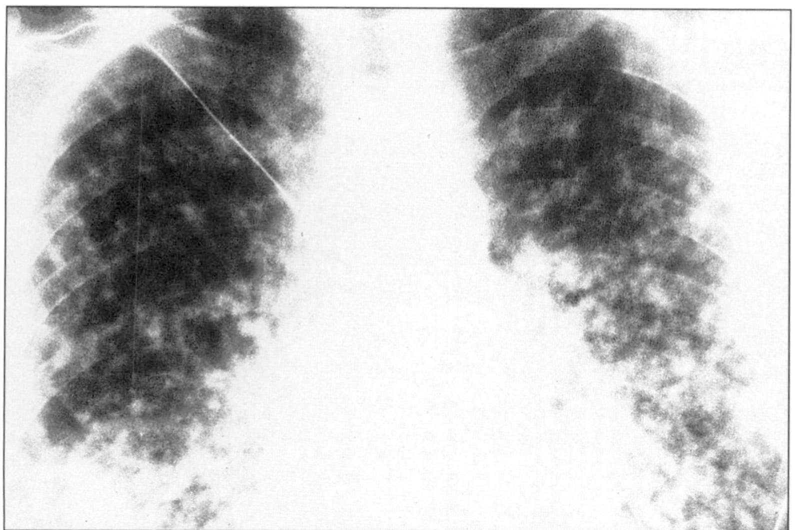

Figure 6-27 Chest radiograph showing diffuse macronodular pulmonary infiltrates in coccidioidomycosis. The individual nodules are larger than miliary nodules, even up to 1 to 2 cm in size. The patient was a 28-year-man with AIDS who lived half of each year in Phoenix, Arizona. He presented with fever and progressive dyspnea. At bronchoscopy, large endobronchial ulcers were seen at the right upper lobe and right middle lobe takeoffs. Endobronchial biopsy specimens showed spherules. Bronchoalveolar lavage was also positive for spherules and was negative for *Pneumocystis carinii* and other pathogens.

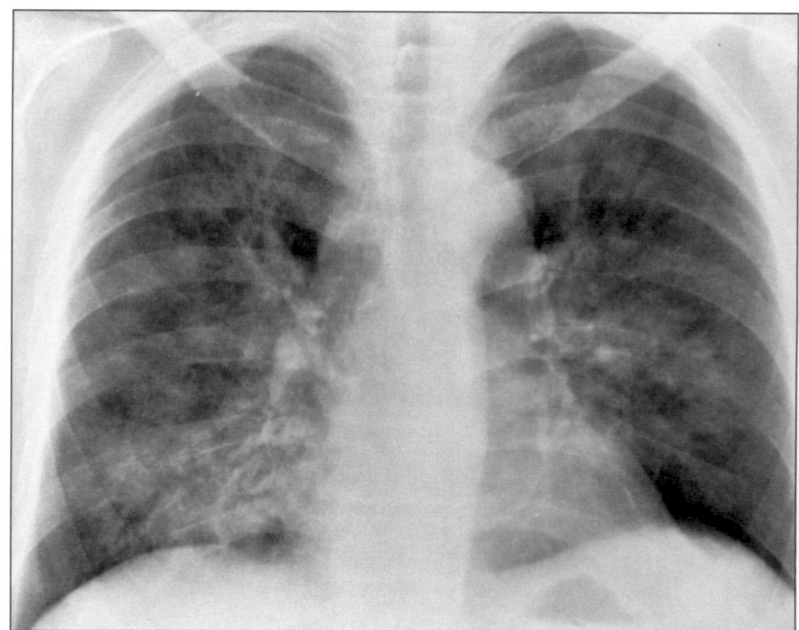

Figure 6-28 Chest radiograph showing diffuse bilateral infiltrates in cryptococcosis. The patient, who was receiving high-dose prednisone for collagen vascular disease, presented with fever and then progressive shortness of breath. Blood cultures were positive for *Cryptococcus neoformans*. Diffuse pulmonary infiltrates from cryptococcal infection are most common in patients with AIDS. AIDS patients with cryptococcal infection, unlike immunocompetent patients, usually have positive cryptococcal antigen in the serum at a titer higher than that in cerebrospinal fluid.

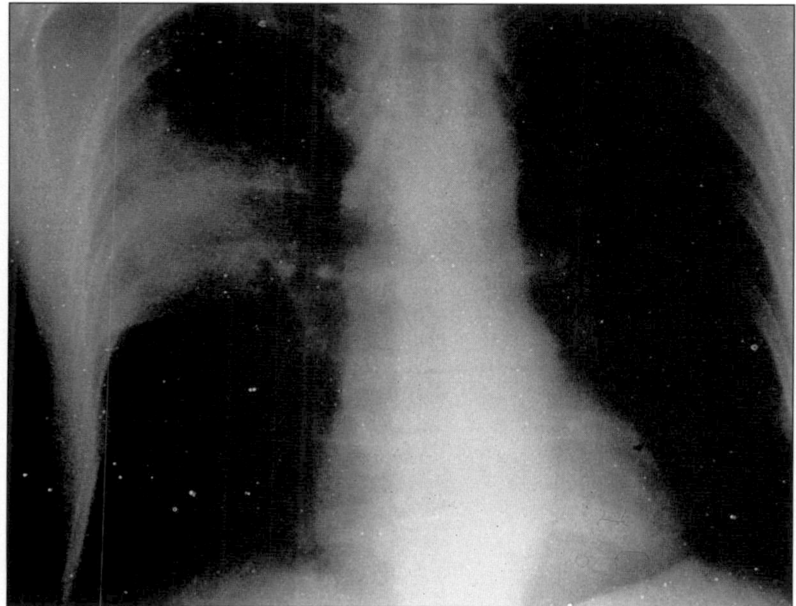

Figure 6-29 Chest radiograph in invasive aspergillosis showing a dense wedge-shaped infiltrate in the right upper lobe. The patient was a 74-year-old man with prolonged neutropenia. Invasive aspergillosis complicates prolonged neutropenia or severe neutrophil dysfunction, including phagocyte dysfunction caused by prolonged therapy with high-dose prednisone. The disease is angioinvasive and can present with a wedge-shaped peripheral infiltrate. Patients can have hemoptysis and pleuritic pain and present with a syndrome resembling pulmonary infarction.

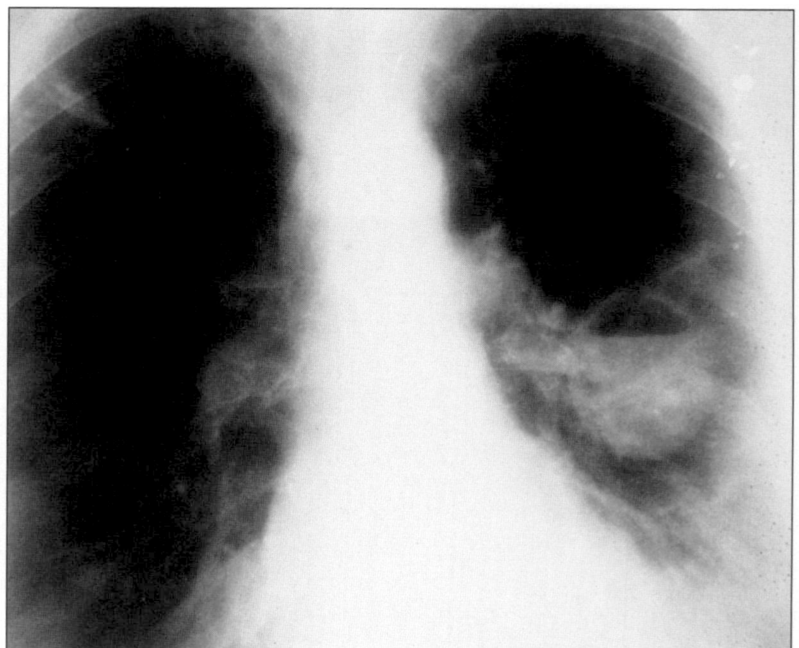

Figure 6-30 Chest radiograph in mucormycosis showing a large cavitary mass in the left lower lobe. The patient was a 60-year-old woman who had idiopathic thrombocytic purpura being treated with high-dose prednisone. She also had diabetes induced by the prednisone and was receiving insulin. She presented with fever and this radiographic mass on chest radiographs. Specimens drawn by transthoracic fine-needle aspiration showed typical hyphae of *Mucor*, and the cultures were also positive. The patient was treated by reducing the prednisone dose and with intravenous amphotericin B and recovered.

Anaerobic Lung Infections, Lung Abscesses, and Nosocomial Pneumonias

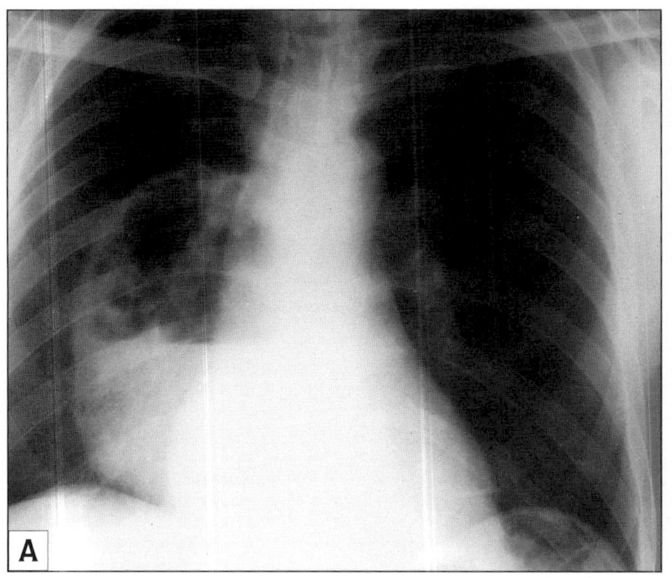

Figure 6-31 **A**, Chest radiograph of right lower lobe abscess in a 60-year-old alcoholic. **B**, Computed tomography scan of the chest, demonstrating the extent of the abscess cavity. A consistent feature of anaerobic lung infections is tissue necrosis resulting in abscess formation, bronchopleural fistulae, and empyemas. Clinically, low-grade fever and foul-smelling sputum are generally present. Anemia and weight loss, as well as associated empyema, are also common. Although successful treatment for this patient involved lobectomy, clinical response is usually obtained with prolonged antimicrobial therapy and postural drainage. Indeed, surgical resection is relatively contraindicated, given the risks of spillage of abscess contents, and is usually reserved for patients with underlying neoplasms. Mortality of lung abscess in most series is 15% or less.

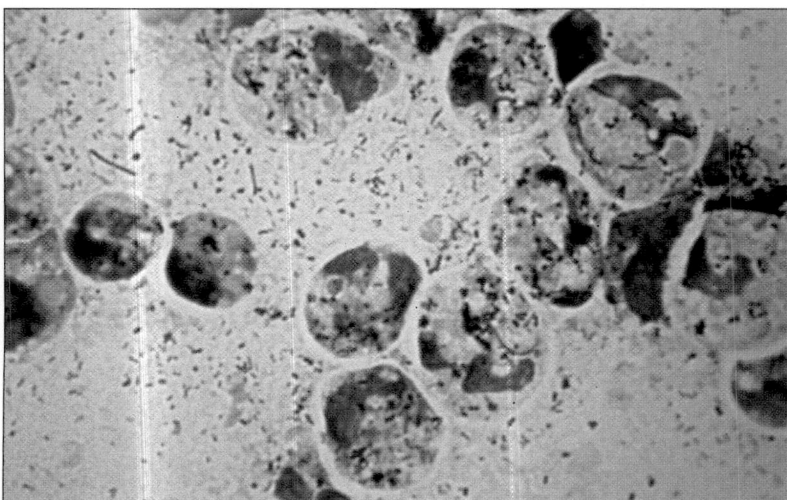

Figure 6-32 Gram stain of expectorated sputum in a patient with an anaerobic lung abscess. Gram-negative bacilli and gram-positive cocci may be seen. Although bacteriologic diagnosis cannot be made from these specimens, the presence of mixed flora, without significant growth of pathogens on routine culture, may suggest anaerobic involvement. In community-acquired aspiration pneumonia and lung abscesses, anaerobic oral flora, including *Prevotella*, *Porphyromonas*, *Peptostreptococcus*, and *Fusobacterium*, predominate. In hospitalized patients, nosocomial pathogens, such as enteric gram-negative bacilli, *Pseudomonas*, and *Staphylococcus aureus*, may also be involved.

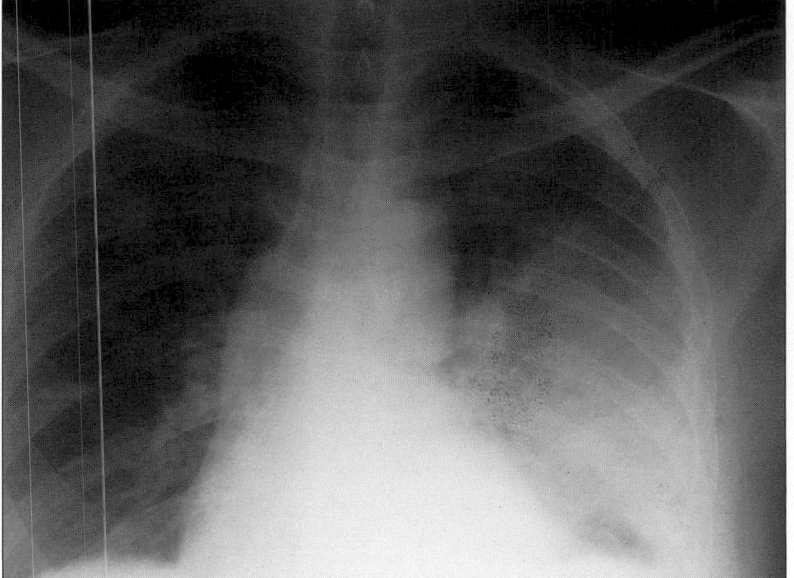

Figure 6-33 Chest radiograph showing anaerobic empyema. Anaerobes now account for 30% to 50% of empyemas. This suppurative complication of anaerobic pneumonitis, or lung abscess with bronchopleural fistula, requires adequate drainage of the pleural space as is indicated for any grossly purulent empyema. Pleural fluid is an easily accessible source for uncontaminated cultures, simplifying isolation of anaerobes.

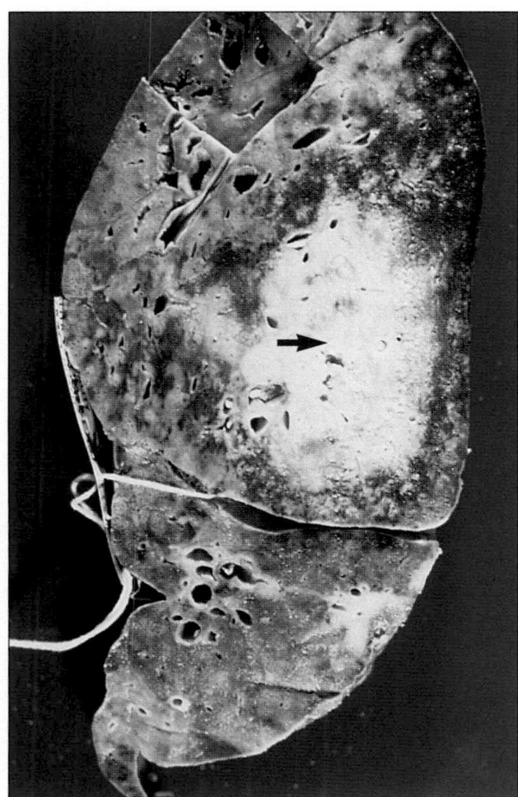

FIGURE 6-34 Autopsy specimen of lung showing necrotizing pneumonia (*arrow*) in a mechanically ventilated patient. Pneumonia causes the most deaths among the nosocomial infections. The mortality rate is estimated at 20% to 50% and is probably higher with some gram-negative isolates (such as *Pseudomonas aeruginosa*). Given the estimated rate of nosocomial pneumonia, as many as 100,000 patients may die annually in the United States from such infections.

VIRAL PNEUMONIAS

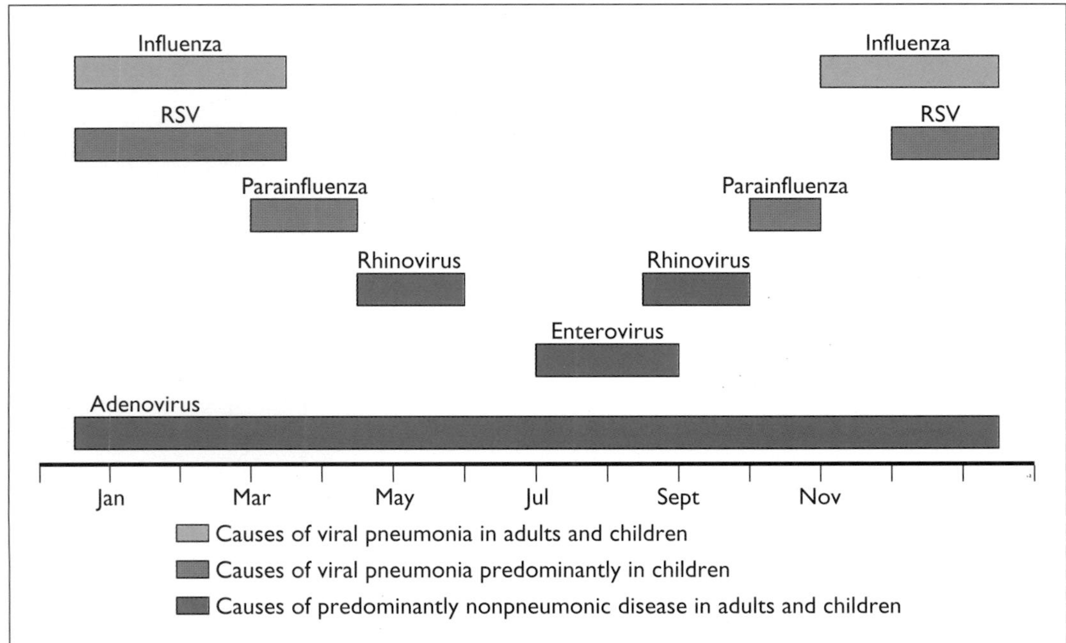

FIGURE 6-35 Seasonal variation in respiratory virus infections. Viral pneumonia is caused by relatively few virus types. Not included in this graph are the viruses that cause primarily rashes (*eg,* measles and varicella) and are occasionally complicated by pneumonia, especially in adults. Each of the viruses has its own season, and outside that season, these viruses are seldom isolated. A concentration of cases of viral pneumonia occurs in the winter, with fewer cases in the spring and fall. Although viral pneumonia in adults is uncommon, it is an important clinical problem, and the clinical course can be severe. During the viral season, when a patient presents severely ill with acute pneumonia that is "atypical" (because no bacterial cause can be identified), the physician often concludes that it must be due to *Legionella pneumophila*. However, cultures of respiratory secretions for virus often will yield virus, usually influenza A or B virus. Although influenza causes pneumonia in children, most cases occur in very young infants. Respiratory syncytial virus (RSV) is more common than influenza and also affects a greater age range. Parainfluenza is also an important pathogen, especially in the immunocompromised child. In the summer, the only virus that causes pulmonary infiltration is the hantavirus (not shown). In contrast to the winter, many of the "atypical" cases of pneumonia in the summer are caused by *Legionella*. In truth, *Legionella* pneumonia really resembles typical pneumonia, except that a bacterial pathogen is not readily identified.

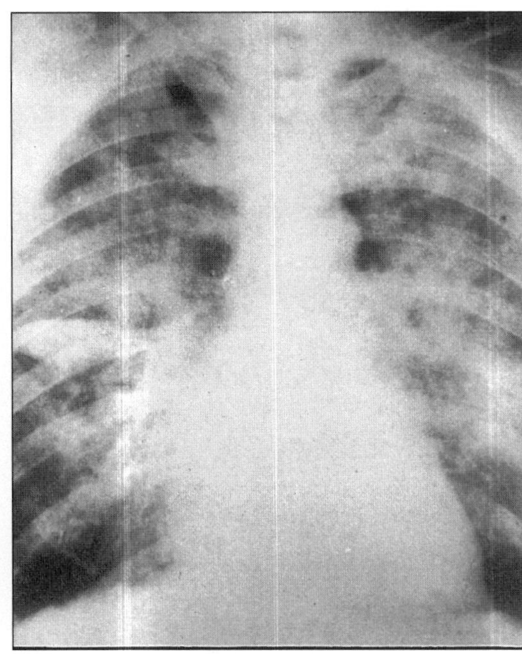

FIGURE 6-36 Admission chest radiograph of a 49-year-old man with primary influenza pneumonia superimposed on rheumatic heart disease with mitral stenosis and insufficiency. The density in the right midlung field represents a loculated interlobar effusion that was present prior to the acute illness. Diffuse interstitial infiltrates are seen bilaterally. This disease is typically associated with significant hypoxemia. (*From* Louria *et al.* [7]; with permission.)

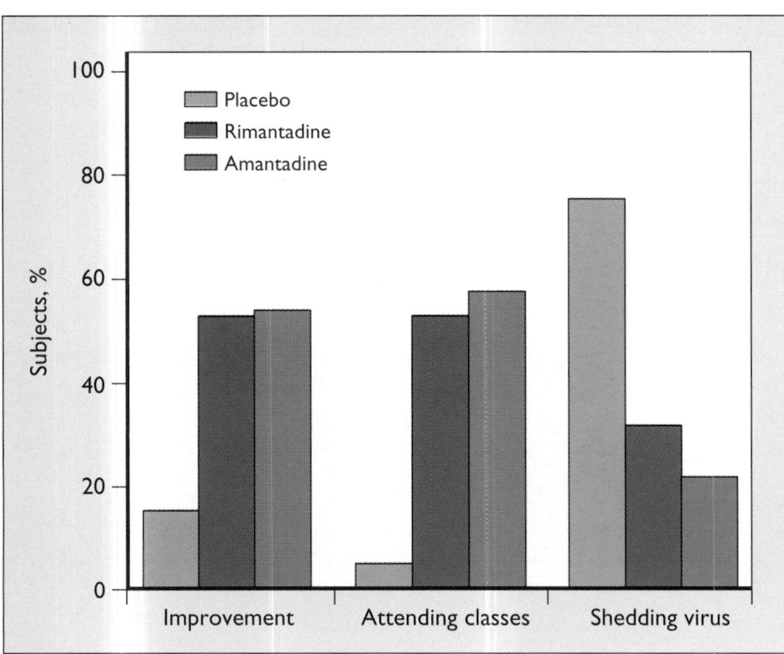

FIGURE 6-37 Treatment of H1N1 influenza with rimantadine versus amantadine in young adults. The first clinical evidence of effective antiviral treatment occurred in the treatment of influenza syndrome. Although outwardly the effect seems small, producing only a modest benefit in duration of fever and improvement in overall feeling of well-being, other evidence in fact suggests there is a greater impact. In a trial comparing rimantadine, amantadine, and placebo, the antiviral recipients not only improved more quickly than did placebo recipients, but also they returned to class more quickly following a bout of culture-proven influenza. Resuming classes (or work) has important economic ramifications, and because the individuals are clinically better, their performance may add to the difference. In addition, improvement was correlated with an antiviral effect. Conceivably, the shorter duration of viral shedding in the antiviral recipients could reduce transmission to susceptible persons, adding a second layer of benefit. (*Adapted from* Van Voris *et al.* [8].)

Frequency of clinical findings in influenza vs RSV

	Influenza	RSV
Fever > 39.4° C	+++†	+
Myalgia	++++	++
Rhinorrhea	+	++++
Sore throat	+++	+
Asthma*	+++	++++
New wheezing	+	++++
COPD*	++++	++++
Diarrhea	–	–

*Exacerbation of these conditions.

†The frequency of occurrence and/or degree of severity is indicated, ranging from none (-) to uncommon/mild (+) to very frequent/severe (++++).

COPD—chronic obstructive pulmonary disease; RSV—respiratory syncytial virus.

FIGURE 6-38 Comparative frequencies of symptoms in elderly patients with proven influenza or respiratory syncytial virus (RSV) infection. Although both influenza and RSV infection can exacerbate asthma or chronic obstructive pulmonary disease, noticeable differences are apparent in the degree of fever (> 103° F), severity of nasal discharge, complaint of sore throat and precipitation of wheezing in an individual who had not previously wheezed. This clinical differentiation between influenza and RSV infection is important in at least two ways. First, in a long-term health care facility, where nearly 100% of the residents have been vaccinated against influenza, it tells physicians that RSV may be causing the outbreak and not be discouraged about their vaccine program. Second, it may forestall the use of an antiviral directed against influenza if the clinical presentation is more characteristic of RSV.

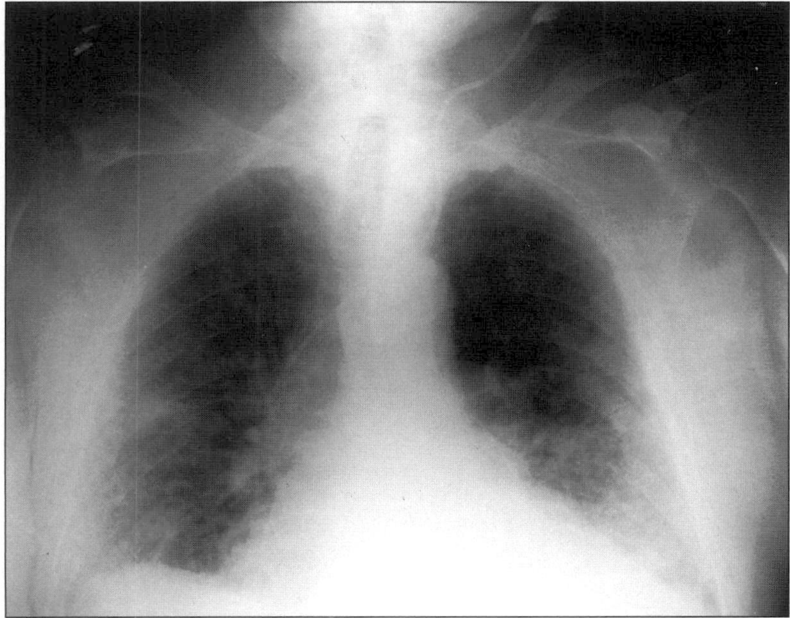

Figure 6-39 Chest radiograph showing respiratory syncytial virus (RSV) pneumonia in an elderly man. This elderly man presented with symptoms and chest findings consistent with congestive heart failure (CHF), but he was febrile. He was given standard therapy for CHF, but he failed to clear his lung fields and remained febrile. When RSV was isolated from a tracheal suction specimen, he was placed on inhaled ribavirin and improved promptly. Conclusions about the role of antiviral therapy in this setting are uncertain; however, in infants with congenital heart disease and unrelenting RSV infection, ribavirin appears to lead to improvement.

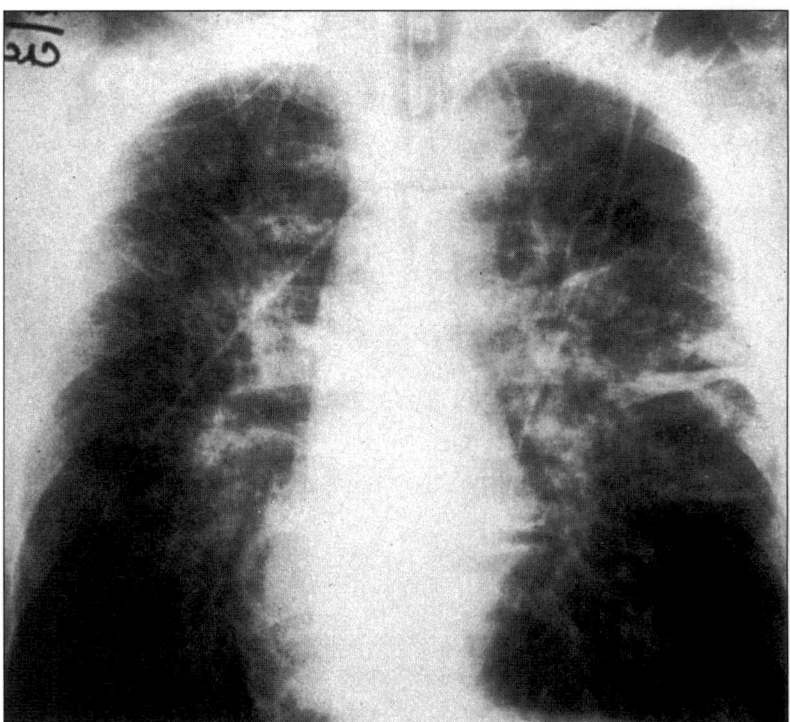

Figure 6-40 Chest radiograph of severe hantavirus pulmonary syndrome. Patients presenting with acute hantavirus pulmonary syndrome often are short of breath yet have a clear chest. Over the next several hours, they evolve rapidly, becoming hypoxic secondary to findings shown in this chest film. (*Courtesy of* G.J. Mertz, MD.)

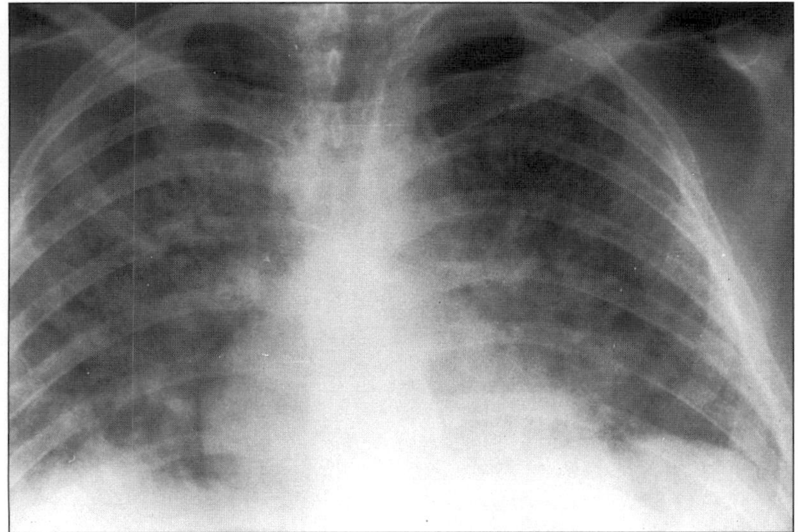

Figure 6-41 Typical diffuse reticulonodular infiltrates of varicella pneumonia in a pregnant woman. Varicella may be more severe in pregnancy. Early treatment with acyclovir has been shown to reduce fever and tachypnea in otherwise healthy adults with varicella pneumonia. (*From* Haake *et al.* [9]; with permission.)

PROTOZOAN AND HELMINTHIC INFECTIONS OF THE LUNGS

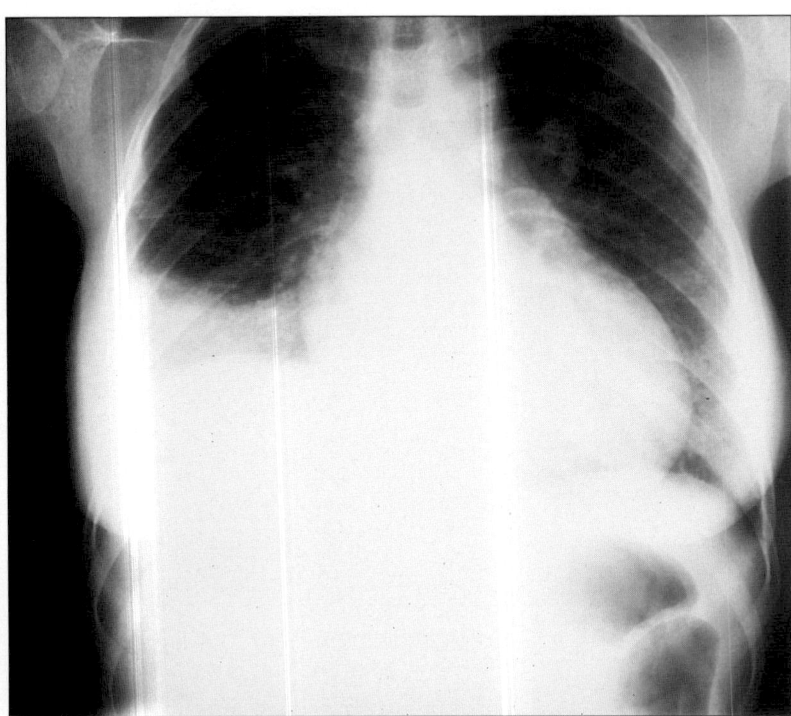

FIGURE 6-42 Chest radiograph of a patient with amebic liver abscess showing elevation of the right hemidiaphragm with pleural effusion. The incidence of pulmonary involvement in *Entamoeba histolytica* liver abscess ranges from 3% to 30%. When the abscess is adjacent to the diaphragm, it leads to its elevation, secondary atelectasis, and reactive pleural transudate. Pleuritic pain referred to the shoulder is typical, and pulmonary symptoms may dominate the clinical presentation. Effective treatment of the liver abscess leads to prompt resolution of the lung disease [10].

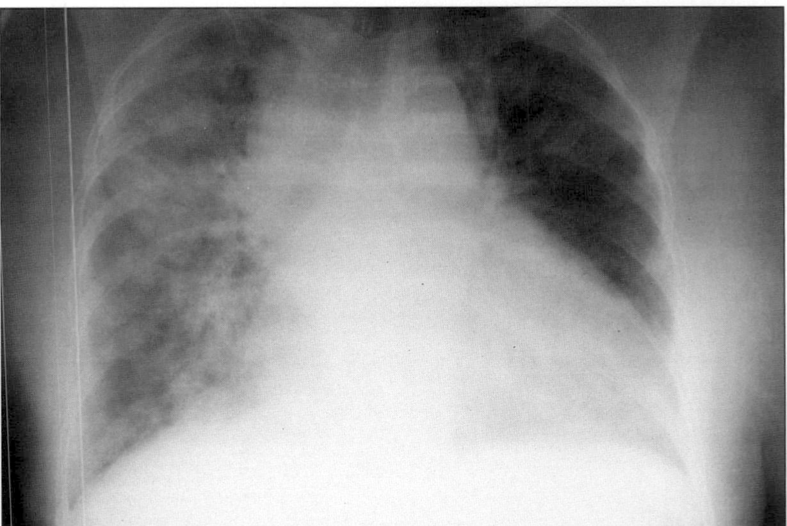

FIGURE 6-43 Disseminated strongyloides related to corticosteroid immunosuppression. Chest radiograph showing acute respiratory distress syndrome (ARDS). A 35-year-old Puerto Rican woman living in New York City who had not been home for 10 years had stage IV lymphoma treated with steroids and chemotherapy. She developed *Escherichia coli* septicemia, ARDS, and worsening diarrhea. *Strongyloides stercoralis* worms of every stage were found in her stool. Disseminated strongyloidiasis may occur in patients immunocompromised from any cause, particularly steroids or immunosuppressive drugs, and has an 85% mortality. It is characterized by ARDS, gram-negative septicemia with meningitis, and diarrhea. Larva currens or purpuric skin lesions in the flanks may be seen. Eosinophilia is absent. In disseminated disease, worms can be seen in BAL fluid and are easily detectable in stool samples [11].

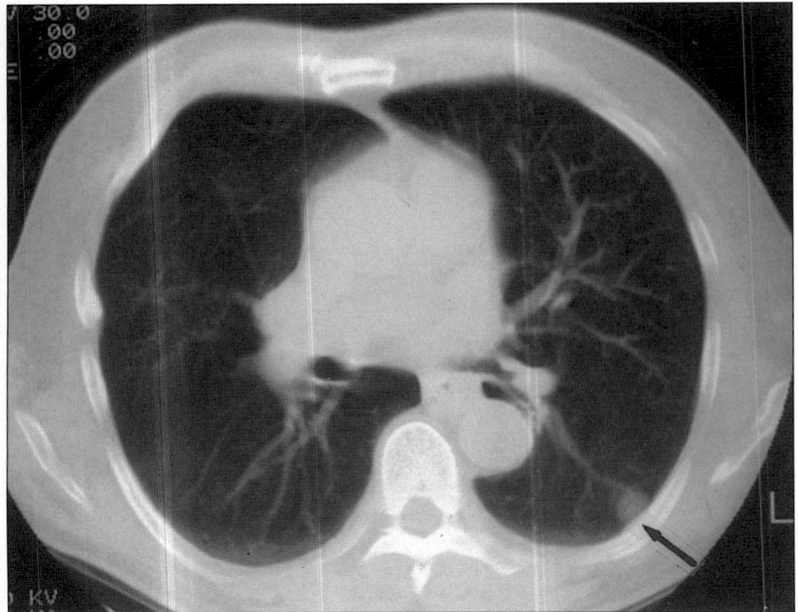

FIGURE 6-44 Computed tomography scan showing pleuropulmonary nodule of dirofilariasis (*arrow*). Immature filariae of *Dirofilaria immitis* migrate from the skin to the pulmonary circulation. Because they cannot mature (accidental infection) in humans, they die causing local vasculitis with pulmonary infarction; a granulomatous reaction may follow. Patients are usually asymptomatic. The coin lesions discovered on routine chest radiographs are frequently mistaken for malignancy. (*Courtesy of* K.L. Green, MD.)

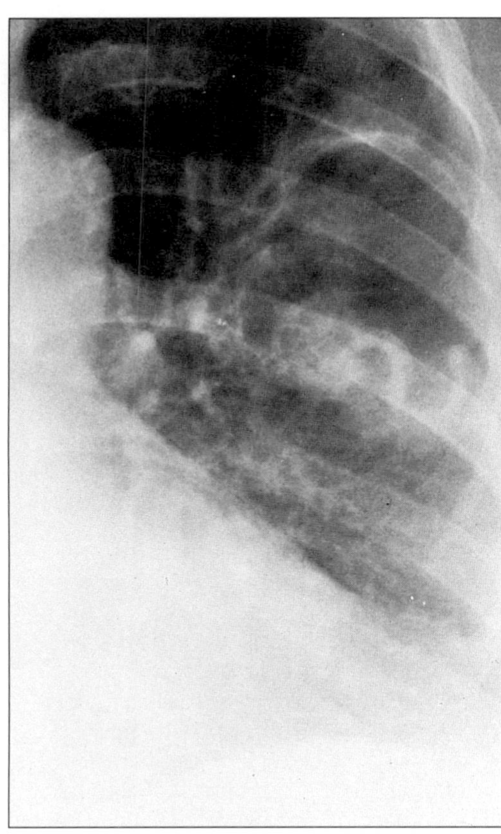

FIGURE 6-45 Chest radiograph showing ruptured hydatid cyst with water-lily or snake sign. This pathognomonic radiologic finding is seen when the cyst ruptures. A double line appears between the ectocyst and pericyst, and the collapsed hydatid membranes float on the surface of residual hydatid fluid and "sand." The patient complains of cough productive of watery sputum streaked with blood. Most tolerate this event, but 5% to 20% suffer anaphylactic shock or severe asthma and urticaria.

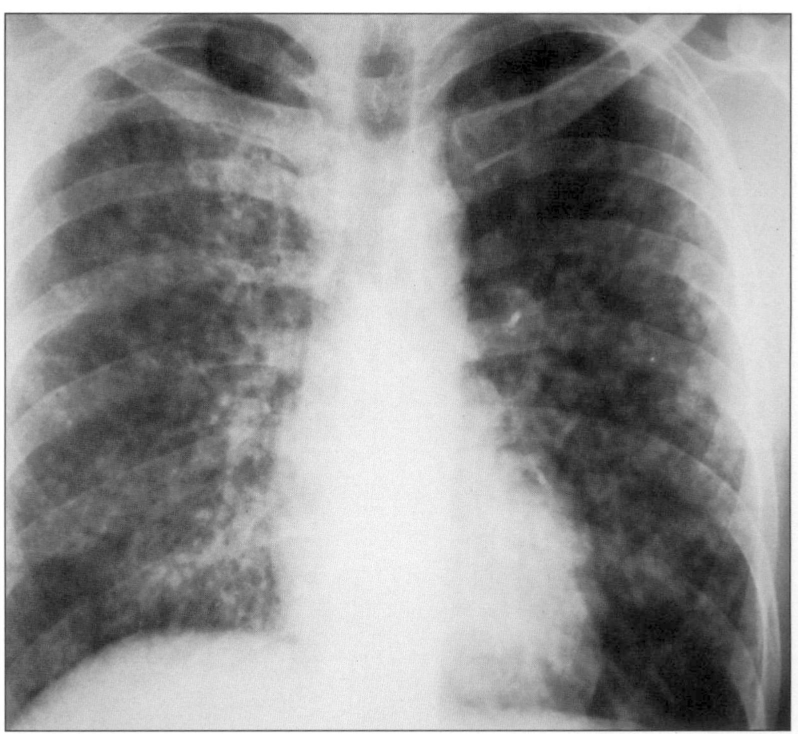

FIGURE 6-46 Chest radiograph showing miliary mottling in *Schistosoma mansoni* infection. Each pair of adult flukes in the mesenteric veins lives from 3 to 10 years and produces 200 to 3000 eggs daily. Most embolize to the liver, but some reach the pulmonary circulation, leading to obstruction to blood flow, arteritis, and granuloma formation followed by fibrous scarring. (*Courtesy of* G. McGuinness, MD.)

PLEURAL EFFUSION AND EMPYEMA

Incidence of pleural effusion and bacterial infection of the pleural space complicating pneumonia

	Incidence	
Infecting organism	**Pleural effusion**	**Infected pleural space**
Streptococcus pyogenes	75%	35%
Streptococcus pneumoniae	50%	3%
Staphylococcus aureus	40%	20%
Haemophilus influenzae	45%	20%
Escherichia coli	40%	80%
Klebsiella pneumoniae	10%	20%
Pseudomonas aeruginosa	50%	40%
Anaerobes	35%	90%
Legionella spp	40%	?
Mycoplasma pneumoniae	10%	NA
Viral, Q fever, psittacosis	Rare	NA

NA—not applicable.

FIGURE 6-47 Incidence of pleural effusion and bacterial infection of the pleural space complicating pneumonia. The frequencies of associated pleural effusion and infections are estimated in a variety of pneumonias. (*Adapted from* Light [12].)

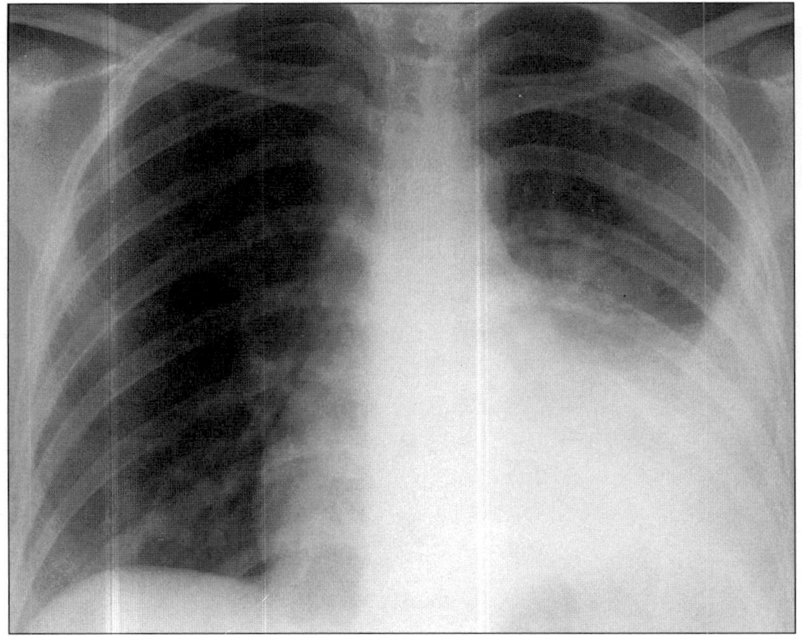

Figure 6-48 Acute community-acquired pneumonia with complicated parapneumonic effusion. Posteroanterior chest radiograph of a 30-year-old woman with fever and cough shows a left lower lobe consolidation. The lateral aspect of the density has the appearance of a pleural effusion, forming a meniscus. Ultrasound study (not shown) was not helpful in delineating the effusion. A computed tomography (CT) scan (also not shown) reveals, however, the loculated pleural effusion and subjacent pulmonary consolidation. Pleural fluid was obtained by CT-guided diagnostic thoracentesis.

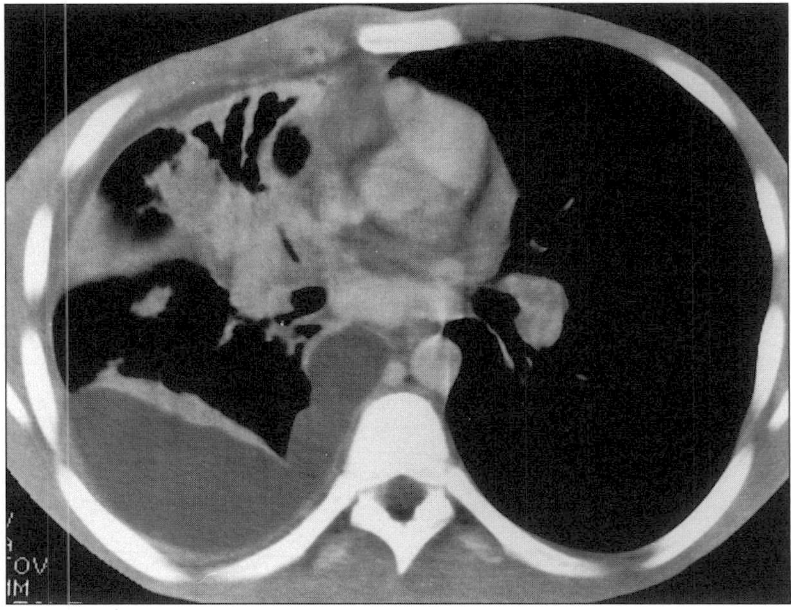

Figure 6-49 Pseudomonas empyema managed with intracavitary urokinase. An 18-year-old man with cystic fibrosis with Pseudomonas pneumonia of the right lung, complicated by effusion, had protracted fever despite appropriate antibiotic coverage. Contrast-enhanced computed tomography scan strongly suggests that the pleural collection, by its restricted configuration of fluid in nondependent locations, contains loculations. The individual septations are invisible because they have the same density as the pleural fluid. The pneumonia is visible anteriorly.

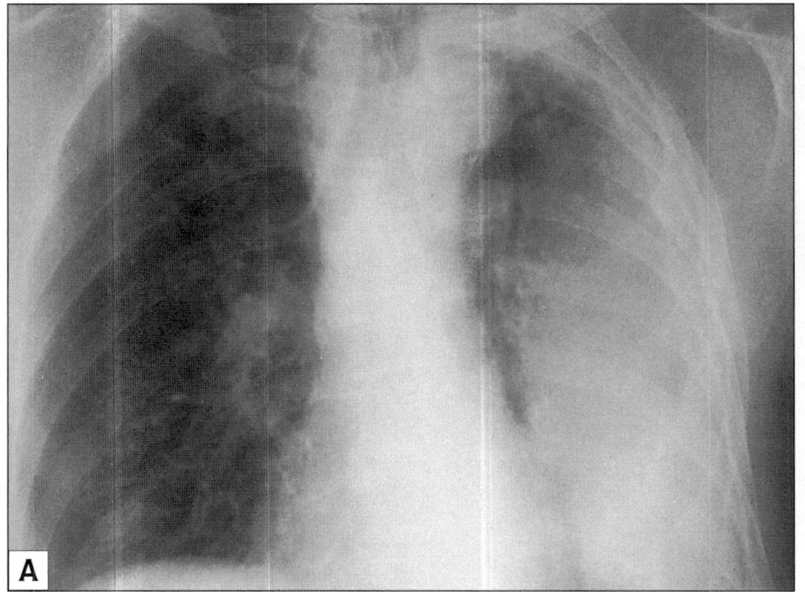

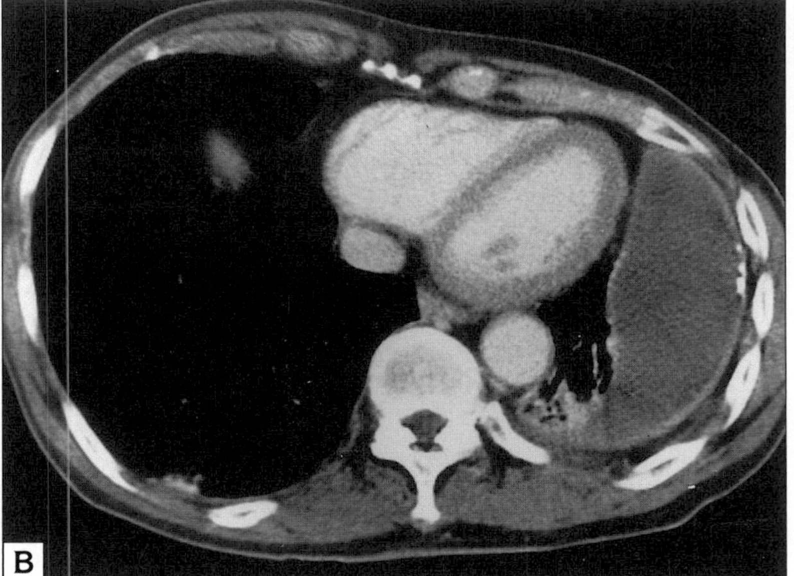

Figure 6-50 Large chronic tuberculous empyema. An asymptomatic 54-year-old man had a remote history of tuberculosis. **A**, The posteroanterior chest radiograph shows extensive thickening of the pleura laterally on the left side. Calcification is present. This radiographic appearance was unchanged during 10 years of observation. The differential diagnosis of unilateral thickened and calcified pleura includes a chronic empyema, most likely to be tuberculous, or a posttraumatic, organized hemothorax. The latter diagnosis is usually associated with healed ipsilateral rib fractures, not seen in the current case. **B**, Contrast-enhanced computed tomography image reveals a large chronic tuberculous empyema. The rib interspaces are narrowed, reflecting volume loss. Marked extrapleural fat hyperplasia is evident, deep to the ribs and superficial to the parietal pleura. Both parietal and visceral pleura are thickened and demonstrate contrast enhancement. Both layers also demonstrate focal calcification. Pleural collections due to tuberculosis can remain clinically quiescent and unchanged for many years. Drainage of such chronic collections is not indicated.

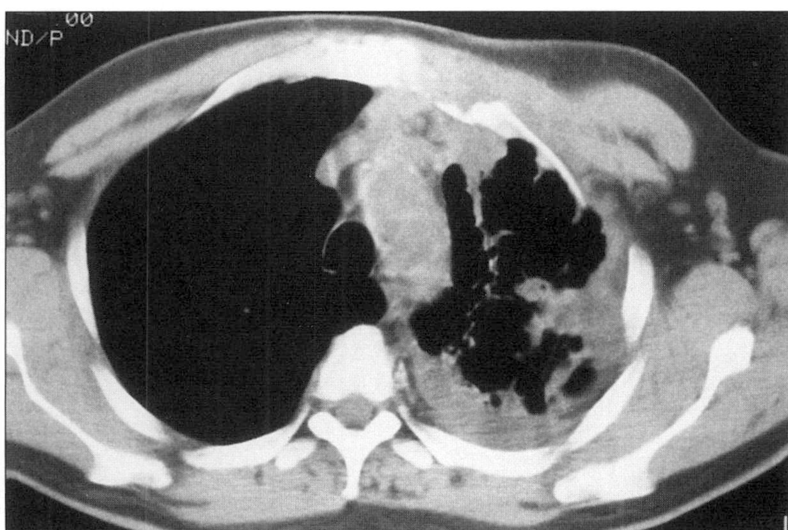

Figure 6-51 Thoracic actinomycosis with involvement of the pleural space, mediastinum, and chest wall. An alcoholic man presented with indolent weight loss, low-grade fever, and chest-wall tenderness and erythema. The computed tomography scan revealed a left upper lobe pneumonia spreading contiguously to involve the adjacent pleura, mediastinum, and chest wall. Edema and an inflammatory mass are evident in the subcutaneous tissues and musculature of the anterior chest wall. Involvement of an anterior rib is seen. Mediastinal lymphadenopathy and a small, dependently layering pleural effusion are also present. The diagnosis was established by fine-needle aspiration of the fluctuant subcutaneous abscess.

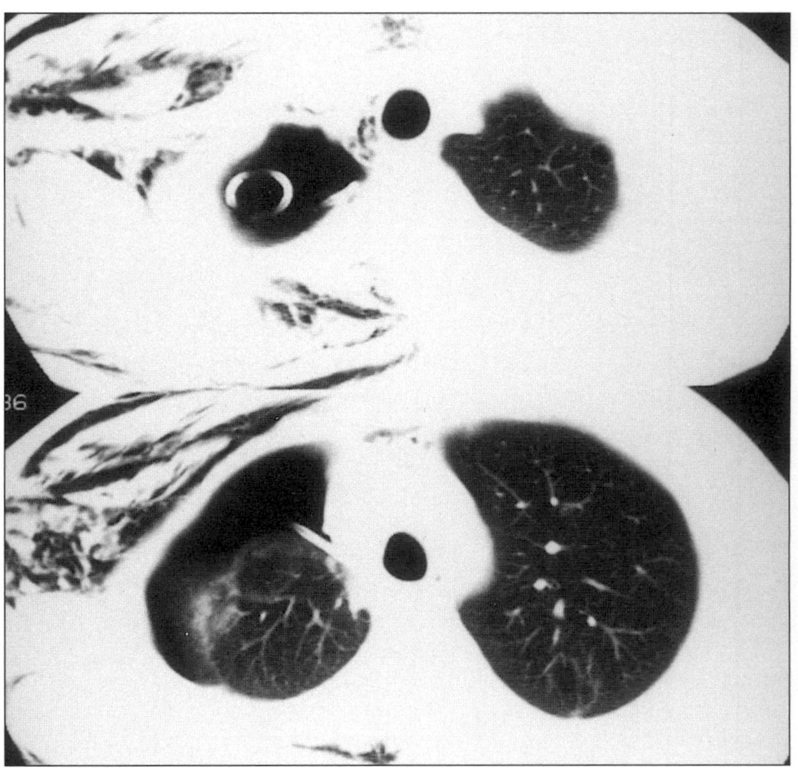

Figure 6-52 Pneumothorax and subcutaneous emphysema. During catheter placement for treatment of a persistent bronchopleural fistula, which followed a segmental pulmonary resection, two computed tomography images show the distal portion of a curved catheter placed in the pleural space. There is marked subcutaneous air from a prior chest tube placement. Air is noted to dissect between fascial planes, highlighting the pectoral muscles.

Pneumonias in Cancer Patients

A. Causes of pneumonias complicating a neutrophil defect

Bacteria	Fungi	Parasites	Viruses
Streptococcus spp	*Aspergillus* spp	—	—
Staphylococcus spp	Mucoraceae		
Enterobacteriaceae	*Trichosporon* spp		
Pseudomonas aeruginosa	*Fusarium* spp		
Bacillus spp	*Candida* spp		
	Pseudallescheria boydii		

Figure 6-53 Causes of pneumonias complicating cancer. **A**, Neutrophil defect (*eg*, cytotoxic chemotherapy, acute leukemia, transplantation). (*continued*)

B. Causes of pneumonia complicating a T-lymphocyte/mononuclear phagocyte defect

Bacteria	Fungi	Parasites	Viruses
Mycobacterium spp	*Cryptococcus neoformans*	*Pneumocystis carinii*	Cytomegalovirus
Nocardia asteroides	*Histoplasma capsulatum*	*Toxoplasma gondii*	Varicella-zoster virus
Legionella spp	*Coccidioides immitis*	*Strongyloides stercoralis*	Measles virus
Rhodococcus equi	*Candida* spp		Adenovirus
Chlamydia pneumoniae	*Penicillium marneffii*		Respiratory syncytial virus

C. Causes of pneumonia complicating a globulin or splenic defect

Bacteria	Fungi	Parasites	Viruses
Streptococcus pneumoniae		*Pneumocystis carinii*	
Haemophilus influenzae			
Neisseria meningitidis			

FIGURE 6-53 (*continued*) **B**, T-lymphocyte/mononuclear phagocyte defect (*eg*, Hodgkin's disease, transplantation, HIV infection). **C**, Globulin or splenic defect (*eg*, multiple myeloma, chronic lymphocytic leukemia, transplantation, splenectomy).

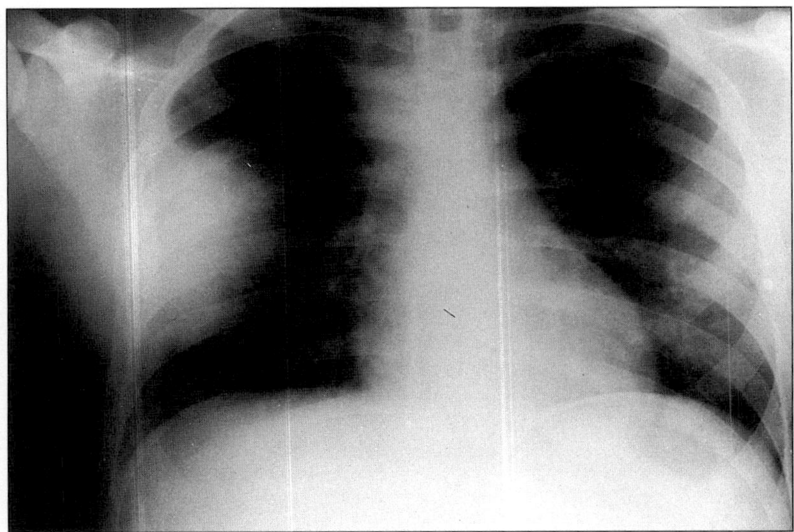

FIGURE 6-54 *Pseudomonas aeruginosa* pneumonia in a neutropenic patient. A chest radiograph shows a typical wedge-shaped infiltrate. Sputum samples in neutropenic patients do not show polymorphonuclear cells, and thus a representative sputum should show the absence of epithelial cells, normal oral flora, and the presence of multiple gram-negative rods.

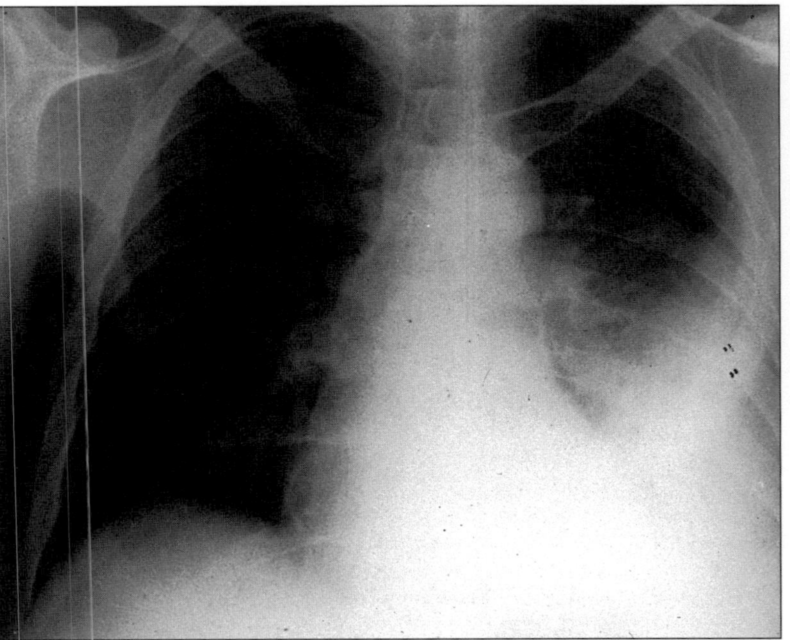

FIGURE 6-55 Chest radiograph of a patient with lymphoma, neutropenia, and a T-cell defect (*Mycobacterium tuberculosis* infection). Acute pneumonia considered to be gram-negative bacillary because of neutropenia turned out to be tuberculosis because of a T-cell defect. Multiple immune defects must be considered in some patients according to underlying disease and types of chemotherapy.

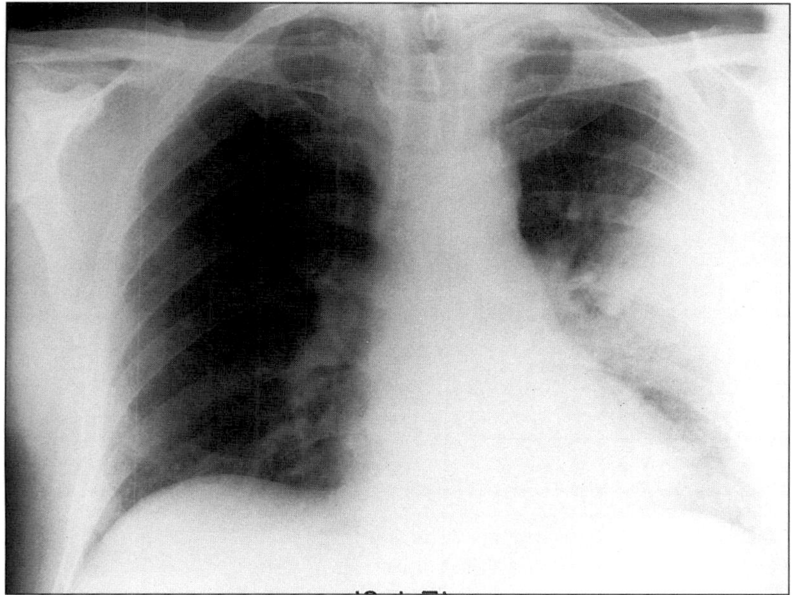

Figure 6-56 Chest radiograph of a patient with neutropenia following cytotoxic chemotherapy, complicated by invasive aspergillosis. The large wedge-shaped infiltrate looks similar to that produced by *Pseudomonas aeruginosa*, and the pathogenesis is similar. Invasion of vessels with clotting and infarction is common with *Aspergillus* species or Mucorales infections in neutropenic patients.

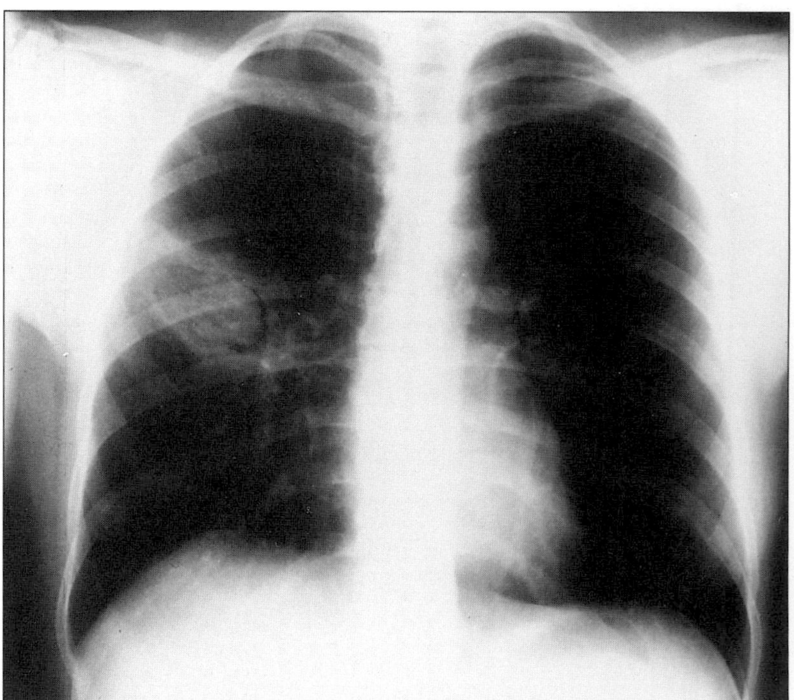

Figure 6-57 Chest radiograph of pulmonary mucormycosis. In this patient, pulmonary lesions suggestive of aspergillosis proved to be due to mucormycosis on open lung biopsy. Progressive pulmonary lesions due to either fungus result in fungus balls in the cavitary lesions.

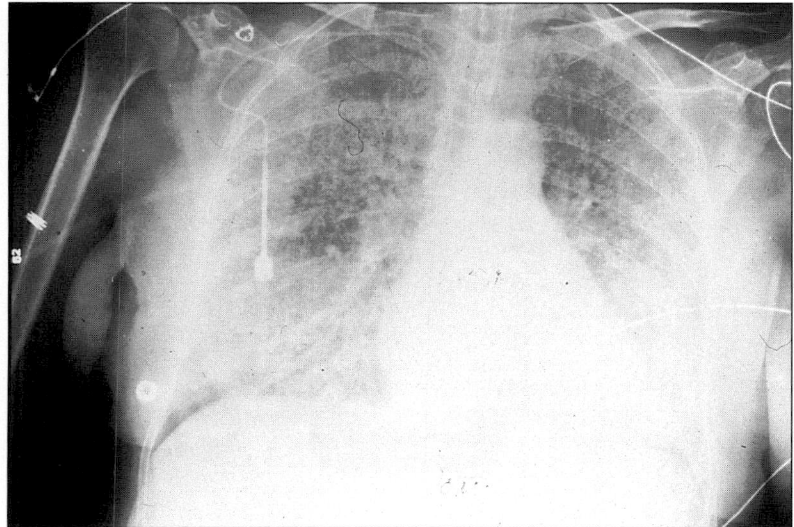

Figure 6-58 Disseminated strongyloidiasis. Disseminated strongyloidiasis or the hyperinfection syndrome with pneumonia is unusual in patients with T-cell defects but is eminently treatable, especially if diagnosed early. Polymicrobic sepsis should suggest the diagnosis, especially in a person with a T-cell defect who is not neutropenic or does not have an indwelling intravenous catheter. Sputum wet mount (not shown) reveals the organism and is the most direct, but late, method of diagnosis. Chest radiograph showing diffuse pulmonary infiltrates. Typically, diffuse alveolar and interstitial infiltrates appear on the radiograph. The patient responded to therapy.

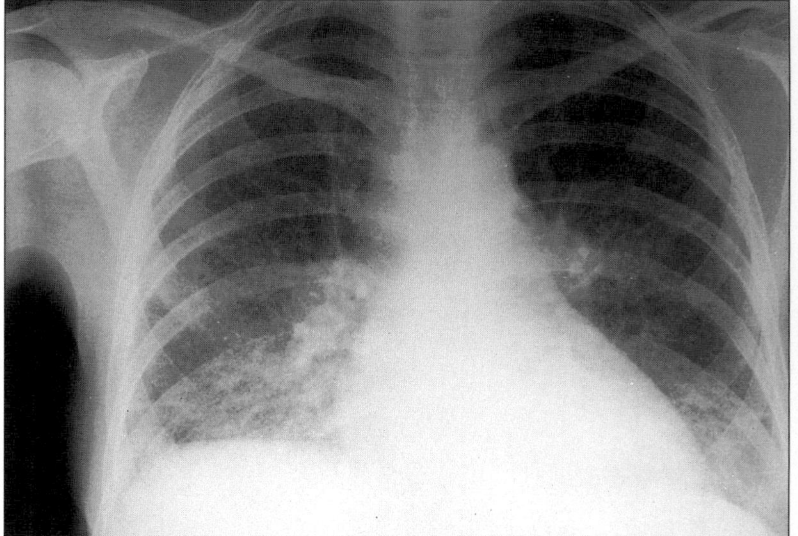

Figure 6-59 Chest radiograph showing a diffuse infiltrate due to cytomegalovirus (CMV) pneumonia in a bone marrow transplant patient. A lung biopsy specimen revealed "owl's eye" inclusions characteristic of CMV infection plus coinfection by *Toxoplasma*. Cancer patients are often susceptible to dual infections because of a specific immune defect, such as a T-cell defect in this patient, but also they often have multiple immune defects broadening their susceptibility. Clinicians must be alert to the possibility of dual infection, and if less invasive procedures do not answer the clinical question, more invasive procedures such as bronchoalveolar lavage or lung biopsy are warranted at the earliest opportunity.

Respiratory Infections in Transplant Recipients

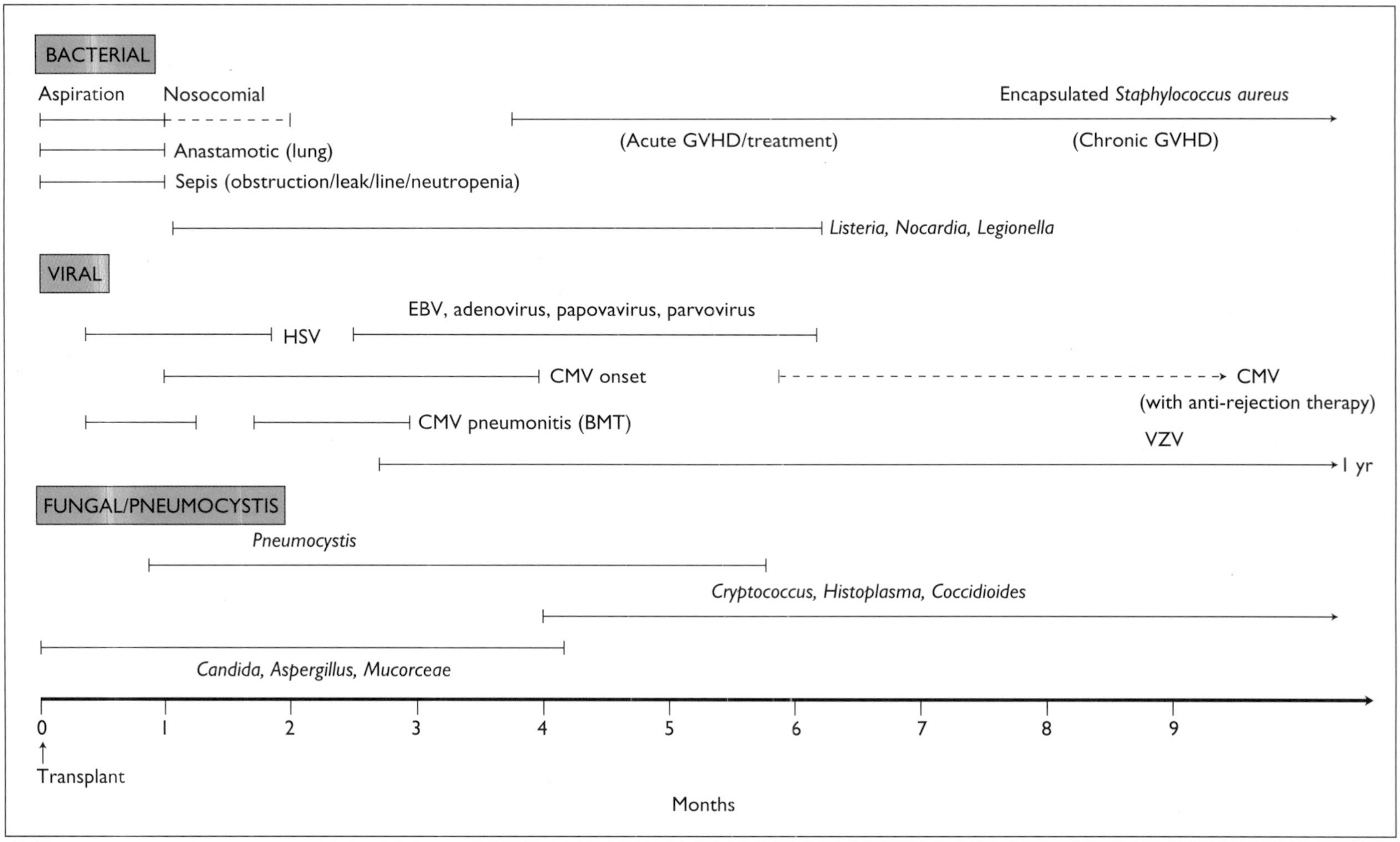

BACTERIAL

Aspiration — Nosocomial

Anastamotic (lung)

Sepis (obstruction/leak/line/neutropenia)

Encapsulated *Staphylococcus aureus*

(Acute GVHD/treatment)

(Chronic GVHD)

Listeria, Nocardia, Legionella

VIRAL

HSV

EBV, adenovirus, papovavirus, parvovirus

CMV onset

CMV (with anti-rejection therapy)

CMV pneumonitis (BMT)

VZV

1 yr

FUNGAL/PNEUMOCYSTIS

Pneumocystis

Cryptococcus, Histoplasma, Coccidioides

Candida, Aspergillus, Mucorceae

0 1 2 3 4 5 6 7 8 9

Transplant

Months

Figure 6-60 Timetable for pulmonary infections following transplantation. Patients' greatest risk for specific infections occurs in a specified sequence after transplantation. Patients who deviate significantly from this pattern may represent increased epidemiologic exposure to a given pathogen or a unique susceptibility (*eg*, increased immune suppression or tissue injury). Technical problems, such as anastomotic leaks or infections of hematomas, are associated with infection in the first month following transplantation but become a source of recurrent disease if uncorrected. (BMT—bone marrow transplant; CMV—cytomegalovirus; EBV—Epstein-Barr virus; GVHD—graft-vs-host disease; HSV—herpes simplex virus; VZV—varicella-zoster virus.) (*Modified from* Rubin *et al.* [13].)

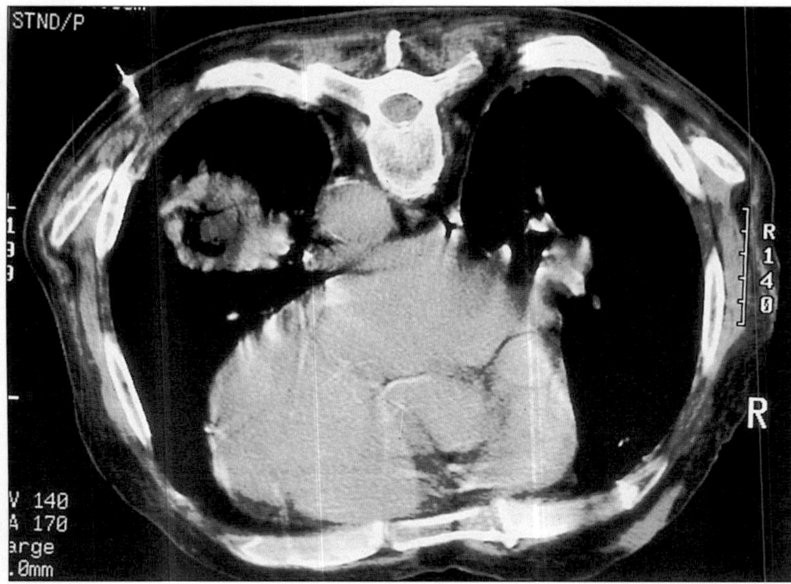

Figure 6-61 Pulmonary mucormycosis presenting as a rapidly progressive, solitary abscess. A 65-year-old man 5 years after cadaveric kidney transplantation presented with a cough and low-grade fever. Initial chest radiograph (not shown) was read as consistent with a new lingular infiltrate, probable pneumonia. Bronchoscopy and examination of bronchoalveolar lavage fluid were unremarkable. Computed tomography scan evaluation showed the lung abscess had doubled in size over 36 hours, despite therapy with broad-spectrum antibiotics and amphotericin B. Examination of an aspirate obtained by percutaneous needle aspiration was negative. However, the clinical appearance was consistent with mucormycosis, and the patient was taken to surgery for resection. At surgery, the lingula and adjacent tissue were friable and gray in appearance and resected en bloc. The resected lung contained a single large abscess cavity containing necrotic tissue and blood. No organisms were detected within the necrotic tissues on frozen section evaluation. *Mucor circinelloides* was found by histopathologic techniques in the perivascular areas of the ischemic lung tissue.

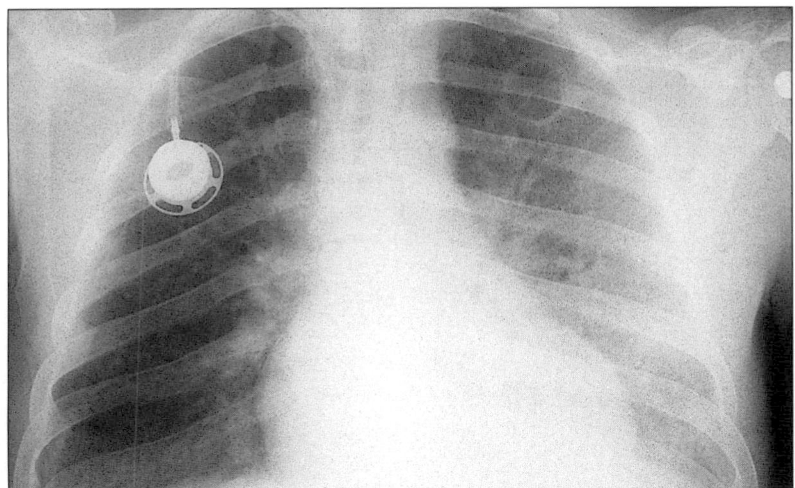

Figure 6-62 Chest radiograph of 27-year-old diabetic after kidney transplantation, showing a pulmonary cavity discovered during taper of corticosteroid therapy. The cavity contained *Aspergillus* and *Pneumocystis carinii*. Dual infections are not uncommon in the lungs of transplant recipients. Failure to respond to optimal therapy for one infection should suggest the presence of a second process (infectious or noninfectious). Cytomegalovirus often coinfects the lungs in bone marrow and lung transplant recipients. Histopathologic documentation of infection should be considered in all immunocompromised patients, particularly those failing to respond to therapy.

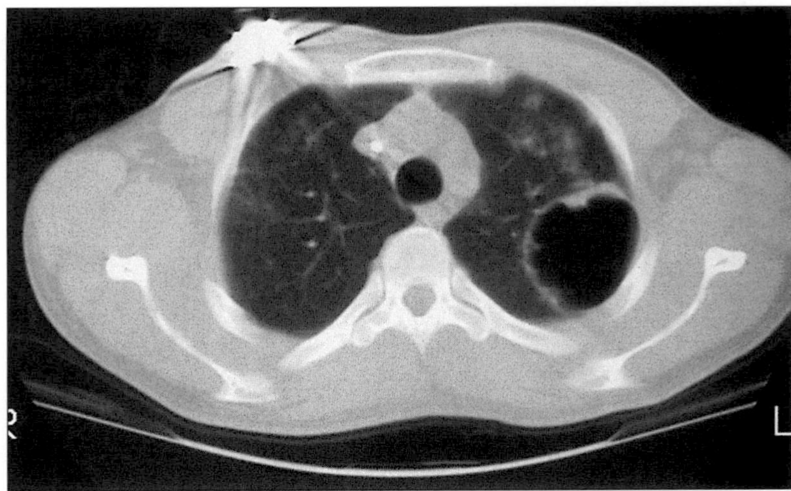

Figure 6-63 Chest computed tomography (CT) scan of the patient in Figure 6-62 with dual infection by *Pneumocystis* and *Aspergillus*. The chest CT is useful to distinguish interstitial processes from invasive disease. Disease masked by corticosteroids or immunosuppression is often seen by CT.

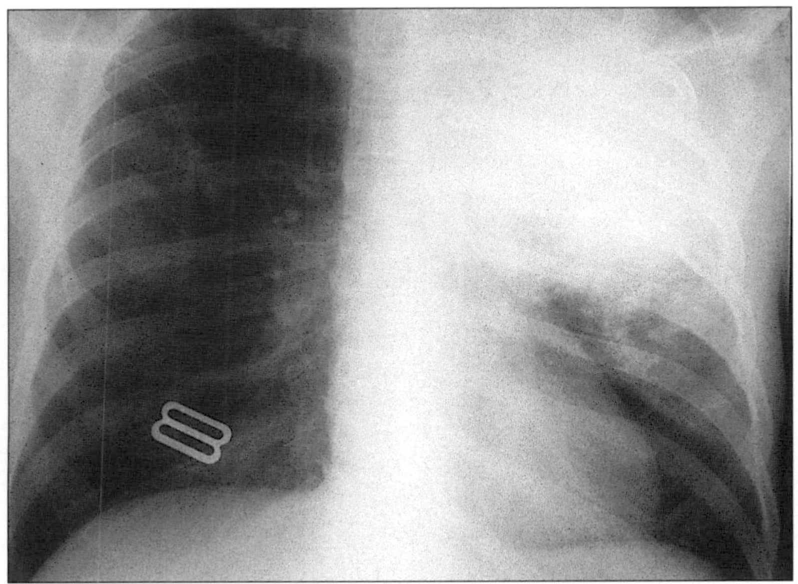

Figure 6-64 Chest radiograph showing *Legionella pneumophila* pneumonia in a renal transplant recipient. The broad defect in cellular immunity seen in transplant recipients predisposes to infection with intracellular pathogens. Because erythromycin may increase serum cyclosporine levels, close follow-up of such levels is advisable during macrolide therapy. Controlled trials have not been completed with newer macrolide agents (azithromycin, clarithromycin), rifampin (in combination with macrolide), trimethoprim-sulfamethoxazole, quinolines, or tetracyclines. *Legionella* urinary antigen detection tests identify approximately 80% of *L. pneumophila* infections, but not infections due to other *Legionella* species. Culture on buffered charcoal yeast extract supplemented with dyes and antibiotics is advantageous. The yield of cultures from good sputum samples is generally equivalent to those of induced or bronchoscopic specimens. Direct fluorescent antibody testing is highly specific (up to 99%) but may miss infections with small numbers of organisms. DNA probes and polymerase chain reaction tests are also available, having high levels of sensitivity and specificity (for the ribosomal messenger RNA of the *Legionella* family).

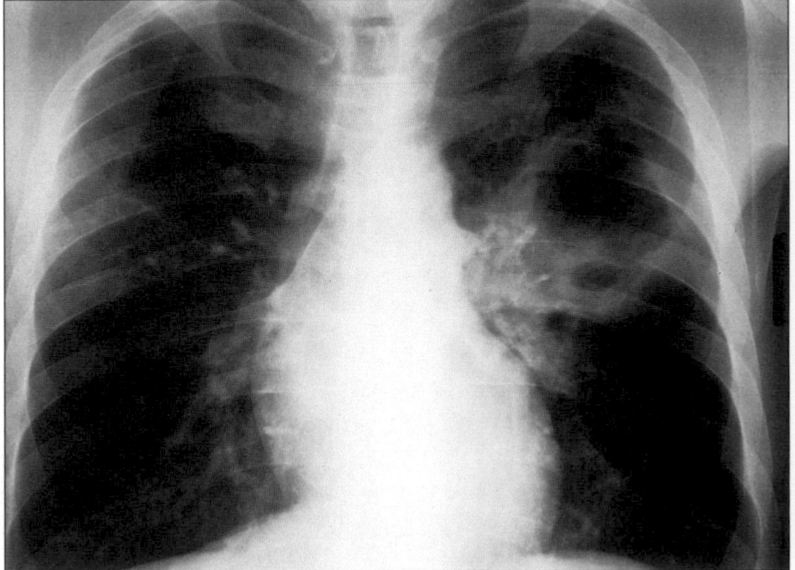

Figure 6-65 Bacterial lung abscess with coinfection by Strongyloides stercoralis in a Vietnamese kidney transplant recipient. Chest radiograph shows a lung abscess due to *Enterobacter* species. Bronchoscopic examination revealed simultaneous *Pneumocystis carinii* and *S. stercoralis* infections. *Strongyloides* is capable of completing its life cycle within the human host but is usually limited to the gastrointestinal tract by the intact immune system. During immunosuppression, infectious complications may be observed in locations through which the nematode passes during acute infection, including the skin, bloodstream, lungs, and gastrointestinal tract. Migration across the wall of the gastrointestinal tract during immunosuppression (hyperinfection) is associated with systemic signs of "sepsis" and central nervous system infection (parasitic and bacterial). Preventative therapy for strongyloidiasis may be useful in patients from endemic regions who are being evaluated for organ transplantation. The activation of systemic infection (hyperinfection) due to *Strongyloides* migrating from the gastrointestinal tract or the anatomic obstruction produced by migration through the lung parenchyma may contribute to life-threatening bacterial infection. The immune mechanisms responsible for the control of *Strongyloides* infection are under investigation.

Pulmonary Manifestations of Extrapulmonary Infection

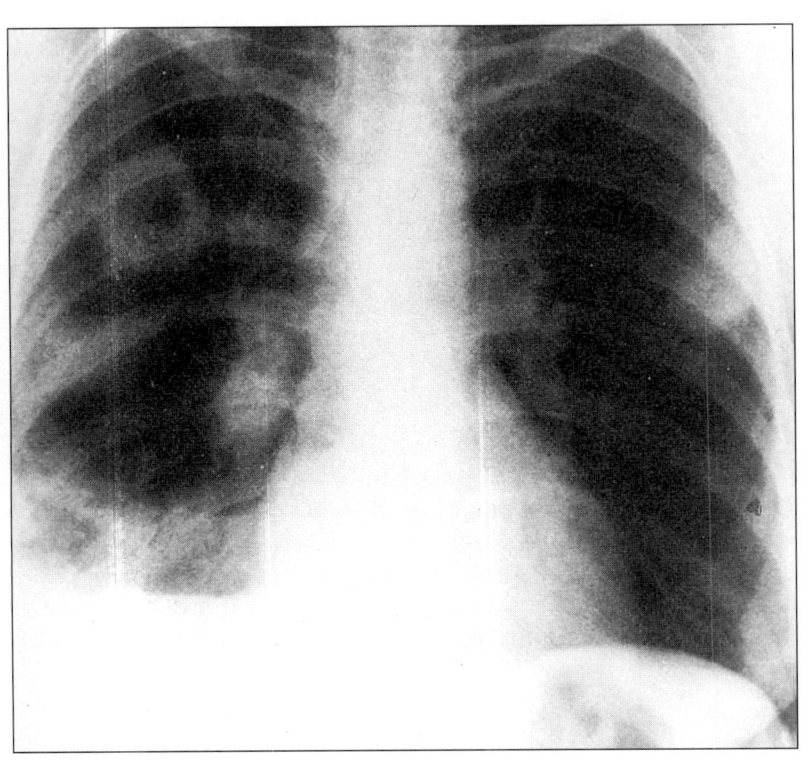

Figure 6-66 *Francisella tularenisis* is a gram-negative, pleomorphic coccobacillary organism that grows poorly on artificial media unless fortified with serum, glucose, and cystine. The organism is associated with a large number of wild animals, especially squirrels and rabbits. The infection is spread among animals via deerflies or ticks or by bites from infected animals. Most human cases are acquired from contact with infected animals, via deerfly or tick bites, or through ingestion of contaminated meat. Chest radiograph of a 51-year-old woman who presented with acute onset of chills, fever, nausea, malaise, myalgia, and headache several days after being bitten by numerous ticks. Respiratory disease often begins with a poorly productive cough, chest pain, and dyspnea. Radiologic changes characteristically include evidence of parenchymal and pleural disease. The pattern is diffuse bronchopneumonia, often with hilar adenopathy. Pleural effusions are not unusual, as demonstrated in this patient. When tularemia is contracted through insect or animal bites, the initial sites of infection demonstrate necrosis, granuloma formation, and local abscesses. Ingestion of infected meat may result in pharyngeal and intestinal involvement with ulceration. Pulmonary infection causes pneumonitis features with mediastinal lymph node enlargement. (*From* Rubin [14]; with permission):

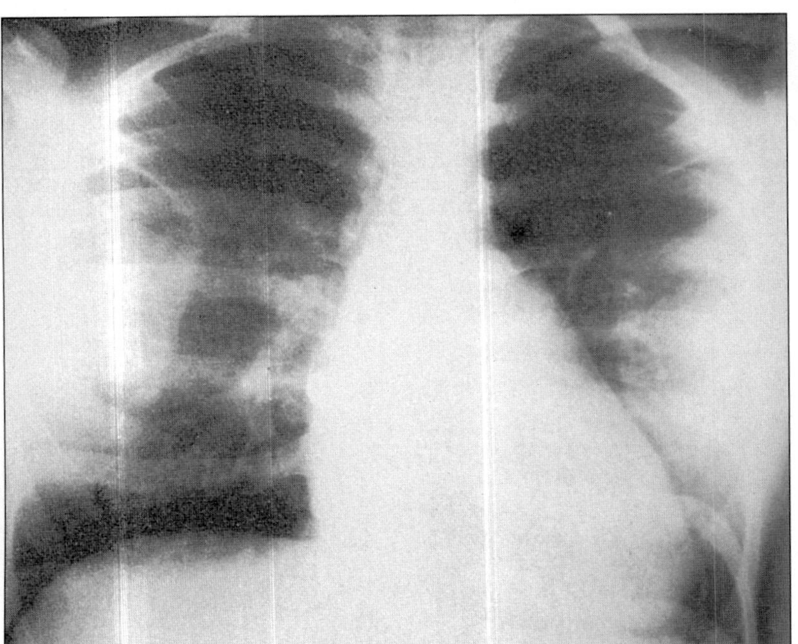

Figure 6-67 Rocky Mountain spotted fever. A chest radiograph demonstrated bilateral infiltrates that progressed to an acute respiratory distress syndrome pattern. The typical presentation of Rocky Mountain spotted fever is that of an acute febrile illness with headache, malaise, myalgia, and a maculopapular rash that begins on the extremities and spreads centrally. In severe cases, there can be multiple organ involvement. (*From* Sacks *et al.* [15]; with permission.)

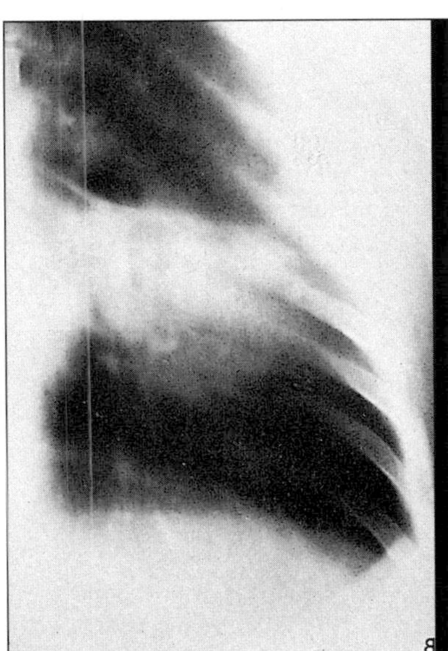

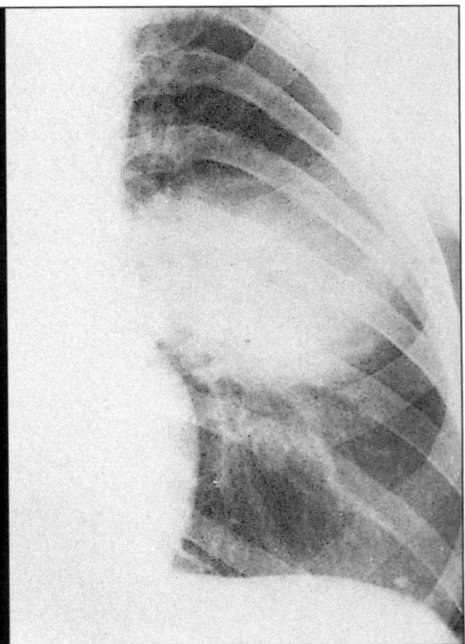

Figure 6-68 Chest radiograph in pulmonary actinomycosis demonstrating an intraparenchymal infiltrate that frequently extends to the chest wall. The typical radiographic pattern of acute actinomycosis consists of airspace pneumonia, without recognizable segmental distribution, commonly in the periphery of the lung and with a predilection for the lower lobes. With appropriate antibiotic therapy, the infection is usually resolved without complications. Without therapy, a lung abscess may develop, or the infection may extend into the pleura and chest wall, with osteomyelitis of the ribs and abscess formation in these areas. (*From* Fraser *et al.* [16]; with permission.)

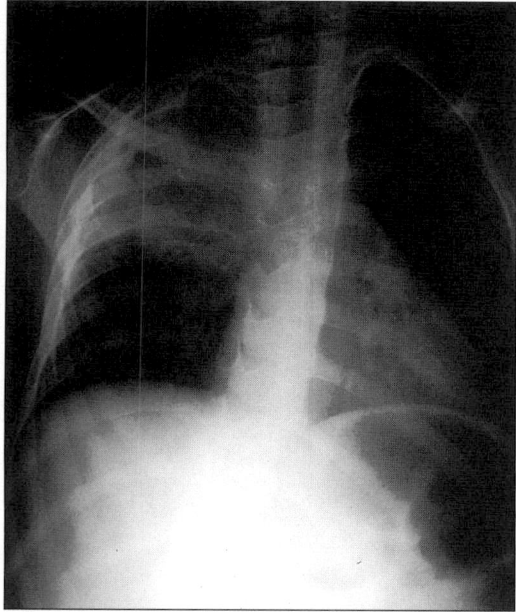

FIGURE 6-69 Chest radiograph showing a consolidating right upper lobe infiltrate in an 8-year-old boy with pulmonary blastomycosis. In contrast with histoplasmosis and coccidioidomycosis, direct, intimate exposure to an infected site (such as an area of construction) is probably necessary for infection with *Blastomyces dermatitidis*. When a person is exposed to a contaminated site, microconidia of the fungus can be inhaled. If infection occurs, an intense neutrophilic response develops. A specific cell-mediated immunologic response occurs within 7 to 14 days. Blastomycosis occurs most frequently in rural areas among individuals with outdoor jobs or interests.

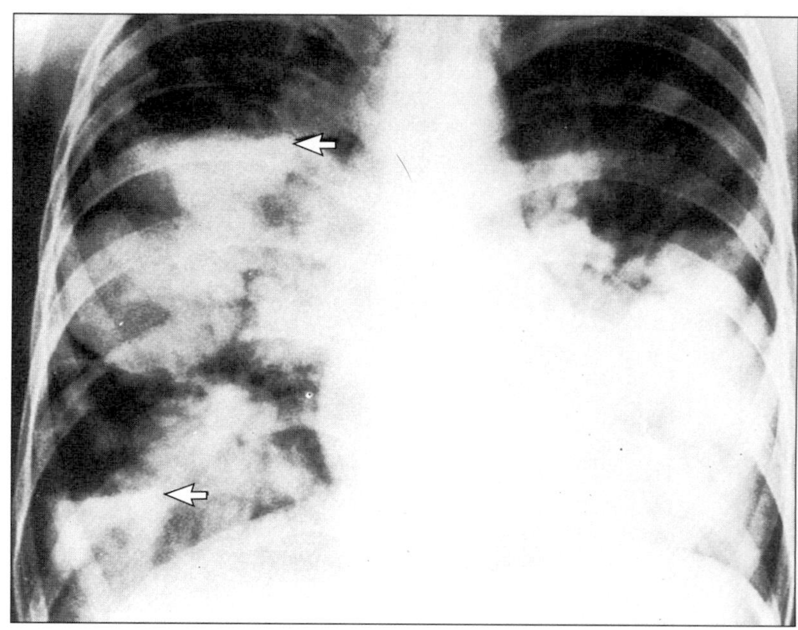

FIGURE 6-70 Chest radiograph of a 14-year-old Iranian girl with multiple hydatid cysts of the lung. The majority of these cysts are intact, but at least four have ruptured into the tracheobronchial tree and show prominent air–fluid levels (*arrows*). The irregular configuration of the air–fluid interface is a result of floating membranes (water-lily sign). Pulmonary echinococcal cysts characteristically present as solitary, sharply circumscribed masses surrounded by normal lung, predominantly in the lower lobes. (Courtesy of Hassan Fateh, MD.)

ACUTE AND CHRONIC BRONCHITIS AND BRONCHIOLITIS

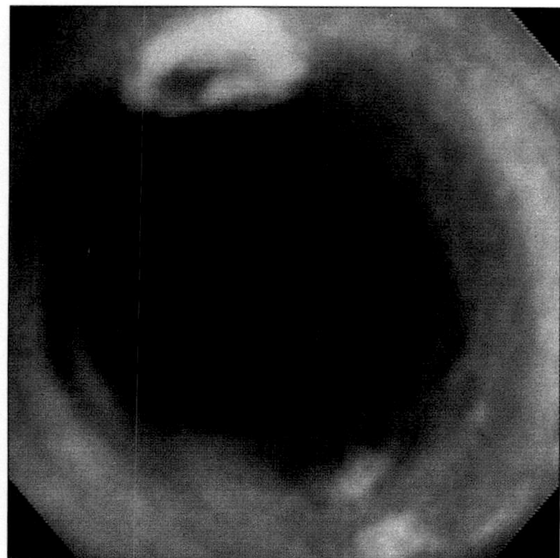

FIGURE 6-71 Bronchoscopic view of tracheobronchial tree showing white plaques due to *Aspergillus* infection. The infectious causes include bacteria, predominantly *Streptococcus pneumoniae*, *Haemophilus influenzae*, *Moraxella catarrhalis*, and *Legionella*; *Mycobacterium tuberculosis*; *Chlamydia* (TWAR strain); *Mycoplasma pneumoniae*; fungi, such as *Candida* spp, *Histoplasma capsulatum*, and *Aspergillus* spp; and a number of viruses. The photograph shows a bronchoscopic view of the tracheobronchial tree of a patient with AIDS. The white plaques proved to be due to *Aspergillus* infection. (*Courtesy of* J. Jagirdar, MD.)

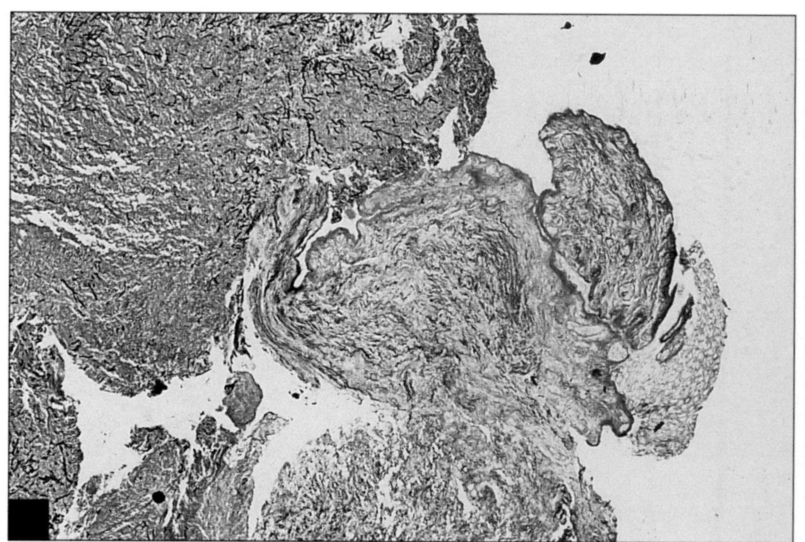

FIGURE 6-72 Histopathologic examination in acute tracheobronchitis due to *Aspergillus*. Gomori methenamine silver stain demonstrates the branched septated hyphae characteristic of *Aspergillus* infection. (*Courtesy of* J. Jagirdar, MD.)

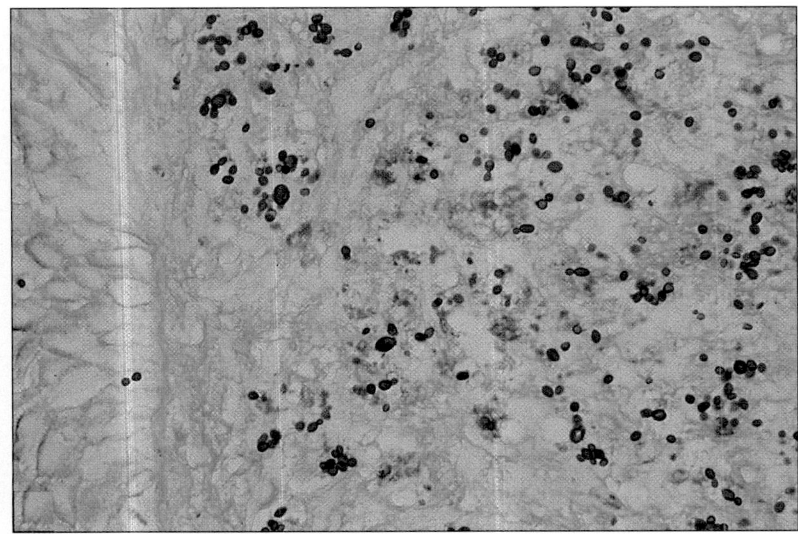

FIGURE 6-73 Histopathologic specimen demonstrating *Histoplasma* tracheobronchitis. Transbronchial biopsy was performed on a Puerto Rican man with AIDS plus cough and shortness of breath. High-power view of the biopsy specimen stained with Gomori methenamine silver shows budding yeasts. Cultures grew *Histoplasma capsulatum*. (*Courtesy of* J. Jagirdar, MD.)

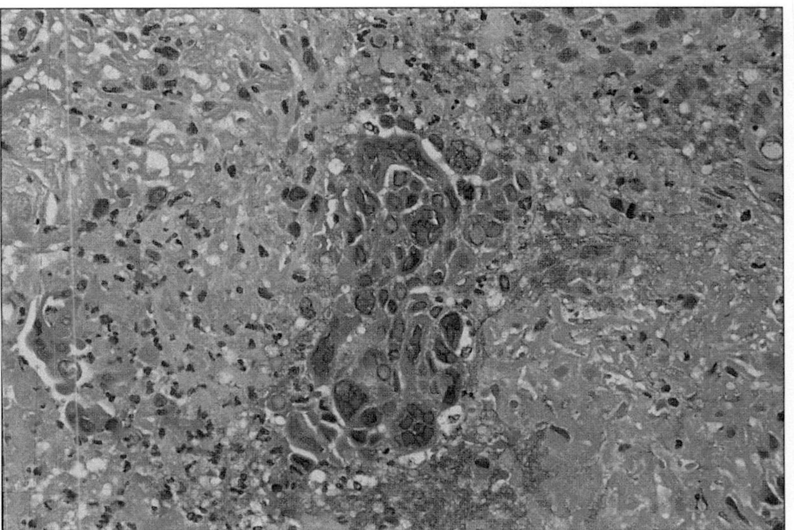

FIGURE 6-74 Histopathologic examination in viral tracheobronchitis. Transbronchial biopsy was performed on a 50-year-old Chinese woman with polymyositis who was treated with prednisone and developed a cough and shortness of breath. An initial biopsy had shown atypical cells suspicious of malignancy, prompting a sleeve resection. This biopsy specimen, also stained with hematoxylin-eosin, demonstrates many cells with intranuclear inclusions suggestive of HSV infection, including multinucleated cells with the characteristic ballooning inclusions. Immunohistochemical staining (not shown)proved that the infection was caused by HSV-1. (*Courtesy of* J. Jagirdar, MD.)

REFERENCES

1. Fang G, Fine M, Orloff J, *et al.*: New and emerging etiologies for community-acquired pneumonia with implications for therapy: A prospective multicenter study of 359 cases. *Medicine* 1990, 69:307–316.
2. Marrie TJ: Community-acquired pneumonia. *Clin Infect Dis* 1994, 18:501–515.
3. Schaffner W: *Chlamydia psittaci* (psittacosis). *In* Mandell GL, Bennett JE, Dolin R (eds.): *Principles and Practice of Infectious Diseases*, 3rd ed. New York: Churchill Livingstone; 1990:1440–1443.
4. Goodwin RA, des Prez RM: Apical localization of pulmonary tuberculosis, chronic pulmonary histoplasmosis, and progressive massive fibrosis of the lung. *Chest* 1983, 83:801–805.
5. Iseman MD, Corpe RF, O'Brien RJ, *et al.*: Diseases due to *Mycobacterium avium-intracellulare*. *Chest* 1985, 87(suppl):139S–149S.
6. Bone RC, *et al.* (eds.): *Pulmonary and Critical Care Medicine. Care Volume*, vol. 2, St. Louis: Mosby; 1993.
7. Louria DB, Blumenfeld HL, Ellis JT, *et al.*: Studies on influenza in the pandemic of 1957–1958: II. Pulmonary complications of influenza. *J Clin Invest* 1959, 38:213–265.
8. Van Voris LP, Betts RF, Hayden FG, *et al.*: Successful treatment of naturally occuring influenza A/USSR/77 H1N1. *JAMA* 1981, 245:1128.
9. Haake DA, Zakowski PC, Haake DL, Bryson YJ: Early treatment with acyclovir for varicella pneumonia in otherwise healthy adults: Retrospective controlled study and review. *Rev Infect Dis* 1990, 12:788–798.
10. Lyche KD, Jensen WA, Kirsch CM, *et al.*: Pleuropulmonary manifestations of hepatic amebiasis. *West J Med* 1990, 153:275–278.
11. Remington JS, Swartz MN (eds.): *Current Clinical Topics in Infectious Disease*, vol 7. New York: McGraw-Hill, 1986:1.
12. Light RW: *Pleural Diseases*. Philadelphia: Lea & Febiger, 1983.
13. Rubin RH, Wolfson JS, Cosimi AB, *et al.*: Infection in the renal transplant recipient. *Am J Med* 1981, 70:405–411.
14. Rubin SA: Radiographic spectrum of pleuropulmonary tularemia. *AJR* 1978, 131:277–281.
15. Sacks HS, Lyons RW, Lahiri B: Adult respiratory distress syndrome in Rocky Moutain spotted fever. *Am Rev Respir Dis* 1981, 123:547–549.
16. Fraser RG, Paré JAP, Paré PD, *et al.*: *Diagnosis of Diseases of the Chest*, 3rd ed. Philadelphia: W.B. Saunders; 1989.

CHAPTER 7

Intra-abdominal Infections, Hepatitis, and Gastroenteritis

Editor
Bennett Lorber

Contributors
Helen Buckley
Sydney M. Finegold
Robert A. Gatenby
Robert M. Genta
David Y. Graham
Richard L. Guerrant
Lionel Rabin
Robert D. Shaw
Rosemary Soave
Samuel E. Wilson

INTRA-ABDOMINAL INFECTIONS AND ABSCESSES

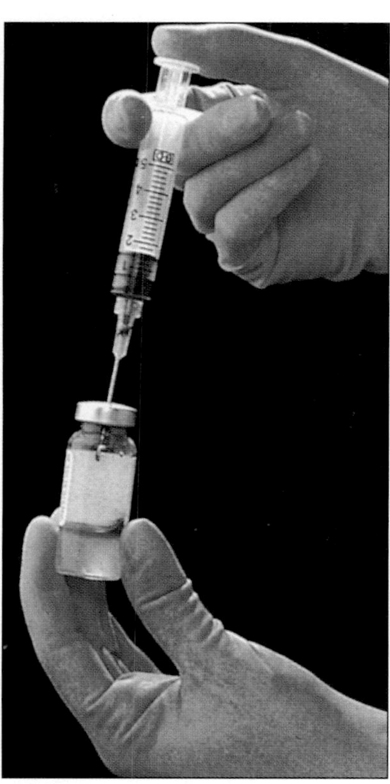

FIGURE 7-1 Injection of the specimen into an anaerobic transport vial. The agar in the bottom of the vial is nonnutritive and contains an oxidation-reduction indicator, such as methylene blue or, preferably, resazurin. Care should be taken not to inject air inadvertently along with the specimen. The specimen should be injected slowly so that it remains on top of the agar. Specimens remain anaerobic in such containers for at least 72 hours, but obviously it is advantageous for the laboratory to culture the material as soon as possible. (*From* Finegold *et al.* [1]; with permission.)

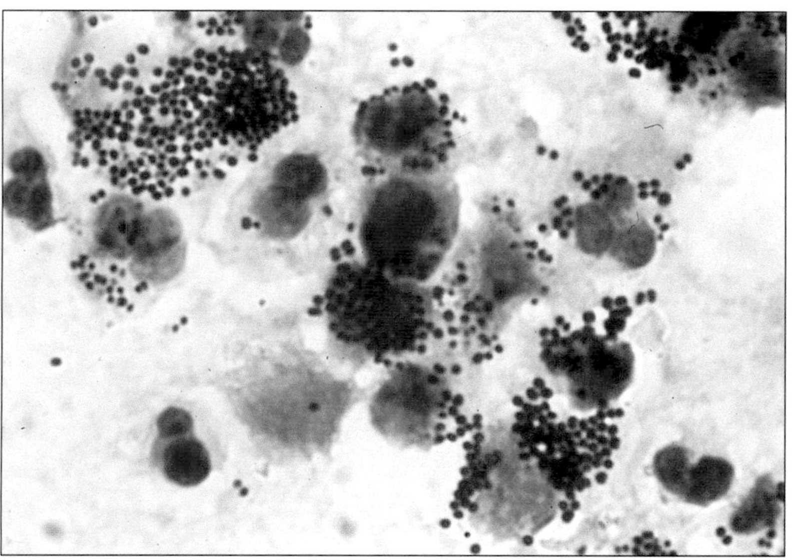

FIGURE 7-2 Gram stain of postoperative abdominal wound infection showing large numbers of intracellular gram-positive cocci in clusters (*Staphylococcus aureus*). Several organisms that may be involved in postoperative infections have distinctive morphology such that one may predict fairly accurately the identity of the organism; this is often true of the anaerobes. Accordingly, quick identification becomes a huge help to the clinician in choosing the most appropriate antimicrobial regimen early in the course of the infection and thereby minimizing the ill effects of the process. Such identification is especially important in the case of infection following bowel surgery, where there may be many different organisms, up to 10 to 20 or more, involved in the infectious process; the microbiology laboratory may need considerable time (sometimes weeks) to isolate each organism in pure culture and identify it. Although the practice is to concentrate on a smaller number of organisms (those known to be important pathogens or resistant to antimicrobial agents and those present in larger numbers), it may still take several days to identify these key organisms. The Gram stain, of course, takes only minutes to prepare and read.

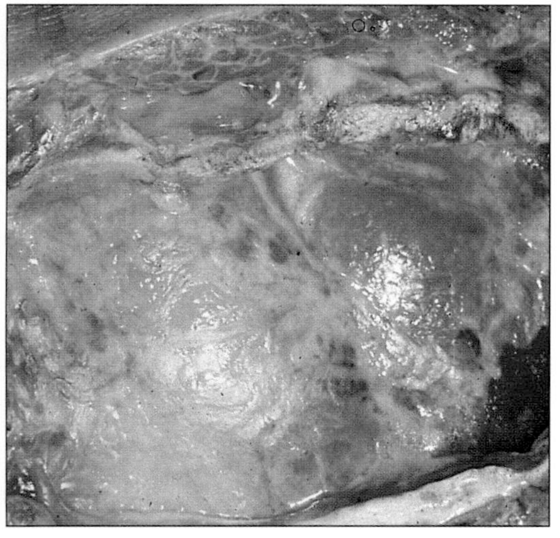

FIGURE 7-3 Necrotizing fasciitis of the abdominal wall. Pus can be seen between the fascia and abdominal wall in the upper part of the figure. The most common bacterial etiology of this entity is group A β-hemolytic streptococci. In the past, this condition was known as hemolytic streptococcal gangrene or hospital gangrene, and it was an extremely common and serious problem in US hospitals during the Civil War and in various hospitals in Europe in the 1800s. A recent upsurge in cases has occurred in the community (it is no longer a hospital problem because of modern sanitation and hospital infection-control measures) related to virulent, toxin-producing strains of *Streptococcus pyogenes* (the "flesh-eating bacteria"). Staphylococci also commonly cause this infection, and anaerobes are not uncommonly involved, particularly in the entity known as Fournier's gangrene, which typically involves the perineal area, especially in diabetics. Among the anaerobes recovered from necrotizing fasciitis are various gram-negative bacilli, including the *Bacteroides fragilis* group, various clostridia, including *Clostridium perfringens,* and anaerobic and microaerophilic streptococci. In many cases in which anaerobes are involved, facultative gram-negative rods and enterococci are also present. This entity may be a postoperative complication, as in the patient pictured, but also occurs after injury, even trivial injury.

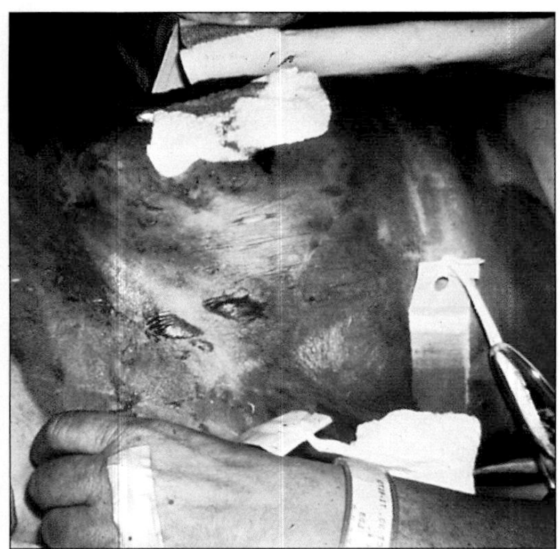

FIGURE 7-4 Clostridial myonecrosis (gas gangrene) of the abdominal wall occurring postoperatively. Note the bronzed discoloration (compare with the color of the hand) and the bullae. Clostridial myonecrosis is one of the most serious of the soft-tissue infections. Pain is one of the hallmarks of the process; it is typically sudden in onset and one of the first things noted by the patient. Accumulations of gas in the soft tissue, never marked in amount, may be detected in most cases, and a peculiar sweetish or mousy smell may be noted. Mental changes are not uncommon, and patients may go into shock. The most common *Clostridium* found in this process is *C. perfringens;* the other species that may be seen include *C. novyi, C. septicum, C. histolyticum, C. bifermentans,* and *C. fallax.*

Common organisms associated with CAPD-related peritonitis

Gram-positive bacteria	60%–70%
Staphylococcus (coagulase-negative)	30%–45%
Staphylococcus aureus	10%–20%
Streptococcus	10%–15%
Enterococcus	3%–5%
Diphtheroids	1%–2%
Gram-negative bacteria	20%–30%
Enterobacteriaceae	10%–20%
Pseudomonas aeruginosa	5%–10%
Other	2%–3%
Fungi	5%–15%
Mycobacteria	0%–3%
Anaerobes, polymicrobial	0%–10%

CAPD—continuous ambulatory peritoneal dialysis.

FIGURE 7-5 Common organisms associated with continuous ambulatory peritoneal dialysis (CAPD)-related peritonitis. Peritonitis remains the most common complication of CAPD and is a primary reason for discontinuing use of this dialysis technique in patients. Overall, the average incidence of peritonitis is 1.3 to 1.4 episodes per patient per year of dialysis, although the rates vary considerably among individual patients and facilities. Peritonitis is usually caused by a single pathogen that originates from the normal flora of the skin or upper respiratory tract. (*Adapted from* Finegold and Johnson [2].)

A. Aerobic and anaerobic species isolated from patients with gangrenous or perforated appendicitis: Aerobic and facultative bacteria

	Gangrenous, % (*n*=27)	Perforated, % (*n*=44)	All, % (*n*=71)
Escherichia coli	70.4	77.3	74.6
Viridans streptococci	18.5	43.2	33.8
Streptococcus group D	7.4	27.3	19.7
Pseudomonas aeruginosa	11.1	18.2	15.5
Enterococcus spp	18.5	9.1	12.7
Staphylococcus spp	14.8	11.4	12.7
Pseudomonas spp	7.4	9.1	8.5
Citrobacter freundii	3.7	6.8	5.6
β-Hemolytic streptococci group F	7.4	4.5	5.6
β-Hemolytic streptococci group C	3.7	4.5	4.2
Enterobacter spp	7.4	2.3	4.2
Klebsiella spp	3.7	4.5	4.2
β-Hemolytic streptococci group G	0	4.5	2.8
Moraxella spp	3.7	2.3	2.8
Corynebacterium spp	0	2.3	1.4
Serratia marcescens	3.7	0	1.4
Eikenella corrodens	0	2.3	1.4
Hafnia alvei	3.7	0	1.4
Haemophilus influenzae	0	2.3	1.4

FIGURE 7-6 Aerobic and anaerobic species isolated from patients with gangrenous or perforated appendicitis. **A**, Aerobic and facultative bacteria. (*continued*)

B. Aerobic and anaerobic species isolated from patients with gangrenous or perforated appendicitis: Anaerobic bacteria

	Gangrenous, % (*n*=27)	Perforated, % (*n*=44)	All, % (*n*=71)
Bacteroides fragilis	70.1	79.5	76.1
B. thetaiotaomicron	48.1	61.4	56.3
Bilophila wadsworthia	37.0	54.5	47.9
Peptostreptococcus micros	44.4	45.5	45.1
Eubacterium spp	40.7	29.5	33.8
B. intermedius	33.3	27.3	29.6
B. vulgatus	18.5	34.1	28.2
B. splanchnicus	25.9	27.3	26.8
Fusobacterium spp	22.2	27.3	25.4
B. ovatus	18.5	27.3	23.9
Microaerophilic streptococci	29.6	20.5	23.9
Peptostreptococcus spp	29.6	18.2	22.5
Lactobacillus spp	22.2	20.5	21.1
B. uniformis	22.2	18.2	19.7
B. distasonis	14.8	20.5	18.3
Clostridium clostridioforme	18.5	18.2	18.3
B. gracilis	11.1	15.9	14.1
Actinomyces spp	11.1	11.4	11.3
C. ramosum	11.1	9.1	9.9
Porphyromonas spp	18.5	2.3	8.5
B. buccae	3.7	6.8	5.6
B. caccae	7.4	4.5	5.6
C. innocuum	7.4	4.5	5.6
B. stercoris	7.4	4.5	5.6
C. sporogenes	3.7	6.8	5.6
Propionibacterium acnes	7.4	4.5	5.6
C. leptum	11.1	0	4.2
Desulfomonas spp	3.7	4.5	4.2
Unidentified gram-negative rod	37.0	36.4	36.6
Unidentified gram-positive rod	14.8	29.5	23.9
Unidentified pigmenting rod	18.5	18.2	18.3

Figure 7-6 (*continued*) **B**, Anaerobic bacteria [3]. (*Adapted from* Finegold and Johnson [2].)

Microorganisms in bile in acute cholecystitis

Aerobes–174 (87%)			
Gram-negative	132 (66%)	Gram-positive	42 (21%)
Escherichia coli	77	*Enterococcus faecalis*	30
Klebsiella	22	β-Hemolytic streptococci	4
Proteus	13	*Staphylococcus epidermidis*	4
Enterobacter	8	Viridans streptococcus	1
Pseudomonas	4		
Anaerobes–25 (13%)			
Gram-negative	2(1%)	Gram-positive	23 (12%)
Bacteroides spp	2	*Clostridium perfringens*	16
		Peptostreptococcus	7

Figure 7-7 Microorganisms in bile in acute cholecystitis. The bacteriologic findings from one study of 199 cases are presented. The bacteria responsible for gallbladder infections reflects the normal bowel flora, particularly the duodenum. The duodenal flora in these patients is not uncommonly abnormal as a result of such factors as achlorhydria, gastric or small bowel obstruction, and small bowel diverticula or blind loops. The infecting flora of biliary tract infections usually includes *Escherichia coli, Klebsiella, Enterobacter*, and enterococci. Anaerobes are found with some frequency, particularly *Clostridium perfringens* and *Bacteroides fragilis.* Anaerobic or polymicrobic infections (involving anaerobes) are seen more often in elderly patients and those who have undergone previous biliary tract surgical procedures or manipulations. These patients usually have more severe symptoms and a higher incidence of complications. (*Adapted from* Keighley [4].)

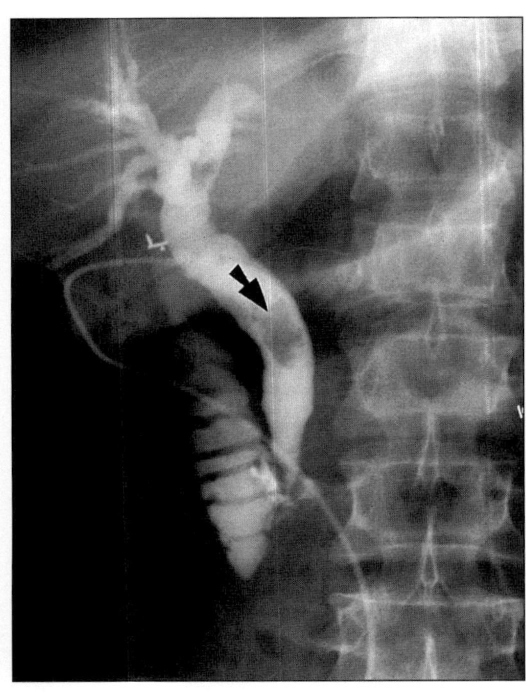

FIGURE 7-8 Acute cholecystitis. Operative cholangiogram with a common bile duct stone (*arrow*).

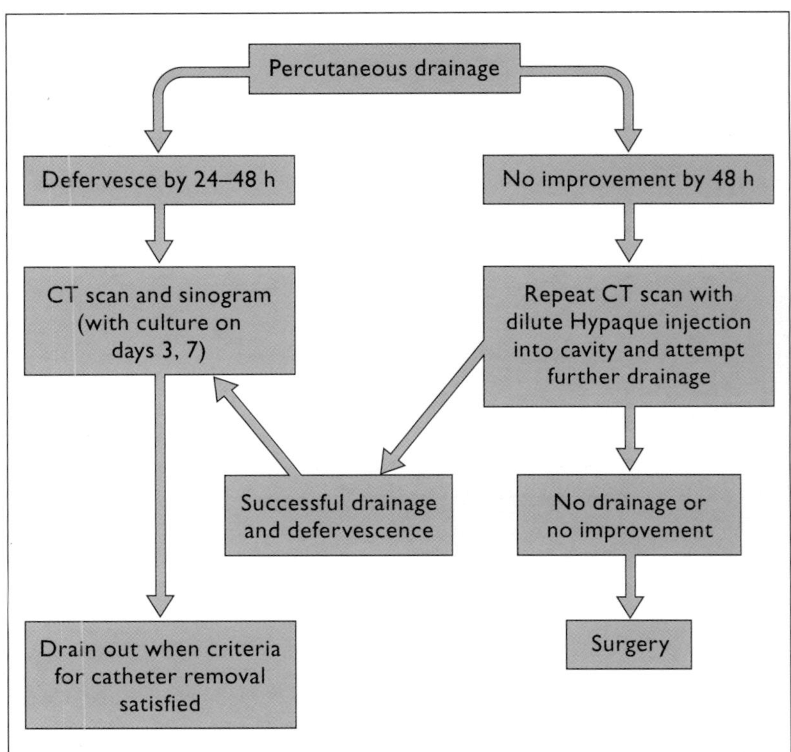

FIGURE 7-9 Algorithm for the management of patients with intra-abdominal abscesses using percutaneous drainage. Antimicrobial therapy should be administered concomitantly [5]. (CT—computed tomography.) (*Adapted from* Rotstein and Simmons [6].)

HEPATITIS

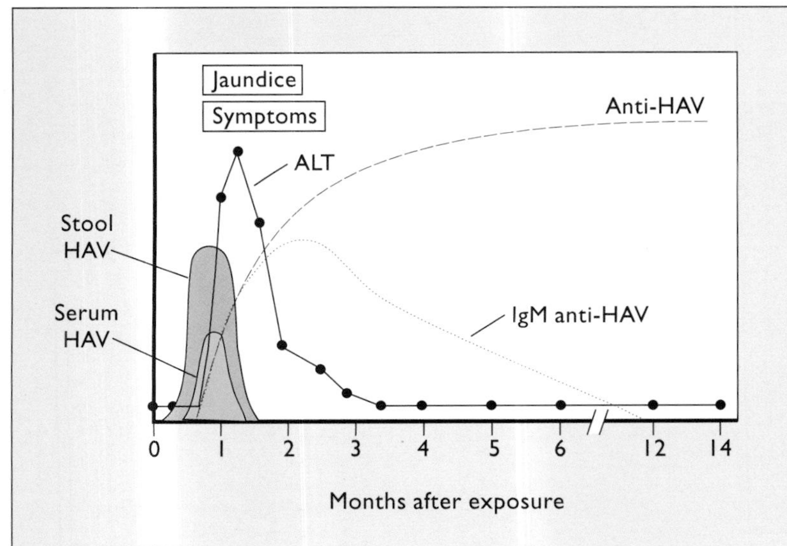

FIGURE 7-10 Typical time course of hepatitis A with emphasis on serologic manifestations. Demonstration of IgM anti–hepatitis A virus (HAV) is diagnostic of hepatitis A infection. IgM anti–HAV occurs at the time of onset of symptoms and may persist for months. (ALT—alanine aminotransferase.)

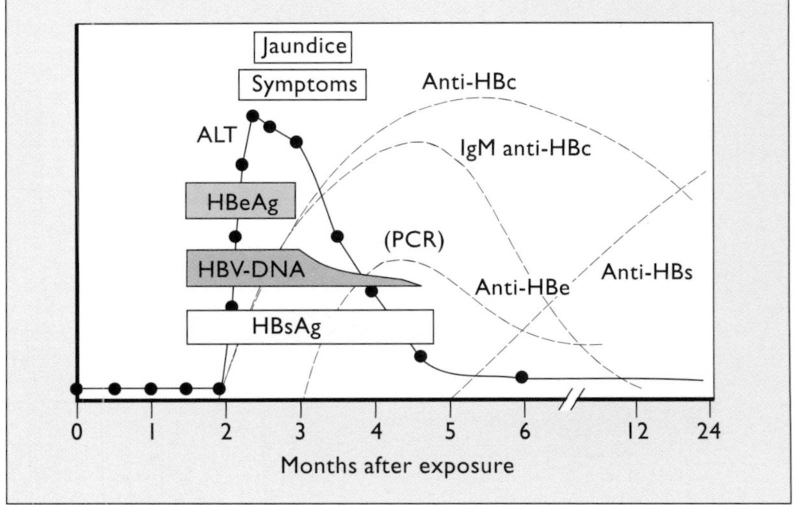

FIGURE 7-11 Typical clinical, serologic, and virologic time course of hepatitis B. (ALT—alanine aminotransferase; HBc—hepatitis B core; HBeAg—hepatitis B e antigen; HBsAg—hepatitis B surface antigen; HBV—hepatitis B virus; PCR—polymerase chain reaction.) (*From* Hsu *et al.* [7].)

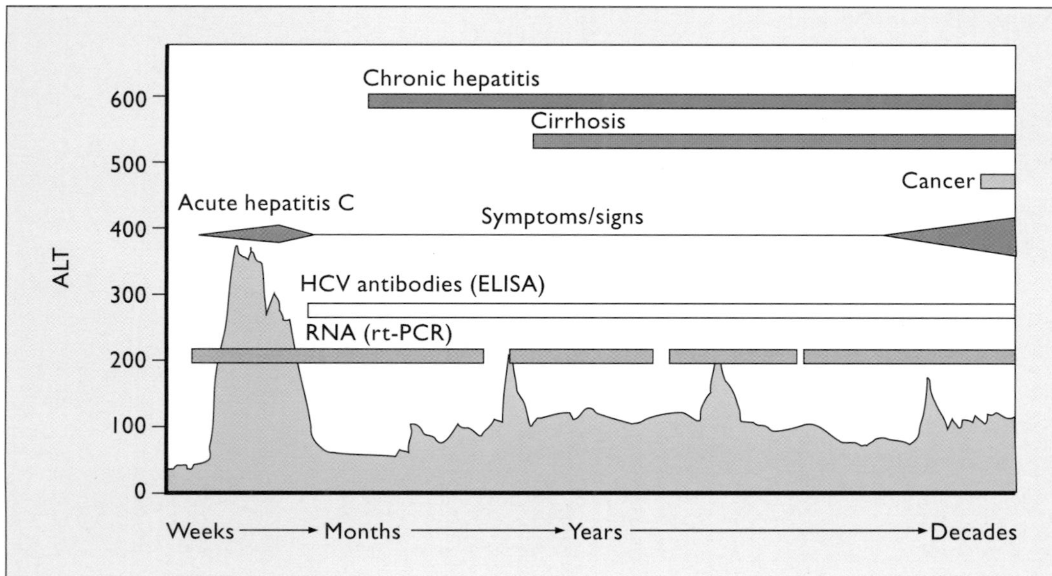

FIGURE 7-12 Natural history of hepatitis C. Chronicity may develop over months, years, or decades and may lead to cirrhosis and an increased risk for hepatocellular carcinoma. (ALT—alanine aminotransferase; ELISA—enzyme-linked immunoassay; HCV—hepatitis C virus; rt-PCR—reverse transcriptase polymerase chain reaction.) (*From* Lemon and Brown [8].)

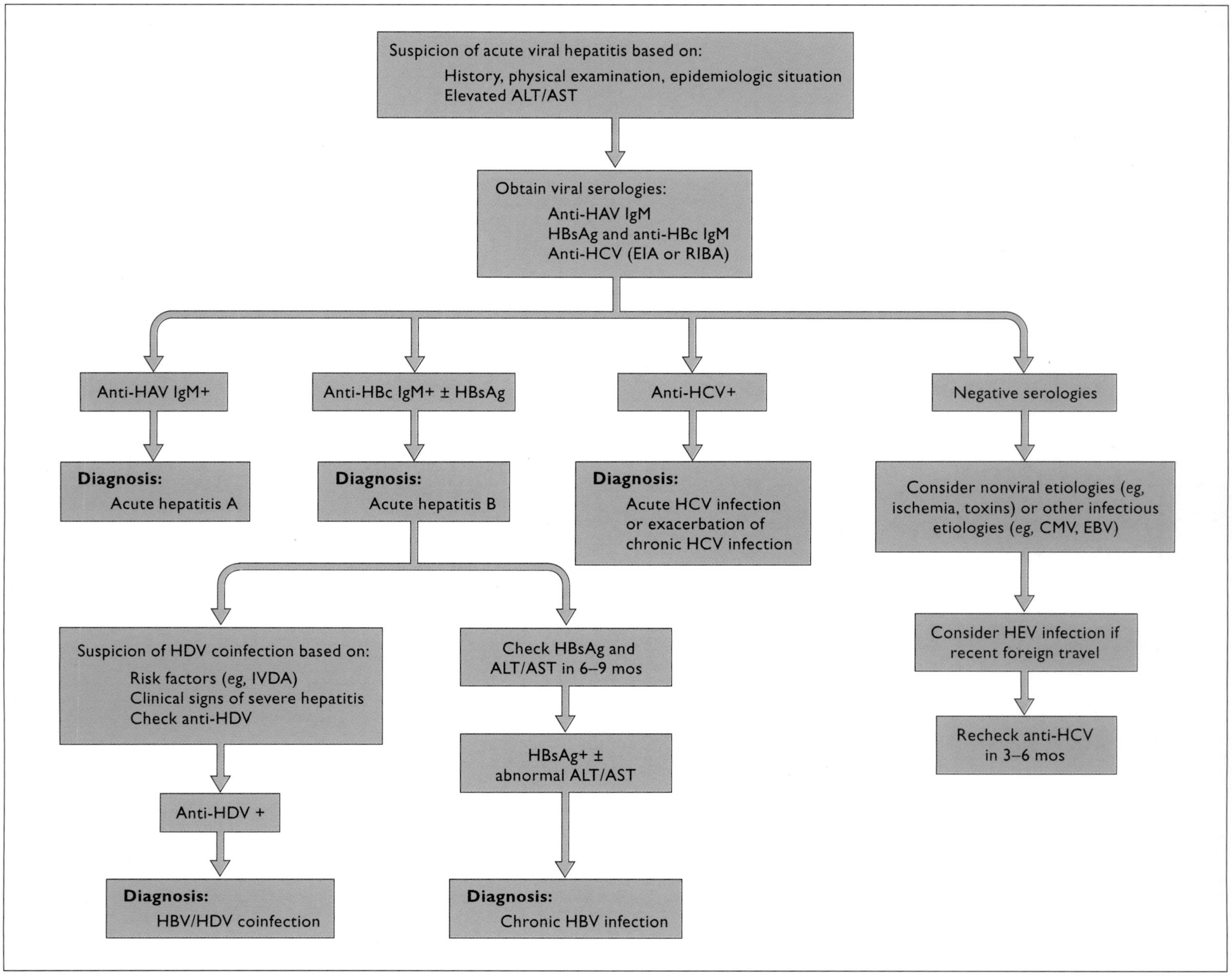

Suspicion of acute viral hepatitis based on:
History, physical examination, epidemiologic situation
Elevated ALT/AST

Obtain viral serologies:
Anti-HAV IgM
HBsAg and anti-HBc IgM
Anti-HCV (EIA or RIBA)

Anti-HAV IgM+
→ **Diagnosis:** Acute hepatitis A

Anti-HBc IgM+ ± HBsAg
→ **Diagnosis:** Acute hepatitis B
→ Suspicion of HDV coinfection based on: Risk factors (eg, IVDA); Clinical signs of severe hepatitis; Check anti-HDV
→ Anti-HDV +
→ **Diagnosis:** HBV/HDV coinfection
→ Check HBsAg and ALT/AST in 6–9 mos
→ HBsAg+ ± abnormal ALT/AST
→ **Diagnosis:** Chronic HBV infection

Anti-HCV+
→ **Diagnosis:** Acute HCV infection or exacerbation of chronic HCV infection

Negative serologies
→ Consider nonviral etiologies (eg, ischemia, toxins) or other infectious etiologies (eg, CMV, EBV)
→ Consider HEV infection if recent foreign travel
→ Recheck anti-HCV in 3–6 mos

FIGURE 7-13 Algorithm for diagnostic investigation of suspected viral hepatitis. The rate of possible coinfection, superinfection, or drug-induced etiologies must also be considered in cases with confusing or atypical clinical and serologic findings. (ALT—alanine aminotransferase; AST—aspartate aminotransferase; CMV—cytomegalovirus; EBV—Epstein-Barr virus; EIA—enzyme immunoassay; HAV—hepatitis A virus; HBc—hepatitis B core; HBsAg—hepatitis B surface antigen; HBV—hepatitis B virus; HCV—hepatitis C virus; HEV—hepatitis E virus; HDV—hepatitis D virus; IVDA—intravenous drug abusers; RIBA—recombinant immunoblot assay.) (*From* Hsu [7].)

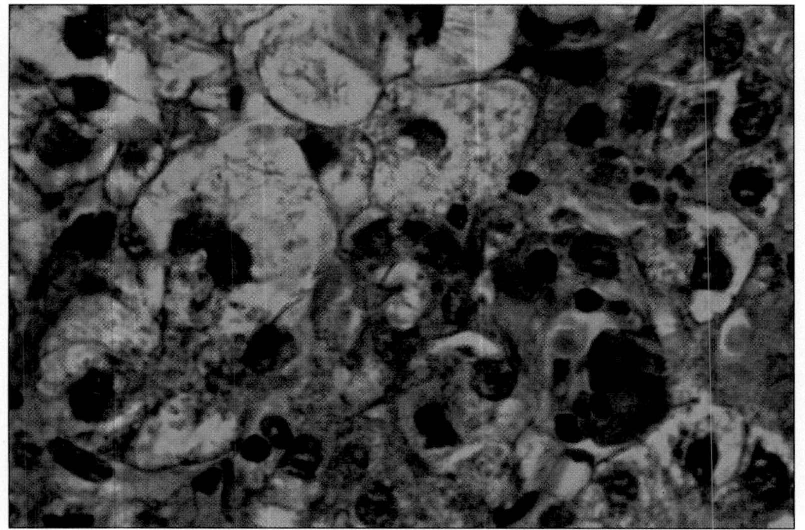

Figure 7-14 Liver histology in acute viral hepatitis, with marked ballooning degeneration of hepatocytes and acidophilic (apoptotic) body formation. Ballooned cells (whether singly, in groups, or diffusely) may undergo necrosis by rupture or lysis. Acidophilic/apoptotic body formation is preceded by acidophilic degeneration characterized by cell shrinkage, increased eosinophilia, increased angularity and loss of attachment to neighboring cells, nuclear pyknosis, karyorrhexis or karyolysis. Portions of a degenerating or dying hepatocyte may break off, forming apoptotic bodies. Acidophilic/apoptotic bodies extruded into sinusoids are eventually phagocytosed by Kupffer cells [9]. (Hematoxylin-eosin stain; original magnification, × 175.)

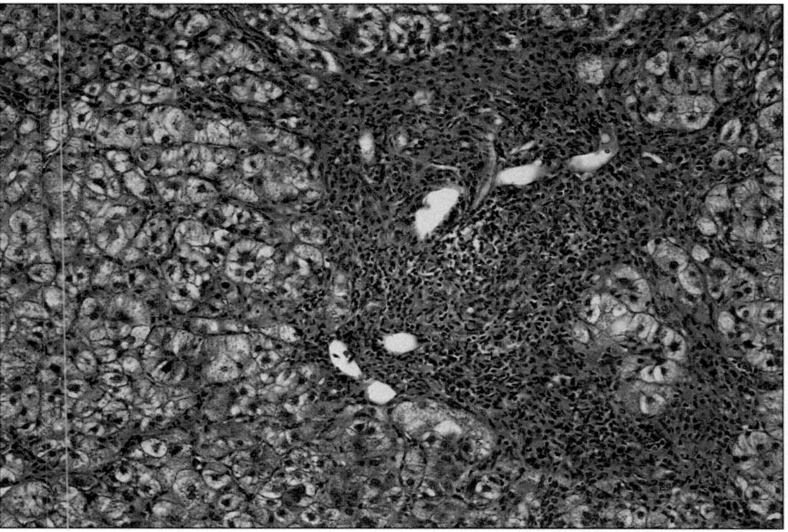

Figure 7-15 Liver histology in chronic hepatitis. An expanded portal area contains a heavy infiltrate of chronic inflammatory cells, focal entrapment of small groups, or individual hepatocytes giving rise to limiting plate irregularity (Hematoxylin-eosin stain; original magnification, × 45.)

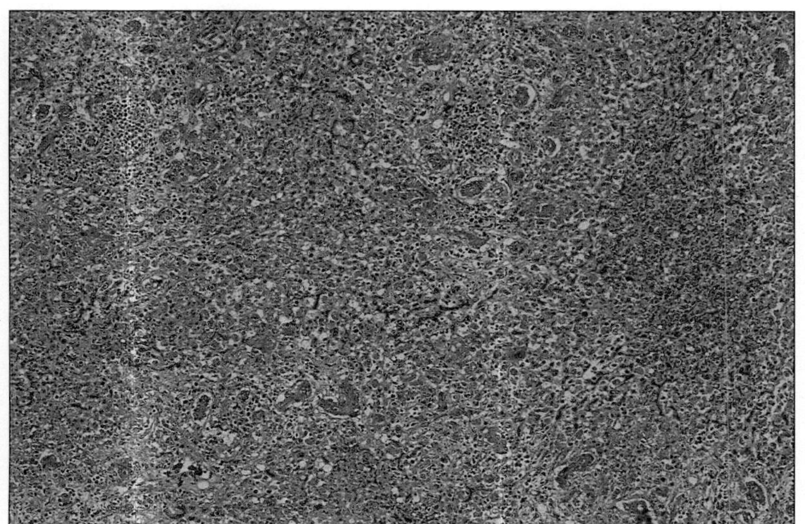

Figure 7-16 Liver histology in fatal fulminant hepatitis. The figure displays acute viral hepatitis with massive necrosis and marked hepatocellular loss. Relatively few remaining islands of liver cells are seen. Reactive ductal (cholangiolar) proliferation is seen in zone 1 (periportal areas). (Hematoxylin-eosin stain; original magnification, × 25.)

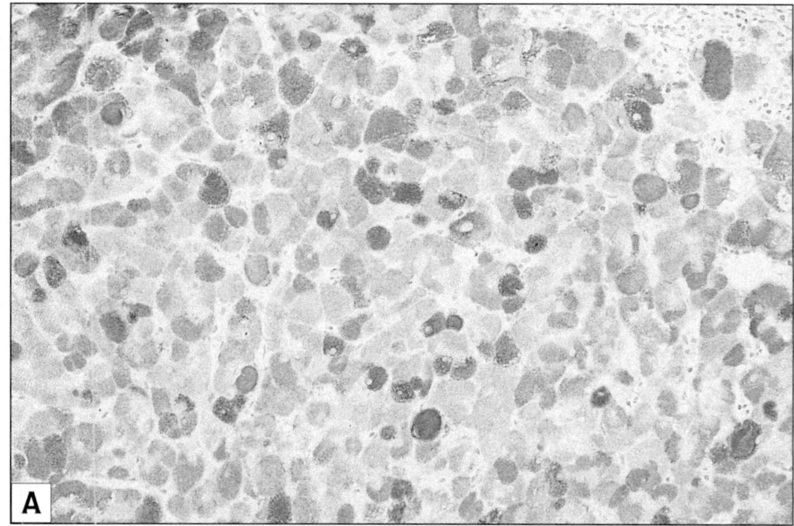

Figure 7-17 Immunoperoxidase stains in chronic hepatitis B. **A,** Immunoperoxidase staining for hepatitis B surface antigen (HBsAg). The immunoperoxidase technique is far more sensitive than Skikata staining methods (Victoria blue, orcein, or aldehyde fuchsin). The figure shows diffuse immunoreactivity for HBsAg, with strongly reactive hepatocytes as well as areas of weak immunoreactivity. Note that nuclei do not contain HBsAg. In some hepatocytes, the staining is membranous. (*continued*)

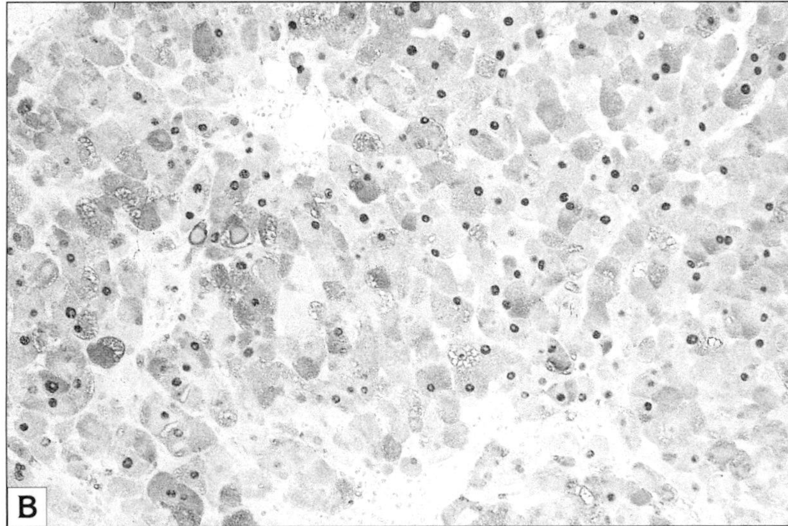

FIGURE 7-17 (*continued*) **B.** Immunoperoxidase staining for hepatitis B core antigen (HBcAg). There is strong immunoreactivity for HBcAg in the nuclei of affected hepatocytes and prominent spillover into the cytoplasm (*Both panels*, original magnification, × 50.)

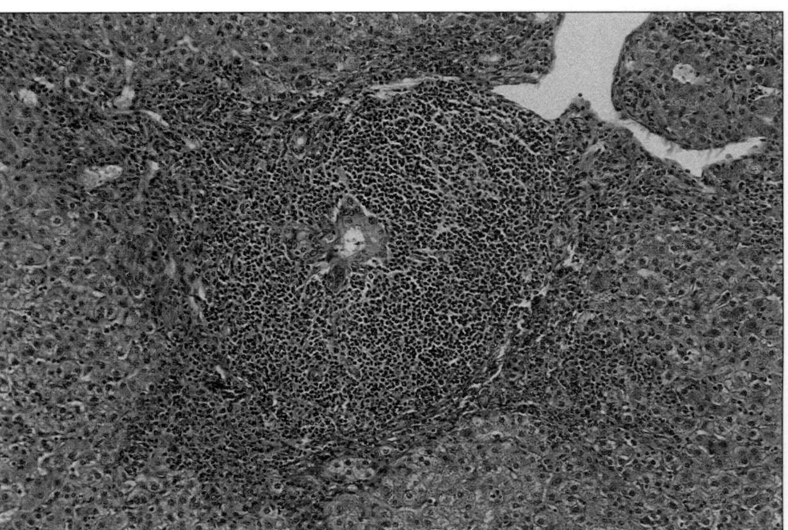

FIGURE 7-18 Liver biopsy in chronic hepatitis C. Note the prominent portal inflammation and occasional peripheral piecemeal necrosis. This section also exhibits a striking chronic nonsuppurative ductal injury (so-called Poulsen lesion), which resembles primary biliary cirrhosis [10]. (Hematoxylin-eosin stain; original magnification, × 33.)

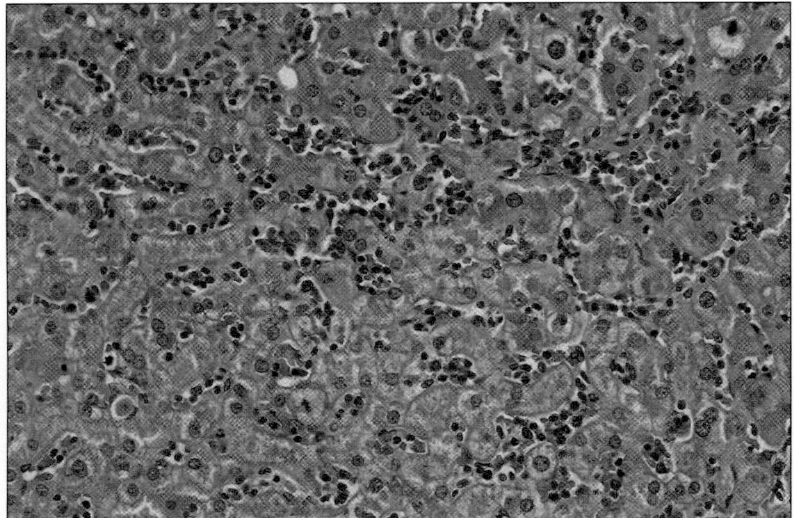

FIGURE 7-19 Sinusoidal beading in infectious mononucleosis. An extensive hepatic sinusoidal chronic inflammatory cell infiltrate, an occasional mitotic figure, and a rare free acidophilic/apoptotic body can be seen. The sinusoidal "beading," or "Indian file" appearance, is characteristic for infectious mononucleosis. The diagnosis was confirmed serologically. (Hematoxylin stain; original magnification, × 50.)

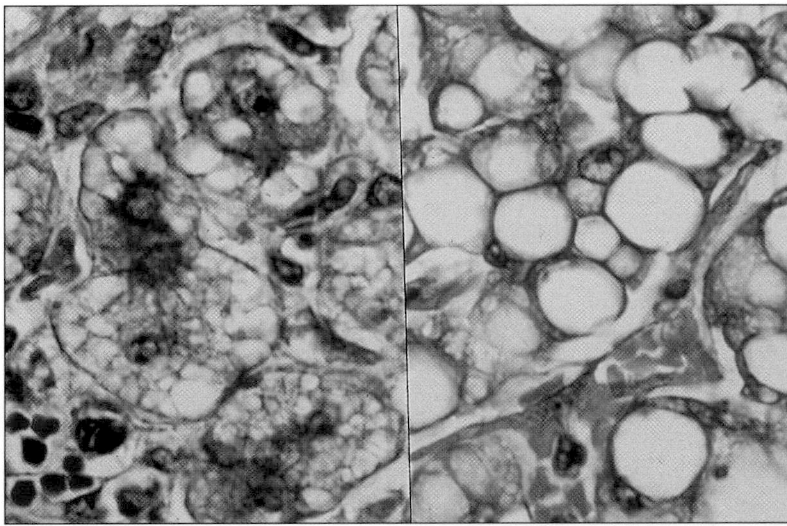

FIGURE 7-20 Reye's syndrome (postviral infection). In early childhood to adolescence, patients appearing to recover from a viral infection (*eg*, chickenpox, influenza) who are treated with aspirin may develop a type of fatty change. *Left*, Swollen hepatocytes with microvesicular steatosis. Microvesicular steatosis, however, also occurs in various other conditions, such as acute fatty metamorphosis of pregnancy, tetracycline or valproate hepatotoxicity, Jamaican vomiting sickness, defects in ureagenesis, and alcoholic foamy degeneration. *Right*, Nonspecific large vacuolar steatosis. This type of fatty change may occur in obesity, alcoholism, diabetes mellitus, or corticosteroid therapy. (Hematoxylin-eosin stain. Original magnification; *left panel*, × 40; *right panel*, × 140.)

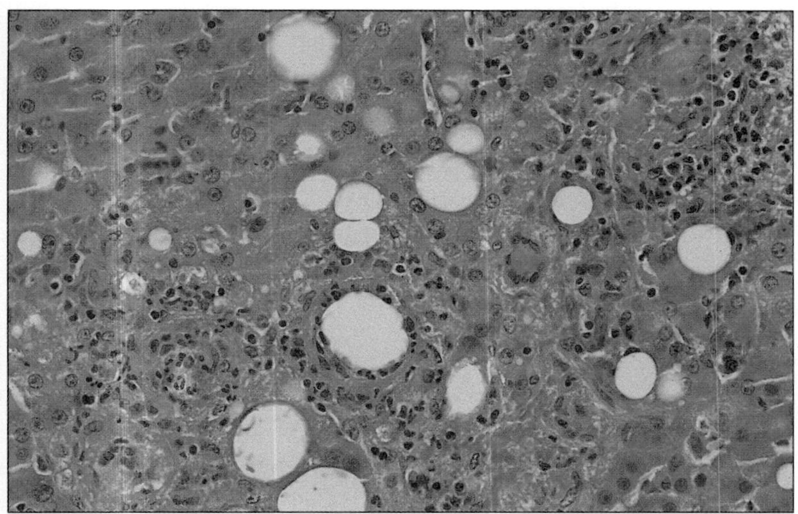

FIGURE 7-21 Liver biopsy specimen with noncaseating granulomata due to Q fever. In the lower center of the field is a doughnut-shaped granuloma with inflammatory cells and a fibrin ring. Although not pathognomonic, fibrin-ring granulomas may be associated with Q fever. (Hematoxylin-eosin stain; original magnification, × 80.)

BACTERIAL ENTERITIS

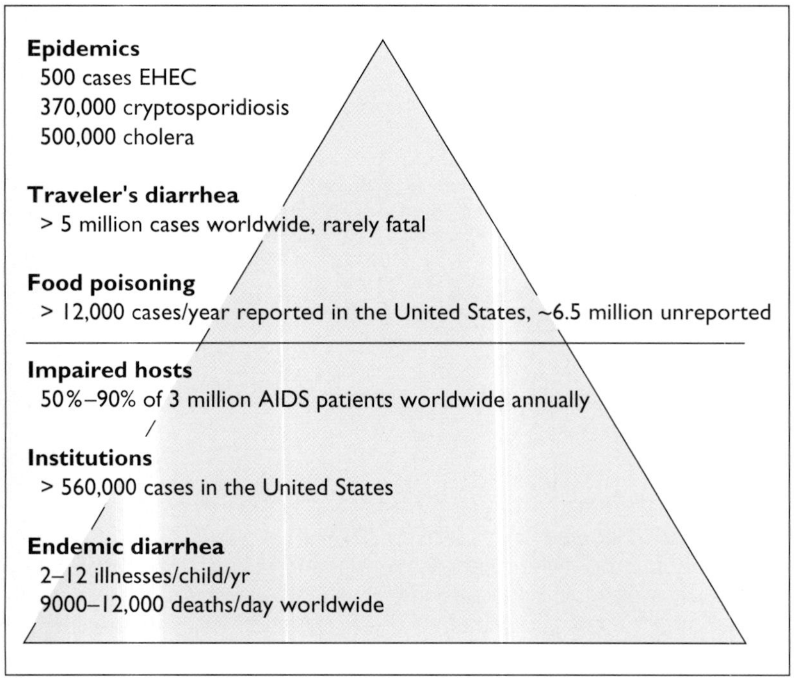

FIGURE 7-22 Six types of microbial diarrhea. Worldwide, diarrheal diseases are second only to cardiovascular disease as a cause of death and are the leading cause of childhood death. Microbial diarrhea occurs in six settings. Reaching the greatest attention are occasional epidemics, such as those caused by enterohemorrhagic *Escherichia coli* (EHEC), water-borne cryptosporidiosis, and global spread of new cholera pandemics; traveler's diarrhea, which affects up to one third of 16 million international travelers each year; and food poisoning. Receiving considerably less attention but responsible for considerably more cases worldwide are diarrheal illnesses in impaired hosts (such as occurs in 50% to 90% of AIDS patients globally each year) and diarrhea in institutions (such as daycare centers, hospitals, and extended care facilities). Finally, there is endemic diarrhea, accounting for two to 12 illnesses per child per year and more than 9000 deaths each day globally [11].

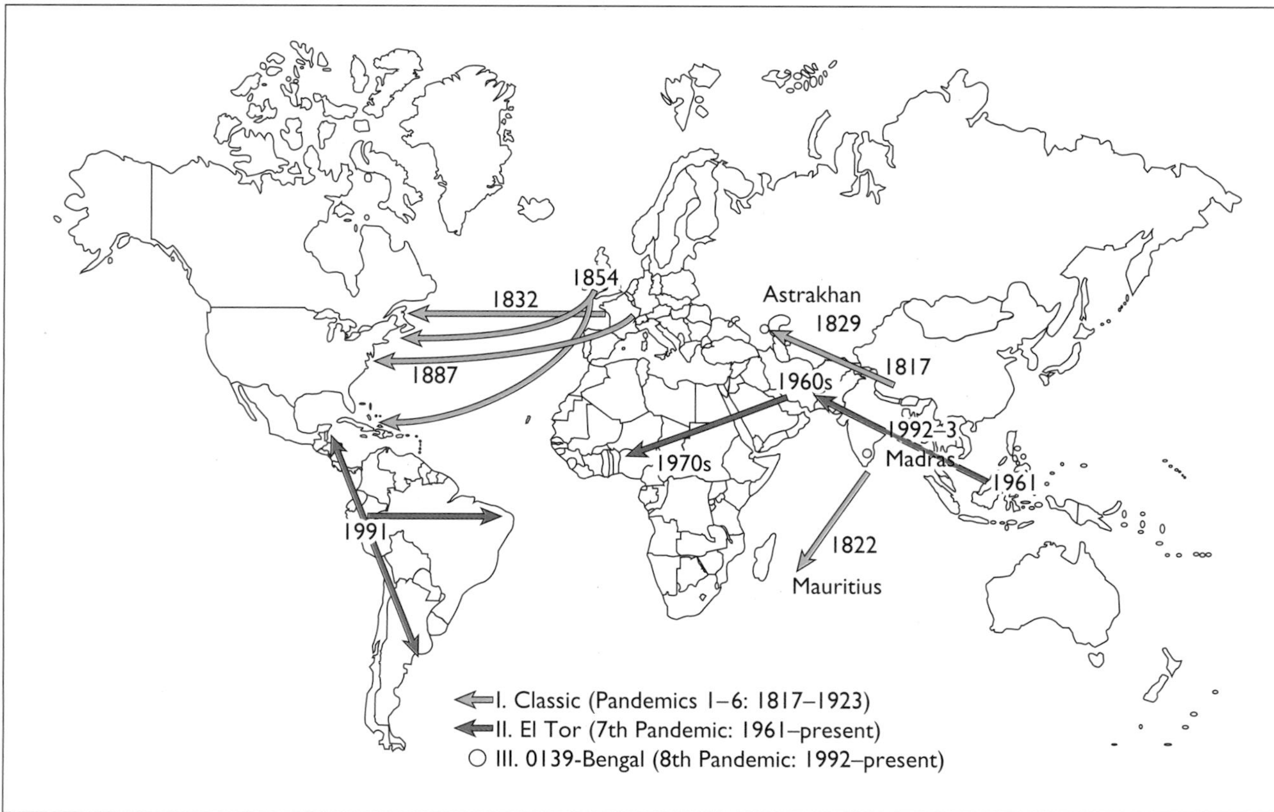

FIGURE 7-23 Collision of the 7th and 8th cholera pandemics. The first six cholera pandemics, which may have been due to classic *Vibrio cholerae* infections, occurred as six waves between 1817 and 1923. The 7th pandemic, with a distinct strain, El Tor, began in the Celebes in 1961 and continues through the present, with extensive spread in Latin America since 1991. Originating in Madras in late 1992, O139 Bengal is yet a third strain of *V. cholerae* that has rapidly become epidemic throughout many areas of South Asia since 1993 and threatens to become the 8th pandemic. (*Adapted from* Guerrant [11].)

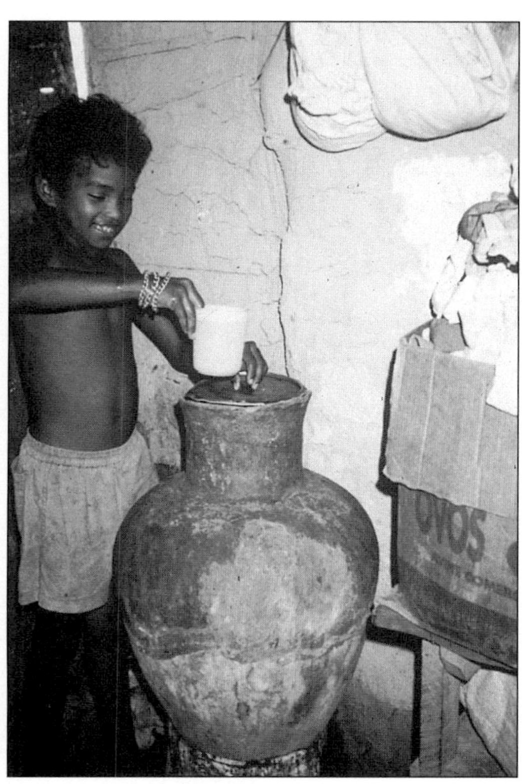

FIGURE 7-24 A child dipping a cup with his hand into the household water supply during a cholera epidemic in Fortaleza, Brazil. This common practice may contribute to the spread of cholera and is the focus of control programs designed to provide improved water sources and storage containers with narrow necks or spigots.

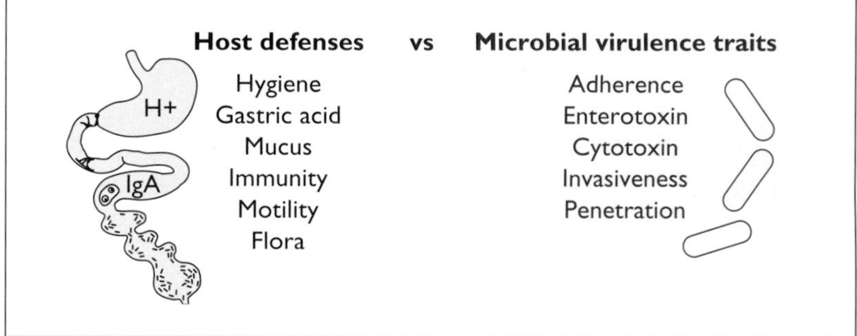

FIGURE 7-25 Host defenses and microbial virulence traits. Several specific enteric host defenses prevent many enteric infections and are often violated or bypassed in individuals who become infected. Normal hygiene usually prevents the acquisition of infectious doses of microbs in hygienic industrialized areas. The neutralization of gastric acid increases one's chances of enteric infections with many agents. Mucosal immunity, normal motility, and normal microbial flora are important barriers to colonization by enteric pathogens as well. Conversely, specific microbial virulence traits—such as adherence in an important region of the bowel, production of secretory enterotoxins or cell-damaging cytotoxins, direct invasiveness such as that seen with *Shigella*, or penetration through intact epithelial cells such as occurs with *Salmonella* infections—are key traits that enable an organism to be a pathogen.

Infectious doses of enteric pathogens	
Shigella	10^{1-2}
Campylobacter jejuni	10^{2-6}
Salmonella	10^{5}
Escherichia coli	10^{8}
Vibrio cholerae	10^{8}
Giardia lamblia	10^{1-2} cysts
Entamoeba histolytica	10^{1-2} cysts

FIGURE 7-26 Infectious doses of enteric pathogens. Most identified enteric pathogens are acquired via the fecal-oral route, emphasizing the role of personal hygiene in host defense. For bacteria such as *Salmonella*, *Escherichia coli*, and *Vibrio cholerae*, a large number of organisms (100,000–100 million) usually must be ingested to overcome host defenses and cause disease (assuming other host defenses are intact). Some other organisms such as *Shigella*, cysts of *Giardia*, *Entamoeba histolytica*, and *Cryptosporidium*, as well as certain strains of *Campylobacter jejuni* appear to be infectious with less than a few hundred organisms or cysts and may be readily transmitted via person-to-person contact, as in daycare centers. (*From* Guerrant [12].)

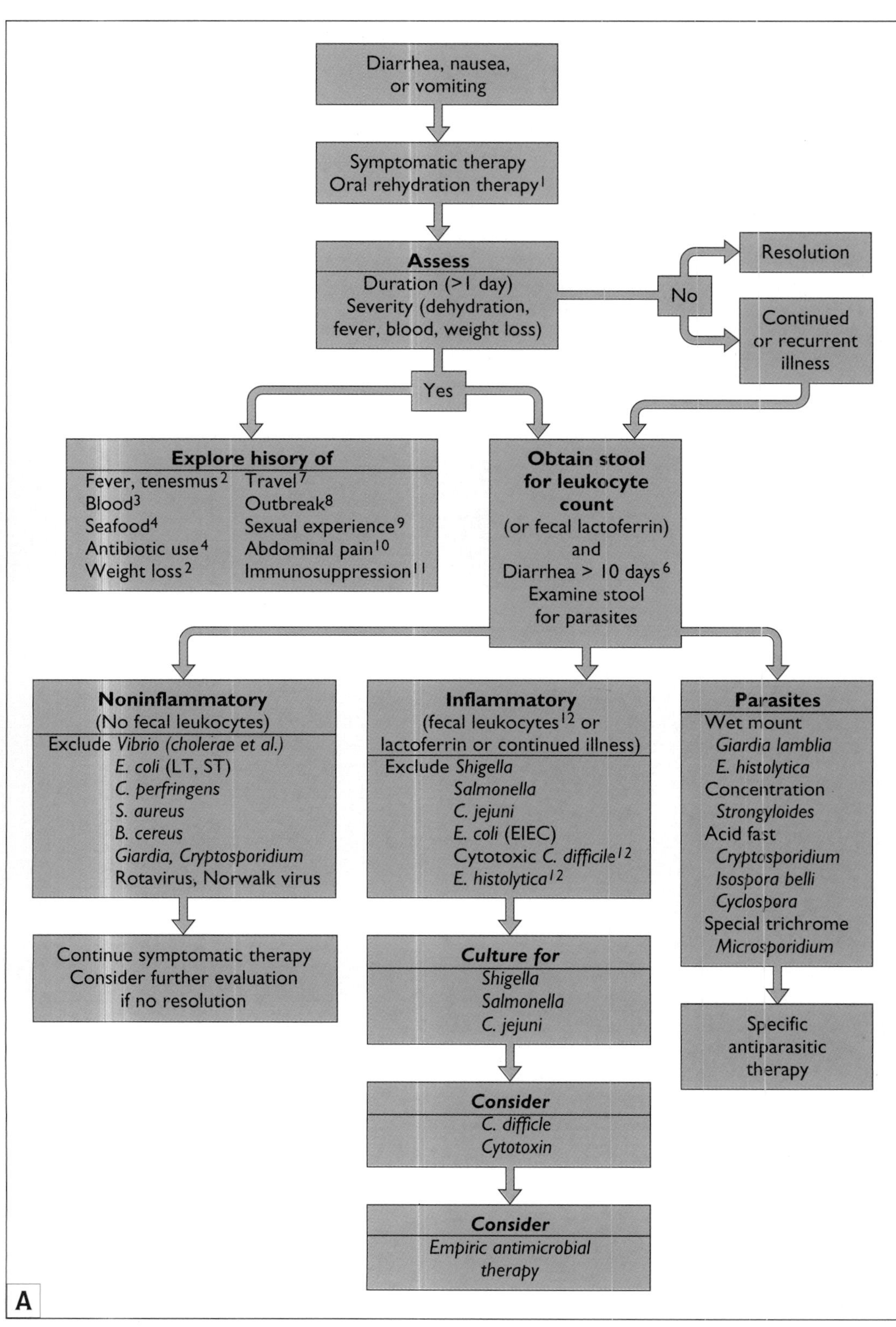

FIGURE 7-27 **A** and **B**, Selective diagnostic and therapeutic approach to diarrhea, nausea, and vomiting. Although all patients with significant gastrointestinal illnesses should receive adequate rehydration, orally if possible, further diagnostic or more specific antimicrobial therapy should be directed by specific findings in the history or stool examination. Diarrhea lasting for > 1 day or associated with severe dehydration, bloody stool, fever, or weight loss warrants additional evaluation of history and stool examination for leukocytes or a leukocyte marker (such as lactoferrin). Diarrhea lasting for 10 days should prompt examination for parasites. (*See panel 27B* for footnotes.) (EIEC—enteroinvasive *E. coli*; LT—heat-labile toxin; ST—heat-stable toxin.) (*Adapted from* Guerrant and Bobak [13].) (*continued*)

B. Diagnosis and management of diarrhea, nausea, or vomiting

1. Oral rehydration solution can be prepared by adding 3.5 g NaCl, 2.5 g $NaHCO_3$ (or 2.9 g Na citrate), 1.5 g KCl, and 20 g glucose *or* glucose polymer (*eg*, 40 g sucrose *or* 4 tbsp sugar *or* 50–60 g cereal flour such as rice, maize, sorghum, millet, wheat, or potato) per liter (1.05 qts) of clear water. This makes approximately Na 90, K 20, Cl 80, HCO_3 30, glucose 111 mmol/L.

   One level tsp of table salt and 8 level tsp of table sugar per liter makes about 86 mmol Na and 30 g sucrose/L, to which one could add 1 cup orange juice or 2 bananas for potassium.
2. Fever or tenesmus suggest an inflammatory proctocolitis.
3. Diarrhea with blood, especially without fecal leukocytes, suggests enterohemorrhagic (Shiga-like toxin–producing) *Escherichia coli* O157 or amebiasis (in which leukocytes are destroyed by the parasite).
4. Ingestion of inadequately cooked seafood should prompt consideration of infections with *Vibrio* or Norwalk-like viruses.
5. Antibiotics should be stopped if possible and cytotoxigenic *Clostridium difficile* considered. Antibiotics may also predispose to other infections, such as salmonellosis.
6. Persistence (> 10 days) with weight loss should prompt consideration of giardiasis or cryptosporidiosis.

   Whereas many stool examinations for ova and parasites are often of low yield, specific requests for *Giardia* and *Cryptosporidium* ELISA (in patients with > 10 days of diarrhea) or, in immunocompromised patients, acid fast stain for *Cryptosporidium, Isospora,* or *Cyclospora* are worth considering.
7. Travel to tropical areas increases the chance of developing enterotoxigenic *E. coli,* as well as viral (Norwalk-like or rotaviral), parasitic (*Giardia, Entamoeba, Strongyloides, Cryptosporidium*), and if fecal leukocytes are present, invasive bacterial infections.
8. Outbreaks should prompt consideration of *Staphylococcus aureus, Bacillus cereus,* anisakiasis (incubation period < 6 h), *Clostridium perfringens,* enterotoxigenic *E. coli, Vibrio, Salmonella, Campylobacter, Shigella,* or enteroinvasive *E. coli* infection. Consider saving *E. coli* for heat-labile toxin, heat-stable toxin, invasiveness, adherence testing, serotyping, and stool for rotavirus, and stool plus paired sera for Norwalk-like virus or toxin testing.
9. Sigmoidoscopy in symptomatic homosexual men should distinguish proctitis in the distal 15 cm only (caused by herpesvirus, gonococcal, chlamydial, or syphilitic infection) from colitis (*Campylobacter, Shigella, C. difficile,* or *Chlamydia* [lymphogranuloma venereum serotypes] infections) or noninflammatory diarrhea (due to giardiasis).
10. If unexplained abdominal pain and fever persist or suggest an appendicitis-like syndrome, culture for *Yersinia enterocolitica* with cold enrichment.
11. In immunocompromised hosts, a wide range of viral (cytomegalovirus, herpes simplex virus, coxsackievirus, rotavirus), bacterial (*Salmonella, Mycobacterium avium-intracellulare*), and parasitic (*Cryptosporidium, Isospora, Strongyloides, Entamoeba,* and *Giardia*) agents should be considered.
12. Some inflammatory, colonic pathogens, such as cytotoxigenic *C. difficile* or *Entamoeba histolytica,* may destroy fecal leukocyte morphology, so a reliable leukocyte marker such as fecal lactoferrin may provide a better screening test.

ELISA—enzyme-linked immunosorbent assay.

FIGURE 7-27 (*continued*).

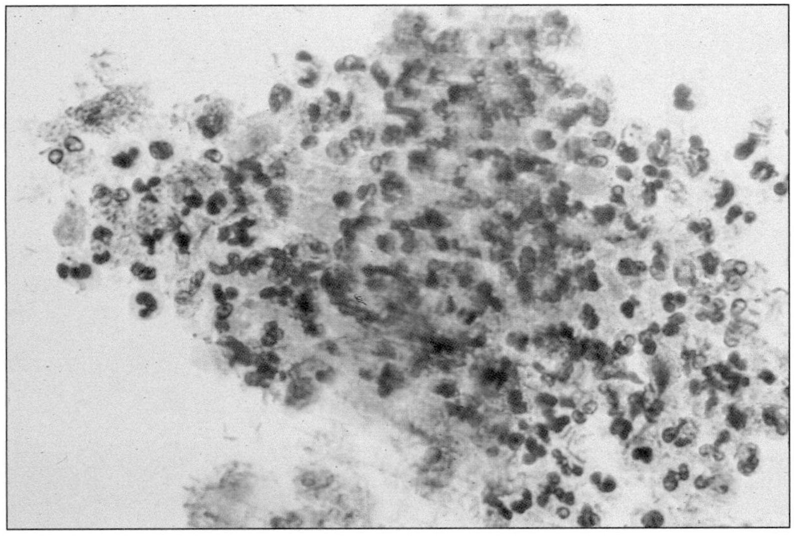

FIGURE 7-28 Fecal leukocytes on wet mount of stool specimen stained with methylene blue. Clumps of numerous polymorphonuclear leukocytes can be seen in a patient with *Shigella* infection. Examination of fresh stool is a potentially helpful screen for colonic mucosal inflammation due to invasive bacteria, such as *Shigella* or *Campylobacter jejuni*, or idiopathic inflammatory disease. However, it requires that a skilled microscopist examine a freshly stained fecal specimen to avoid false-positive and false-negative readings.

Etiologies of traveler's diarrhea*

Characteristics	Latin America	Africa	Asia
Duration of stay, *d*	21 (2–42)	28 (28–35)	(28–42)
Attack rate, %	52 (21–100)	54 (36–62)	(39–57)
Percentage with			
Enterotoxigenic *Escherichia coli*	46 (28–72)	36 (31–75)	(20–34)
Shigella	0 (0–30)	0 (0–15)	(4–7)
Salmonella	—	0 (0–0)	(11–15)
Campylobacter jejuni	—	—	(2–15)
Vibrio parahaemolyticus	—	—	(1–13)
Rotavirus	23 (0–36)	0 (0–0)	—

*Data given as the median (range) from 26 studies.

FIGURE 7-29 Etiologies of traveler's diarrhea. Numerous studies of travelers to Latin America, Africa, or Asia all show a 21% to 100% attack rate over a usual 2- to 4-week travel. By far, the predominant associated pathogens in one third or more of cases are enterotoxigenic *Escherichia coli* that produce either the heat-labile or heat-stable toxins or both. Other pathogens vary with the location visited. (*From* Guerrant and Bobak [14].)

Safe and unsafe foods in developing tropical regions

Low-risk foods and beverages	High-risk foods and beverages
Any item served steaming hot (> 59° C)	Foods that are moist and served at room temperature, especially those at a buffet
Foods that are dry (*ie*, bread and crackers)	Fruits and vegetables with skin intact—strawberries, tomatoes, grapes
Items with very high sugar content (syrups and jellies)	Salads and other uncooked vegetables
Fruits and vegetables that have been peeled	Sauces and dressings in open containers on the table
Peanut butter	Milk (other than powdered milk that is constituted with previously boiled water or irradiated milk kept refrigerated after preparing or opening)
Any fresh food item properly washed and prepared by the traveler	Tap water or ice
Bottled carbonated drinks including mineral water, soft drinks, and beer	

FIGURE 7-30 Safe and unsafe foods in developing tropical regions. The usual adage of "boil it, peel it, cook it, or forget it" is the safest policy for travelers. Especially important to avoid are tap water and foods that are served at room temperature, having been left out for an unknown period. Although some authors may suggest prophylactic antimicrobial for travelers at special risk, attempts at use of prophylactic agents might provide only a false sense of security for travelers at high risk, such as those with immunocompromise, for infections that would not be prevented by prophylactic antibiotics (such as *Cryptosporidium*, which requires fastidious attention to food and water advisories). The potential risks of prophylactic antibiotics therefore might well outweigh their potential benefit in preventing only readily treatable infections. The author (RLG) recommends careful precautions with prompt treatment with either bismuth subsalicylate, other bismuth preparations, or prompt antimicrobial therapy with an agent such as a quinolone (for adults) or sulfamethoxazole-trimethoprim (for children). (*From* DuPont [15].)

Possible causes of diarrhea in AIDS patients

Pathogen	Diarrhea, % (n = 181)	No diarrhea, % (n = 28)
Cytomegalovirus	12–45	15
Cryptosporidium	14–26	0
Microsporidium	7.5–33	0
Entamoeba histolytica	0–15	0
Giardia lamblia	2–15	5
Salmonella spp	0–15	0
Campylobacter spp	2–11	8
Shigella spp	5–10	0
Clostridium difficile toxin	6–7	0
Vibrio parahaemolyticus	4	0
Mycobacterium spp	2–25	0
Isospora belli	2–6	0
Blastocystis hominis	2–15	16
Candida albicans	6–53	24
Herpes simplex	5–18	40
Chlamydia trachomatis	11	13
Strongyloides	0–6	0
Intestinal spirochetes	11	11
One or more pathogens	55–86	39

Figure 7-31 Possible causes of diarrhea in patients with AIDS. One or more identifiable pathogens can usually be identified in 65% to 86% of patients with diarrhea and AIDS. This list is led by cytomegalovirus, followed by *Cryptosporidium*, *Microsporidium*, and numerous other potential pathogens, some of which may respond to specific therapy and should be sought. This diagnosis usually can be accomplished by noninvasive special methods. (*From* Guerrant and Bobak [14].)

Helicobacter pylori Infection

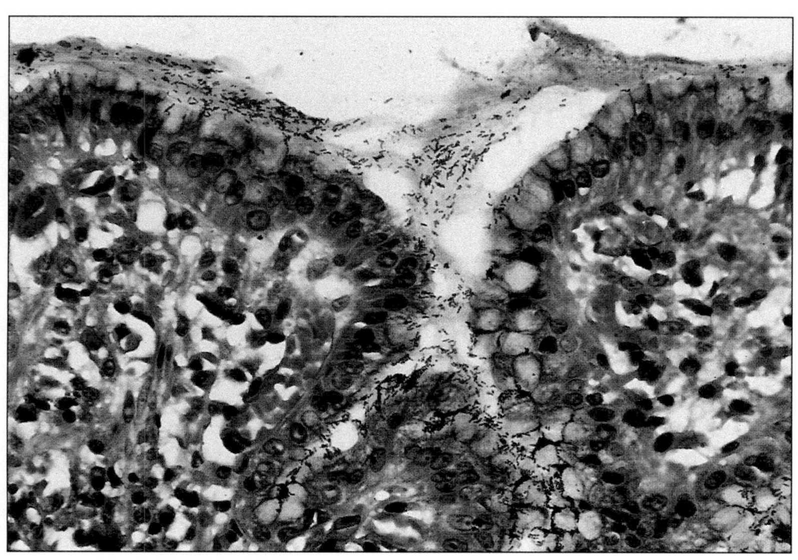

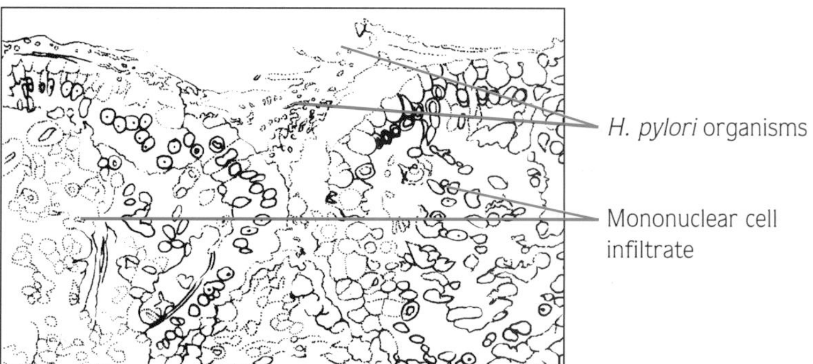

Figure 7-32 Heavy *Helicobacter pylori* infection of the gastric antrum. Large numbers of bacteria are seen within the mucus and foveolae. The surface epithelium has lost its orderly arrangement, and the mucin component of the superficial cells is greatly reduced. The inflammatory infiltrate in the lamina propria is predominantly mononuclear.

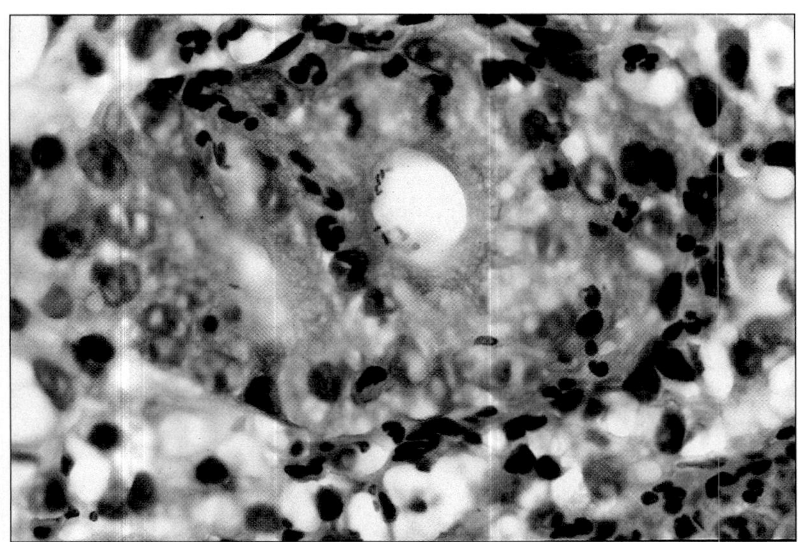

FIGURE 7-33 Antral gland with severe neutrophilic infiltration and few *Helicobacter pylori* within its lumen. Contrary to widespread belief, there is often little relationship between the location and intensity of the inflammatory infiltrate and the location and density of *H. pylori*.

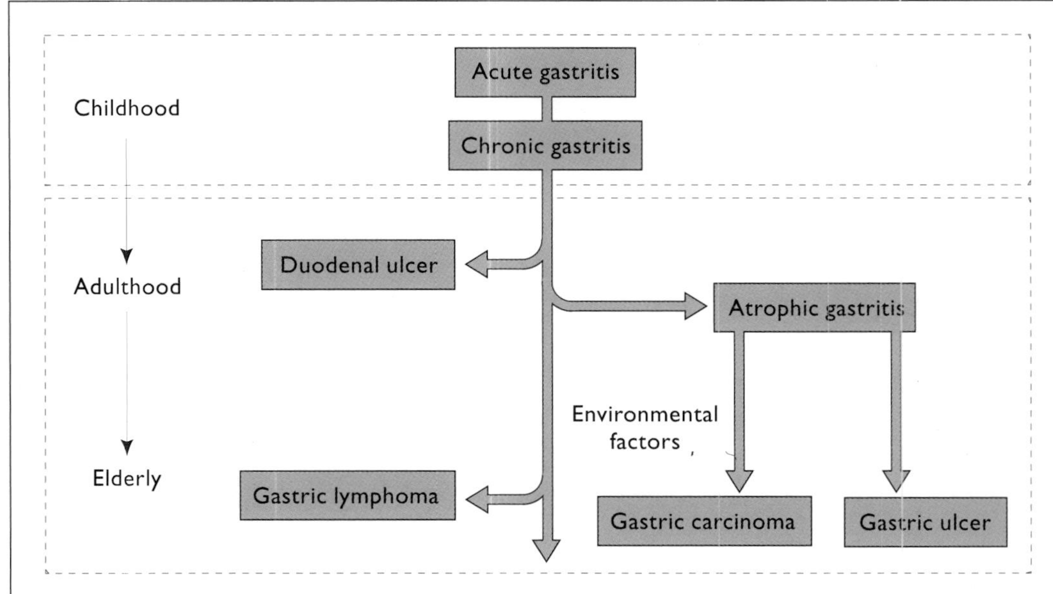

FIGURE 7-34 Time course of *Helicobacter pylori* infection and resultant diseases. *H. pylori* infection is typically acquired in childhood, and the pattern of acute and chronic inflammation is maintained throughout life. One in six infected persons develops peptic ulcer, with duodenal ulcer appearing at an earlier average age than gastric ulcer. Gastric adenocarcinoma is usually a very late event and may require environmental factors to bring about the transition from chronic atrophic gastritis to one with advanced stages of intestinal metaplasia. Gastric lymphoma can occur in any of the histologic types and is probably a chance occurrence related to the chronic stimulation of the chronic inflammatory reaction to the infection; in some cases, remission has been achieved with cure of the *H. pylori* infection. (*Adapted from* Graham [16].)

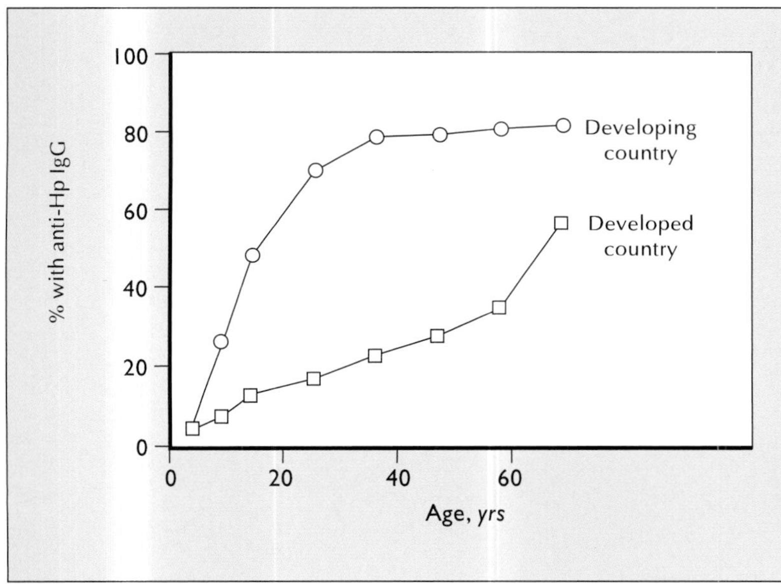

FIGURE 7-35 Differing prevalence of *Helicobacter pylori* (*Hp*) infection in developed versus developing countries. When prevalence rates for *H. pylori* infection in the different regions of the world are averaged, it shows the striking difference between developed and developing countries. This different epidemiologic pattern of *H. pylori* infection is due to the difference in rate of acquisition of the infection in childhood. (*Adapted from* Graham [16].)

Epidemiologic associations between gastritis and *Helicobacter pylori* infection

Factor	Gastritis	*H. pylori*
Age	✔	✔
Lower socioeconomic class	✔	✔
Duodenal ulcer	✔	✔
Gastric ulcer	✔	✔
Gastric cancer	✔	✔
Pernicious anemia	✔	—
Gender	—	—
Smoking or alcohol use	—	—
NSAID use	—	—

NSAID—nonsteroidal anti-inflammatory drug.

FIGURE 7-36 Comparison of epidemiologic associations in gastritis and *Helicobacter pylori* infection. The epidemiologic associations of gastritis and *H. pylori* infection are identical, with the exception of the lack of a clear role for *H. pylori* in pernicious anemia. By 1973, the epidemiology of gastritis had been fairly well defined, and the identification of *H. pylori* as a cause of gastritis allowed rapid progress and confirmed that most previous associations with gastritis could be transferred to *H. pylori*.

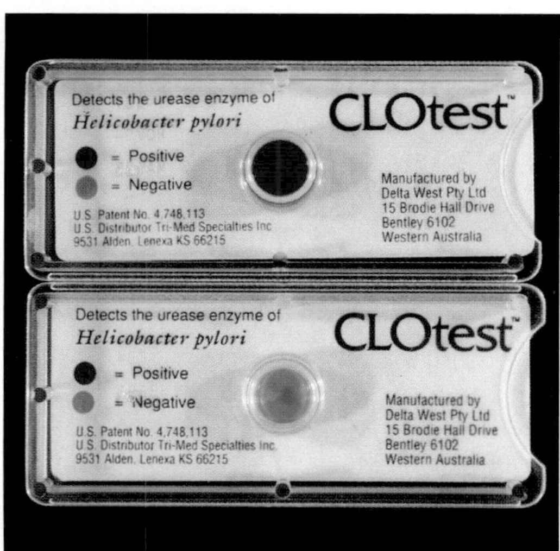

Figure 7-37 Rapid urease tests. Three commercially available rapid urease tests are shown. The rapid urease tests have a sensitivity and specificity of approximately 90% (95% confidence intervals for either false-positive or false-negative tests are 1%–13%). Both false-positive and false-negative tests occur, although false-negative tests outnumber false-positive ones. False-positive results are more common if one interprets the test in the afternoon or evening. The CLOtest (Delta West Pty. Ltd., Australia) relies on a gastric biopsy specimen placed in a gel containing urea and a pH indicator. Production of ammonia increases pH and changes the color. The initial pH of the medium is lower for hp*fast* and theoretically excludes false-positive tests from other microorganisms with urease activity. (*From* Graham [16]; with permission.)

Figure 7-38 Culture of *Helicobacter pylori* on brain-heart infusion agar. The typical clear, glistening *H. pylori* colonies, approximately 1 mm in diameter, can be seen on freshly made brain-heart infusion agar with 7% horse blood. The rate of primary isolation is highest on this media. Culture is done at 37° C in 12% CO_2 with 100% humidity.

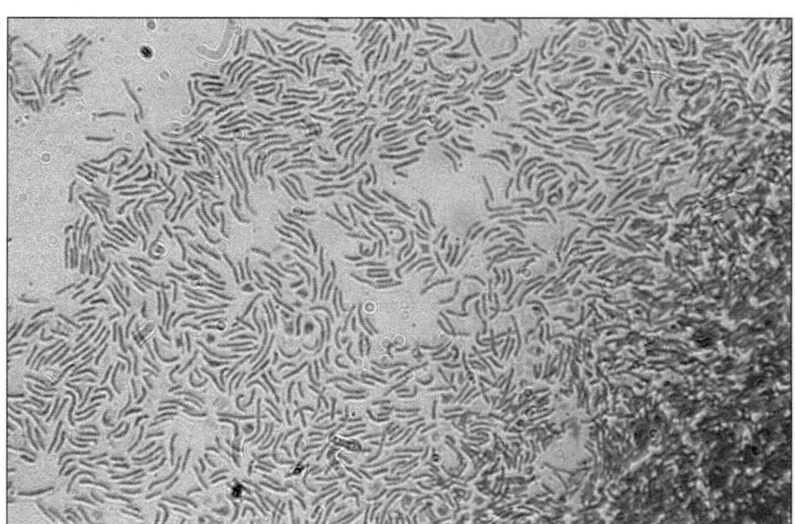

Figure 7-39 Gram stain of cultured *Helicobacter pylori* showing typical morphology.

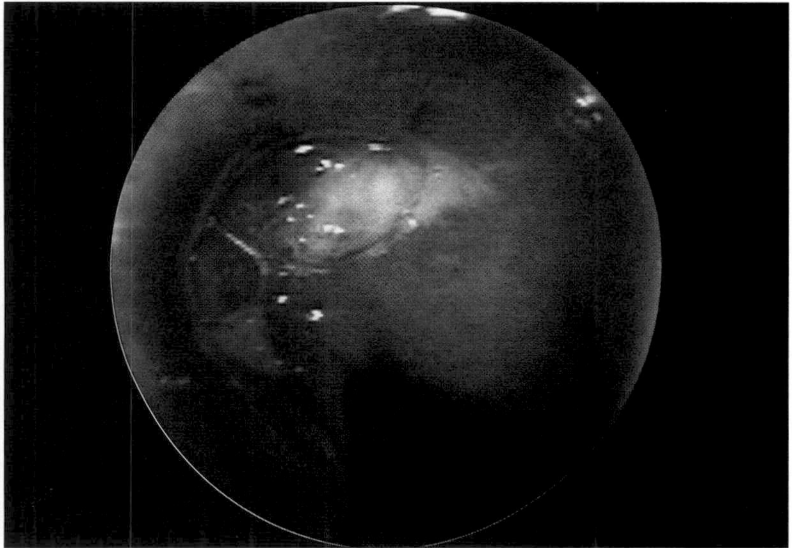

Figure 7-40 Endoscopic view showing deep, 1-cm duodenal ulcer prior to therapy. This is a typical ulcer at the apex of the bulb with deep excavation.

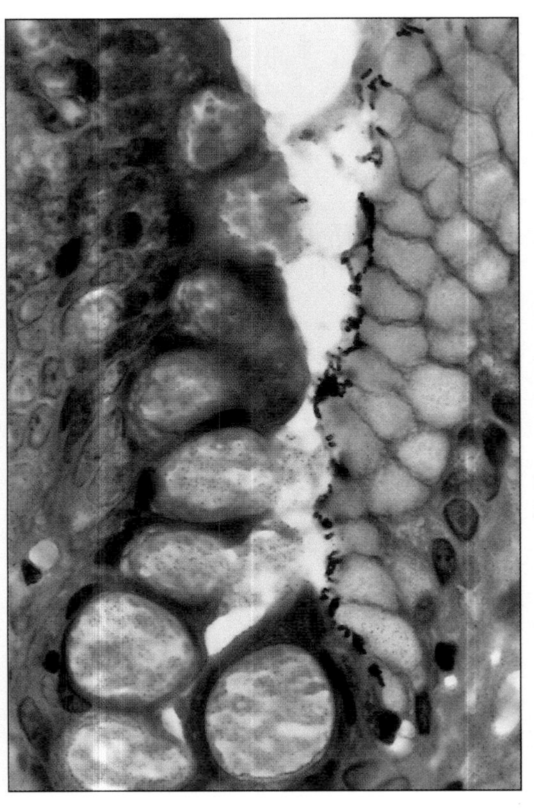

FIGURE 7-41 High-power microscopic view of intestinal metaplasia involving a gastric foveola. Intestinal metaplasia appears to create a hostile environment for *Helicobacter pylori*. Although there is heavy bacterial colonization in the *right* portion of this gastric foveola, no *H. pylori* are present in the *left* portion, which is entirely lined by intestinal-type epithelium. In some patients, however, *H. pylori* have been detected attached to areas of intestinal metaplasia.

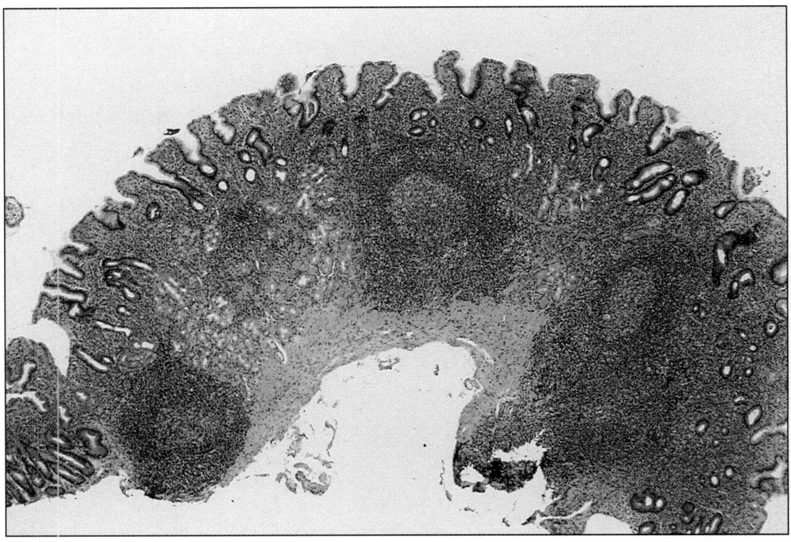

FIGURE 7-42 Low-power photomicrograph of antral biopsy specimen with three prominent lymphoid follicles. Lymphoid follicles are a constant inflammatory response in *Helicobacter pylori* gastritis. In some biopsy specimens, one may find several large and apparently confluent lymphoid follicles, which make the distinction from low-grade lymphomas arising from mucosa-associated lymphoid tissue difficult and sometimes impossible.

VIRAL ENTERITIS

Important agents of viral enteritis
Rotavirus
Groups A, B, C
Caliciviruses
Small round-structured viruses including Norwalk, Hawaii, Snow Mountain agents
Enteric adenovirus
Astrovirus

FIGURE 7-43 Important agents of viral enteritis. Rotaviruses are the leading cause of severe gastroenteritis in infants and young children worldwide. Small round-structured viruses (SRSVs), including the Norwalk virus, are known to be caliciviruses, which are a leading cause of epidemic outbreaks among adults. The SRSVs also include the agents previously known as Norwalk-like viruses.

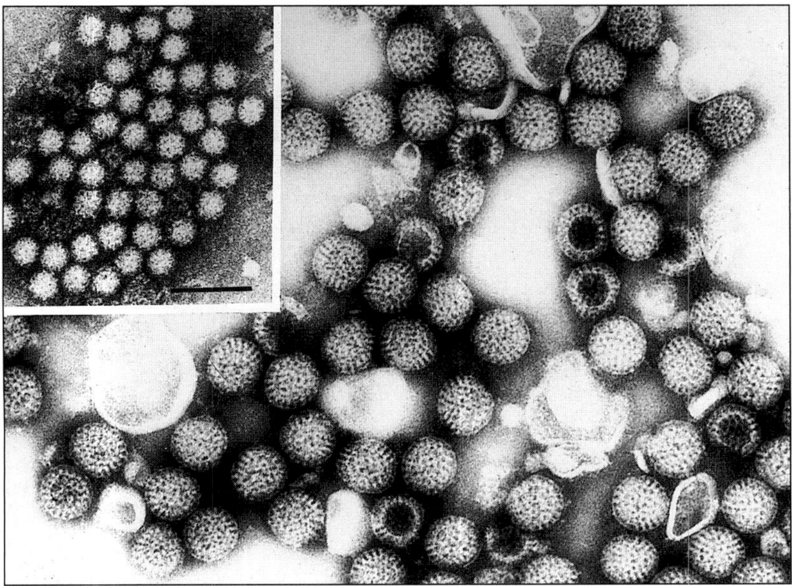

FIGURE 7-44 Human rotavirus particles in a stool filtrate prepared from an infant with gastroenteritis. Rotavirus was first identified as a human pathogen in 1973 by direct visualization with electron microscopy. This electron micrograph, first published in 1974, shows the classic double capsid particles thought to resemble wheels with spokes. This image explains the name of the virus, after the Latin *rota*, meaning wheel. (*From* Kapikian [17]; *inset from* Kapikian [25]; with permission.)

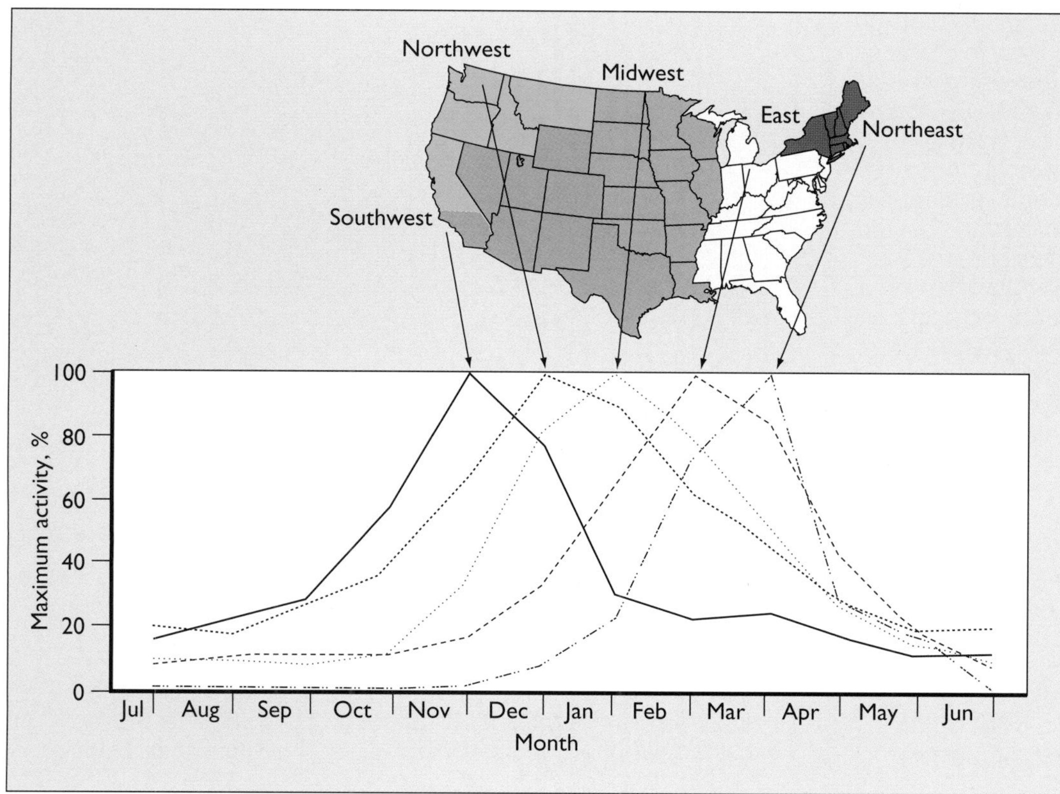

FIGURE 7-45 Regional rotavirus activity by month in the United States between 1984 and 1988. Data were collected in a 5-year retrospective survey of sentinel laboratories in the United States, covering the period 1984 to 1988. Results showed that rotavirus infections occur as epidemics predominantly in the winter months. The earliest outbreaks of each season tend to be in the western states in the fall months, with a wave-like progression across the continent toward the northeast, where the peak incidence of outbreaks is in the late winter and early spring [18].

Clinical features of group A rotavirus gastroenteritis in children

Symptoms	Frequency, %
Diarrhea	98
Diarrhea > 10 × daily	28
Vomiting	87
Vomiting > 5 × daily	51
Fever	84
Abdominal pain	18
Gross blood in stool	1
Hospitalization	39

FIGURE 7-46 Clinical features of group A rotavirus gastroenteritis in children. Rotavirus-induced gastroenteritis in infants and young children most commonly presents with watery diarrhea, fever, vomiting, and occasional dehydration. There is no blood or mucus in the stools; leukocytes may be detected in the feces of a small percentage of patients [19].

Clinical features of rotavirus gastroenteritis in adults

Symptoms	Adults, *n*
Diarrhea	14
Abdominal cramps	11
Vomiting	4
Upper respiratory symptoms	3
Fever	2
Nausea	1

FIGURE 7-47 Clinical features of rotavirus gastroenteritis in adults. Rotaviruses are less commonly a cause of severe diarrhea in adults than in infants and young children. Outbreaks of rotavirus gastroenteritis in adults have been reported in nursing home and hospital settings. Adult contacts of children with symptomatic rotavirus infection usually develop asymptomatic infection and shed rotavirus in their feces. In this prospective family study, of the 11 patients having abdominal cramps, three of these subjects had no diarrhea. The three patients with upper respiratory tract symptoms had no gastrointestinal symptoms [20].

Clinical and epidemiologic features of calicivirus infections

Epidemiology	Epidemics of vomiting and diarrhea in older children and adults
	Occurs in families, communities, nursing homes, cruise ships
	Often associated with shellfish, other food, water
Signs/symptoms	Vomiting, diarrhea, fever, myalgia, headache
	Lasts 24–48 hours
Diagnosis	Immunoassay, immune electron microscopy, rt-PCR

rt-PCR—reverse transcription and polymerase chain reaction genomic amplification.

FIGURE 7-48 Clinical and epidemiologic features of calicivirus infections. This group of viruses is responsible for a large number of previously undiagnosed outbreaks. The diversity and prevalence of these agents is becoming better known with more widespread use of new molecular tools for diagnosis and epidemiologic studies.

PARASITIC ENTERITIS

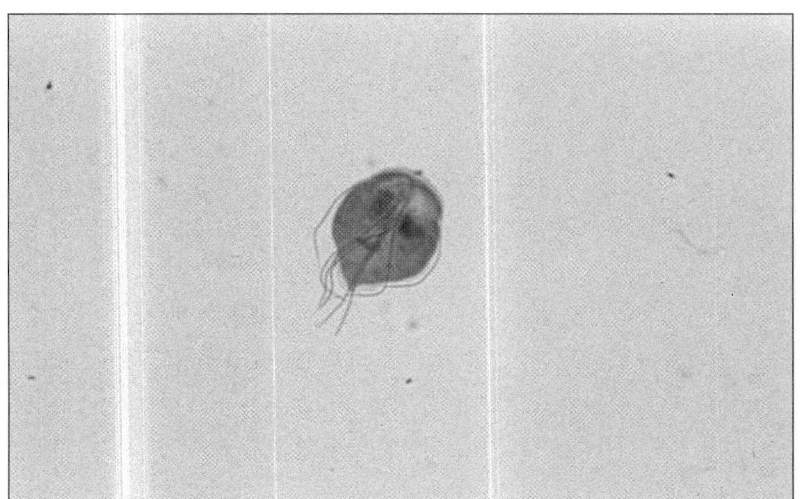

FIGURE 7-49 *Giardia lamblia* trophozoite. Trophozoites are pear-shaped, bilaterally symmetrical bodies and measure 9 to 21 × 5 to 15 μm. Characteristic structures include four pairs of flagella and two nuclei in the area of the sucking disc. Trophozoites move by oscillating about the long axis, producing motion said to resemble a falling leaf. (Giemsa stain.) (*Courtesy of* M. Scaglia, MD.)

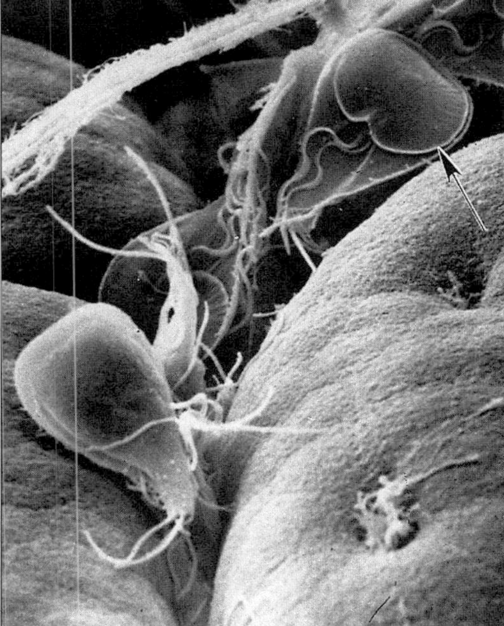

FIGURE 7-50 Scanning electron micrograph of *Giardia lamblia* trophozoites in a crevice over human jejunal villus. On the ventral surface of the organism, note the slightly concave attachment disc (*arrow*). The irregular dorsal surface of the *Giardia* is seen in the organism to the lower left. (× 2000.) (*Courtesy of* R. Owen, MD; *from* Owen, Fogel *et al.* [21]; with permission.)

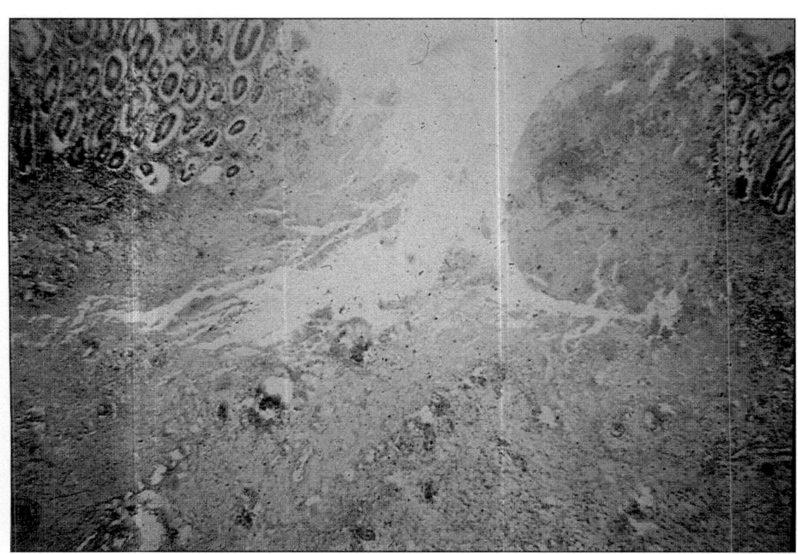

FIGURE 7-51 Colonic biopsy specimen from a patient with amebic dysentery. The specimen shows a flask-shaped ulcer with necrosis and an inflammatory exudate. This pathologic finding indicates amebic invasion into the submucosa. (Periodic acid–Schiff stain.)

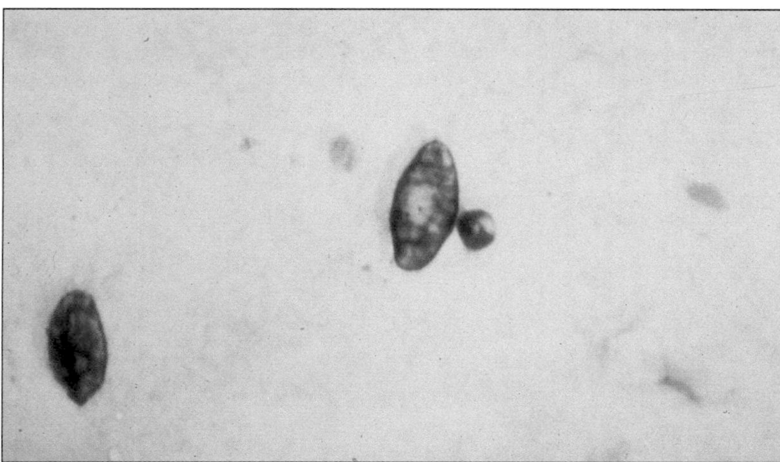

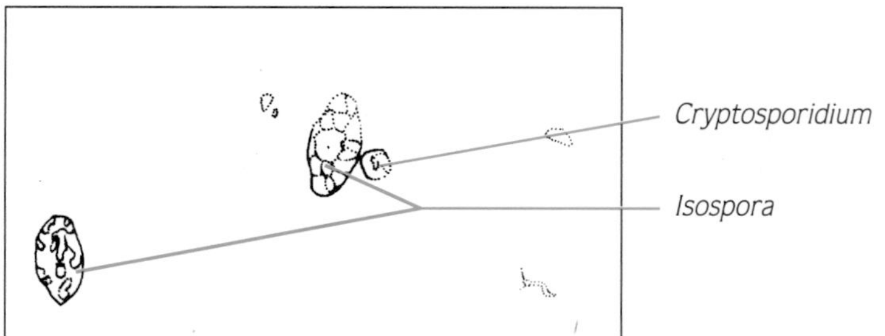

Figure 7-52 Fecal smear from an AIDS patient who was dually infected with *Cryptosporidium* and *Isospora*. (Modified Kinyoun acid-fast stain; × 450.) (*Courtesy of* M. Boncy.)

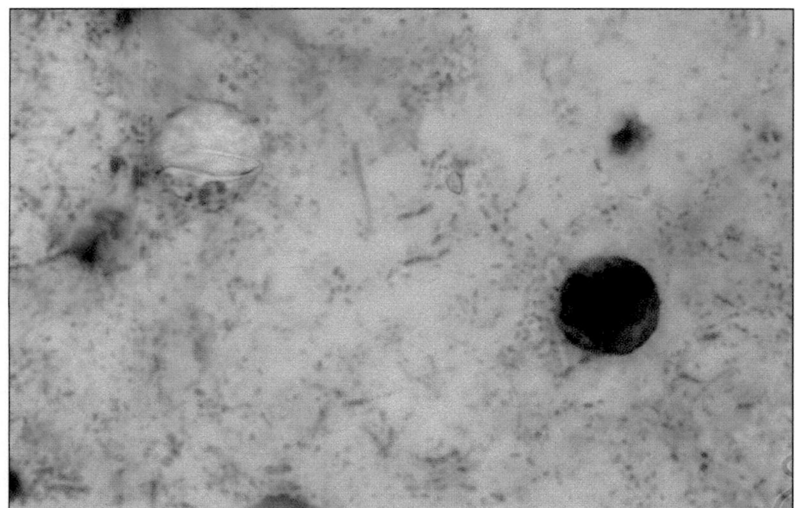

Figure 7-53 Fecal smear showing acid-fast and unstained *Cyclospora* oocysts. Variability in staining is typical for this organism. (Modified Kinyoun stain; × 1000.)

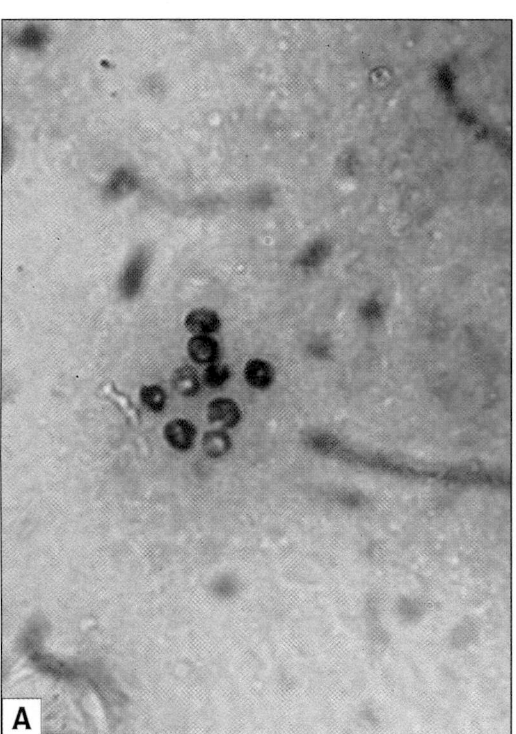

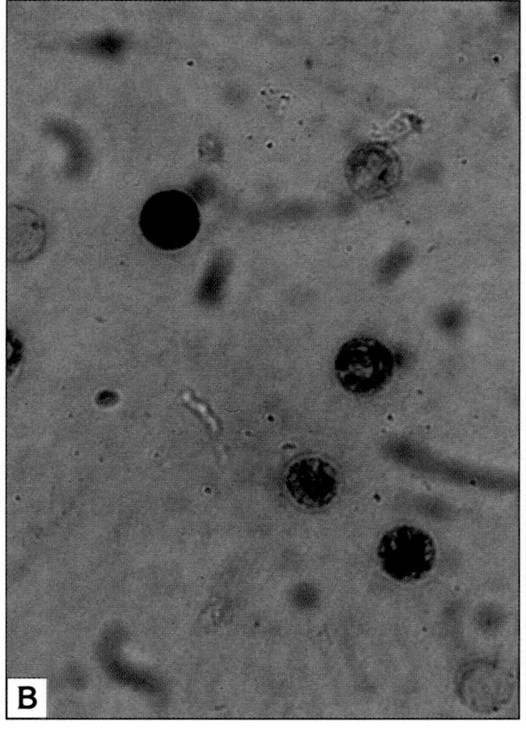

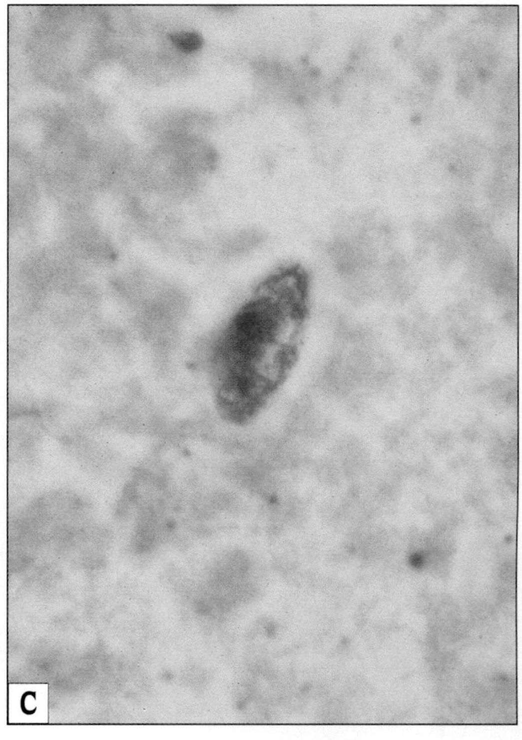

Figure 7-54 Comparative staining patterns of coccidians on fecal smears. **A–C**, *Cryptosporidium* (*panel 54A*), *Cyclospora* (*panel 54B*), and *Isospora* (*panel 54C*) are easily detected with acid-fast–stained smears of fecal specimens. The three organisms can be differentiated by their morphologic features: *Cryptosporidium* are 4 µm, round, and sometimes crescent-shaped; *Cyclospora* are 8 µm and round; *Isospora* are elliptical, 23 to 33 µm long × 10 to 19 µm wide. Enteritis caused by the three organisms is clinically indistinguishable. (Modified Kinyoun stain; × 630.)

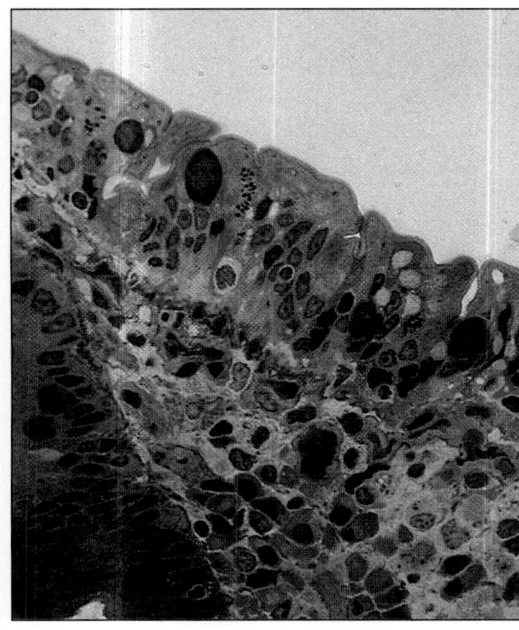

Figure 7-55 Duodenal biopsy specimen from a patient with AIDS, showing lightly stained oval parasites (*Enterocytozoon bieneusi*). Clusters of densely stained spores and intraepi thelial lymphocytes are also apparent. (Methylene blue-azure II, basic fuchsin stain; × 640.) (*From* Orenstein [22]; with permission.)

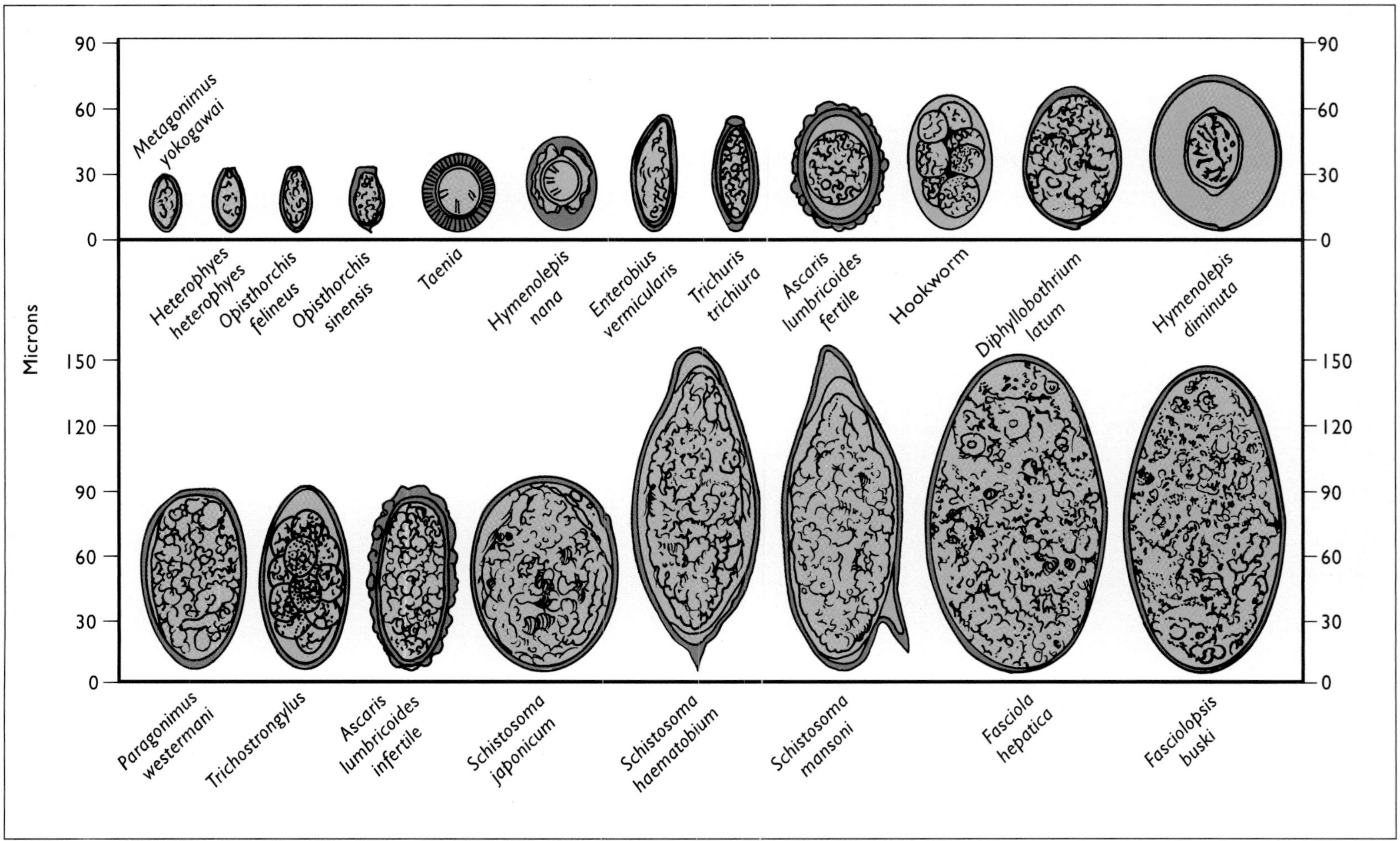

Figure 7-56 Relative sizes of helminth eggs. Diagnosis of helminthic infection most commonly depends on careful examination of stool or urine for eggs [23].

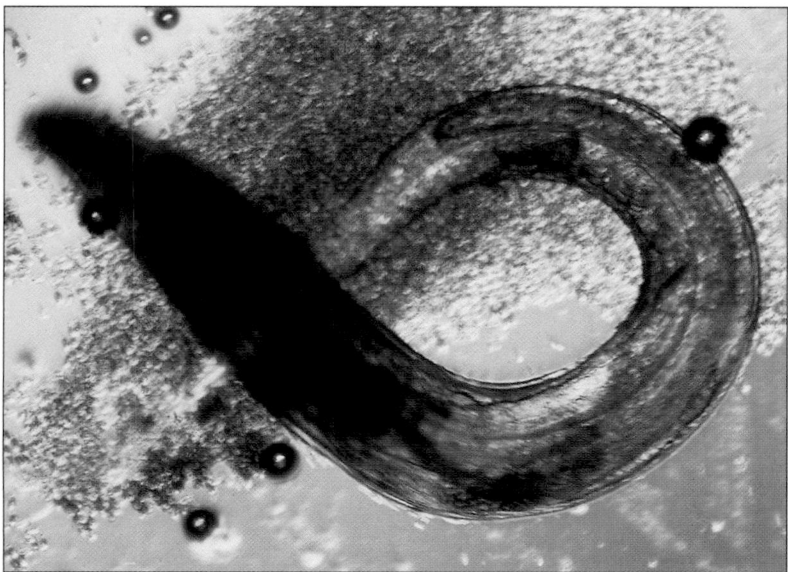

Figure 7-57 Pinworm spewing its eggs. *Enterobius vermicularis* is prevalent throughout the world but occurs more commonly in temperate climates. There are an estimated 42 million cases in the United States. The name is derived from the long, sharply pointed tail of the female worm. Gravid females contain an average of 11,000 ova, which they deposit in the perianal and perineal areas during their nightly migrations. Resultant anal pruritus is the most common symptom of this infection. (*From* the collection of B.H. Kean, MD.)

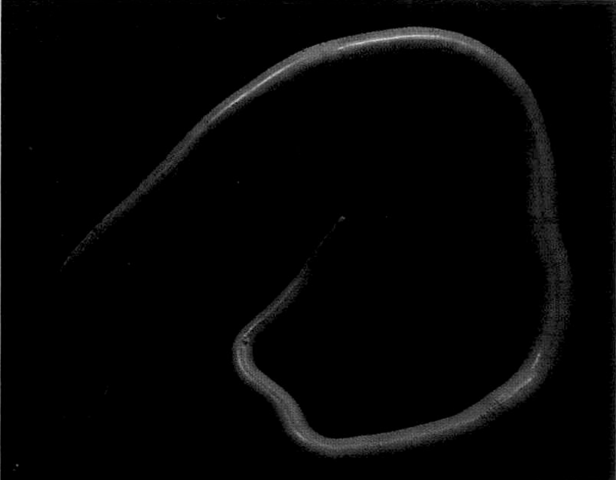

Figure 7-58 Adult *Ascaris lumbricoides* worm. Female worms may be as thick as a pencil and range from 20 to 35 cm in length, whereas males are slender and usually < 30 cm long. Ascariasis is the most common helminthic infection worldwide, with an estimated prevalence of 1 billion. Because virtually 100% of individuals living in areas of inadequate sanitation are infected, and each individual may be carrying hundreds of worms, the worm burden for our planet is staggering. (*From* the collection of B.H. Kean, MD.)

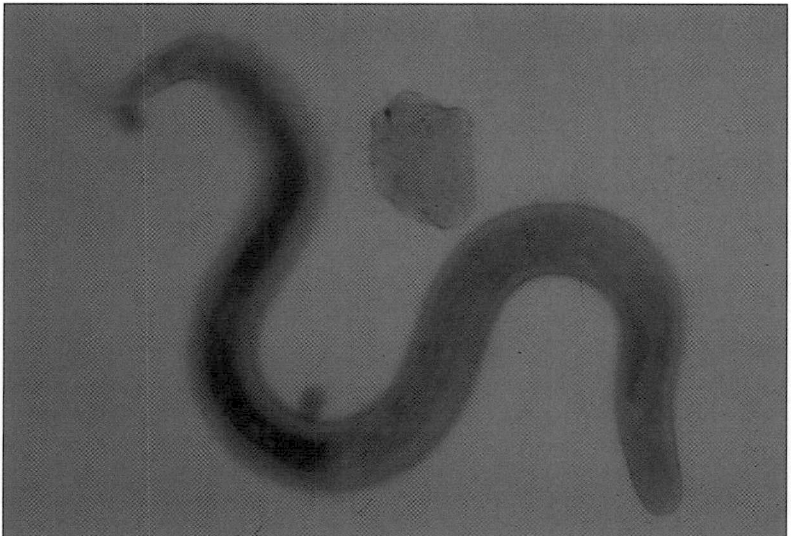

Figure 7-59 *Strongyloides* larva in bronchoalveolar lavage fluid of a bone marrow transplant patient who presented with bilateral pulmonary infiltrates. Autoinfection is probably the mechanism that allows for persistent infection in those individuals from an endemic area. Parasite and host are able to survive without problems until the host is immunosuppressed, at which time the larvae then begin to proliferate and disseminate to multiple organs. Mortality is very high in the hyperinfection syndrome. (Iodine stain.)

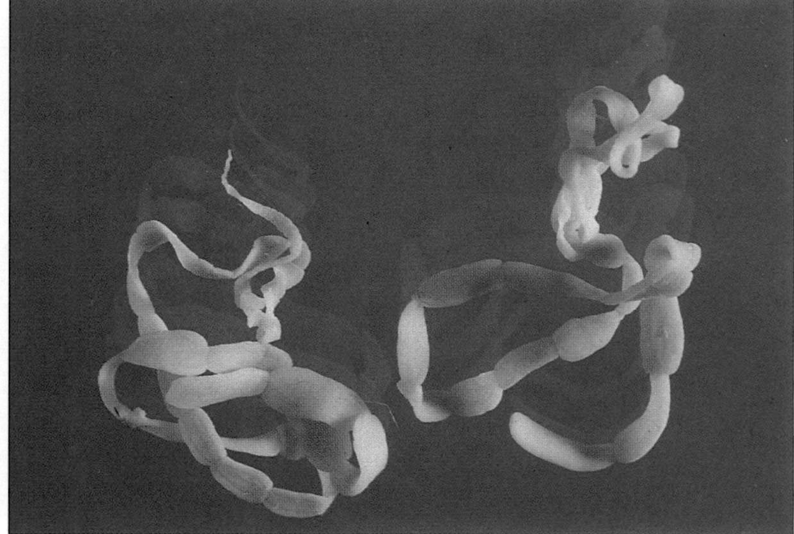

Figure 7-60 *Taenia saginata* proglottids. (*Courtesy of* M. Scaglia, MD.)

FUNGAL ENTERITIS

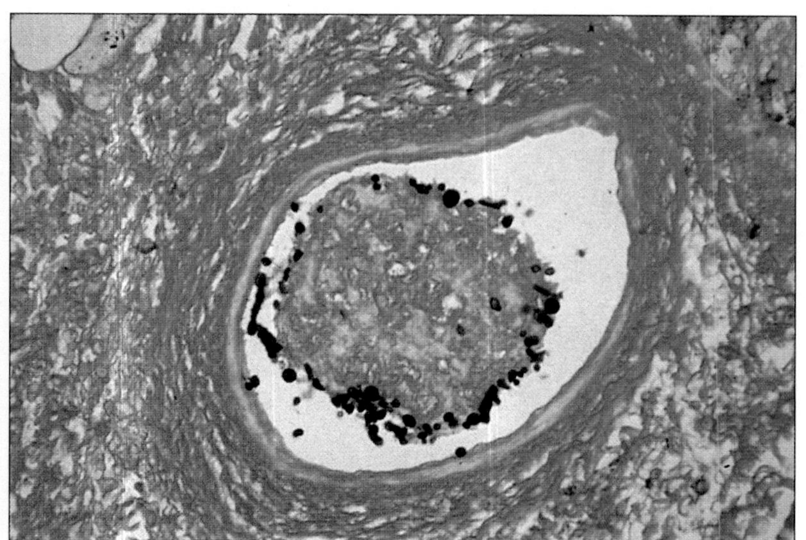

FIGURE 7-61 Mesenteric artery embolus seen in a severely neutropenic patient who had hematogenously disseminated candidiasis involving the liver and spleen. Note the presence of yeast cells and hyphae of candida within the embolus. Candidiasis represents a spectrum of infections caused by *Candida* species. The disease manifestations are protean and range from mucosal and superficial, to acute life threatening, to chronic disease. *Candida albicans* is part of the gastrointestinal flora of humans, and disease caused by this species is usually endogenous in origin. Other candidal species, such as *C. tropicalis, C. parapsilosis, C. lusitania, C. krusei, C. guilliermondii*, and *C. glabrata*, are generally thought to be exogenously acquired. Many factors will determine the development of these protean clinical manifestations and include local, physiological, and iatrogenic ones. Candida blood infections are common in university hospitals and most likely as a result of medical progress. (Gomori methenamine silver stain; × 100.) (Courtesy of M. Rinaldi, PhD.)

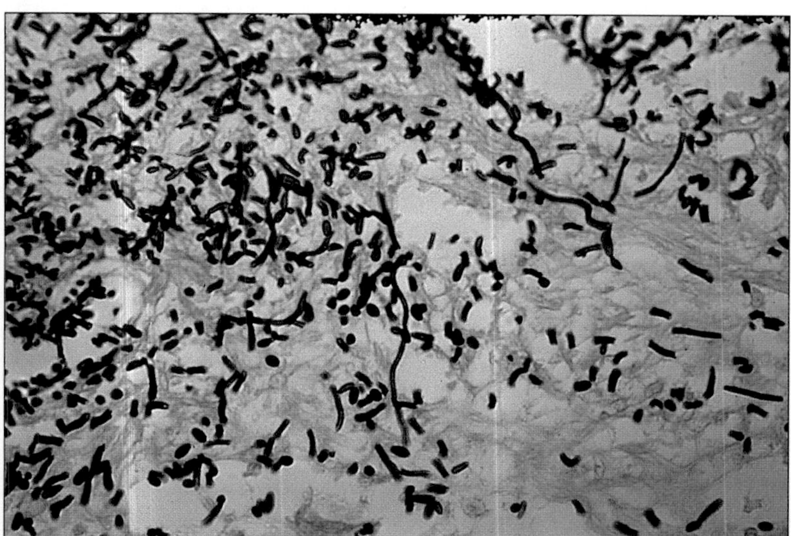

FIGURE 7-62 Gastric tissue section demonstrating disseminated candidiasis. This case of fatal disseminated *Candida* infection occurred in a leukemia patient. The organism is seen in gastric tissue, demonstrating budding yeasts, pseudohyphae of varying lengths, and true hyphae. Most cases of life-threatening candidal infections are seen in the immunosuppressed, and esophageal lesions are a great source of morbidity in patients with AIDS and those undergoing chemotherapy. (Gomori methenamine silver stain; × 400.) (*Courtesy of* M. Rinaldi, PhD.)

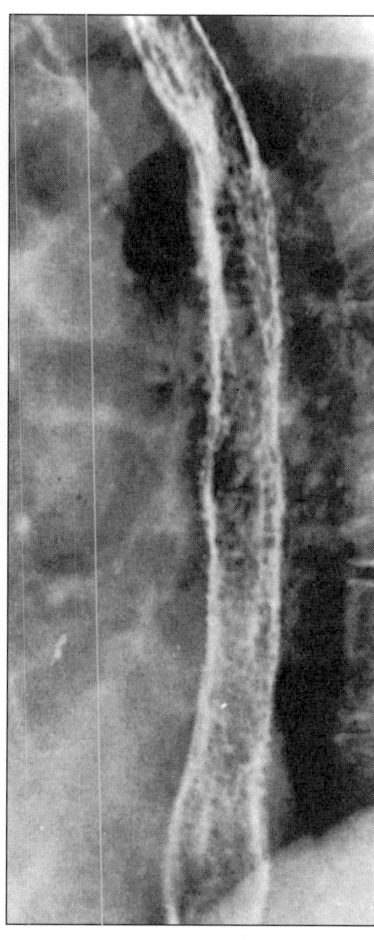

FIGURE 7-63 Barium contrast esophagograms of *Candida* esophagitis. Esophagogram shows a markedly irregular esophagus due to multiple plaques in a patient with AIDS and severe odynophagia. (*From* Polis [24]; with permission.)

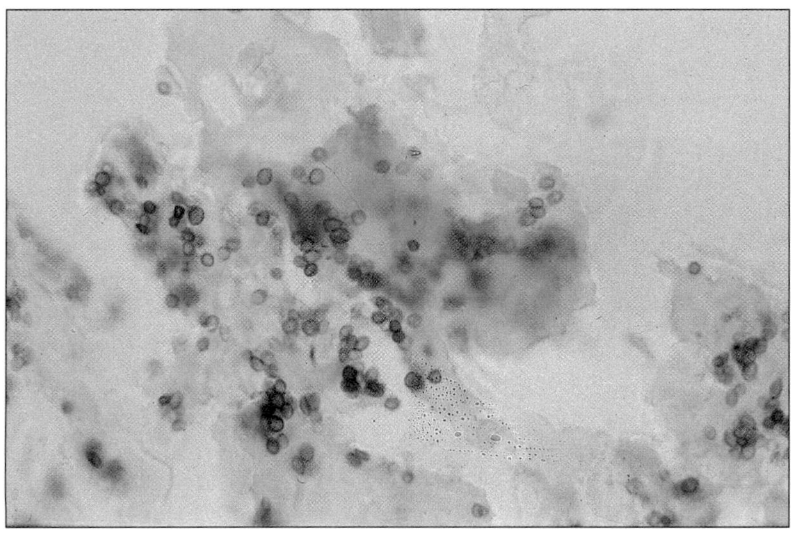

Figure 7-64 Gastric mucosa specimen showing intracellular yeast cells in disseminated histoplasmosis. The specimen is from the autopsy of a patient with AIDS who developed disseminated histoplasmosis. *Histoplasma capulatum* is a mold that lives in soil and accumulates in the presence of feces from blackbirds, chickens, or bats. The organism is acquired by inhalation, and most cases are subclinical, not requiring hospitalization. This is a dimorphic organism, the infective form being the mold phase, and once inhaled, it converts to the yeast phase within the alveolar macrophages. Silver stain readily demonstrating the yeast phase of *Histoplasma* in the gastric mucosa. Note that the cells of *Histoplasma* are relatively uniform in size. (× 1000.) (*Courtesy of* M. Rinaldi, PhD.)

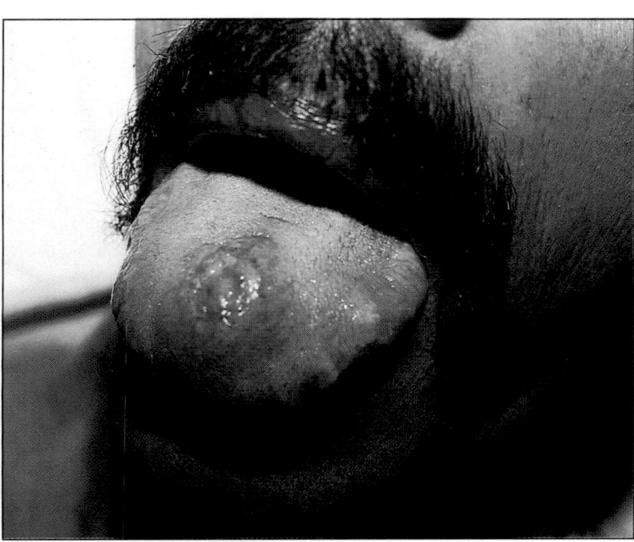

Figure 7-65 Oral ulcer of disseminated histoplasmosis in a patient with AIDS. (*Courtesy of* E.J. Bottone, PhD.)

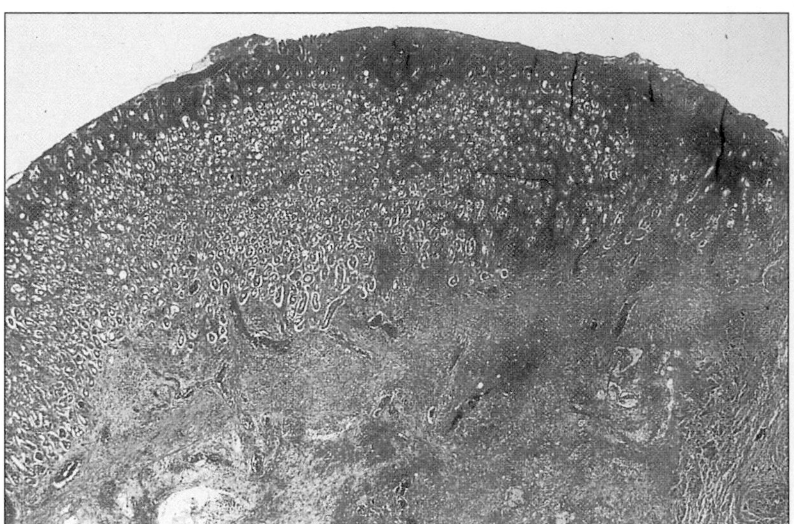

Figure 7-66 Hemorrhagic necrosis of the gastric mucosa in disseminated *Rhizopus* infection. Tissue is usually hemorrhagic in disseminated mucormycosis. This specimen is from an autopsy of a severely immunocompromised patient who died of disseminated disease caused by *Rhizopus*. (Hematoxylin-eosin stain; × 50.) (*Courtesy of* W. Merz, PhD.)

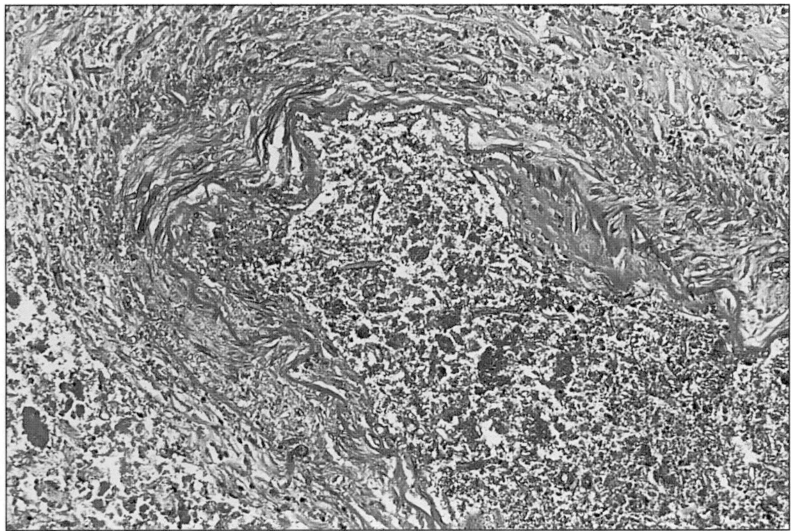

Figure 7-67 Blood vessel invasion in mucormycosis. Pathology is characterized by blood vessel invasions. The hematoxylin-eosin–stained section, from the same case as Figure 7-66, shows blood vessel invasion with thrombosis by fungal elements. (× 200.) (*Courtesy of* W. Merz, PhD.)

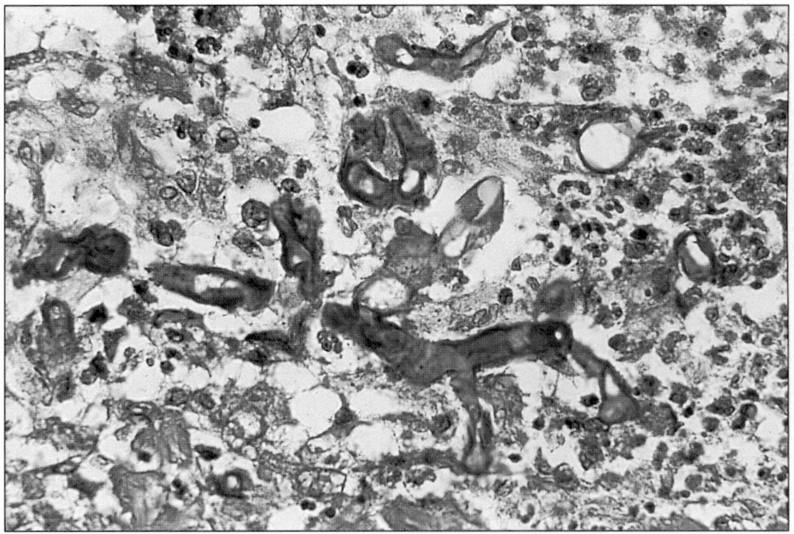

Figure 7-68 Periodic acid–Schiff-staining of a tissue section shows large nonseptate hyphae with 90° angle branching typical of *Rhizopus*. Note the ribbon appearance of the hyphae, which occurs because the hyphae fold when cut. (× 400.) (*Courtesy of* W. Merz, PhD.)

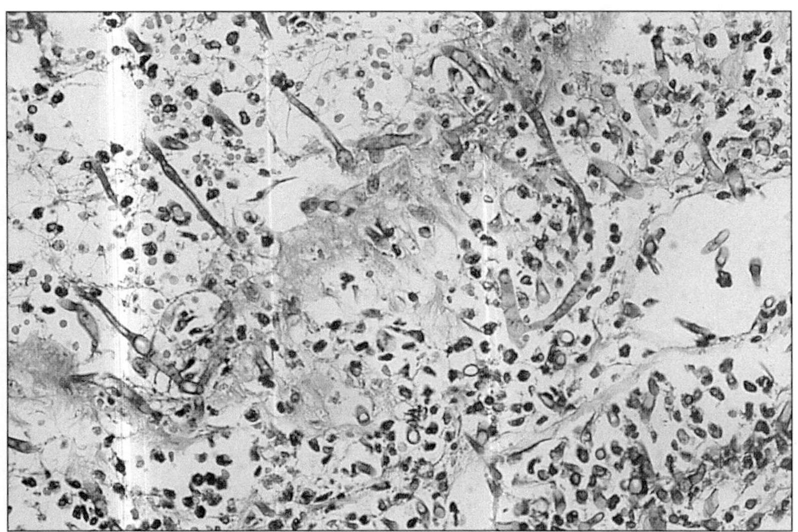

FIGURE 7-69 Tissue section showing *Aspergillus.* The organism in tissue is characterized by having septate hyphae and 45° angle (dichotomous) branching. Note that the organism is within the vessel wall. (Hematoxylin-eosin stain; × 400.)

DIAGNOSTIC IMAGING

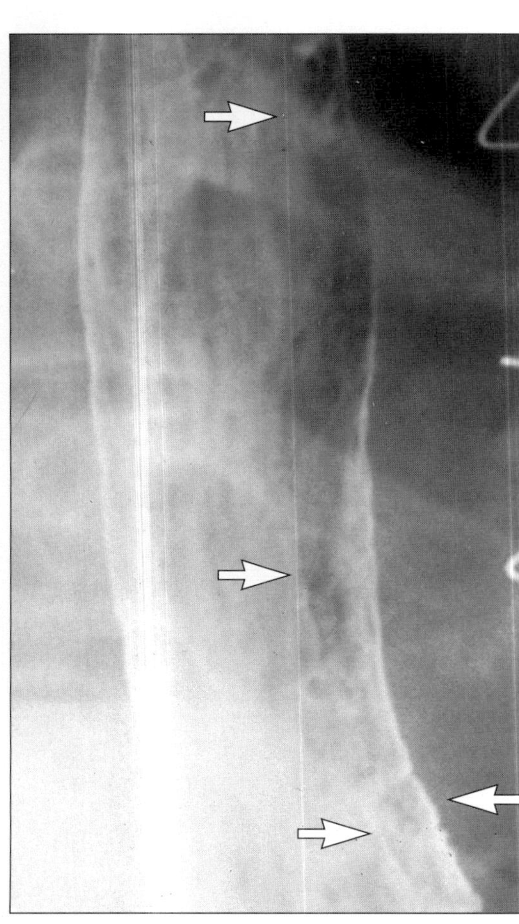

FIGURE 7-70 Herpes simplex esophagitis. A double-contrast esophagogram in a patient following heart transplantation shows multiple shallow ulcers (some of which are linear) in the distal esophagus (*arrows*) with intervening normal mucosa. Biopsies demonstrated herpes virus.

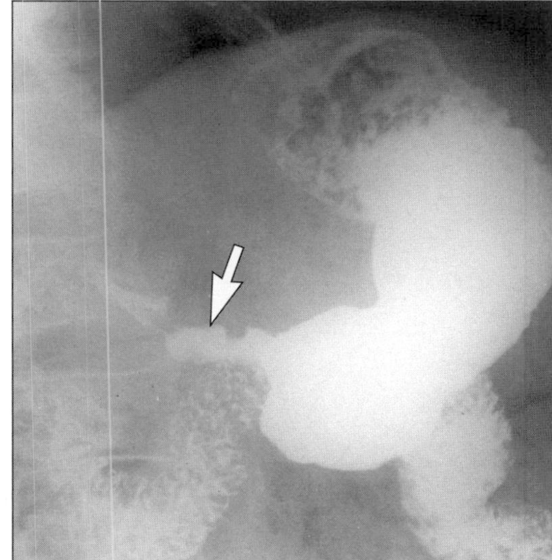

FIGURE 7-71 Antral syphilis. A barium examination of the stomach demonstrates thickening and narrowing (*arrow*) of the antrum. This appearance and location are typical of gastrointestinal involvement by syphilis, now rarely seen.

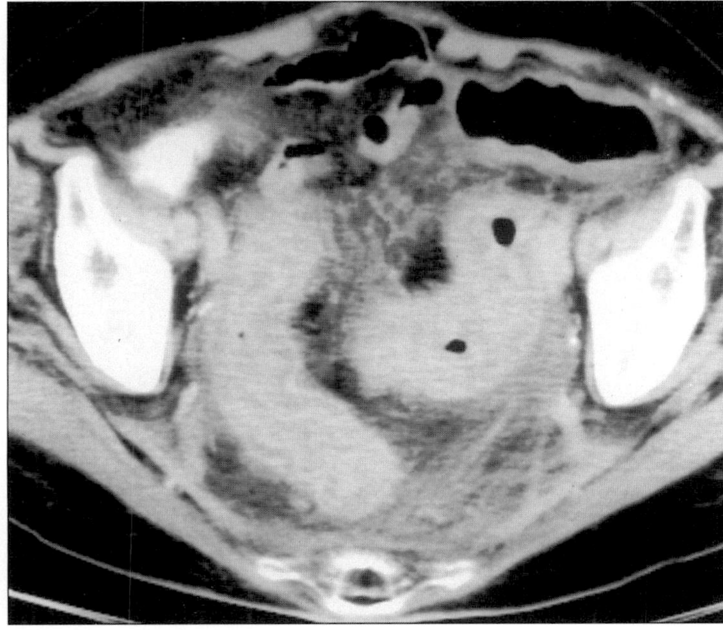

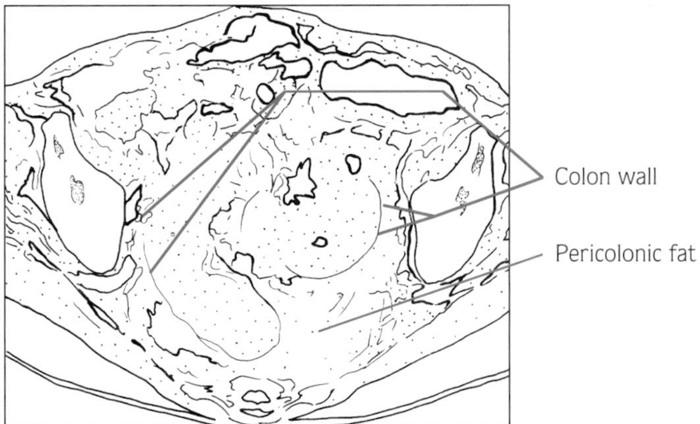

FIGURE 7-72 Pseudomembranous colitis. Computed tomography scan of the abdomen shows marked thickening of the wall of the entire colon. There is evidence of intense inflammation with spiculated increased soft tissue in the pericolonic fat. This presentation is the characteristic appearance of *Clostridium difficle* colitis in a patient who previously had received clindamycin therapy.

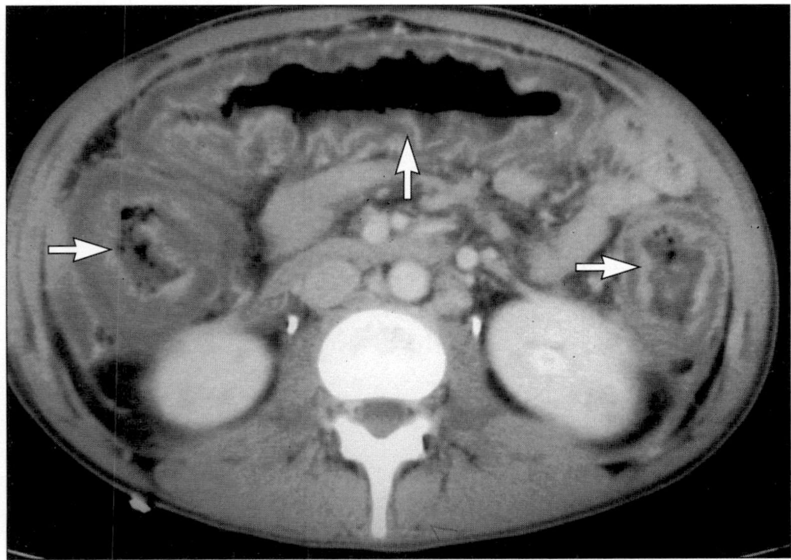

FIGURE 7-73 Cytomegalovirus colitis. A computed tomography scan of the abdomen demonstrates marked thickening of the wall of the entire colon (*arrows*) in a patient with severe diarrhea and AIDS. Biopsy done via colonoscopy demonstrated cytomegalovirus.

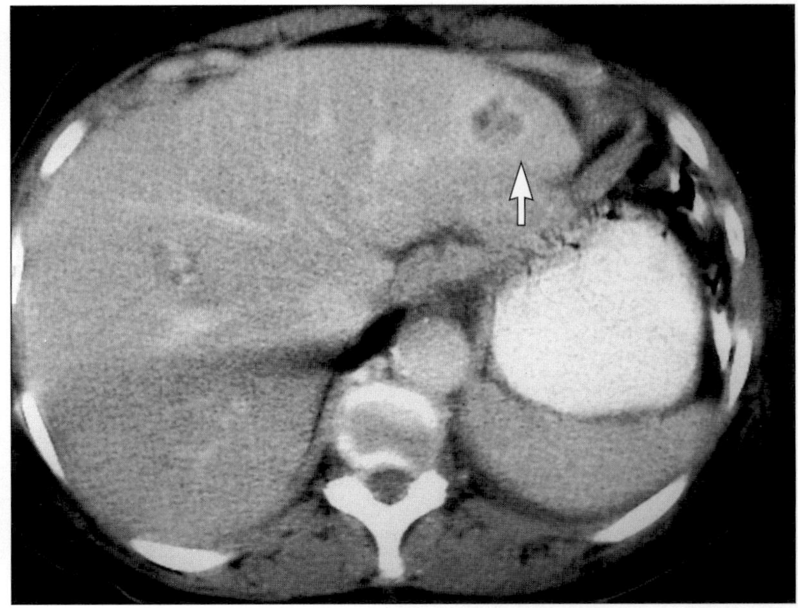

FIGURE 7-74 Hepatic abscess. A computed tomography scan with oral and intravenous contrast material demonstrates a low-density lesion in the left lobe of the liver with an enhancing edge (*arrow*). This lesion proved to be a polymicrobial abscess in this patient with diverticulitis. Enhancement in the periphery of the abscess after intravenous injection of contrast material is a common finding in hepatic abscess, distinguishing it from a simple cyst or hepatic tumor.

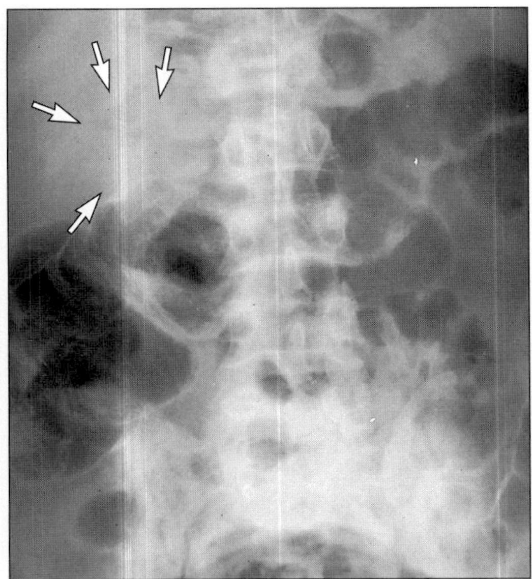

FIGURE 7-75 Emphysematous cholecystitis. Plain film of the abdomen shows a rounded air collection in the right upper quadrant (*arrows*).

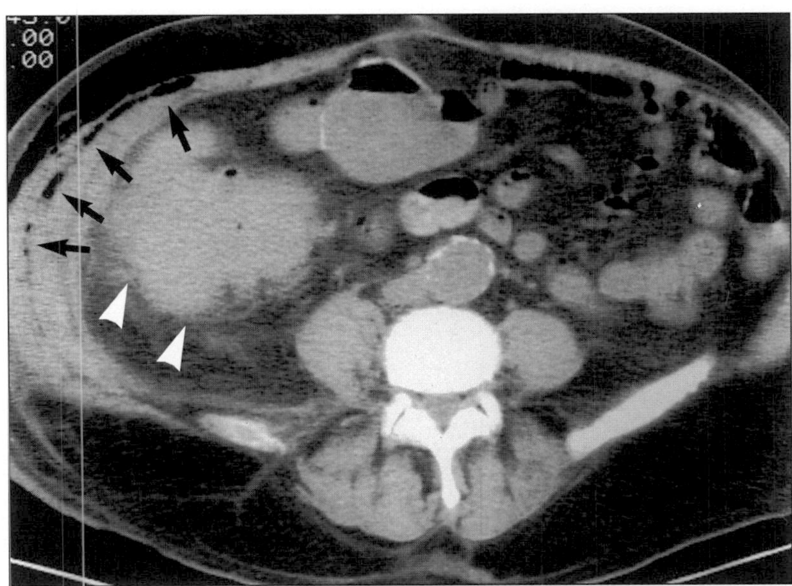

FIGURE 7-76 Necrotizing fasciitis. Computed tomography scan of a patient presenting with extensive edema demonstrates air in the subcutaneous tissues (*arrows*) along the right flank due to necrotizing fasciitis. The scan also demonstrates an unsuspected mass in the right colon (*arrowheads*), which extends into the pericolonic fat; it was found to be a primary adenocarcinoma of the cecum.

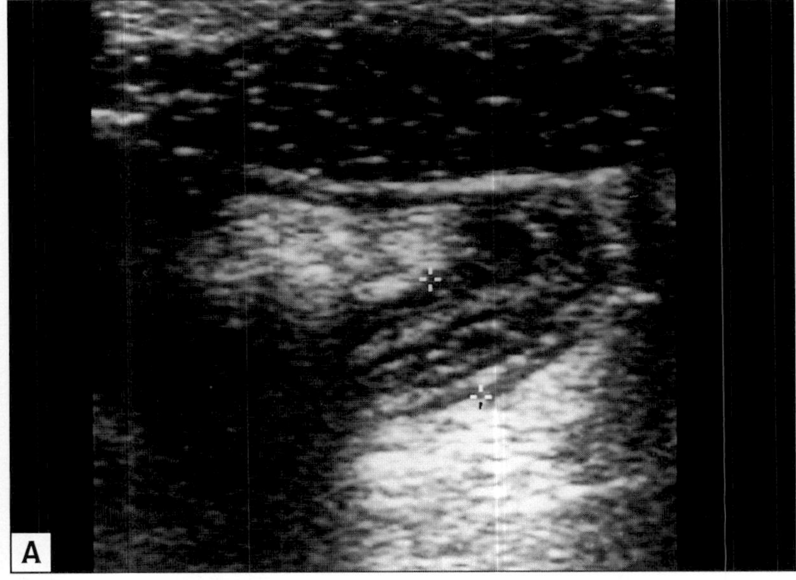

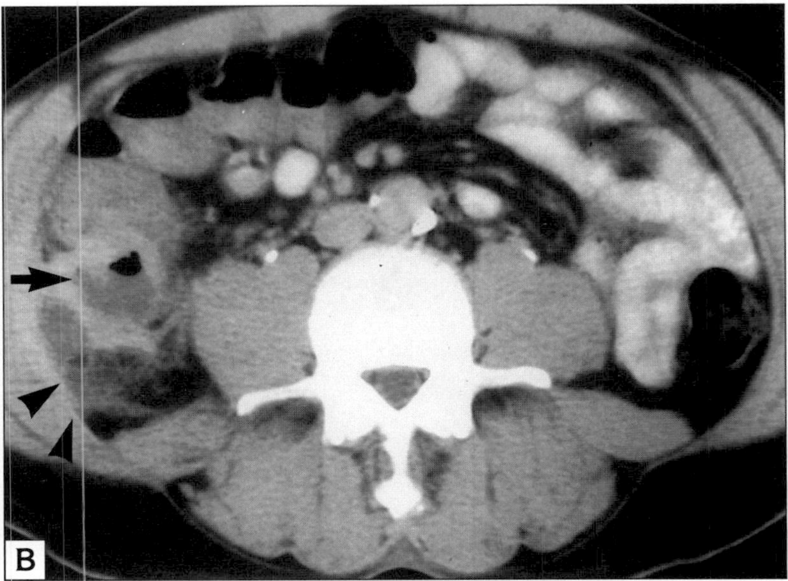

FIGURE 7-77 Appendicitis. Ultrasound of the appendix is accomplished by compressing the rectus muscle against the psoas muscle, entrapping the appendix between them. **A**, An appendiceal diameter > 6 mm is diagnostic of appendicitis. **B**, Computed tomography (CT) scans are equally accurate in the diagnosis. Characteristic findings include spiculation of pericecal fat, appendicolith, and thickening of the appendix (although the appendix is frequently not visible). This CT scan demonstrates spiculation in the pericecal fat (*arrowheads*) with a thick-walled, air–fluid collection (*arrow*), indicating a periappendiceal abscess.

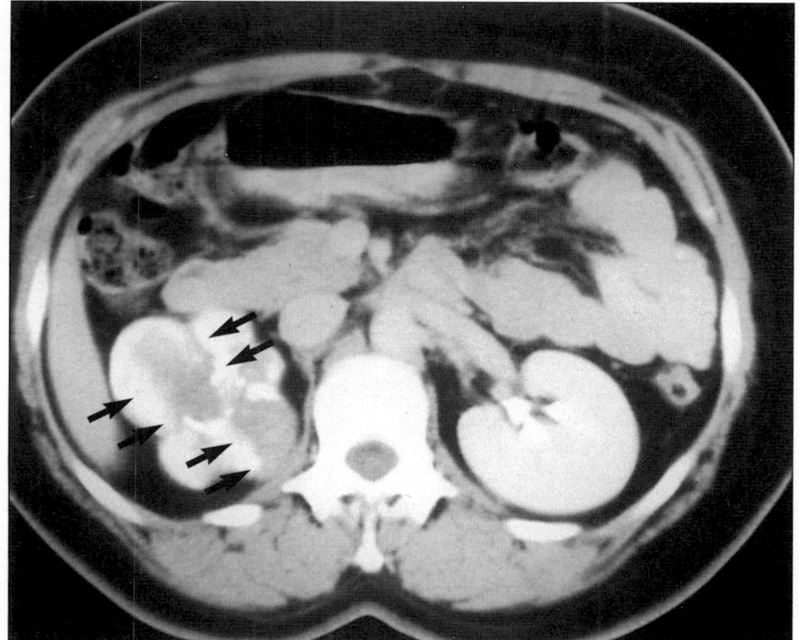

Figure 7-78 Renal abscesses. Computed tomography scan through the kidneys shows two well-defined right renal masses (*arrows*) with thick irregular walls surrounding central areas of diminished density. This appearance is characteristic of renal abscesses.

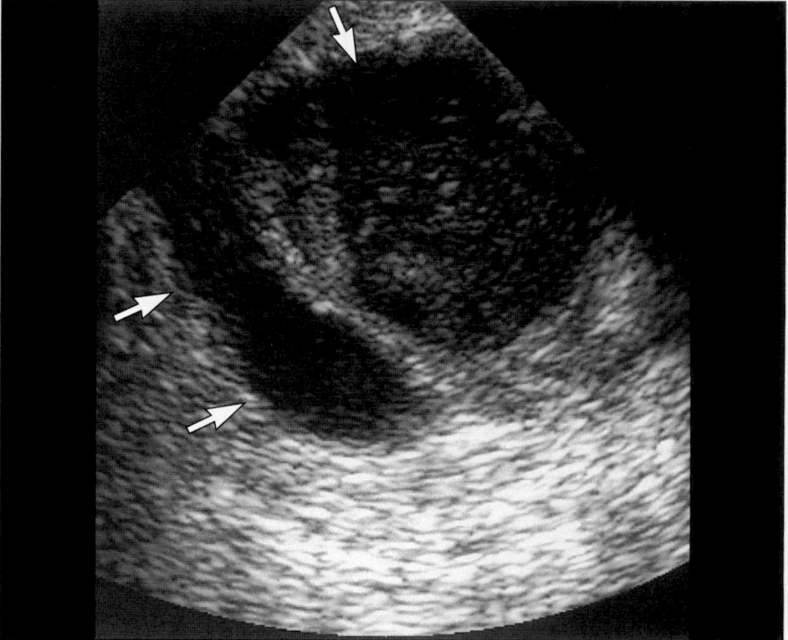

Figure 7-79 Pelvic inflammatory disease and tuboovarian abscess. Transabdominal ultrasound demonstrates dilatation of the fallopian tube (*arrows*) to the level of the ovary, as typically seen in pelvic inflammatory disease.

References

1. Finegold SM, Baron EJ, Wexler HM: *A Clinical Guide to Anerobic Infections.* Princeton Scientific Publishing/Star Publishing Co.; 1992.
2. Finegold SM, Johnson CC: Peritonitis and intraabdominal infections. *In* Blaser MJ, Smith PD, Ravdin JI, *et al.* (eds.): *Infections of the Gastrointestinal Tract.* New York: Raven Press; 1995:369–403.
3. Bennion RS, Thompson JE, Baron EJ, Finegold SM: Gangrenous and perforated appendicitis with peritonitis—treatment and bacteriology. *Clin Ther* 1990, 12:31–44.
4. Keighley MR: Micro-organisms in bile: A preventable cause of sepsis after biliary surgery. *Ann R Coll Surg Engl* 1977, 59:328.
5. Rotstein OD: Peritonitis and intra-abdominal abscesses. *In* Wilmore DW (ed.): *Care of the Surgical Patient*, vol 2, sect IX, ch 8. New York: Scientific American, Inc.: 1989:3–24.
6. Rotstein OD, Simmons RL: Intraabdominal abscesses. *In* Gorbach SL, Bartlett JG, Blacklow NR (eds.): *Infectious Diseases.* Philadelphia: W.B. Saunders; 1992:668.
7. Hsu HH, Feinstone SM, Hoofnagle JH: Acute viral hepatitis. *In* Mandell GL, Bennett JE, Dolin R (eds.): *Principles and Practice of Infectious Diseases*, 4th ed. New York: Churchill Livingstone; 1995:1136–1153.
8. Lemon SM, Brown EA: Hepatitis C virus. *In* Mandell GL, Bennett JE, Dolin R (eds.): *Principles and Practice of Infectious Diseases*, 4th ed. New York: Churchill Livingstone; 1995:1474–1486.
9. Ueda N, Shah SV: Apoptosis. *J Lab Clin Med* 1994, 124:169–177.
10. Poulsen H, Christofferson P: Abnormal bile duct epithelium in chronic aggressive hepatitis and cirrhosis. *Hum Pathol* 1972, 3:217–225.
11. Guerrant RL: Lessons from diarrheal diseases: Demography to molecular pharmacology. *J Infect Dis* 1994, 169:1206–1218.
12. Guerrant RL: Principles and syndromes of enteric infection. *In* Mandell GL, Bennett JE, Dolin R (eds.): *Principles and Practice of Infectious Diseases*, 4th ed. New York: Churchill Livingstone; 1995:945–962.
13. Guerrant RL, Bobak DA: Bacterial and protozoal gastroenteritis. *N Engl J Med* 1991, 325:327–340.
14. Guerrant RL, Bobak DA: Nausea, vomiting, and noninflammatory diarrhea. *In* Mandell GL, Bennett JE, Dolin R (eds.): *Principles and Practice of Infectious Diseases*, 4th ed. New York: Churchill Livingstone; 1995:965–978.
15. DuPont HL: Traveler's diarrhea. *In* Blaser MJ, Ravdin JI, Smith PD, *et al.* (eds.): *Infections of the Gastrointestinal Tract.* New York: Raven Press; 1995:302.
16. Graham DY: *An Update on Helicobacter pylori* [AGA educational slide/lecture program]. Alexandria, VA: American College of Gastroenterology; 1996.
17. Kapikiam AZ: Acute viral gastroenteritis. *Prev Med* 1974, 3:535–542.
18. LeBaron CW, Lew J, Glass RI, *et al.*: Annual rotavirus epidemic patterns in North America: Results of a 5-year retrospective survey of 88 centers in Canada, Mexico, and the United States. Rotavirus Study Group. *JAMA* 1990, 264:983.
19. Uhnoo I, Olding SE, Kreuger A: Clinical features of acute gastroenteritis associated with rotavirus, enteric adenoviruses, and bacteria. *Arch Dis Child* 1986, 61:732–738.
20. Wenman WM, Hinde D, Feltham S, Gurwith M: Rotavirus infection in adults: Results of a prospective family study. *N Engl J Med* 1979, 301:303–306.
21. Owen R, Fogel R, *et al.*: Girardiasis and traveler's diarrhea [clinical conference]. *Gastroenterology* 1980, 78:1602–1614.
22. Orenstein JM, Tenner M, Cali A, Kotler DP: A microsporidian previously undescribed in humans, infecting enterocytes and macrophages, and associated with diarrhea in an acquired immunodeficiency syndrome patient. *Hum Pathol* 1990, 21:475–481.
23. Brooke MM, Melvin DM: Morphology and Diagnostic Stages of Intestinal Parasites of Man. Atlanta: Centers for Disease Control and Prevention; 1972. [DHEW publication no. (PHS) 72-H116.]
24. Polis M: Esophagitis. *In* Mandell GL, Bennett JE, Dolin R (eds.): *Principles and Practice of Infectious Diseases*, 4th ed. New York: Churchill Livingstone; 1995:962–965.
25. Kapikian AZ, Wyatt RG, Dolin R, *et al.*: Visualization by immune electron microscopy of a 27-nm particle associated with acute infectious nonbacterial gastroenteritis. *J Virol* 1972, 10:1075–1081.

Chapter 8

External Manifestations of Systemic Infections

Editor

Robert Fekety

Contributors

Donald Armstrong
Neil Barg
Bruce H. Clements
Adnan S. Dajani
J. Stephen Dumler
Janine Evans
Thomas G. Evans
Patricia Ferrieri
Janet R. Gilsdorf
Barney Graham
Clark Gregg
David Gregory
Carol A. Kauffman
Philip E. LeBoit
Stephen Malawista
Steven M. Opal
Richard D. Pearson
David H. Persing
C.J. Peters
David A. Relman
P.E. Rollin
W. Michael Scheld
David M. Scollard
Thomas Shope
Anastacio de Q. Sousa
S.R. Zaki
Stephen H. Zinner

Viral Exanthems of Childhood

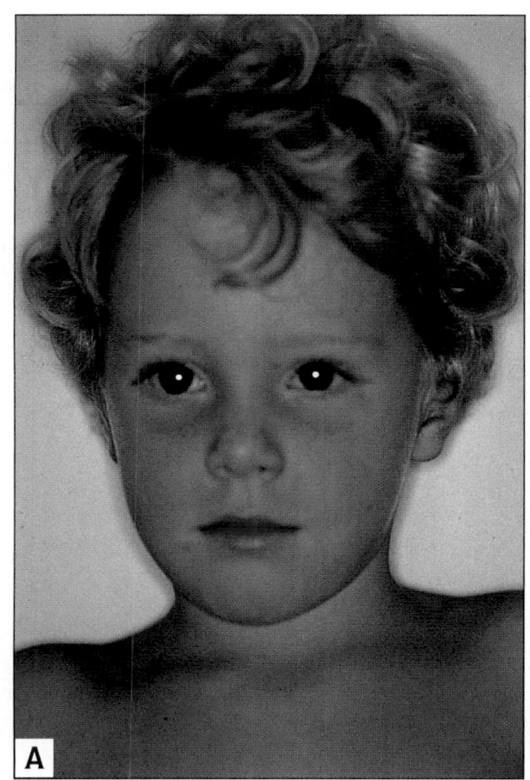

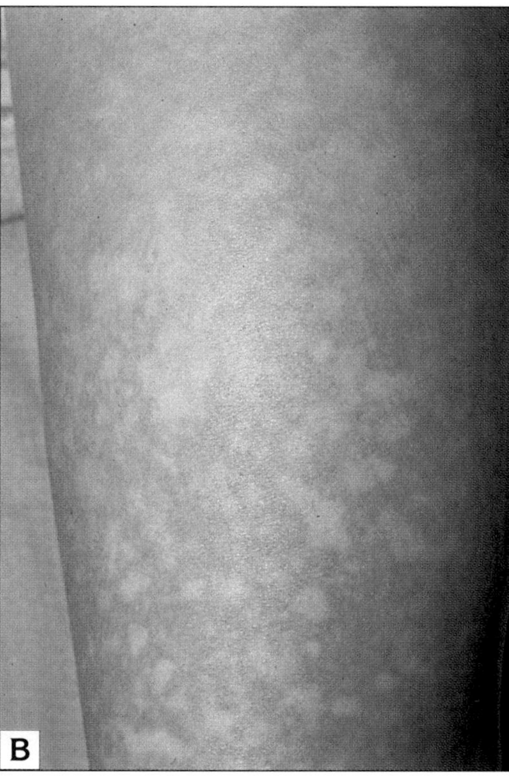

Figure 8-1 Cutaneous rash of erythema infectiosum. **A**, The initial cutaneous manifestation of erythema infectiosum, which occurs during the recovery phase of the infection and is thought to be immunologically mediated, is a malar flush, giving the characteristic appearance of "slapped cheeks" and circumoral pallor. **B**, The macular erythematous rash then spreads to the arms, trunk, and extremities, where it may fade with a reticulated or lacy pattern.

Clinical features of erythema infectiosum (fifth disease)

Etiology	Parvovirus B19
Incubation period	4–14 days
Epidemiology	Outbreaks in elementary and junior high schools Household spread common
Nature of rash	Symmetric, intensely red, flushed "slapped cheeks" appearance, with caudal spread to arms, trunk, buttocks, and thighs, often in a reticular pattern Macular erythemic rash may be intermittent, recurring over several months Rash may fluctuate in intensity depending on environmental conditions, such as temperature, sun exposure, exercise, and stress
Other signs and symptoms	Low-grade fever in 15%–30% of patients Prodrome of mild headache and URI symptoms Arthritis and arthralgias, more common in adult women Infection during early pregnancy may result in fetal hydrops and death
Laboratory findings	Aplastic crisis in patients with high red cell turnover Elevated parvovirus-specific IgM antibody during illness

URI—upper respiratory infection.

Figure 8-2 Clinical features of erythema infectiosum. Erythema infectiosum (fifth disease) is caused by the DNA-containing parvovirus B19, which infects primarily erythroid precursors. Although principally an infection of school-aged children, the virus may cause illness in people of all ages, from fetuses to the elderly.

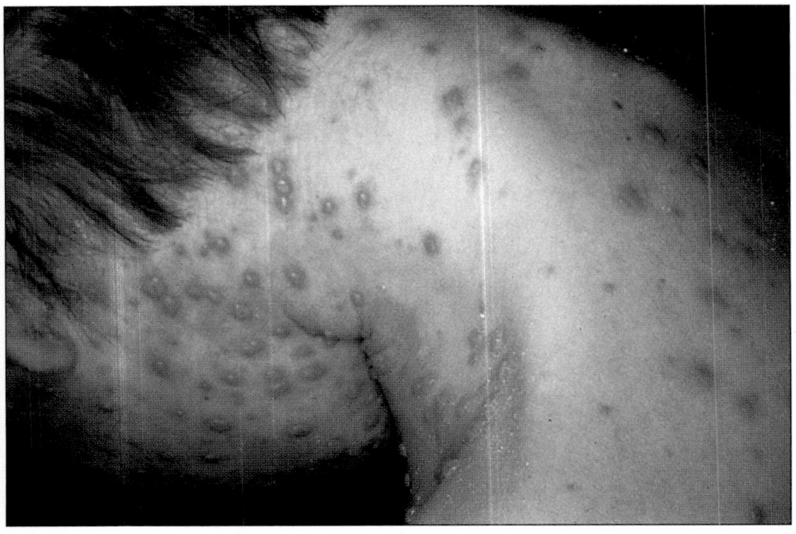

FIGURE 8-3 Vesicular lesions of chickenpox. Chickenpox results from a patient's first infection with the varicella-zoster virus. The characteristic vesicular lesions on an erythematous base, resembling a dew drop on a rose petal, develop around the hair line and on the face.

Clinical features of chickenpox

Etiology	VZV (Herpesviridae)
Incubation period	Usually 14–15 days from exposure to appearance of vesicles (range, 10–20 days)
Epidemiology	Annual epidemics occur from fall to spring Preschool and school-aged children most often infected Transmission by close contact
Nature of eruption	Vesicular lesions on erythematous base, progressing to pustular, then crusting over at 3–5 days
Other signs and symptoms	Enanthem on palate and nasopharynx of most children during the first days of rash Mild fever in early phase of illness Malaise, pruritus, anorexia, listlessness
Laboratory findings	Culture of vesicular fluid yields virus VZV-specific IgM antibody in single serum specimen or ≥ 4-fold rise in antibody titer on two serum specimens Direct fluorescent antibody staining of scrapings from vesicular lesions

VZV—varicella-zoster virus.

FIGURE 8-4 Clinical features of chickenpox. The varicella-zoster virus is a DNA virus belonging to the Herpesviridae family. The illness is contagious over several days preceding the rash, so the actual moment of exposure is seldom known. Chickenpox occurs in annual epidemics, often beginning in the fall and extending through to the next spring. Preschool and school-aged children are usually infected, with 3 to 4 million cases occurring each year. Infection is associated with close contact, with exposure over 20 to 30 minutes being most efficient. Secondary attack rates within classrooms approximate 20%, but within households it is 70% to 90%. With the introduction of vaccine, the epidemiology will change, but illness will continue to affect those who remain susceptible.

Therapy and prevention of varicella

Acyclovir	Approved for use in management of chickenpox and herpes zoster in normal and immunocompromised patients
Varicella-zoster immune globulin	May prevent or alleviate chickenpox in exposed susceptible person if given within 72 hours of exposure
Varicella vaccine	Recommended for routine use in all healthy children who are susceptible and who are > 1 year of age Infants and children < 13 years of age require a single dose; those ≥ 13 require two doses separated by at least 1 month

FIGURE 8-5 Therapy and prevention of varicella. Acyclovir, a guanine derivative, is activated through phosphorylation by the virus-specified thymidine kinase and selectively inhibits the viral DNA polymerase. Varicella zoster immune globulin (VZIG) is derived from individuals recovering from zoster. Candidates for VZIG include certain susceptible immunocompromised individuals under age 15 years, susceptible women in pregnancy, and neonates exposed within 5 days before delivery or 48 hours postpartum. Varicella vaccine, licensed in March 1995, is now recommended as routine for all healthy children who are susceptible to chickenpox and who are past their first birthday.

Clinical features of childhood herpes simplex

Etiology	HSV (Herpesviridae) types 1 and 2
Epidemiology	Childhood, usually HSV-1 with oropharyngeal entry Adolescence and early adulthood: usually HSV-2 with sexual transmission Neonatal infection: usually acquired during delivery, predominantly HSV-2
Nature of eruption	Clear fluid-filled vesicles, with a narrow base of erythema, appear in clusters Vesicles progress to cloudy, then umbilicated, then crusted lesions Lasts 7–10 days
Other signs and symptoms	Vary widely, may show visceral involvement
Laboratory findings	Vesicular fluid and nasopharangeal secretions yield virus on culture Viral antigens demonstrated by direct fluorescent antibody staining of vesicle scrapings or enzyme immunoassay detection in vesicular fluid

HSV—herpes simplex virus.

FIGURE 8-6 Clinical features of childhood herpes simplex. Herpes simplex virus (HSV) is a DNA virus belonging to the Herpesviridae family. HSV type 1 is the most frequent cause of infection during childhood, usually by way of an oropharyngeal portal of entry. Type 2 is the most frequent cause of infection during adolescence and early adulthood, usually by way of anal/genital contact. Neonatal infection is most frequently acquired during delivery and therefore predominantly HSV type 2, although type 1 causes 10% to 20% of the infections. Illness may begin within hours of birth but generally appears 5 to 10 days after birth. Early symptoms are variable and include respiratory distress syndrome, sepsis syndrome, and convulsions. Only two thirds of neonatal herpes infections involve the skin, and only one third present with skin lesions as the initial indication of infection.

Clinical variants of cytomegalovirus infection in infants and children

Congenital	Potential for serious illness with chronic sequelae, including isolated microcephaly with mental retardation and other learning impairment
Perinatal	Often benign illness, occasionally with subtle long-term sequelae Potential for recrudescent illness
Acquired	
Normal host	Often benign illness, may present as mononucleosis syndrome, but most cases are asymptomatic Potential for serious illness with chronic active disease
Immunocompromised host	Particularly problematic in HIV-infected, transplant, and cancer chemotherapy populations
Recrudescent illness	Replication and illness occurs with change in host immune responsiveness

FIGURE 8-7 Clinical variants of cytomegalovirus infection in infants and children. Infection in normal individuals is followed by recovery, but the virus remains sequestered in latent form. Occasionally, especially when the individual's immune response is compromised, the latent genomes reactivate, virus replicates, and new episodes of illness (recrudescence) occur. This illness may take the form of interstitial pneumonitis, hepatitis, chronic gastroenteritis, retinitis, or central nervous system disease.

Clinical spectrum of infection with coxsackieviruses and echoviruses*

	Coxsackievirus group A	Coxsackievirus group B	Echovirus
Illness associated with many enteroviruses			
Asymptomatic infection	+	+	+
Febrile illness with or without respiratory symptoms	+	+	+
Aseptic meningitis	1–11, 14, 16–18, 22, 24	1–6	All except 24, 26, 29, 32
Encephalitis	2, 5, 6, 7, 9	1–3, 5, 6	2–4, 6, 7, 9, 11, 14, 17–19, 25
Paralysis	4, 6, 7, 9, 11, 14, 21	1–6	1–4, 6, 7, 9, 11, 14, 16, 18, 19, 30
Illness more characteristic of particular groups or serotypes			
Herpangina	2–6, 8, 10, 22		
Exanthem	2, 4, 5, 9, 16	1, 3–5	Especially 9, 16; also 1–8, 11, 14, 18, 19, 25, 30, 32, 33
Hand, foot, mouth syndrome	5, 7, 9, 10, 16		
Pleurodynia		1–5	
Lymphonodular pharyngitis	10		
Pericarditis		1–5	
Myocarditis		1–5	
Generalized disease of newborns		1–5	4, 6, 7, 9, 11, 12, 14, 19, 21, 51
Epidemic conjunctivitis	24		
Neonatal diarrhea			11, 14, 18
Chronic meningoencephalitis (in agammaglobulinemics)			2, 3, 5, 9, 11, 19, 24, 25, 30, 33
Etiologic role undefined			
Diarrhea	+	+	+
Hemolytic-uremic syndrome	4	2, 4	22
Myositis	9	2, 6	9, 11
Guillain-Barré syndrome	2, 5, 9		6, 22
Reye syndrome	+	+	
Mononucleosis-like syndrome	5, 6	5	+
Infectious lymphocytosis	+		25
Diabetes mellitus		+	

*Implicated serotypes are listed.

+—serotype not specified.

FIGURE 8-8 Clinical spectrum of infection with coxsackieviruses and echoviruses. The enteroviruses are capable of causing a vast array of clinically different illnesses. This figure lists the viruses more commonly associated with specific enteroviral infections. (*Adapted from* Modlin [1]; with permission.)

Clinical features of infectious mononucleosis syndrome	
Etiology	Heterophile-positive: EBV Heterophile-negative: EBV (especially in young children); also cytomegalovirus, toxoplasmosis, viral hepatitis, rubella, streptococcal pharyngitis, HIV-1
Incubation period	4–5 wks for EBV-induced illness
Epidemiology	EBV infection occurs in ~ 50% of individuals by age 5 years, with a second wave during adolescence and early adulthood Peak incidence of infectious mononucleosis is in people 15–24 year of age
Nature of eruption	Eruption in absence of ampicillin is rare Rash usually appears on all parts of body within 24 hrs after antibiotic, disappears over subsequent days when drug is stopped
Other signs and symptoms	None
Laboratory findings	None

EBV—Epstein-Barr virus.

Figure 8-9 Clinical features of infectious mononucleosis syndrome. The eruption rarely occurs in the absence of ampicillin, and the usual onset occurs in association with administration of the antibiotic, usually within the initial 24 hours but occasionally delayed (even sometimes after antibiotic has been stopped). The rash is thought to be secondary to breakdown of ampicillin to toxic subproducts. There are no associated signs and symptoms that accompany the rash, and erythema recedes over a short time.

Infective Endocarditis

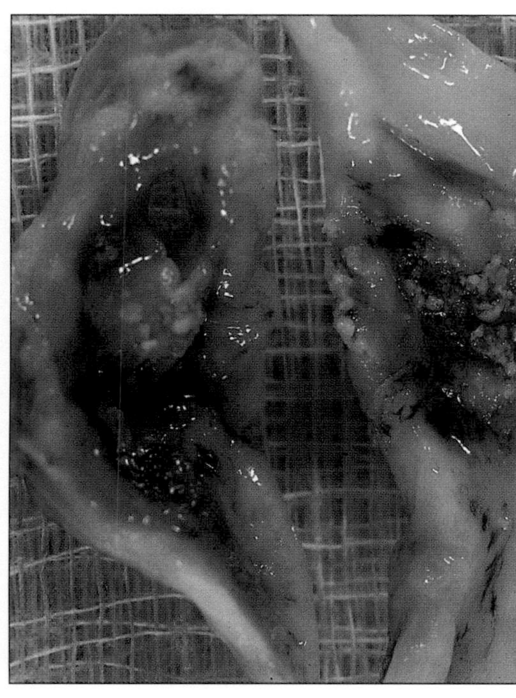

Figure 8-10 Gross specimen from a patient with *Staphylococcus aureus* endocarditis. The patient, a man aged 63 years, developed an acute syndrome characterized by fever, rigors, myalgias, and the rapid onset of shortness of breath. *S. aureus* was isolated from multiple blood cultures, and pulmonary edema was evident on the chest radiograph. At surgery, a bicuspid aortic valve was resected with multiple vegetations. Perforation of this bicuspid valve also is evident, resulting in severe and acute congestive heart failure.

Etiologic agents in infective endocarditis

	Cases, %
Streptococci	60–80
Viridans streptococci	30–40
Enterococci	5–18
Other streptococci	15–25
Staphylococci	20–35
Coagulase-positive	10–27
Coagulase-negative	1–3
Gram-negative aerobic bacilli	1.5–13
Fungi	2–4
Miscellaneous bacteria	< 5
Mixed infections	1–2
"Culture negative"	< 5–24

Figure 8-11 Etiologic agents in infective endocarditis. Gram-positive cocci are the major etiologic agents isolated from cases of infective endocarditis. Streptococci account for 60% to 80% of cases in multiple series. Viridans streptococci remain important. Enterococci, including *E. faecalis* and *E. faecium*, are responsible for 5% to 18% of cases. *Staphylococcus aureus* accounts for 10% to 27% of infective endocarditis on native valves and is a major cause in intravenous drug users. *Staphylococcus epidermidis* is the major cause of prosthetic valve endocarditis but is isolated rarely in native valve disease. A wide variety of gram-negative aerobic bacilli have been isolated. Members of the HACEK group have been recognized with increasing frequency and include organisms belonging to the genera *Haemophilus, Actinobacillus, Cardiobacterium, Eikenella*, and *Kingella*. Miscellaneous bacteria, rarely implicated in endocarditis in the present era, include gram-negative cocci, gram-positive bacilli, anaerobic organisms, and multiple other agents. Fungal endocarditis usually is seen in narcotic addicts, patients after reconstructive cardiovascular surgery, and after prolonged intravenous and/or antibiotic therapy and is usually due to species of *Candida* or *Aspergillus*. Other fungi have been implicated rarely. Mixed infections are unusual, and culture-negative endocarditis occurs with variable frequency in published series. (*From* Scheld and Sande [2].)

Clinical manifestations of infective endocarditis: Signs

	%
Fever	90
Heart murmur	85
Changing murmur	5–10
New murmur	3–5
Embolic phenomenon	> 50
Skin manifestations	18–50
Osler nodes	10–23
Splinter hemorrhages	15
Petechiae	20–40
Janeway lesion	< 10
Splenomegaly	20–57
Septic complications (pneumonia, meningitis, etc.)	20
Mycotic aneurysms	20
Clubbing	12–52
Retinal lesion	2–10
Signs of renal failure	10–15

Figure 8-12 Clinical manifestations of infective endocarditis: Signs. The physical findings relate to fever, heart murmur, and the consequences of emboli or immunopathologic manifestations. Infective endocarditis should be considered in any patient with a fever and heart murmur. Changing murmurs are unusual but of particular importance in the evaluation of a patient with known cardiac risk factors. Older designations of infective endocarditis as "acute or subacute" should be abandoned in favor of classification schemes dependent on isolation of the etiologic agent. (*From* Scheld and Sande [2]).

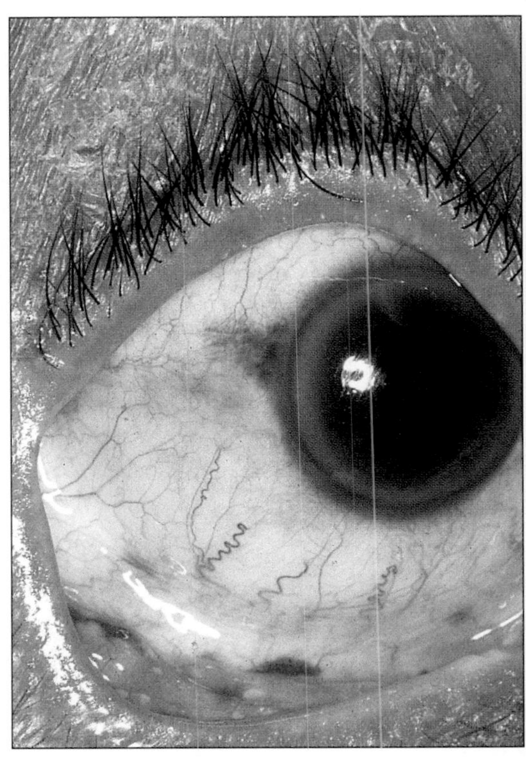

Figure 8-13 Conjunctival hemorrhages in a patient with *Staphylococcus aureus* endocarditis.

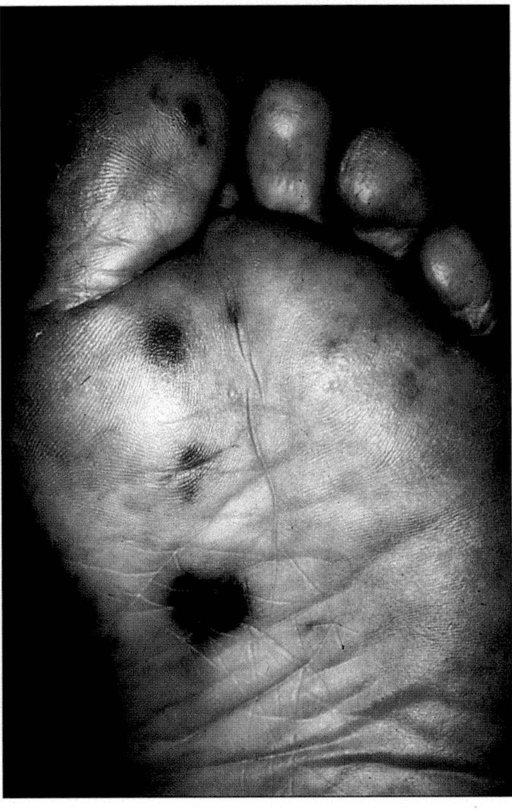

Figure 8-14 Janeway lesions in a patient with *Staphylococcus aureus* endocarditis. Janeway lesions are generally painless, flat, and occasionally hemorrhagic, as in this case. Embolic in origin with microabscess formation in the dermis, they are almost pathognomonic of *S. aureus* endocarditis. (*From* Sande and Strausbaugh [3]; with permission.)

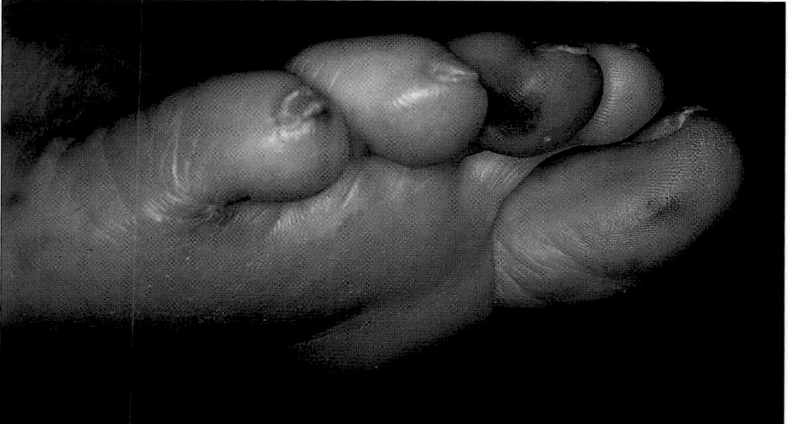

Figure 8-15 Osler's nodes in patients with infective endocarditis. These lesions usually occur in the tufts of the fingers or toes and are painful and evanescent. They likely are mediated by immunopathologic factors.

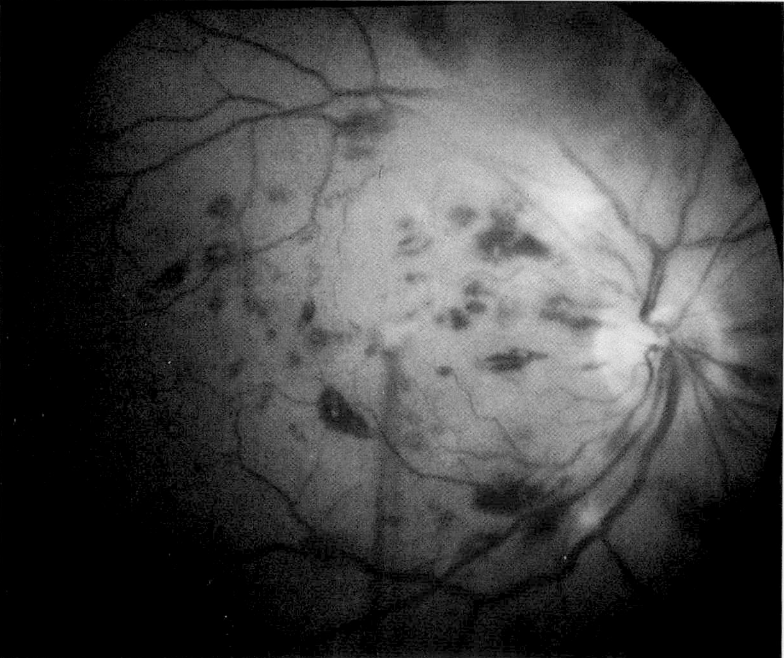

Figure 8-16 Roth spots in infective endocarditis. Of uncertain pathogenesis, these lesions usually are characterized by a central clear area surrounded by hemorrhage.

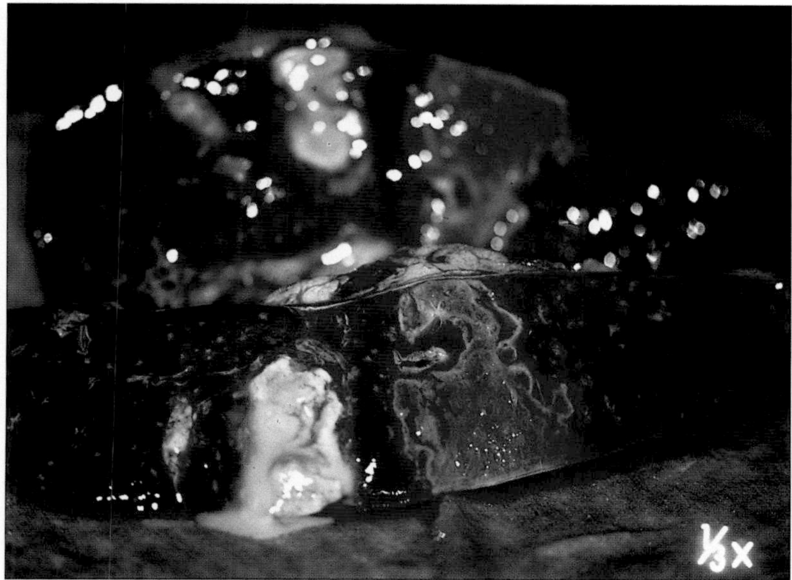

Figure 8-17 Gross specimen of spleen resected from a patient with *Staphylococcus aureus* endocarditis. The patient developed acute left upper quadrant pain and tenderness, and a computed tomography scan documented multiple filling defects within the spleen. This gross specimen demonstrates both bland infarct and abscess formation, with visible pus following emboli to the organ.

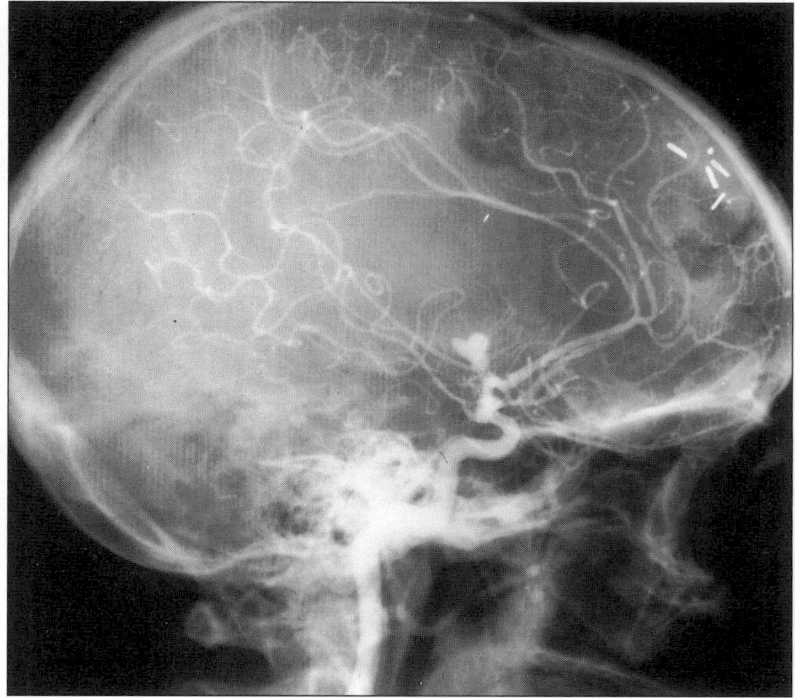

Figure 8-18 Angiogram showing intracerebral mycotic aneurysms. Mycotic aneurysms typically involve the branch points of small, secondary arteries (the site of the clip on the angiogram). Since the clipping, a larger, multilobulated aneurysm has developed at the bifurcation of the internal carotid artery.

Proposed new criteria for diagnosis of infective endocarditis
Definite infective endocarditis
Pathologic criteria
Microorganisms: demonstrated by culture *or* histology in vegetation, or in vegetation that has embolized, or in intracardiac abscess; *or*
Pathologic lesions: vegetation or intracardiac abscess present, confirmed by histology showing active IE
Clinical criteria (*see* definitions in Fig. 2-48)
Two major criteria, *or*
One major and three minor criteria, *or*
Five minor criteria
Possible infective endocarditis
Findings consistent with IE that fall short of *definitive* but not *rejected*
Rejected
Firm alternative diagnosis explaining evidence of IE, *or*
Resolution of endocarditis syndrome with antibiotic therapy for ≤ 4 days, *or*
No pathologic evidence of IE at surgery or autopsy, after antibiotic therapy for ≤ 4 days
IE—infective endocarditis.

Figure 8-19 Proposed new criteria for the diagnosis of infective endocarditis. New criteria for the diagnosis of infective endocarditis have been proposed by Durack *et al.* that are based largely on the presence of typical microorganisms for endocarditis from blood cultures and characteristic findings on echocardiography. These new criteria have been validated by several other groups in recent years. (*Adapted from* Durack *et al.* [4]; with permission.)

Sepsis and Bacteremia

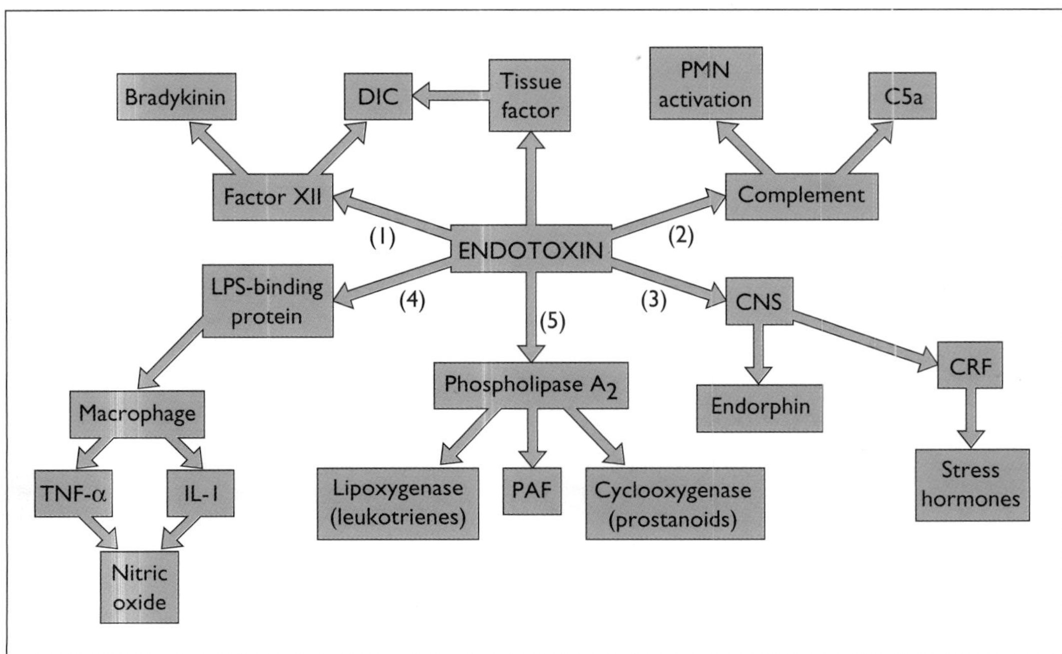

Figure 8-20 Systemic effects of endotoxin. Bacterial endotoxin (such as lipopolysaccharide [LPS] in gram-negative bacteria) activates a cascade of inflammatory mediators from various systems, including the coagulation and fibrinolytic systems (*1*), complement system (*2*), neuroendocrine system (*3*), and eicosanoid pathway (*4*). LPS also activates the monocyte/macrophage cell line (*5*) to release interleukin-1 (IL-1) and tumor necrosis factor-α (TNF-α) via a carrier protein, a LPS-binding protein. *1*, Factor XII in concert with circulating high-molecular-weight (tissue) kininogen converts prekallikrein to kallikrein, which catalyzes kininogen breakdown to the vasoactive peptide bradykinin. Activated factor XII and tissue factor (factor III) further activate the entire coagulation cascade and fibrolytic system, ultimately resulting in disseminated intravascular coagulation (DIC). *2*, Complement activation leads to the release of anaphylatoxins, such as C3a and C5a, which contribute to vasomotor instability in sepsis. *3*, Endotoxin also activates the stress hormone response and β-endorphins, which centrally mediate hypotension. *4*, The eicosanoids are a family of vasoactive cyclic endoperoxides that contribute to the systemic inflammatory response. *5*, The monocyte-macrophage components are the principal elaborators of the inflammatory cytokines, IL-1, IL-6, IL-8, IL-12, and TNF. Shock or hypotension itself is directly produced by cytokine-induced nitric oxide synthesis and release, platelet-activating factor (PAF), bradykinin, complement components, and perhaps other host-derived mediators [2,3]. (CNS—central nervous system; CRF—corticotropin-releasing factor; PMN—polymorphonuclear leukocytes.)

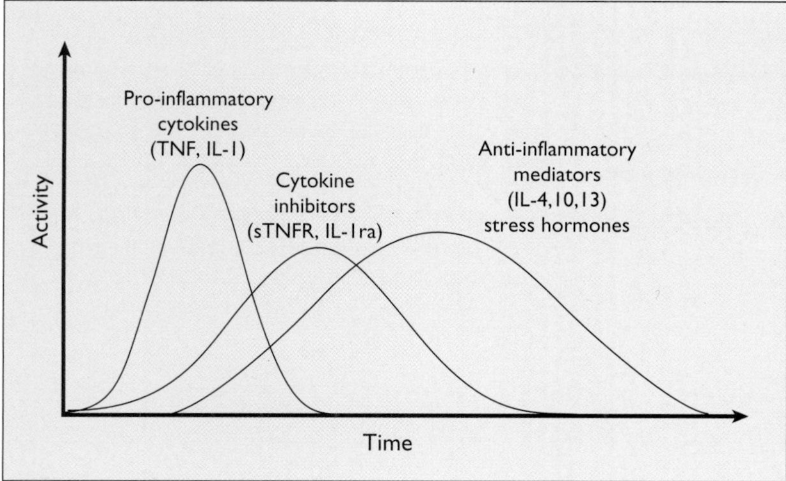

FIGURE 8-21 Sequence of cytokine responses to infection over time. The initial response to an infectious stimulus is the generation of the proinflammatory cytokines tumor necrosis factor-α (TNF-α) and interleukin (IL)-1. Other cytokines, such as IL-6, IL-8, and IL-12, may also participate. Soon, specific cytokine inhibitors are released, such as soluble TNF receptor (sTNFR) and IL-1 receptor antagonist (IL-1ra), which downregulate cytokine activity. Subsequently, anti-inflammatory cytokines, such as IL-4, IL-10, and IL-13, and stress hormones (epinephrine, glucocorticoids) further modulate the response [5].

Clinical signs and symptoms of sepsis
Fever, chills, hypotension
Hypothermia
Hyperventilation
Alteration in mental status
Bleeding or oozing from wounds or puncture sites
Evidence of infection in lung, urinary tract
Ecthyma gangrenosum, petechiae, bullae
Evidence for organ failure: jaundice, cyanosis, oliguria/anuria, heart failure

FIGURE 8-22 Common clinical signs and symptoms associated with bacterial sepsis. Some patients may present with very subtle signs early in their course. For example, hyperventilation or altered mental status may be the only manifestation in some patients. Others, notably neutropenic patients, may present with only fever. Eventually, there is evidence of infection at some body site or in association with specific evidence for organ failure.

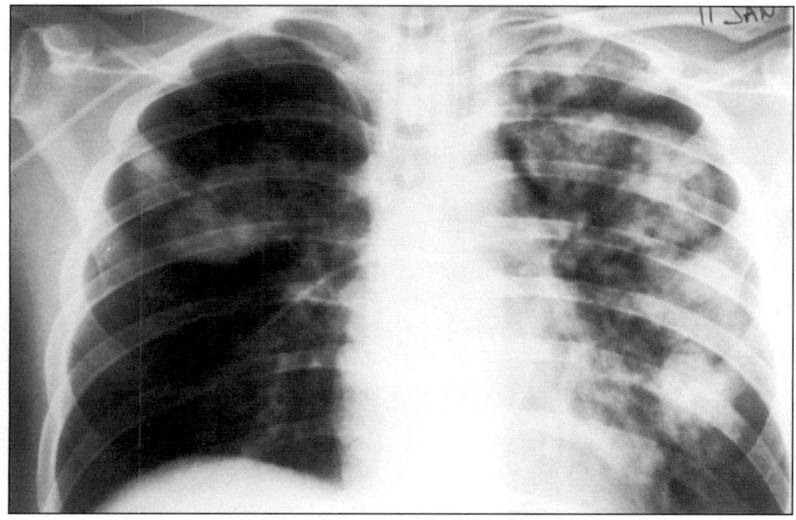

FIGURE 8-23 Chest radiograph showing multiple septic pulmonary emboli in a patient with suppurative phlebitis at the site of an intravascular catheter insertion. *Staphylococcus aureus* was cultured from the blood and the removed catheter tip. Right-sided bacterial endocarditis should be considered in patients with similar presentations. (*Courtesy of* S. Lowry, MD.)

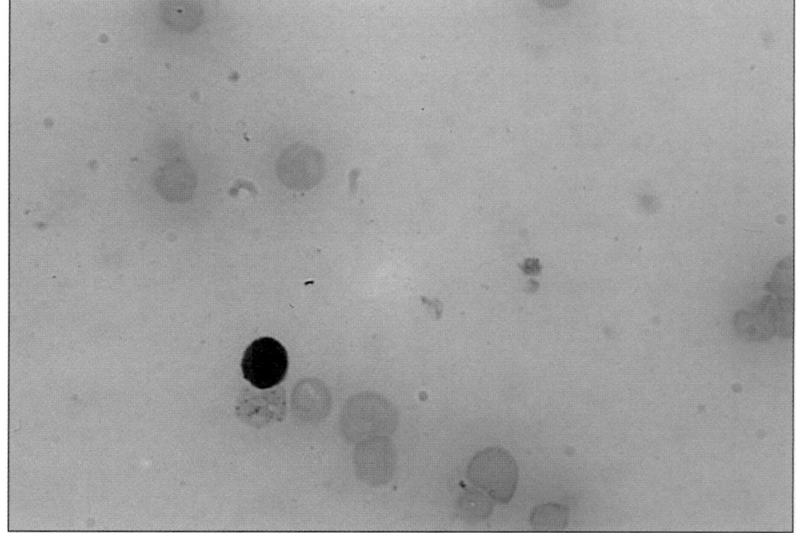

FIGURE 8-24 Wright-stained smear of peripheral blood in clostridial sepsis. Peripheral blood smear shows a paucity of intact erythrocytes and platelets indicative of massive intravascular hemolysis. This hemolysis is due to the generation of clostridial alpha-toxin, which has phospholipase activity that destroys cell membranes. Exchange transfusions have been used with some success to control intravascular hemolysis in these patients.

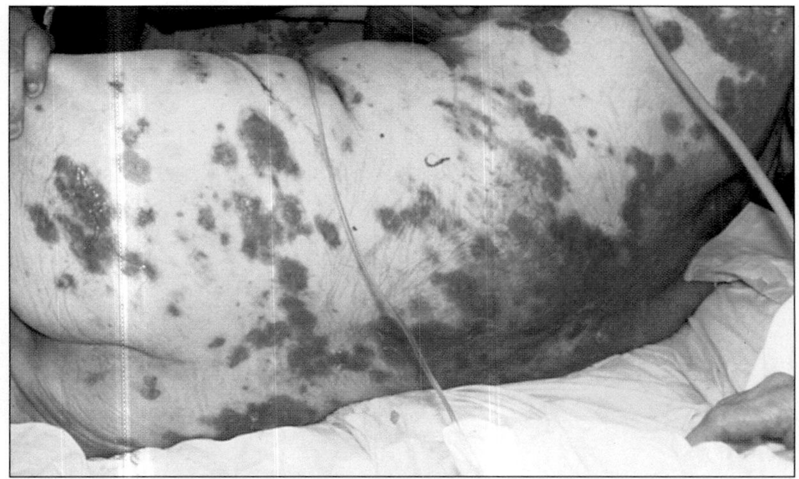

Figure 8-25 Erythematous sedulations in early meningococcemia. Approximately 5 days into the course of meningococcemia, an adult with meningitis caused by *Neisseria meningitidis* shows the characteristic cutaneous necrosis. These lesions are the result of intravascular coagulation induced by direct activation of the coagulation and thrombolytic pathways. The lesions may heal over several weeks, but terminal digits may necrose completely and slough. (*Courtesy of* H. Levy, MD.)

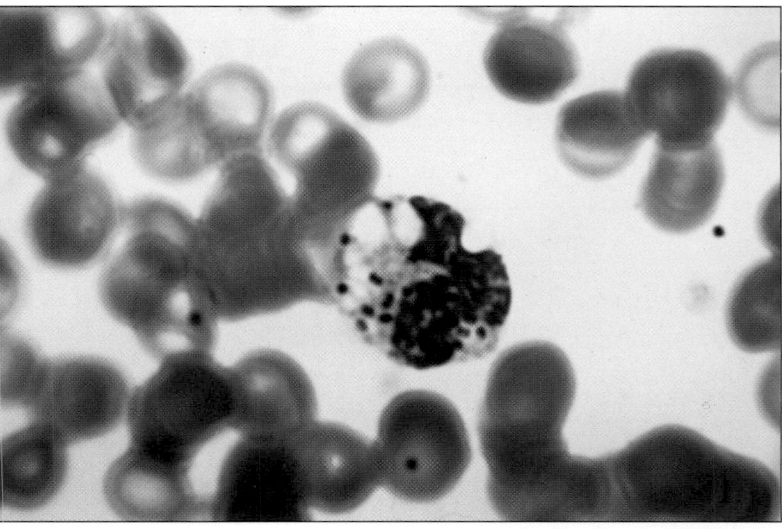

Figure 8-26 Wright-stained smear of peripheral blood in fulminant *Neisseria meningitidis* bacteremia. Note the presence of extracellular and intracellular gram-negative diplococci. Direct visualization of meningococci on unspun peripheral blood is quite unusual. However, similar smears can be obtained by direct aspiration of necrotic skin lesions.

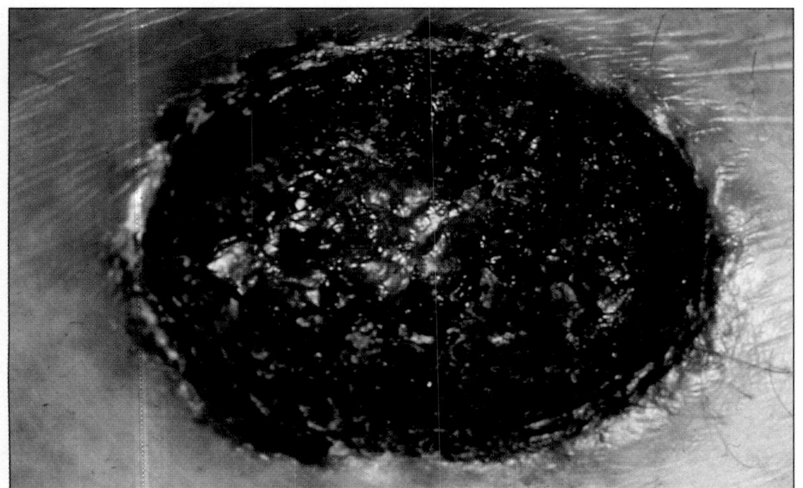

Figure 8-27 Late manifestations of ecthyma gangrenosum. In an immunocompromised patient with *Pseudomonas aeruginosa* bacteremia, a late lesion of ecthyma shows discrete borders and a necrotic center. It is unusual to find more than 6 to 10 such lesions widely scattered over the body. Aspiration of the necrotic center usually reveals necrotic debris, bacteria, and a notable absence of granulocytes. (*Courtesy of* A. Cross, MD.)

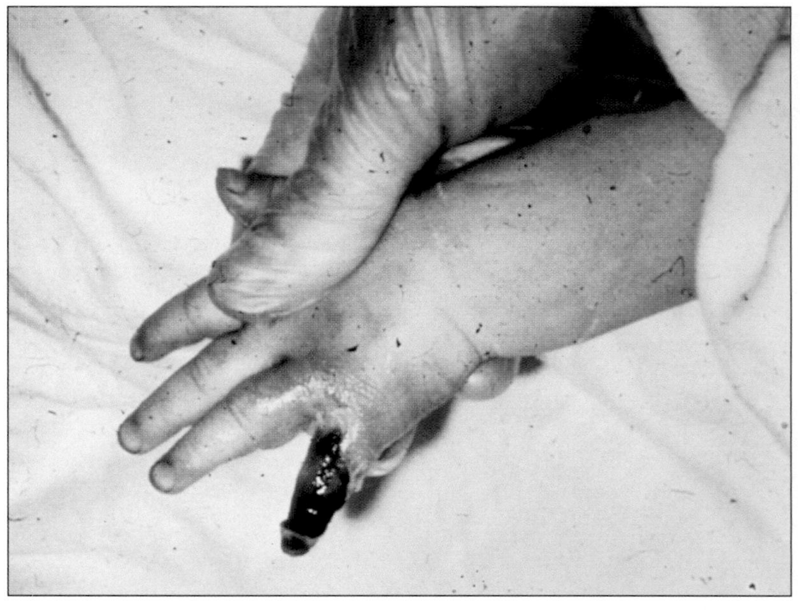

Figure 8-28 Digital necrosis and sloughing in a child with *Pseudomonas aeruginosa* bacteremia. The bacteremia developed following rupture of a gangrenous appendix. This is an unusual manifestation of sepsis given the current antibiotics active against gram-negative bacteria. This patient presented before the availability of specific antipseudomonal antibiotics and did not survive.

Treatment of bacterial sepsis
Maintain airway and venous access
Intravenous antibiotics directed to likely pathogens
Monitor systemic arterial pressure, pulmonary wedge pressures, oxygenation, respiratory status
Fluid and electrolyte replacement to maintain tissue perfusion
Surgical drainage of purulent collections

Figure 8-29 General approach to the treatment of septic patients. As with other emergency conditions, it is critical to establish a patent airway and intravenous access. Antibiotics directed against the likely pathogens must be started promptly after diagnostic blood cultures are obtained. Because many of the complications of sepsis involve organ failure, it is crucial to maintain tissue perfusion with pressure monitoring and fluid and electrolyte management. Prompt surgical drainage is indicated for any suspected purulent collections.

Streptococcal Infections

Group A streptococcal suppurative/invasive diseases

Tonsillopharyngitis	Bone/joint infections
Soft-tissue infections	Osteomyelitis
Impetigo	Pyogenic arthritis
Necrotizing fasciitis	Sinusitis
Cellulitis	Mastoiditis
Lymphangitis	Pulmonary infections
Lymphadenitis	Pneumonitis
Thrombophlebitis	Empyema
Abscess formation	Postpartum infections
Septicemia	Puerperal sepsis
Toxic shock–like syndrome	Myometritis
Meningitis	Breast abscesses

Figure 8-30 Group A streptococcal suppurative/invasive diseases.

Group A streptococcal constituents or extracellular products that may contribute to pathophysiology of sepsis and shock

Constituent/product	Pathogenic property
M protein	Antiphagocytic (anti-M antibody promotes bacterial opsonization, uptake, and PMN killing)
Pyrogenic exotoxins A, B, C	Pyrogenicity
	Suppresses Ig production
	Induces monokines (*eg*, interleukin-1β, TNF-α)
	T-cell mitogen
	Alters reticuloendothelial cell function
	Inhibits neutrophil chemotaxis through TNF-α
	Enhances delayed hypersensitivity, leading possibly to skin findings
Hyaluronidase	Cleaves hyaluronic acid in tissue matrix
Protease	Proteolytic, damaging to proteins
Streptolysin O	May act synergistically with exotoxin to influence monocyte and macrophage monokine production

PMN—polymorphonuclear cells; TNF—tumor necrosis factor.

Figure 8-31 Group A streptococcal constituents or extracellular products that contribute to pathophysiology of sepsis and shock. Group A streptococci produce large numbers of extracellular products. Some of these have been shown to play a role in the pathophysiology of disease production.

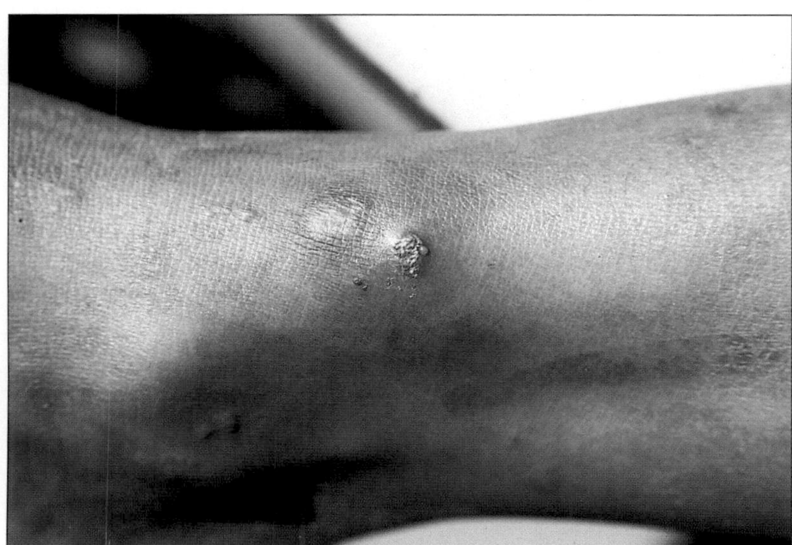

Figure 8-32 Three-day-old lesion of streptococcal impetigo with amber, crumbly crust. Cultures during this stage yield either group A streptococci alone or mixed streptococci and staphylococci.

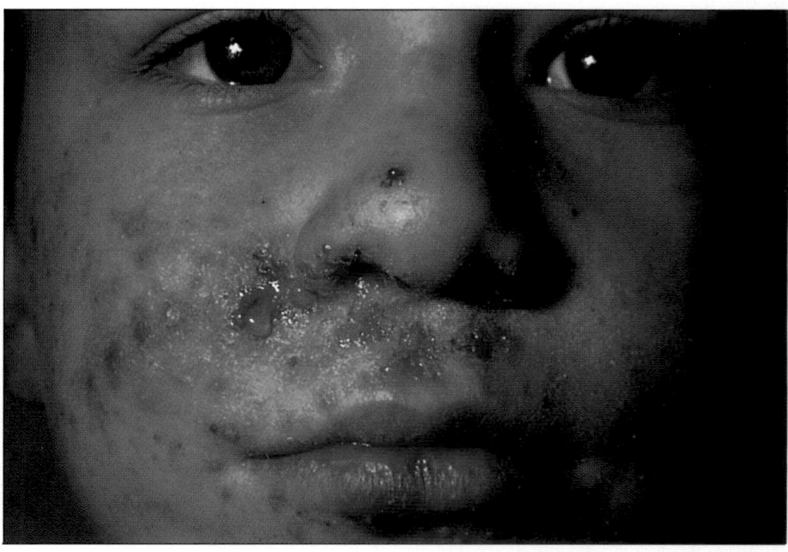

Figure 8-33 Facial impetigo 3 days after onset. Serous, oozing, honey-yellow crusts with a "stuck-on" appearance below the nares and pustules below the lips are apparent in this child aged 5 years with classic impetigo. Culture yielded group A streptococci. (*Courtesy of* A.M. Margileth, MD.)

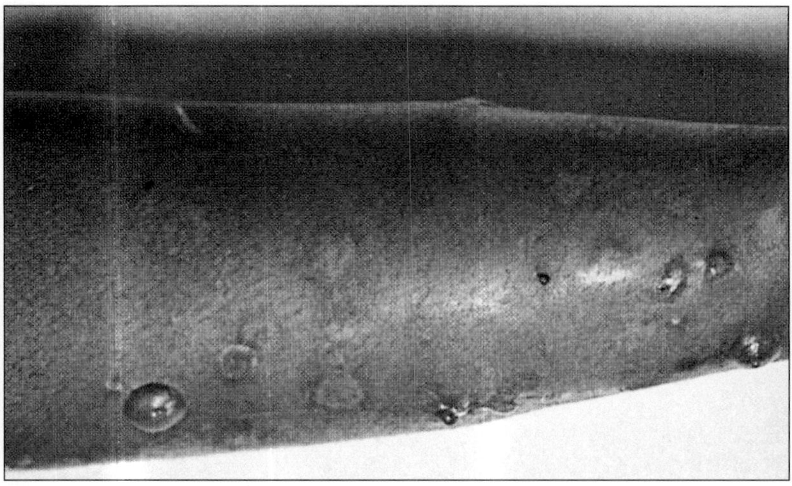

FIGURE 8-34 Staphylococcal impetigo. *Staphylococcus aureus* also may cause impetigo, and recent studies suggest that staphylococcal impetigo may be more common than the streptococcal variety. Clinically, staphylococcal impetigo presents in two forms: In the first form (shown here), bullous impetigo appears as thin-walled, fluid-filled lesions that vary in size from a few millimeters to several centimeters. Bacteria can be recovered from the fluid. In the second form (not shown), lesions have thin, varnishlike, eight-brown crusts.

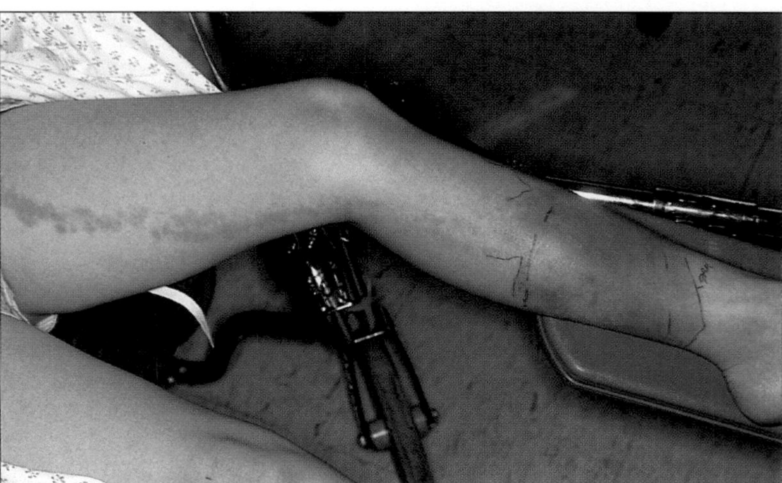

FIGURE 8-35 Streptococcal cellulitis. Group A streptococci are a common cause of cellulitis. Infection is often secondary to blunt or penetrating injury, usually on exposed skin. Infection may spread to involve a large area. Phlebitis or lymphangitis also may be noted. Infections may be very extensive and result in tissue necrosis and gangrene.

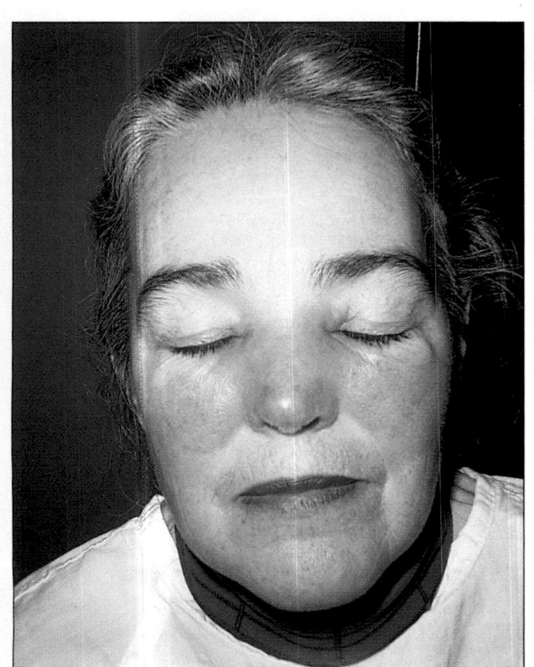

FIGURE 8-36 Erysipelas. Erysipelas is a form of streptococcal cellulitis that usually occurs on the face. There is commonly a leading edge of the infection as it spreads from the involved area. Constitutional symptoms (fever, malaise, chills) are not uncommon.

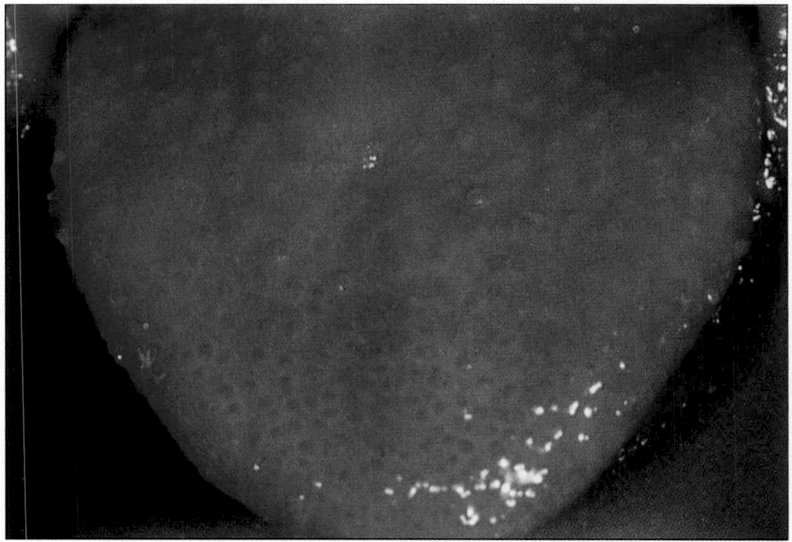

FIGURE 8-37 Strawberry tongue. Strawberry tongue is sometimes seen in cases of scarlet fever. During the first few days of illness, the tongue is covered with a thick white material through which the enlarged red papillae protrude. The white material peels in a few days, resulting in the red strawberry stage shown here. Strawberry tongue also is seen in patients with Kawasaki disease.

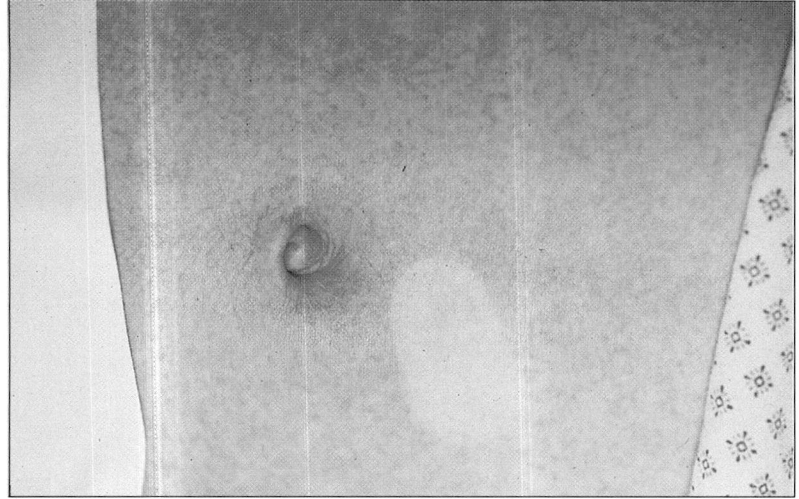

FIGURE 8-38 Blanching of petechial rash in streptococcal toxic shock syndrome. Sudden onset of high fever (to 40° C, 104° F), erythroderma, petechial rash, conjunctival hemorrhages, pharyngitis, and abdominal pain is typical of toxic shock syndrome, as seen in this girl aged 13 years 6 hours after onset. Shock may develop along with hypotension, very poor capillary filling, marked malaise, lethargy, and jaundice. In this patient, a throat culture was positive for group A streptococci and her antistreptolysin titer was elevated to 1:1360 (although most cases of toxic shock syndrome are due to *Staphylococcus aureus*). Desquamation of her fingers and toes developed after 3 to 7 days on antibiotic therapy, with recovery following. (*Courtesy of* A.M. Margileth, MD.)

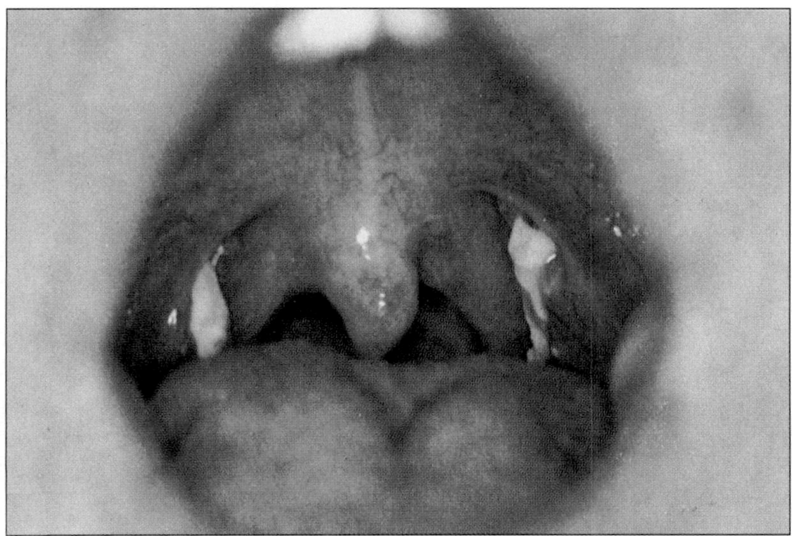

Figure 8-39 Viral causes in the differential diagnosis of streptococcal pharyngitis. Other common causes of pharyngitis include a number of viruses. Infectious mononucleosis is caused by Epstein-Barr virus. In addition to the pharynx, multiple other organs also are involved.

Staphylococcus aureus Infections

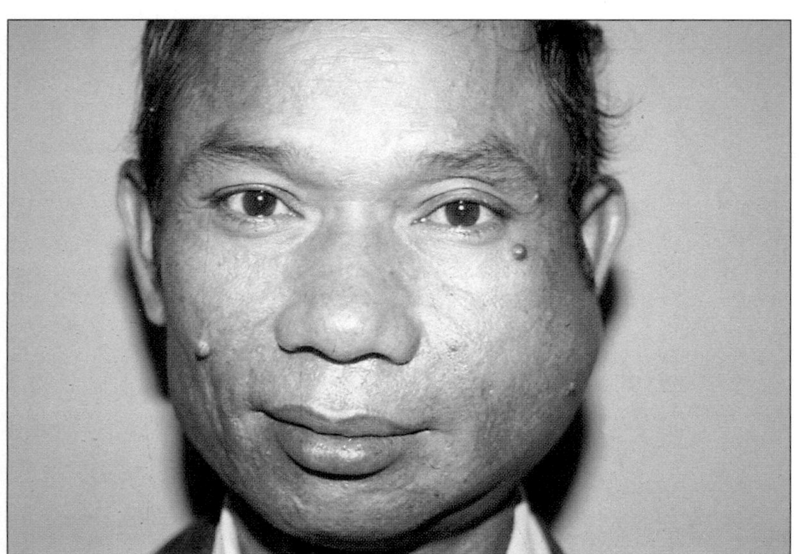

Figure 8-40 Acute staphylococcal parotitis. This disorder usually is hospital-acquired in debilitated patients but occasionally occurs in an ambulatory patient whose parotid gland duct system is unobstructed. Drying of oral secretions by anticholinergic drugs or other conditions that decrease the salivary output of the glands, such as head and neck irradiation or Sjögren's syndrome, may predispose to these abrupt infections. For patients having these problems, frequent drinking of liquids or sucking on hard candies maintains salivary flow and prevents the illness.

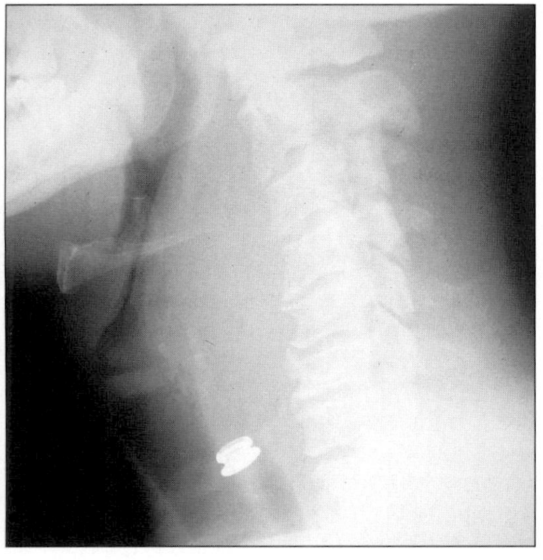

Figure 8-41 Retropharyngeal abscess in a man with diabetes. The patient, aged 39 years, was a type II diabetic (insulin-dependent) injecting drug user with a 1-week history of sore throat and 1 day of muffled speech and neck swelling. A lateral radiograph of the neck soft tissue shows a retropharyngeal space infection. Incision and drainage yielded free pus, which grew a pure culture of *Staphylococcus aureus*. Subsequently the patient developed osteomyelitis of the anterior body of the fifth cervical vertebra, with an abscess in the prevertebral space. Both diabetics who use insulin and drug abusers who inject drugs are subjected to *S. aureus* infections by the use of needles. Particularly in drug abusers, bacteremia often leads to right-sided endocarditis. Sustained bacteremia associated with right-sided endocarditis is probably the cause of metastatic infections. Diabetics are more likely to succumb to serious *S. aureus* infections. Sustained elevations of serum glucose qualitatively diminish neutrophil function, the primary defense against *S. aureus* infections.

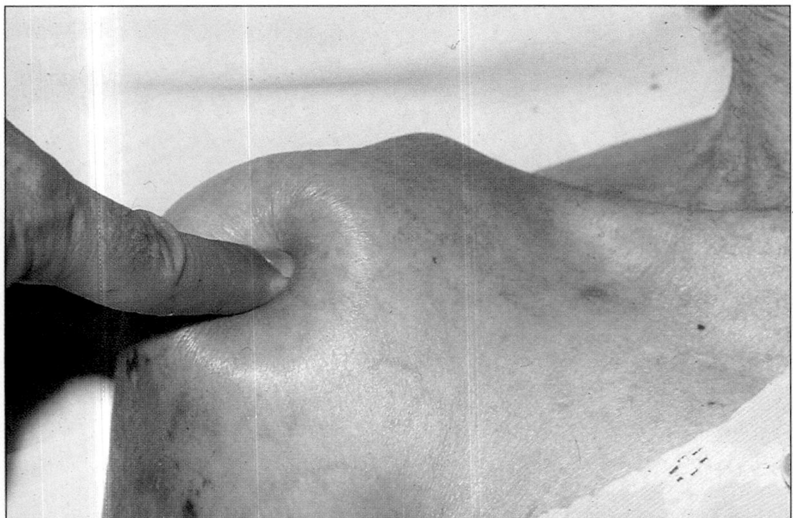

Figure 8-42 Septic arthritis affecting the right shoulder. This patient's coronary artery bypass surgery was complicated by a staphylococcal sternal wound infection. A few weeks later, she was readmitted with fever, right shoulder pain, and lumbar back pain. A radiograph of her lumbar spine showed erosion and sclerosis of two adjacent lumbar vertebrae with disc-space narrowing. Needle aspiration of the right shoulder and of the intervertebral disc revealed staphylococci. The patient was treated with repeated aspiration of the joint and 6 weeks of intravenous oxacillin, 2 g every 4 hours. Radiographs repeated 4 weeks later showed no further destruction of the bony structures.

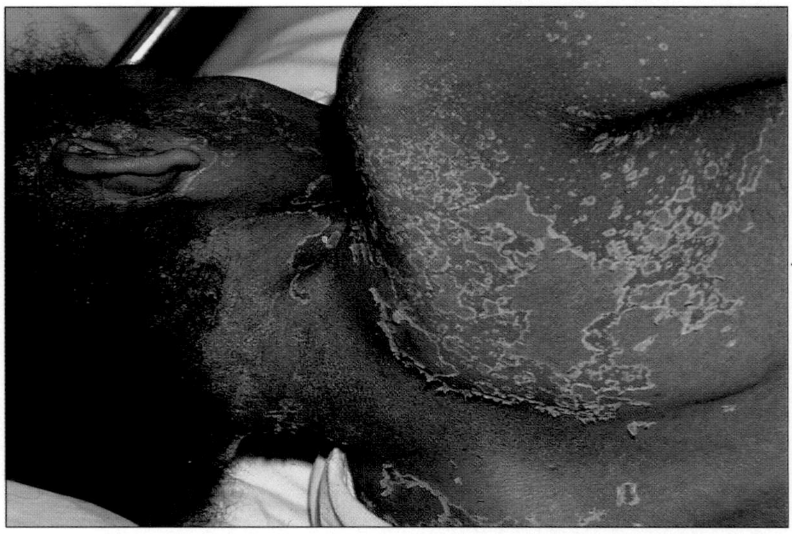

Figure 8-43 Exfoliative rash postinfection. This patient, after a high fever related to staphylococcal bacteremia, developed exfoliation of the superficial layers of the epidermis. No hypotension or other organ dysfunction was observed. This is an example of staphylococcal scarlet fever. Treatment of the underlying staphylococcal infection is sufficient to permit recovery. Staphylococcal strains isolated from these patients may elaborate exfoliative toxins.

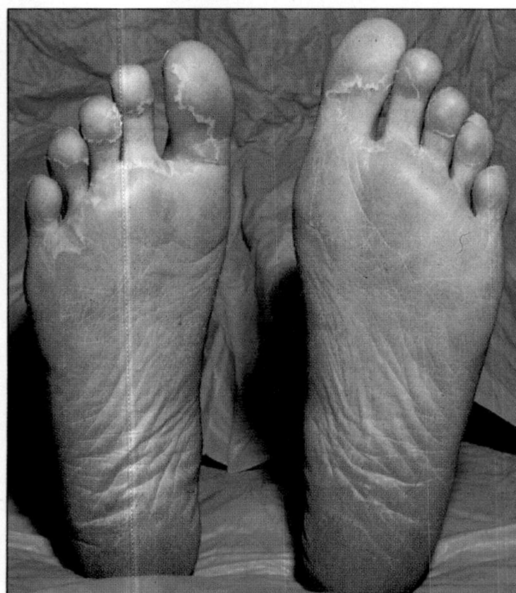

Figure 8-44 Desquamative rash of the soles in toxic shock syndrome. Such a rash affecting the soles (and palms) is characteristic of toxic shock syndrome. The rash is notable for peeling in the creases of the palms and soles and occurs 10 to 14 days after the acute illness. This is in contrast to the rash of staphylococcal scarlet fever, in which rash occurs 2 to 4 days after the acute illness.

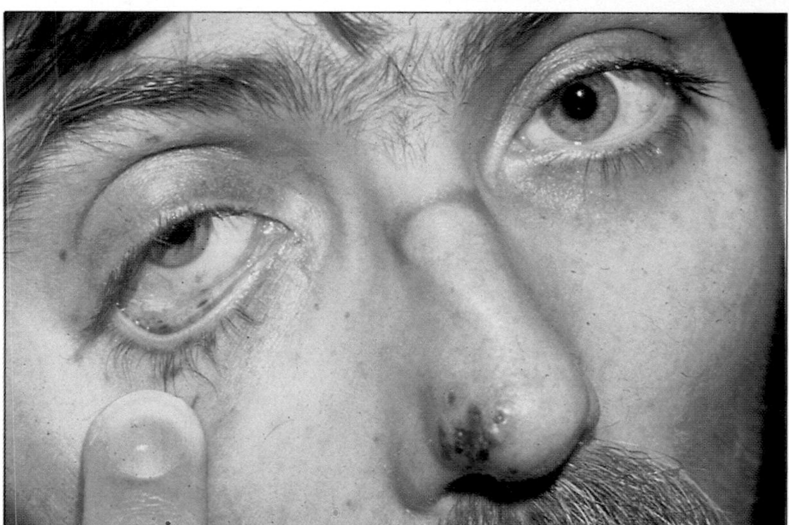

Figure 8-45 Conjunctival hemorrhage in a patient with staphylococcal endocarditis. Hemorrhages of this nature often indicate high-grade and sustained staphylococcal bacteremia. A fundoscopic examination in such patients would be prudent, because endophthalmitis can occur with sustained bacteremia.

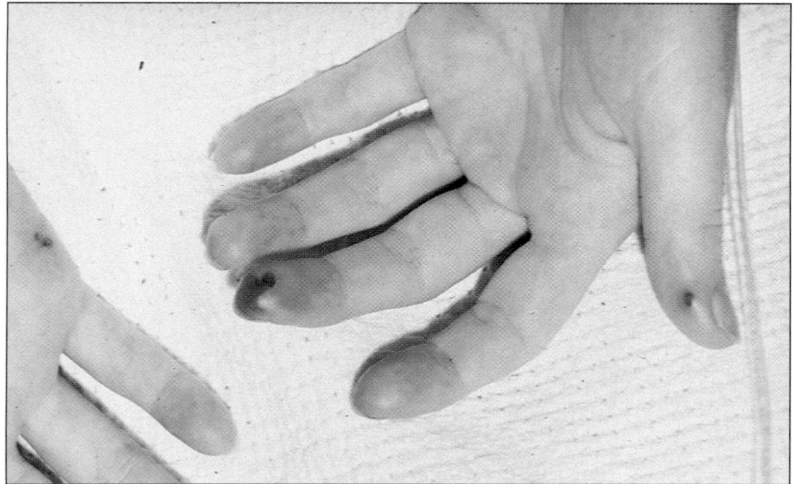

Figure 8-46 Osler's nodes and Janeway lesions on the hands in a patient with infective endocarditis. A young woman, experiencing her fifth episode of staphylococcal endocarditis secondary to intravenous drug abuse, developed painful Osler's nodes on her digits. Also note the Janeway lesion on her right palm. Osler's nodes and Janeway lesions are not commonly seen in the antibiotic era, but patients with a significant delay in the onset of effective antimicrobial therapy are likely to exhibit these manifestations of endocarditis.

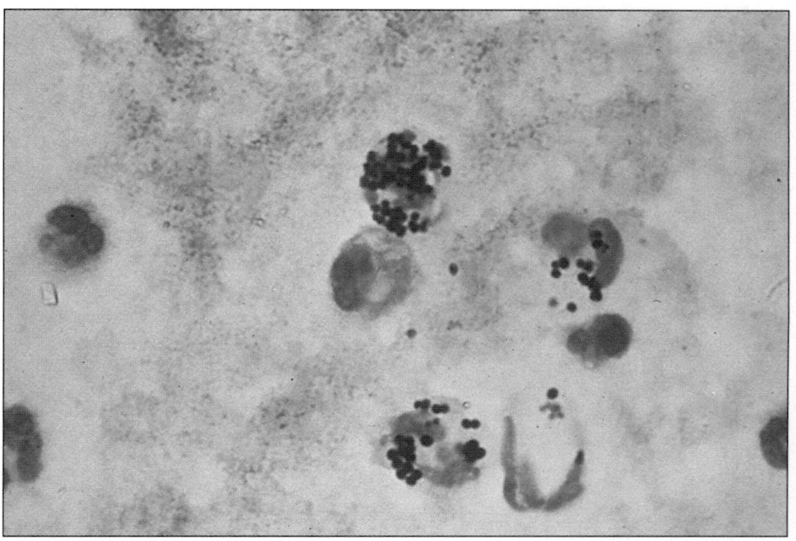

Figure 8-47 Gram stain of *Staphylococcus aureus* colonies. Within purulent material obtained from an abscess caused by *S. aureus*, it is common to find numerous gram-positive cocci in clusters, often within neutrophils. Staphylococci eventually lyse the neutrophil.

Lyme Disease

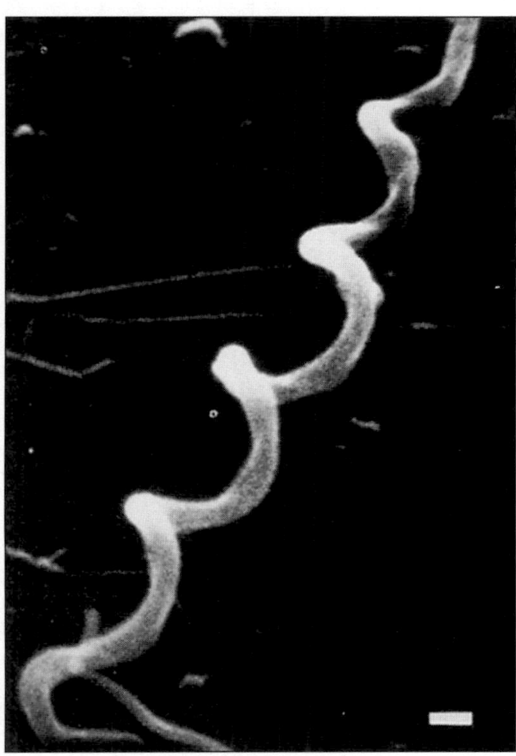

Figure 8-48 Scanning electron micrograph of the spirochete, *Borrelia burgdorferi*, the causative agent of Lyme disease. Note the left-handed coiling of the spirochete. Several strains of *B. burgdorferi* have been isolated, which may account for some differences in disease expression in the United States and Europe. (Bar=0.5 μm.) (*From* Johnson *et al.* [2]; with permission.)

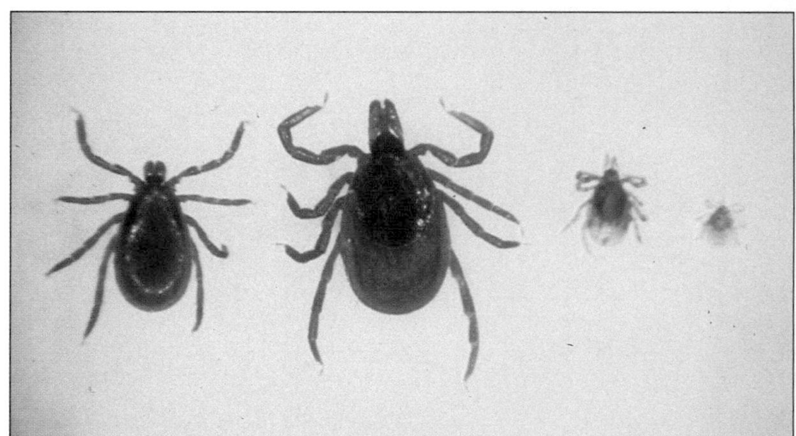

Figure 8-49 Larva, nymph, and adult female and male *Ixodes dammini* ticks (from *right* to *left*). The larva (*far left*) is approximately 1 mm in diameter. *I. dammini* is the principal vector for transmission of Lyme disease in the eastern and midwestern United States. (*From* Rahn [6]; *Courtesy of* Marge Anderson, Pfitzer Central Research, Gronton, CT.)

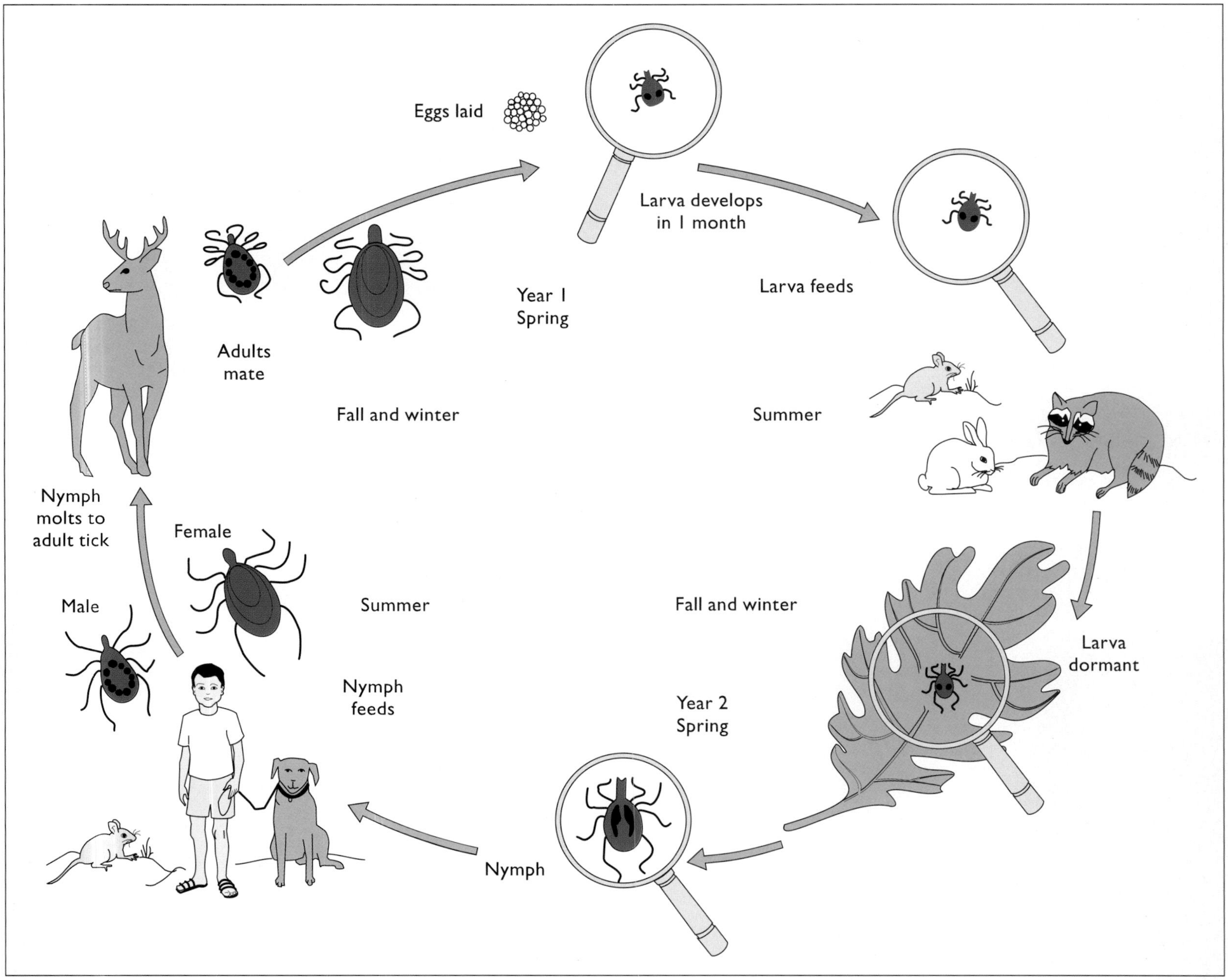

Eggs laid
Larva develops in 1 month
Year 1 Spring
Larva feeds
Adults mate
Fall and winter
Summer
Nymph molts to adult tick
Female
Male
Summer
Fall and winter
Larva dormant
Nymph feeds
Year 2 Spring
Nymph

FIGURE 8-50 Two-year life cycle of *Ixodes dammini* in the northeastern United States. Larvae are born in the spring uninfected and acquire *Borrelia burgdorferi* after feeding on their preferred host, the white-footed mouse. The following spring, larvae molt into nymphs that feed once again on small mammals (or occasionally humans), transmitting the infection to naive hosts. In the late summer and early fall, nymphs molt into adult male and female ticks. Adults mate in early fall, and eggs are laid. Humans and other animals are incidental hosts for *I. dammini* and not required for maintenance of the tick's life cycle. (*Adapted from* Rahn and Malawista [7]; with permission.)

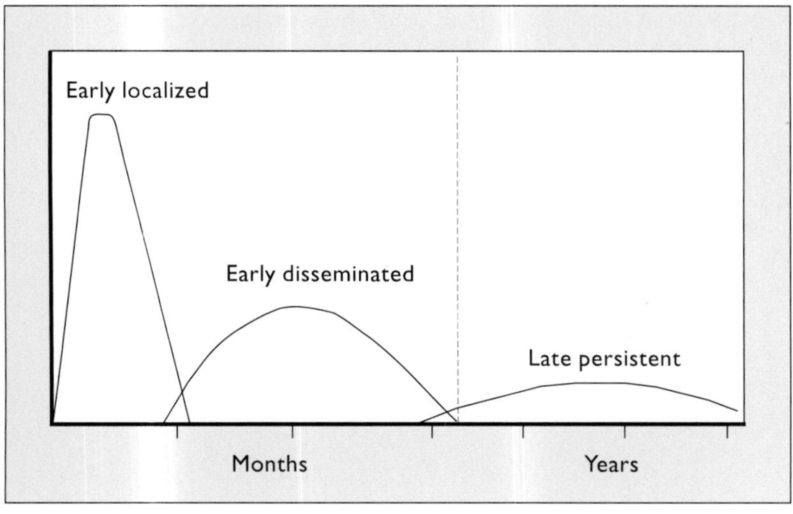

FIGURE 8-51 Clinical stages of Lyme disease. Clinical features of Lyme disease are typically divided into three general stages, termed *early localized*, *early disseminated*, and *late persistent*. Overlap of these stages may occur, and most patients do not exhibit all stages. Early localized disease occurs 3 to 32 days (mean, 7 days) after a tick bite. Symptoms of early disseminated disease appear several weeks after initial infection and coincide with hematologic and lymphatic dissemination of the spirochete. Late persistent infection typically begins months to several years following a tick bite.

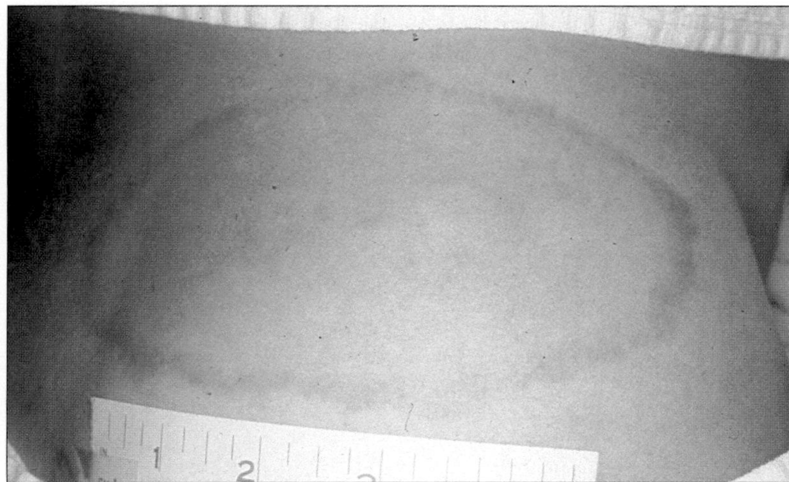

Figure 8-52 Erythema (chronicum) migrans. Erythema migrans (EM), the pathognomonic skin lesion of Lyme disease, appears as an expanding erythematous lesion, often with central clearing, around the site of the tick bite. Rare lesions of EM can have erythematous and indurated centers resembling streptococcal cellulitis or vesicular and necrotic centers. EM is reported in 60% to 80% of patients. Common sites are the thigh, groin, trunk, and axilla. (*From* Steere *et al.* [8]; with permission.)

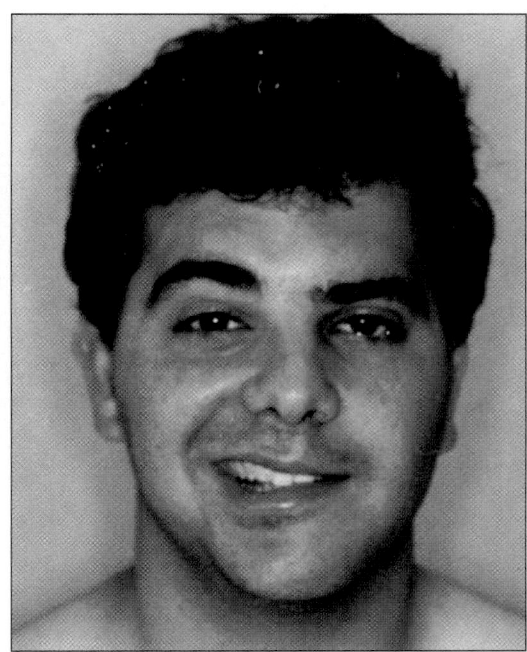

Figure 8-53 Left facial palsy (Bell's palsy) in early Lyme disease. The left facial droop reflects a seventh nerve palsy (Bell's palsy), an early neurologic manifestation of Lyme disease, and one that may be bilateral. Other neurologic manifestations include lymphocytic meningitis or meningoencephalitis and other cranial or peripheral neuritis. They typically occur 2 to 8 weeks after infection. (*From* Klempner [9]; with permission.)

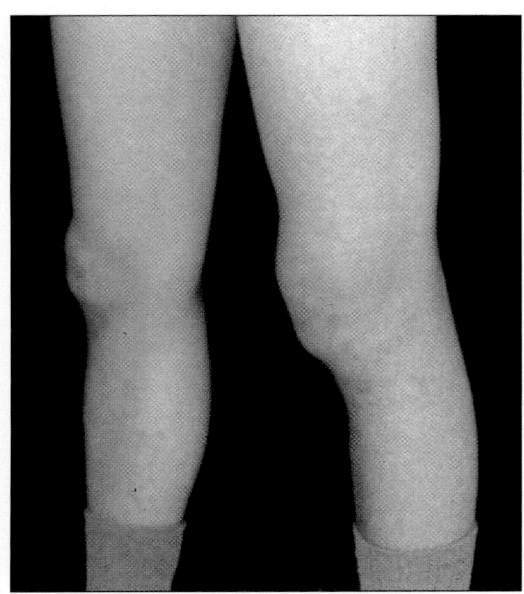

Figure 8-54 Lyme arthritis affecting a unilateral knee. Lyme arthritis occurs in 60% of untreated patients with Lyme disease. The most common presentation is intermittent inflammatory arthritis of one or more large joints, particularly the knee, occurring months to years after erythema migrans. Approximately 10% of these patients develop chronic arthritis. (*From* Steere [10]; with permission.)

A. Treatment recommendations in Lyme disease: Early Lyme disease

Drug	Dosage
Amoxicillin	500 mg three times a day × 21 days
Doxycycline	100 mg twice a day × 21 days
Cefuroxime axetil	500 mg twice a day × 21 days
Azithromycin	500 mg every day × 7 days

Figure 8-55 Treatment recommendations in Lyme disease. **A**, Early Lyme disease. Recommendations apply to Lyme disease without neurologic, cardiac, or joint involvement. For early Lyme disease limited to a single erythema migrans lesions, 10 days is sufficient duration of treatment, rather than the usual 21 days. In addition to amoxicillin, some experts advise the addition of probenecid, 500 mg three times a day. Azithromycin is considered less effective than other agents, but experience with this agent is limited; the optimal duration of therapy is unclear. (*continued*)

B. Treatment recommendations in Lyme disease: Neurologic manifestations

Bell's palsy (no other neurologic abnormalities)
Oral regimens for early disease suffice
Meningitis (± radiculoneuropathy or encephalitis)

Ceftriaxone	2 g/d × 14–28 days
Penicillin G	20 MU/d × 14–28 days
Doxycycline	100 mg twice a day, orally or intravenously, × 14–28 days
Chloramphenicol	1 g four times a day × 14–28 days

C. Treatment recommendations in Lyme disease: Lyme arthritis

Amoxicillin + probenecid	500 mg four times a day × 30 days
Doxycycline	100 mg twice a day × 30 days
Ceftriaxone	2 g/d × 14–28 days
Penicillin G	20 MU/d × 14–28 days

Figure 8-55 (*continued*) **B**, Neurologic manifestations. Optimal duration of therapy in meningitis has not been established; there are no controlled trials of therapy longer than 4 weeks for any manifestation of Lyme disease. There is no published experience in the United States with doxycyclin for treating meningitis. **C**, Arthritis. In patients with Lyme arthritis, an oral regimen should be selected only if there is no neurologic involvement. Amoxicillin is generally, administered three times a day, but the only trial of this agent in Lyme arthritis used a four-times-daily regimen. (*Adapted from* Rahn and Malawista. [11].)

Ehrlichiosis and Babesiosis

Classification of ehrlichiae by 16S ribosomal genotype and/or serologic groups

Genetic group	Major host(s)	Predominant host cell	*In vitro* cultivation	Vector	Geographic distribution	Diagnostic tests
***Ehrlichia canis* group**						
E. canis	Dogs	Mononuclear cells	Yes	Tick	Worldwide	Serology, peripheral blood smear
E. chaffeensis	Humans	Mononuclear cells	Yes	Tick	North America, Europe (?), Africa (?)	Serology, PCR, immunohistology
E. ewingii	Dogs	Granulocytes	No	Tick (?)	North America	Serology, peripheral blood smear
E. muris	Mice	Mononuclear cells	Yes	?	Japan	
Cowdria ruminantium	Cattle, goats	Endothelial cells	Yes	Tick	Africa, Caribbean	Serology, brain biopsy
***E. phagocytophila* group**						
E. phagocytophila	Sheep, goats, cattle	Granulocytes	No	Tick	Europe, Asia (?), Africa (?)	Peripheral blood smear, serology
E. equi	Horses, dogs	Granulocytes	Yes	Tick (?)	North America, Europe (?)	Peripheral blood smear, serology, ELISA
Human granulocytic *Ehrlichia*	Humans	Granulocytes	Yes	Tick (?)	North America, Europe	Peripheral blood smear, serology, PCR, immunohistology
E. platys	Dogs	Platelets	No	?	North America	Serology, ELISA, DFA
Anaplasma marginale	Cattle	Erythrocytes	Yes	Tick	Africa, North America, Europe	Peripheral blood smear
***E. sennetsu* group**						
E. sennetsu	Humans	Mononuclear cells	Yes	?	Japan, Malaysia	Serology, culture
E. risticii	Horses	Mononuclear cells	Yes	?	North America, Europe (?)	Serology, ELISA, PCR
Neorickettsia helminthoeca	Dogs, bears	Mononuclear cells	Yes	Fluke (?)	North America	

DFA—direct fluorescent antibody; ELISA—enzyme-linked immunosorbent assay; PCR—polymerase chain reaction.

Figure 8-56 Classification of ehrlichiae by 16S ribosomal genotype and/or serologic groups. Until 1987, infections by members of the genus *Ehrlichia* were recognized mainly in animals, especially dogs (canine ehrlichiosis), and in humans only in foci in the Orient (sennetsu ehrlichiosis, in western Japan and Malaysia). Human ehrlichiosis was first recognized in the United States in 1986, in a man aged 51 years who became ill 12 to 14 hours after tick bites in rural Arkansas.

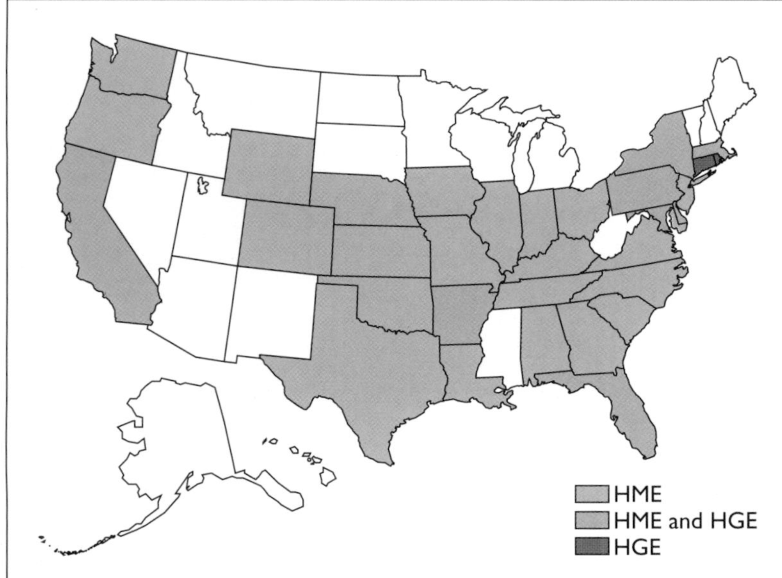

Figure 8-57 Geographic distribution of recognized cases of human monocytic ehrlichiosis (*Ehrlichia chaffeensis* infection) and human granulocytic ehrlichiosis (*E. equi*–like agent) in the United States through 1994. Most cases of human monocytic ehrlichiosis (HME) occur in areas where Rocky Mountain spotted fever is frequently recognized, whereas human granulocytic ehrlichiosis (HGE) occurs mostly where Lyme borreliosis and deer ticks (*Ixodes* spp) are also frequent. The distribution of HME cases overlaps the geographic distribution of the Lone Star tick, *Amblyomma americanum*, the probable major vector of human monocytic ehrlichiosis in the United States. (HME data *courtesy of* J.E. Dawson.)

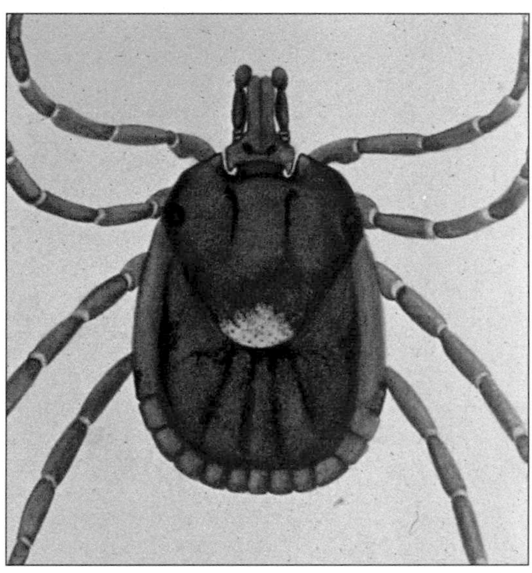

Figure 8-58 The Lone Star tick, *Amblyomma americanum*. *A. americanum* is known to harbor *Ehrlichia chaffeensis* and is probably the major vector of monocytic ehrlichiosis in the United States. This tick is often recognized by the prominent, light-colored "Lone Star" spot located centrally on the dorsal surface of the tick. The presence of *E. chaffeensis* infections in regions outside the range of this tick implicates additional tick vectors, including the American dog tick *Dermacentor variabilis*. Both adult *A. americanum* and *D. variabilis* will bite large and medium-sized animals, and suspected mammalian reservoirs include deer, foxes, and perhaps other canids including dogs [12]. (*Courtesy of* D. Sonenshine, PhD.)

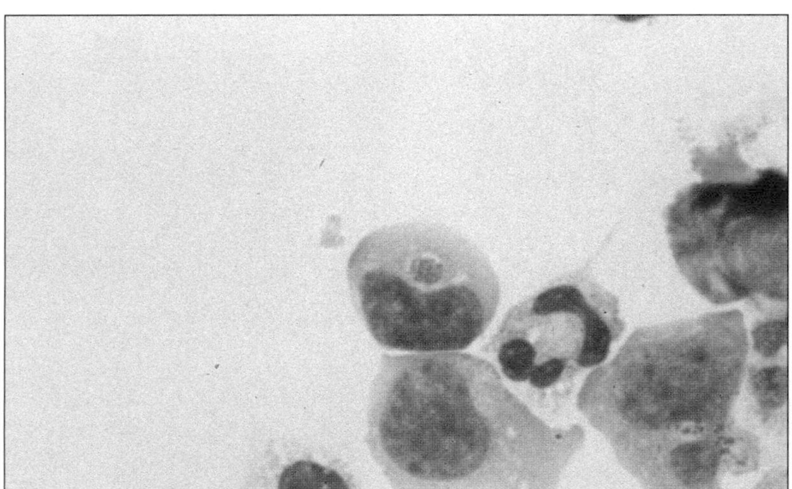

Figure 8-59 *Ehrlichia chaffeensis* morula within a mononuclear cell present in the cerebrospinal fluid of a patient with monocytic ehrlichiosis. The morula measures approximately 3 to 7 µm in diameter and is composed of a phagosome containing multiple ehrlichial bacteria, which stain basophilic with Wright-Giemsa stains. Although patients infected with *E. chaffeensis* may have morulae present in peripheral blood leukocytes, especially monocytes, these are infrequently detected in stained blood smears. *E. chaffeensis* rarely infects granulocytes. The diagnosis is best achieved by the demonstration of a seroconversion in convalescence or by polymerase chain reaction amplification of specific *E. chaffeensis* nucleic acids present in acute phase blood or leukocytes [13]. (Wright stain; original magnification, × 1200.)(*Courtesy of* B.E. Dunn, MD.)

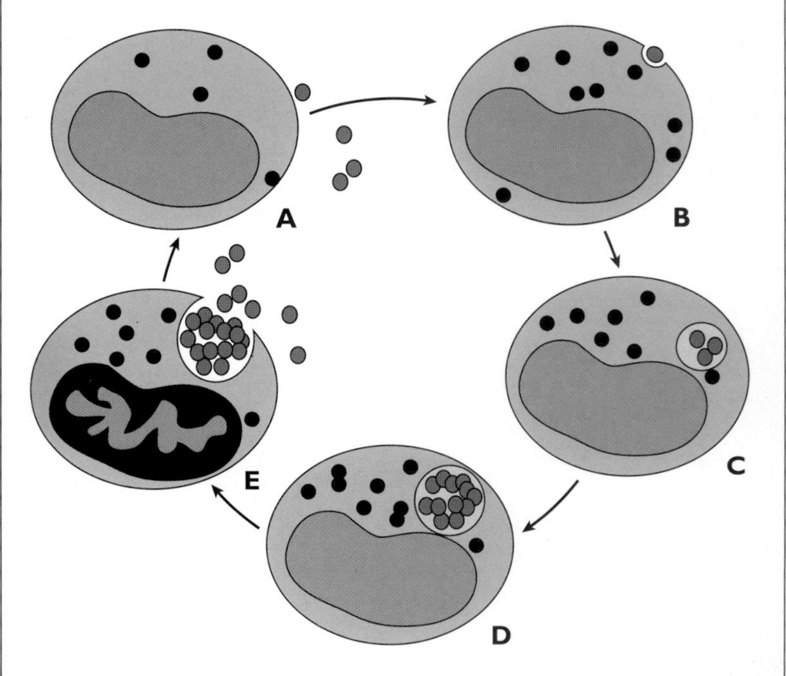

Figure 8-60 Schematic diagram depicting the course of infection of phagocytic cells by ehrlichiae. The depicted cell represents a monocyte or macrophage but could easily be represented by a neutrophil. Ehrlichiae attach to the cell surface via bacterial and host cell protein ligands (*A*). The attached ehrlichia is engulfed (*B*) and inhibits phagolysosome fusion by active bacterial protein synthesis (*C* and *D*). After proliferation, the ehrlichiae are released from the dying cell to infect other susceptible cells (*E*). Active replication of ehrlichiae may be abrogated by interferon-γ, which is probably a necessary component of intact host immunity to recovery and reinfection [14].

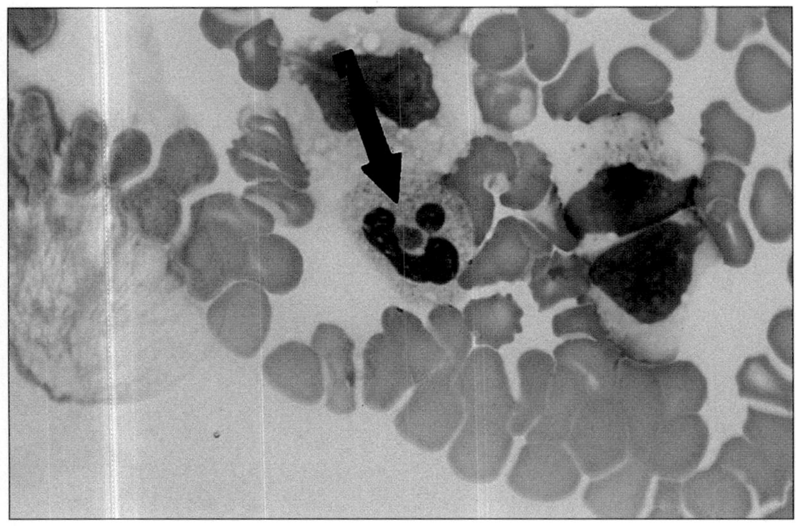

Figure 8-61 Peripheral blood band neutrophil with a morula (*arrow*) from a patient with fatal granulocytic ehrlichiosis. The specific identity of this agent is not known, but it is very closely related to the granulocytic ehrlichiae *Ehrlichia phagocytophila* (in Europe) and *E. equi* (in the United States) only known to cause veterinary diseases. Unlike monocytic ehrlichiosis, ehrlichiae that infect granulocytes may appear in large numbers in peripheral blood. Infection is predominantly restricted to neutrophils and bands. Diagnosis is strongly suggested when morulae are observed only in peripheral blood neutrophils or bands. The diagnosis may be confirmed by polymerase chain reaction amplification of specific granulocytic ehrlichia nucleic acids from acute phase blood; by immunocytologic demonstration of granulocytic ehrlichiae with *E. equi* antibodies in peripheral blood, buffy coat smears, or tissues; or by the demonstration of a serologic reaction with *E. equi* in convalescence [15,16]. (Wright stain; original magnification, × 1200.)

Abnormal laboratory findings in ehrlichiosis

	Monocytic ehrlichiosis, %	Granulocytic ehrlichiosis, %
Leukopenia	60–74	53
Thrombocytopenia	72	88
Anemia (hemoglobin or hematocrit)	50	38
Elevated serum AST	86–88	92

AST—asparate aminotransferase.

Figure 8-62 Abnormal laboratory findings in ehrlichiosis. The percentage of patients with ehrlichiosis who developed specific laboratory abnormalities at any time during the course of illness is presented. Important laboratory features are mild to moderate leukopenia, thrombocytopenia, and elevated serum hepatic transaminases [17–19].

Comparison of clinical features in Lyme disease and babesiosis

	Lyme disease (*n*=224)	Babesiosis (*n*=10)	Both (*n*=26)
Fatigue	49	60	81
Headache	42	60	77
Erythema migrans	85	0	62
Fever	42	80	58
Sweats	11	20	46
Chills	23	50	42
Myalgia	31	20	38
Anorexia	14	10	31
Arthralgia	36	50	27
Emotional lability	7	0	23
Nausea	5	10	23
Neck stiffness	21	30	23
Multiple erythema migrans	14	0	19
Cough	10	20	15
Sore throat	9	20	15
Conjunctivitis	3	0	12
Splenomegaly	0	10	8
Vomiting	4	0	8
Joint swelling	3	0	4

Figure 8-63 Comparison of clinical features in Lyme disease and babesiosis. Babesiosis may vary widely in clinical presentation, from a potentially life-threatening hemolytic disease in persons predisposed to severe infection by old-age, asplenia, or immune suppression, to an occult disease process with few known sequelae that occurs in younger, normosplenic, immunocompetent persons. Little is known about the course of subclinical infection during which the numbers of circulating parasites is likely to be much lower than in clinically apparent cases. A history of tick bite is not consistently obtained from infected patients, but in most cases, a history of travel to an endemic area is present. In addition, because patients with serologically confirmed Lyme disease are, by definition, at increased risk for concurrent babesiosis, patients failing to respond to antimicrobial agents directed at *Borrelia burgdorferi* may be suffering from underlying babesial infection. (*Adapted from* Krause *et al.* [20].)

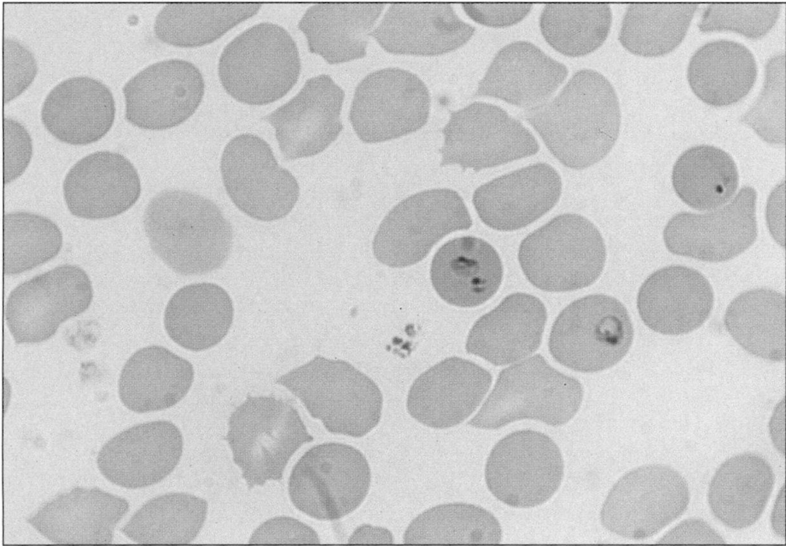

FIGURE 8-64 Peripheral smear of human red blood cells infected with *Babesia microti*. The patient was a man aged 62 years from Minnesota with a several-week history of severe fatigue, malaise, weight loss, and night sweats [21].

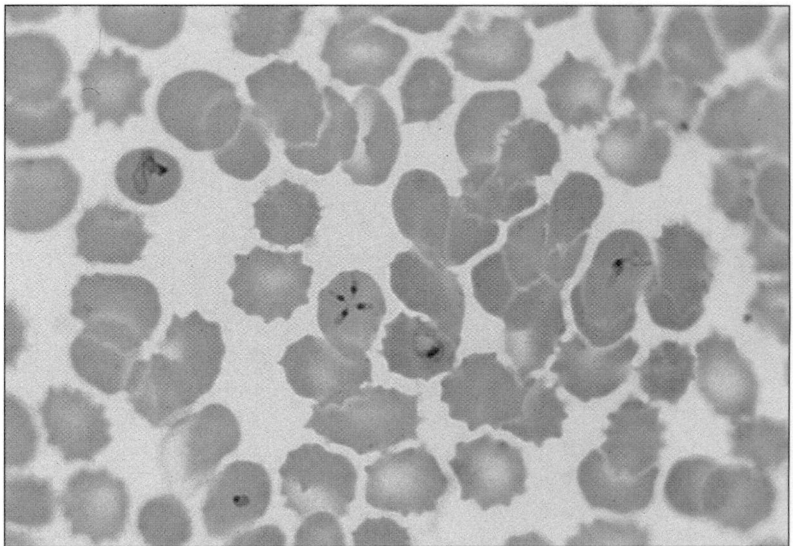

FIGURE 8-65 Peripheral smear of human red blood cells containing a newly identified piroplasm acquired in the Western United States. The patient, an asplenic man aged 41 years, had a several-day history of fever, chills, sweats, headache, body aches, nausea, fatigue, and dark urine. This organism is morphologically similar to *Babesia microti* (*see* Fig. 8-64) but is genetically and antigenically distinct [22]. This infection is caused by an unnamed organism genetically related to the WA1 piroplasms [23,24] and *Babesia gibsoni*, a cause of severe hemolytic anemia in dogs that is often confused with autoimmune hemolytic anemia. This group of related organisms is also phylogenetically related to members of the genus *Theileria*, even to the exclusion of some members of the genus *Babesia* itself [20].

BARTONELLA INFECTIONS

Microbiologic and clinical features associated with pathogenic *Bartonella* species

	B. henselae	*B. quintana*	*B. bacilliformis*
Clinical syndrome	BA, BP, BE, bacteremia/fever, cat scratch disease	Trench fever, bacteremia/fever, BA, BE, BP	Bartonellosis (Oroya fever, verruga peruana)
Vector	?	Louse	Sandfly
Reservoir	Cats	?	?
Detection	Cell-free growth, serum IFA, PCR, immunohistochemistry	Cell-free growth, serum IFA, PCR, immunohistochemistry	Cell-free growth, PCR
Treatment	Macrolides, doxycycline	Macrolides, doxycycline, others	Tetracycline, penicillin

BA—bacillary angiomatosis; BE—bacterial endocarditis; BP—bacillary peliosis; IFA—immunofluorescent assay; PCR—polymerase chain reaction.

FIGURE 8-66 Microbiologic and clinical features associated with pathogenic *Bartonella* species. Both *B. henselae* and *B. quintana* have been associated with bacillary angiomatosis; *B. henselae* is also associated with most cases of cat scratch disease [25]. Bacillary angiomatosis (only *B. henselae*–associated cases) and cat scratch disease are associated with cat scratches and bites, because cats are a reservoir for *B. henselae* [26]. It is unclear whether transmission of bacillary angiomatosis is also dependent on an arthropod vector (possibly cat fleas). *B. quintana* has been responsible for some outbreaks of "urban trench fever" in the past few years associated with chronic alcoholism [27].

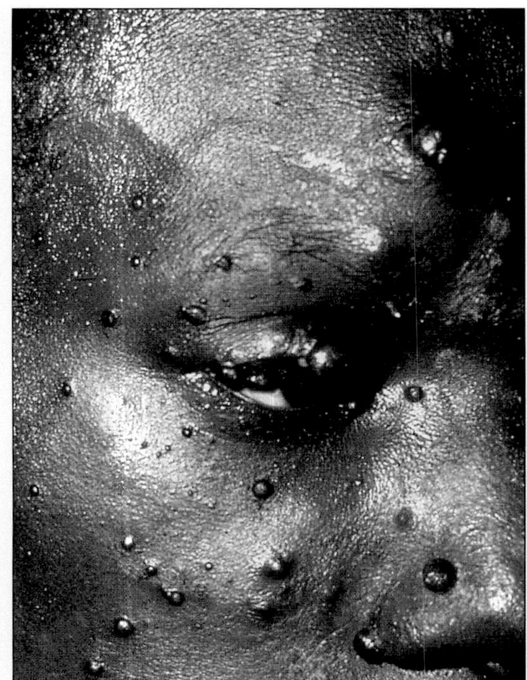

Figure 8-67 Disseminated cutaneous papules in cutaneous bacillary angiomatosis. The range of appearances of cutaneous bacillary angiomatosis is broad. This patient with HIV disease and disseminated cutaneous papules has many lesions clustered on the skin of the eyelids. This distribution is also seen in the disseminated papular form of bartonellosis, called *forma milliar*.

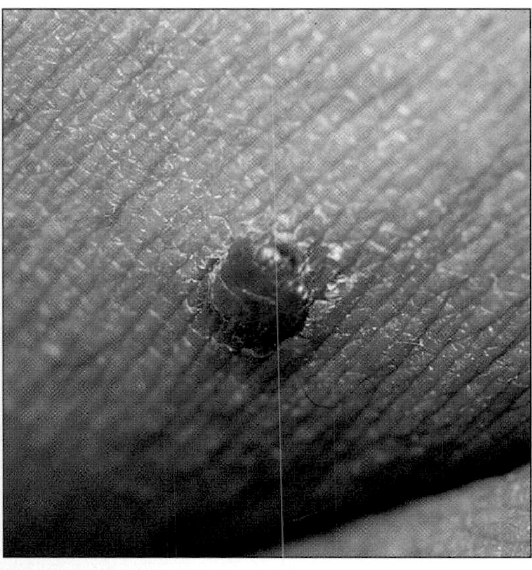

Figure 8-68 Cutaneous bacillary angiomatosis lesion on an HIV-seropositive hispanic man. This lesion is older and has a "collarette" of scale around the periphery.

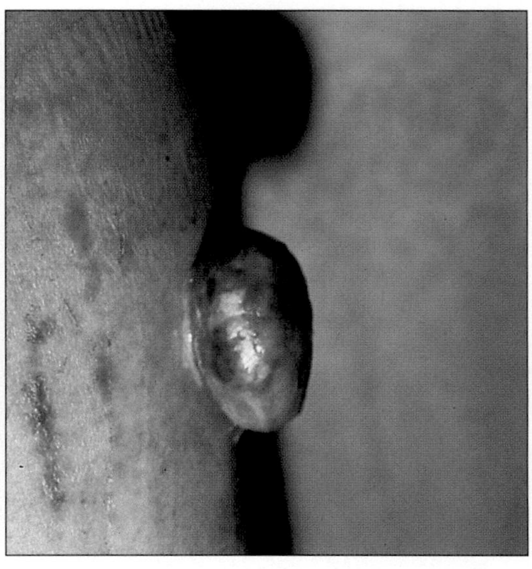

Figure 8-69 A pedunculated cutaneous lesion of bacillary angiomatosis on an HIV-seropositive patient. Pedunculation is a less frequent feature of cutaneous lesions.

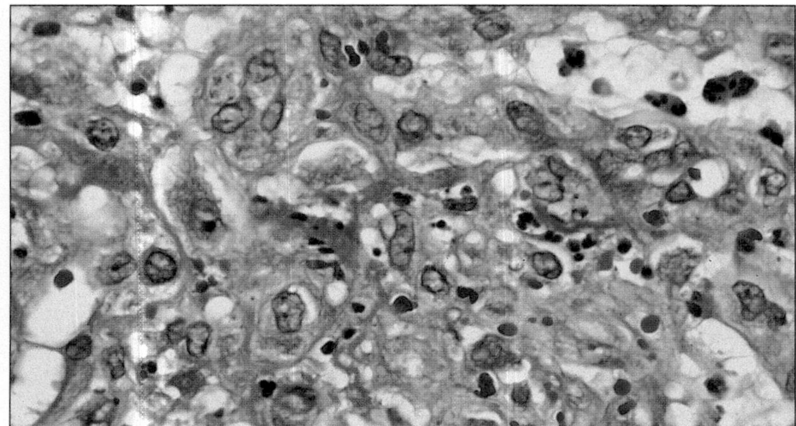

Figure 8-70 Histopathology of cutaneous bacillary angiomatosis. Endothelial cells can be seen with large clear nuclei that have irregular nuclear membranes. The presence of small purplish clusters of bacilli surrounded by neutrophils and neutrophilic nuclear dust is a valuable clue to the pathologist who otherwise could mistake these changes for those of a vascular neoplasm. Histopathologic criteria can distinguish bacillary angiomatosis from Kaposi's sarcoma, pyogenic granuloma, angiosarcoma, and angiolymphoid hyperplasia with eosinophilia [28]. (Hematoxylin-eosin stain.)

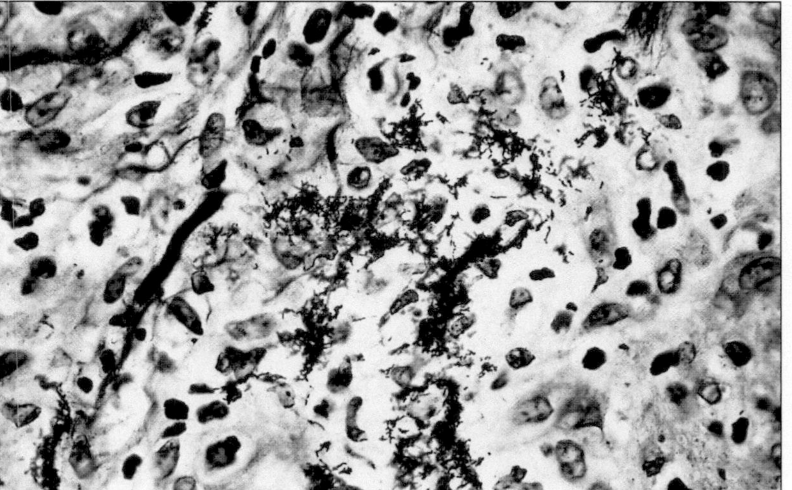

Figure 8-71 Warthin-Starry silver stain of cutaneous bacillary angiomatosis demonstrating tangled masses of bacilli. Note that the nuclei of cells in the background are delicately outlined by silver; this "internal control" is useful in determining the technical adequacy of the stain. Warthin-Starry and related silver stains are technically difficult to perform, and without optimal background staining of cells, the absence of bacteria should not be interpreted as ruling out the disease.

Clinical features of cat scratch disease
Most common presentation is solitary cervical or axillary lymphadenopathy, with stellate necrotizing granulomatous response; duration, 2 wks–8 mos
Preceding inoculation papule
Oculoglandular syndrome of Parinaud seen in 2%–10%
Complications: central nervous system seizures, encephalitis; hepatitis; bone marrow involvement; optic neuritis, retinitis

Figure 8-72 Clinical features of cat scratch disease.

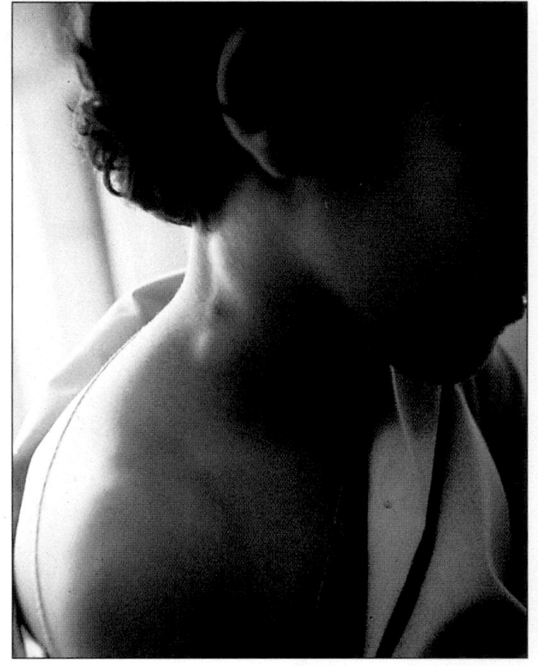

Figure 8-73 Child with posterior cervical lymphadenopathy typical of cat scratch disease. The cervical region is the second most common site for the development of regional lymphadenopathy in cat scratch disease; the axilla is the most common site.

Diagnosis of *Bartonella*-associated disease
Clinical findings and histology ± Warthin-Starry silver stain
Serology: immunofluorescent assay or enzyme-linked immunoassay (4 × ↑ or ↓)
Polymerase chain reaction, immunohistochemistry, culture (research/reference)

Figure 8-74 Diagnosis of *Bartonella*-associated disease. The diagnosis in many cases can be made with clinical and histologic findings alone. Serologic techniques (immunofluorescent antibody or enzyme-linked immunoassay) can be used to corroborate these findings, especially when a concurrent fourfold or greater rise or fall in antibody titer is documented. Polymerase chain reaction assays, immunohistochemistry tests, or culture methods are available in reference or research laboratories only at present [29].

Treatment of *Bartonella*-associated disease	
Cat scratch disease	
Localized (immunocompetent)	None
Disseminated or immunocompromised	Gentamicin, 5 mg/kg/d, *or* ciprofloxacin, 500 mg twice a day (*or* rifampin, TMP-SMX?) × 10–14 days
Other *Bartonella* infection	
Bacteremia, bacterial endocarditis, bacillary angiomatosis, bacillary peliosis	Erythromycin, 500–1000 mg four times a day; *or* tetracycline, 500 mg four times a day; *or* doxycycline, 100 mg twice a day (*or* azithromycin, clarithromycin, rifampin?)
For cutaneous bacillary angiomatosis	Given orally, × 2–3 mos
For visceral or relapsing disease	Given intravenously or orally, 4+ mos

TMP-SMX—trimethoprim-sulfamethoxazole.

Figure 8-75 Treatment of *Bartonella*-associated disease. Uncomplicated cat scratch disease is a self-limited infection and does not require treatment, whereas systemic disease usually requires treatment. Gentamicin and ciprofloxacin are effective therapies, with rifampin and trimethoprim-sulfamethoxazole as possible alternatives [30]. Systemic *Bartonella* disease in an immunocompromised host always requires antibiotic therapy, sometimes for prolonged periods.

Leprosy

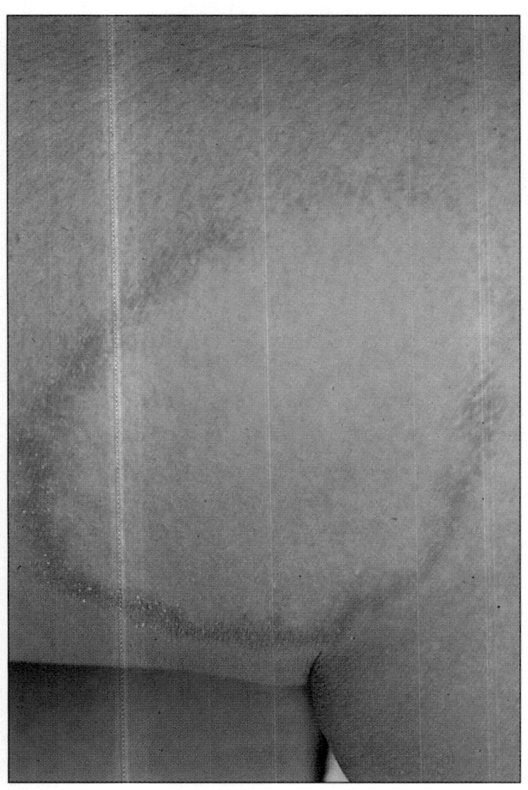

Figure 8-76 Polar tuberculoid leprosy lesion on the thigh. A large, anesthetic, hypopigmented lesion with erythematous borders is seen on the patient's thigh. Many of these lesions will heal without treatment, indicating that the patient possesses a high degree of immunity. With diagnosis, treatment of 6 to 12 months is adequate, with little fear of reactive episodes occurring in this polar form of the disease.

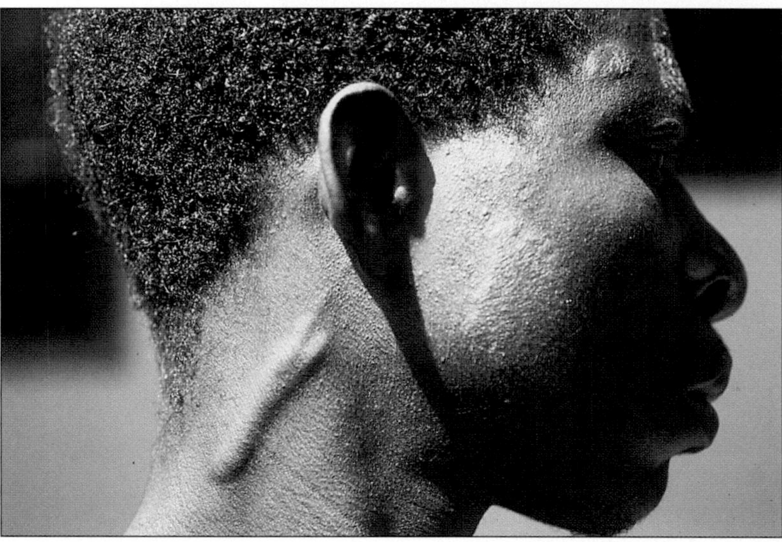

Figure 8-77 Enlarged greater auricular nerve in borderline tuberculoid leprosy. Other branches of the facial nerve are also enlarged in the neck of this patient. Skin lesions can be seen on the cheek and forehead. The nerves may or may not be tender, and any branch of a peripheral nerve may be enlarged and palpable.

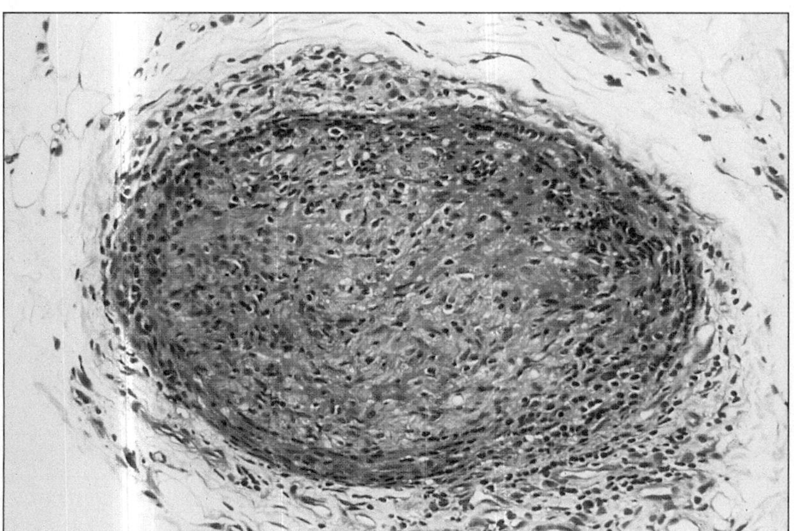

Figure 8-78 Histologic section showing involvement of cutaneous nerves in borderline tuberculoid disease. Inflammation and enlargement of cutaneous nerves are characteristic in borderline tuberculoid leprosy, but nerves may be less extensively enlarged than in tuberculoid lesions. (Hematoxylin-eosin stain.)

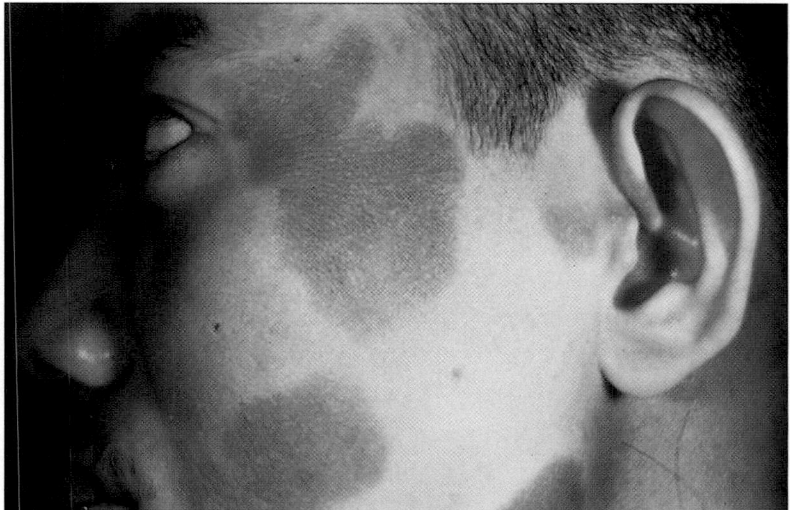

Figure 8-79 Multiple large hyperpigmented lesions of midborderline leprosy on a man's face. Lesion borders range from vague to well demarcated. Other lesions, some anesthetic and some with normal sensation, appear on the trunk and extremities of this patient. Inside the lesions, skin scrapings show a bacteriologic index of 2+ to 3+. Treatment with a three-drug regimen for at least 2 to 3 years is recommended for this multibacillary case.

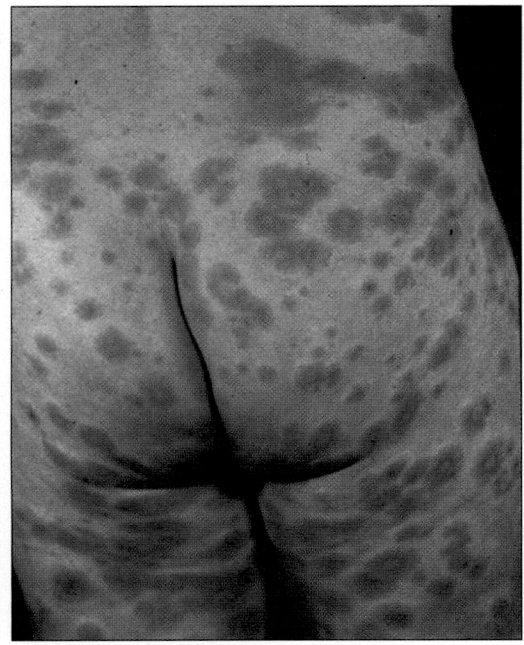

Figure 8-80 Multiple medium-sized lesions of borderline lepromatous leprosy covering a patient's buttocks and thighs. Multiple medium-sized lesions with central clearing with skin scrapings of 3+ to 4+ covered almost the entire body of this man.

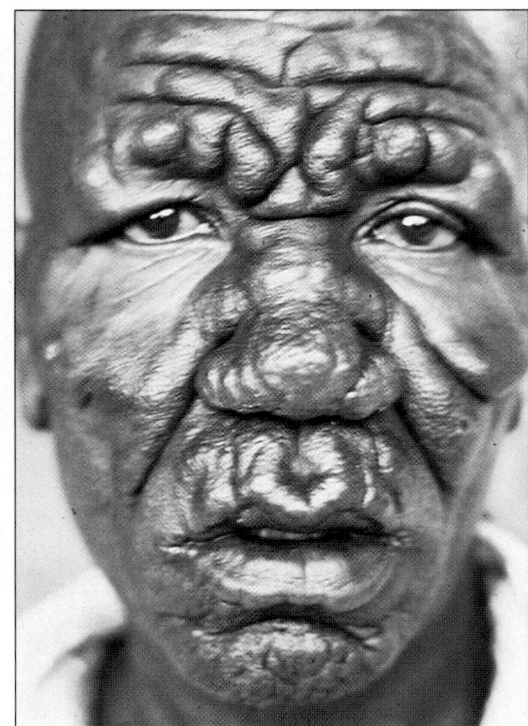

Figure 8-81 Lepromatous leprosy causing leonine facies. Far-advanced, untreated, polar lepromatous leprosy can result in the leonine facies shown in this patient. He has madarosis (loss of eyebrows), partial collapse of the nose, and nasal congestion, with a heavy bacterial load of 6+ anywhere on his body. Also, he has a loss of sensation in his distal extremities. Without treatment, this patient, with a high morphologic index indicating many solid-staining *Myobacterium leprae*, is considered a reservoir of infection. Treatment with multidrug therapy for 2 to 3 years is indicated. These patients are at risk for a type 2 reaction, called *erythema nodosum leprosum*.

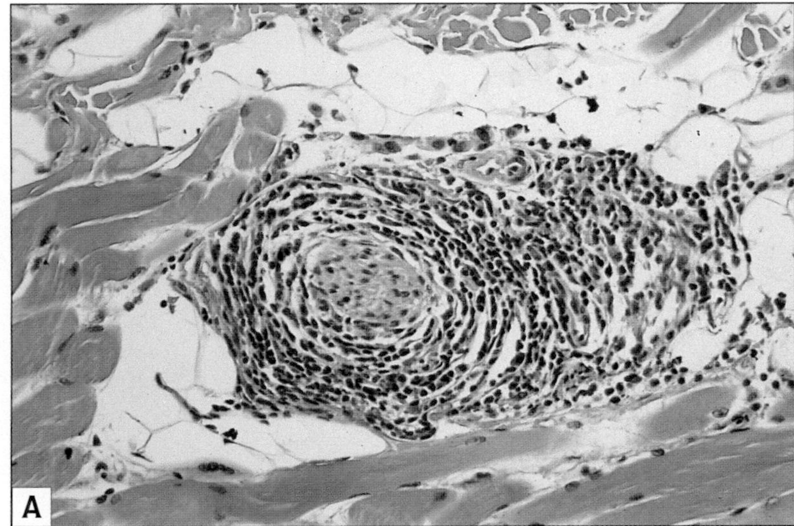

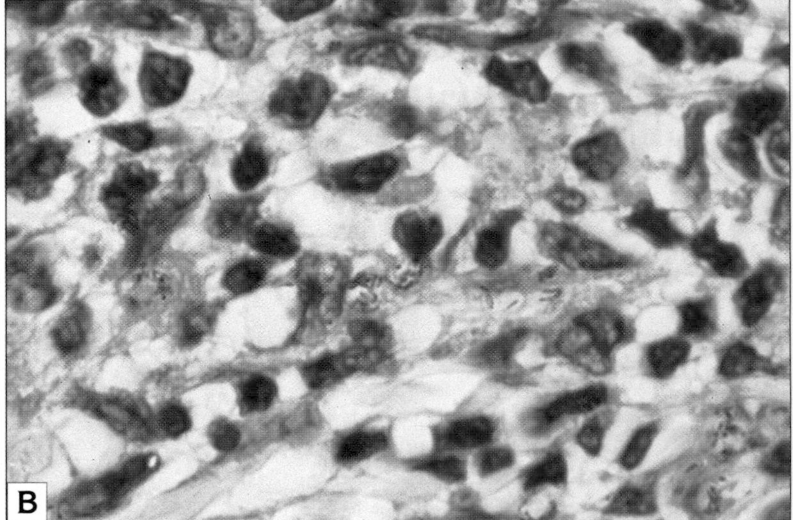

Figure 8-82 Histopathologic sections showing cutaneous nerve involvement in borderline lepromatous leprosy. **A**, The inflammatory involvement of cutaneous nerves is often accompanied by laminar, concentric thickening of the perineurium and epineurium, resulting in an "onion skin" appearance. (Hematoxylin-eosin stain.) **B**, On Fite staining, *Myobacterium leprae* are present in moderate to large numbers in histiocytes and in both the intraneural and epineural components of the nerves.

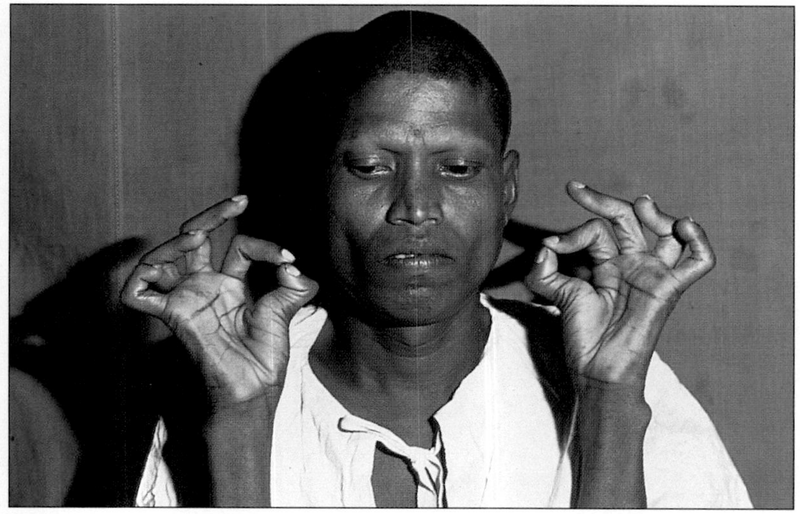

FIGURE 8-83 Bilateral median and ulnar nerve paralysis. Although this patient was classified as having borderline lepromatous leprosy, the loss of eyebrows suggests lepromatous leprosy. In any event, treatment for borderline lepromatous and lepromatous leprosy is the same. In this case, these hands can be helped by surgery.

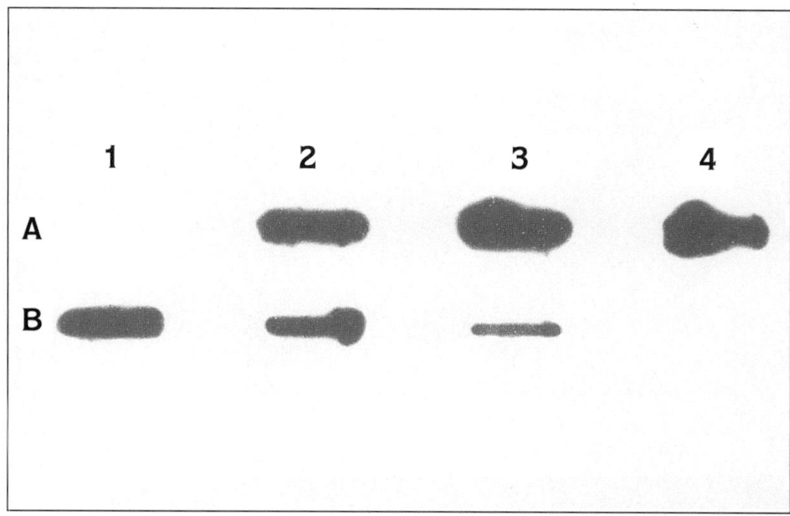

FIGURE 8-84 Polymerase chain reaction (PCR) technique used for confirming diagnosis of leprosy in nonspecific cases. PCR can be used to identify *Mycobacterium leprae* in tissues using primers and probes for a 360-basepair fragment of an 18-kDa protein gene of the organism. The technique is most useful in determining the identity of the organisms when clinical and/or histopathologic features present inconsistencies. Results of PCR amplification and slot-blot hybridization show negative control (*A1*), replicate tests of the biopsy sample showing positive bands for the *M. leprae* gene (*A2–4*), and positive controls (*B1–4*). Positive controls represent the PCR product from 330, 33, 3, and 0.3 bacilli, respectively. Although PCR theoretically can identify very rare organisms, in practice the results indicate that if *M. leprae* cannot be found by standard histologic examination in specimens highly suspect for leprosy, then only approximately 50% of these specimens will yield a positive PCR result [31]. (*Courtesy of* T. Gillis, MD.)

VIRAL HEMORRHAGIC FEVERS

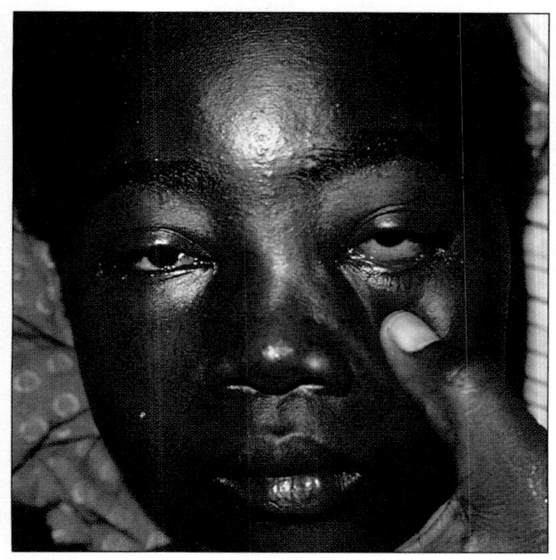

FIGURE 8-85 Conjunctival suffusion in hemorrhagic fever. One of the early signs of abnormal vascular regulation is conjunctival suffusion, seen here in a patient with Lassa fever. This suffusion may be both bulbar and palpebral. Erythema of the oropharyngeal mucous membranes also may be noted. (*Courtesy of* M. Monson, MD.)

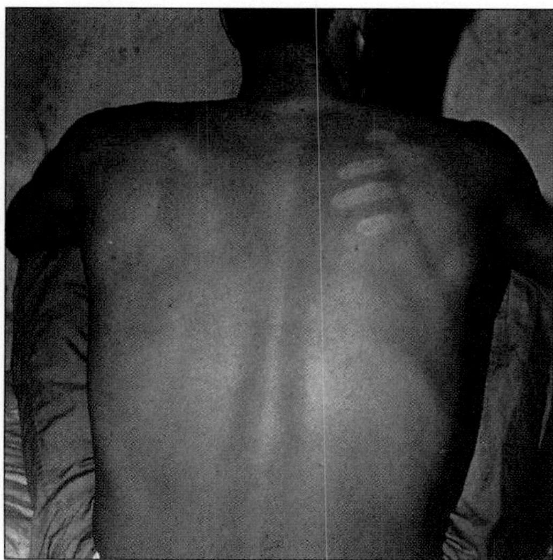

FIGURE 8-86 Acute erythema with blanching in Bolivian hemorrhagic fever. There is often a diffuse erythematous suffusion over the face, anterior thorax (often on the upper part or V-area around the neck), and posterior thorax, which blanches to pressure. These cutaneous or mucous membrane signs usually do not appear in hantavirus pulmonary syndrome, perhaps reflecting the compartmentalization of the pathologic process within the thorax or a different spectrum of mediators. (*Courtesy of* K. Johnson, MD.)

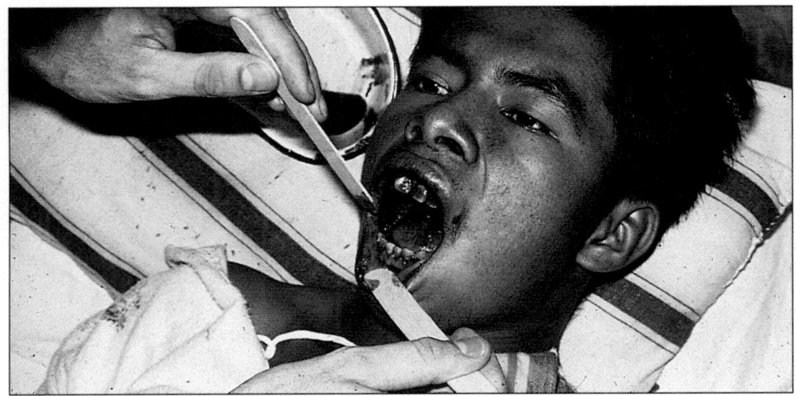

FIGURE 8-87 Gingival hemorrhages occur commonly in hemorrhagic fever, as seen in this patient with Bolivian hemorrhagic fever. Severe hemorrhage is usually manifest by bleeding from mucosal surfaces (particularly the oropharynx, gastrointestinal tract, and female genital tract) or by ecchymoses. (*Courtesy of* K. Johnson, MD.)

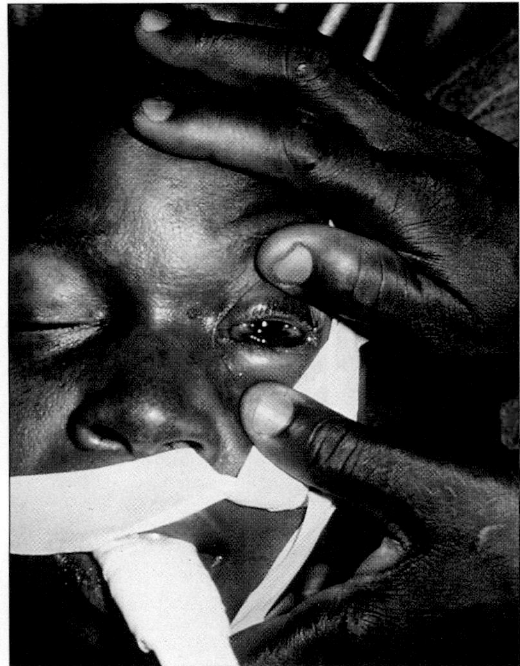

FIGURE 8-88 Facial edema. Periorbital edema, chemosis, and subconjunctival hemorrhage are seen in patient with Lassa fever. (*Courtesy of* M. Monson, MD.)

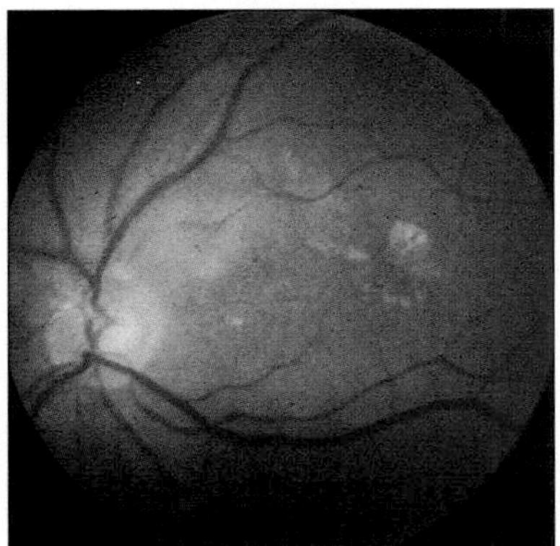

FIGURE 8-89 Retinal lesions in Rift Valley fever. Retinal lesions develop in 1% to 10% of patients with Rift Valley fever and are helpful in recognizing virus epidemics. These retinal photographs show the different characteristics, which consist of hemorrhage, infarct, and inflammation. The prognosis for recovery follows from the type of lesion encountered. Most described retinopathy is macular, but it is not known if this is because patients with macular lesions seek medical attention more commonly. (*Courtesy of* J. Meegan, PhD.)

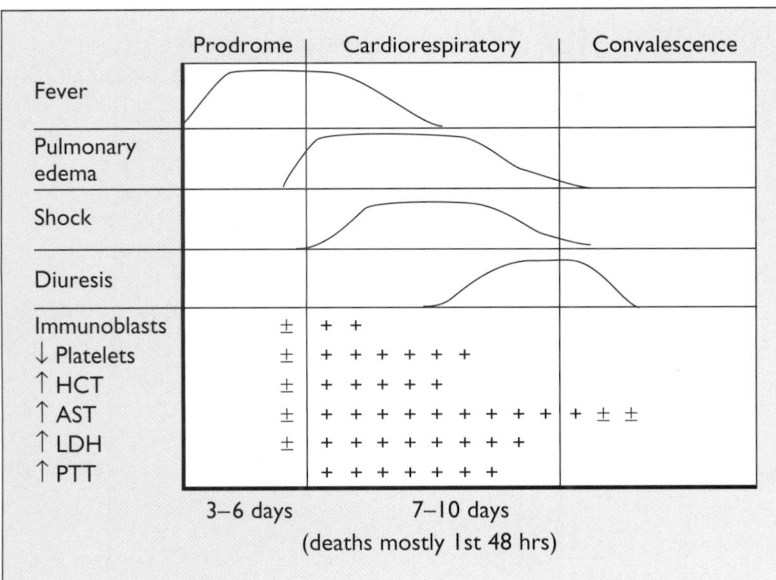

FIGURE 8-90 Clinical course of hantavirus pulmonary syndrome (HPS). The course of HPS differs from that for hemorrhagic fever with renal syndrome. Both show a febrile prodrome that leads to hypotension and end-organ failure. In both diseases, the onset of the immune response precedes severe organ failure, which is thought to be immunopathologic in nature. In the case of HPS, the hypotension does not result in shock until the onset of respiratory failure, but this may reflect the severe physiologic impact of the lung edema. (AST—aspartate aminotransferase; HCT—hematocrit; LDH—lactate dehydrogenase; PTT—partial thromboplastin time.)

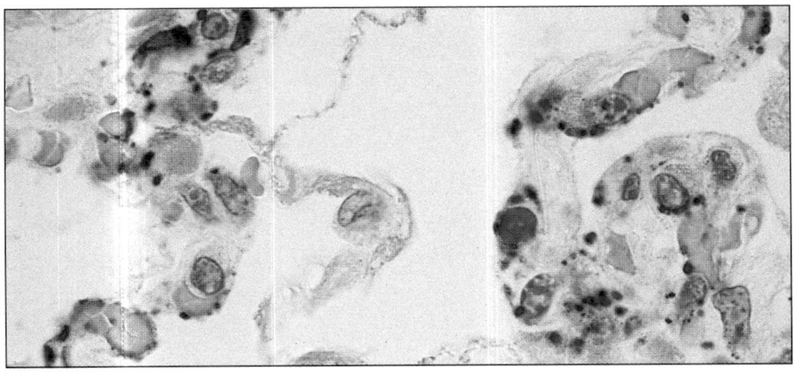

Figure 8-91 Microscopic features of hantavirus pulmonary syndrome. Immunohistochemical stain showing hantaviral antigens predominantly within endothelial cells of the pulmonary microvasculature. The acute pulmonary edema of hantavirus pulmonary syndrome correlates with the abundant hantaviral antigen selectively found in pulmonary capillary endothelium as well as the presence of CD4+ and CD8+ lymphoblasts and activated macrophages. Protein-rich fluid floods into the interstitium and alveoli, without any morphologic lesion in the blood-gas barrier at the light-microscopic level. The pathogenesis differs from that of the neutrophil-mediated lesion of classic adult respiratory distress syndrome, just as the hantavirus pulmonary syndrome differs in its detailed clinical, pathologic, and radiologic picture.

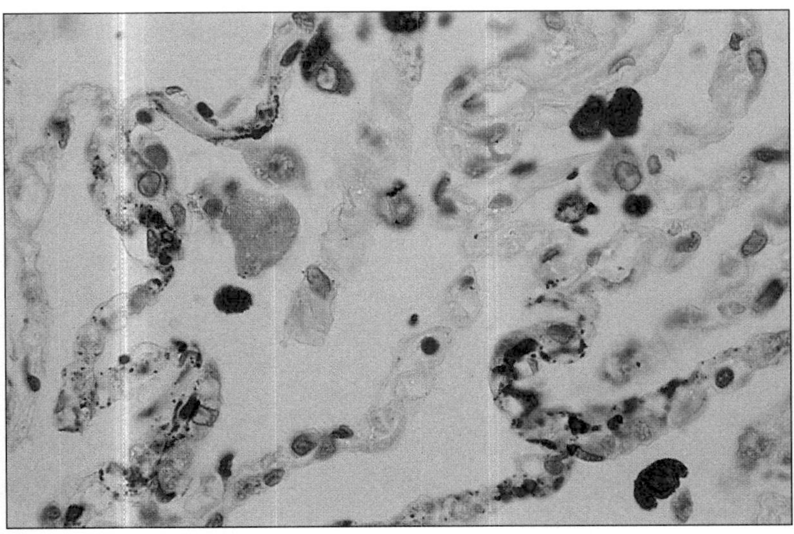

Figure 8-92 Viral antigens in lung tissue in a fatal case of viral hemorrhagic fever. The finding of viral antigens in capillary endothelia is not a unique feature of hantavirus pulmonary syndrome (HPS) and can be seen in a number of viral hemorrhagic fevers. In this figure, Ebola virus antigens are seen in infected endothelium, but, in contrast to HPS, they also can be seen in macrophages, fibroblasts, and other parenchymal cells of this lung section. In such cases, the organ dysfunction and the vasculopathy appear to be a consequence of a direct cytolytic injury and the elaboration of soluble mediators of inflammation.

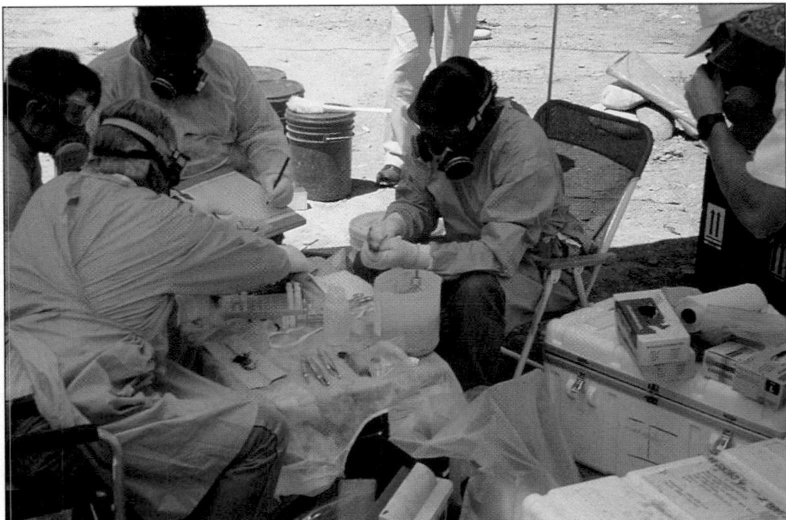

Figure 8-93 Rodent collection in the US southwest. When investigating the reservoirs of hazardous rodent-borne viruses, workers should take extensive precautions, as seen with this team of ecologists and mammalogists working in the southwestern United States. Respiratory protection against small-particle aerosols is provided by fitted respirators, and eye protection is worn. Materials are present for weighing, measuring, obtaining blood samples, and removing tissue samples. In the background, the red buckets are used for copious cleansing of instruments between uses, so that virus isolation and polymerase chain reaction tests on samples are not contaminated by carryover between animals.

Systemic Fungal Infections

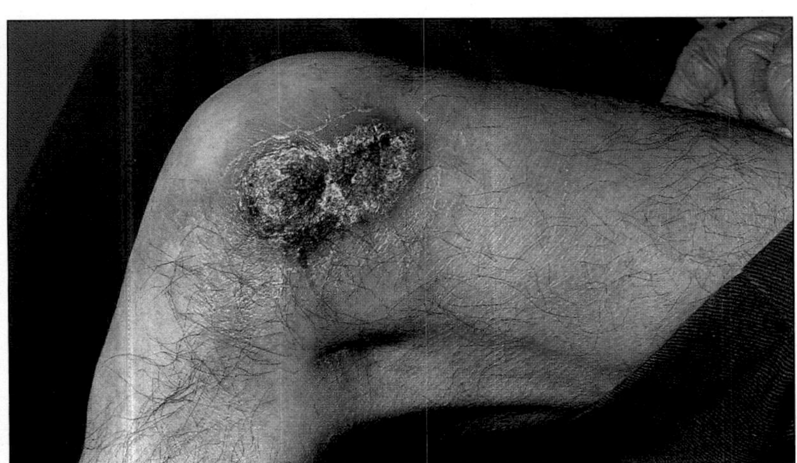

Figure 8-94 Large verrucous skin lesion of blastomycosis on the lateral aspect of the knee. The patient, a man aged 72 years, ran a sawmill in southern Michigan. This lesion was nontender and had been present for at least 6 months. Biopsy revealed large, thick-walled, broad-based budding yeasts typical of *Blastomyces dermatitidis*.

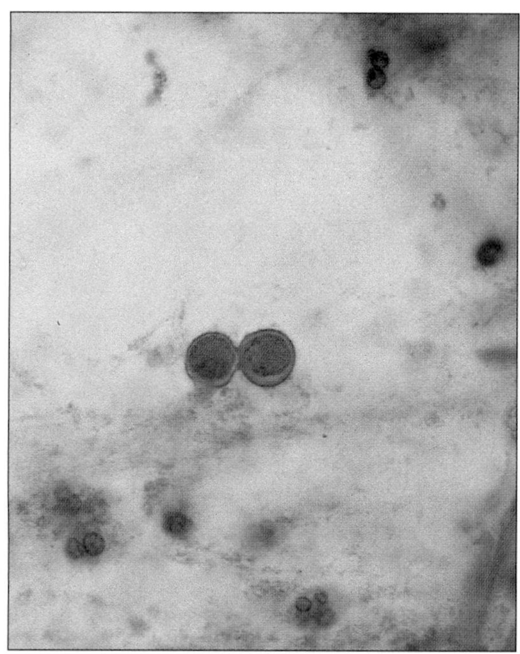

Figure 8-95 Papanicolaou-stained sputum smear in blastomycosis. Sputum was obtained from the patient in Figure 11-9 and stained with Papanicolaou stain. The appearance of this organism is diagnostic for blastomycosis. The organisms are large (8–20 µm) and thick-walled, and the daughter bud is attached to the mother cell by a broad base.

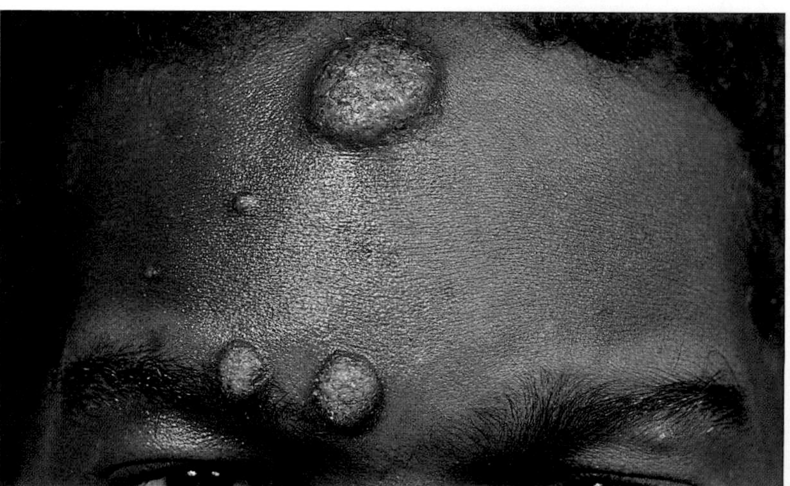

Figure 8-96 Multiple nodular skin lesions in blastomycosis. This man aged 40 years had fever, chills, and shortness of breath and developed more than 100 nodular skin lesions within the course of 2 weeks. At 2 weeks, the patient shows enlargement of all preexisting lesions and development of several new lesions.

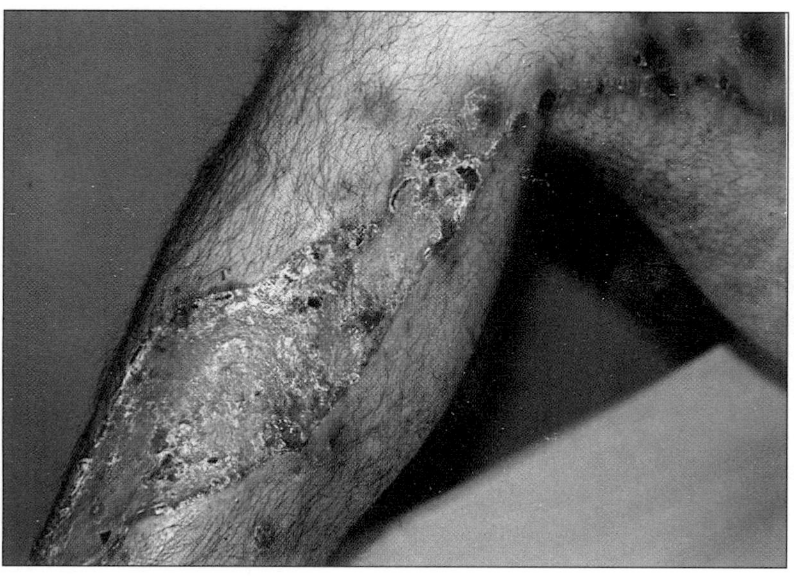

Figure 8-97 Multiple ulcerating and nodular lesions of cutaneous sporotrichosis on the lower leg. Multiple cutaneous lesions developed after a dirt bike accident in a man aged 22 years. The lesion on the lower leg had been skin-grafted several weeks previously, and then new lesions arose at the borders of the graft. Culture of the material removed at operation yielded *Sporothrix schenckii*, and the patient ultimately responded to oral azole therapy.

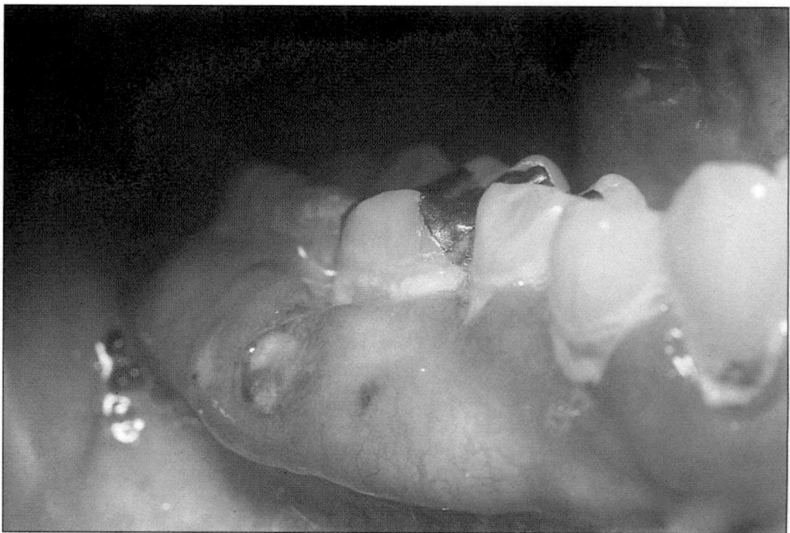

Figure 8-98 Oropharyngeal ulcer of disseminated histoplasmosis. An ulcerated lesion is seen on the gum below the molar teeth in a man aged 65 years who complained of sore mouth, weight loss, and night sweats. Biopsy of this lesion showed small budding yeasts with a morphology typical of *Histoplasma capsulatum*, and the organism grew in culture. (*From* Kauffman [32]; with permission.)

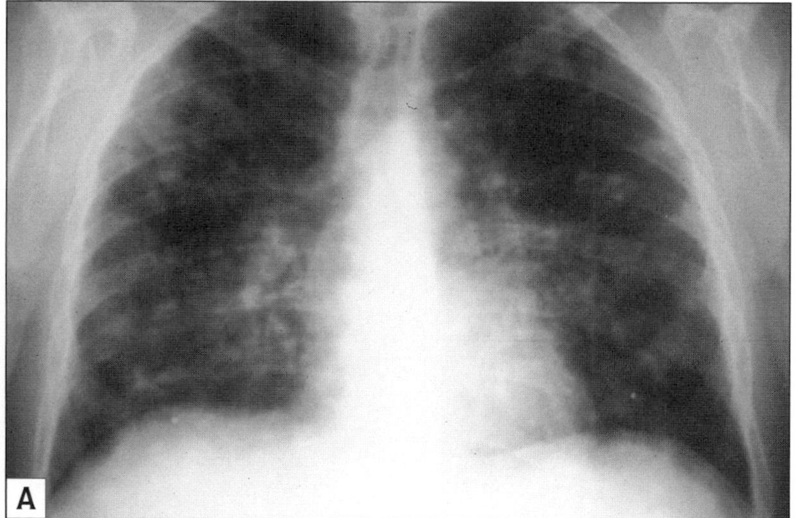

Figure 8-99 Pulmonary coccidioidomycosis. **A**, A chest radiograph of a man aged 40 years with HIV infection. The patient was from Michigan but had previously lived in Phoenix. He had fevers, weight loss, fatigue, dyspnea, and cough. Radiograph shows extensive bilateral nodular infiltrates. Culture of bronchoalveolar lavage fluid yielded *Coccidioides immitis*. (*continued*)

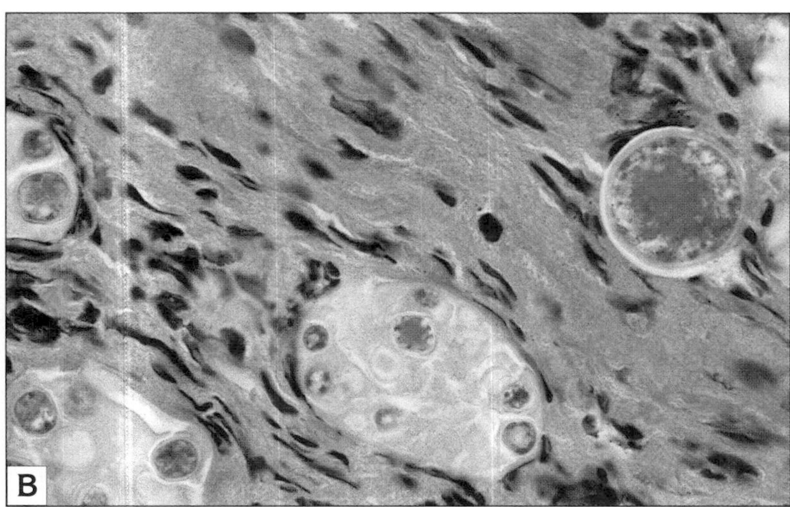

Figure 8-99 (*continued*) **B**, A lung biopsy specimen shows numerous large spherules (50–80 µm) with endospores typical of *Coccidioides immitis*. (Hematoxylin-eosin stain.)

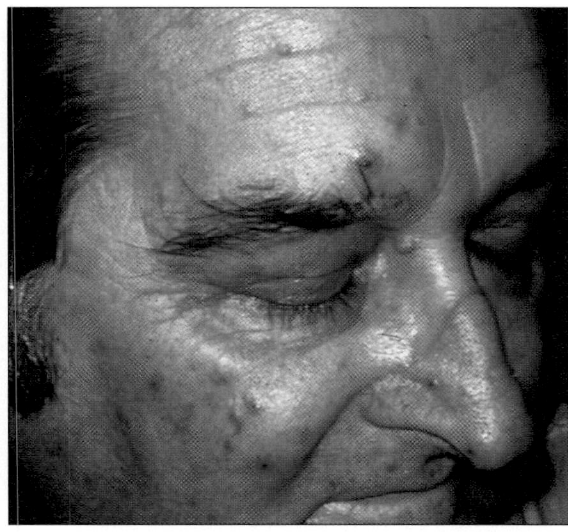

Figure 8-100 Multiple, painless skin lesions due to cryptococcosis. A man aged 50 years with Hodgkin's disease developed fever, shortness of breath, and multiple nontender skin lesions. Lesions on his face arose over the course of a week.

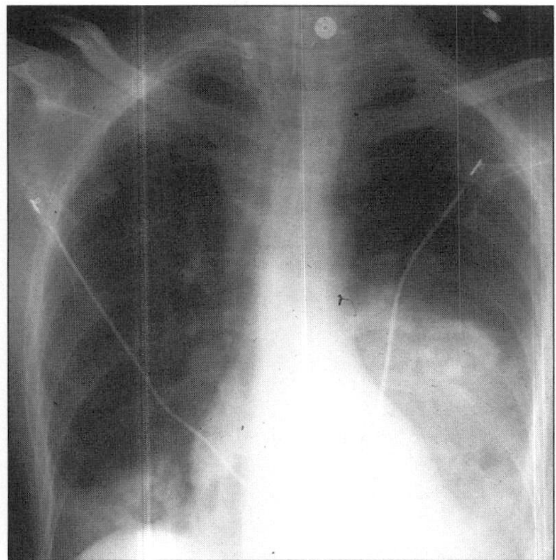

Figure 8-101 Chest radiograph showing cavitary lesions in pulmonary aspergillosis. A patient with sarcoidosis on high-dose prednisone for 2 months came to the hospital with acute dyspnea, pleuritic chest pain, fever, and confusion. Cavitation is obvious in the lesion in the right lower lobe.

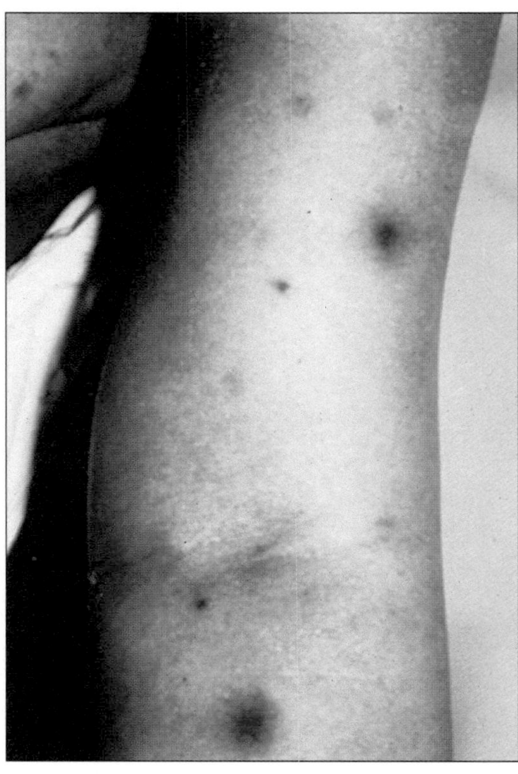

Figure 8-102 Skin lesions of disseminated candidiasis in a young woman with acute leukemia who was neutropenic and on broad-spectrum antibiotics. These lesions have an erythematous base and necrotic center. Aspirate from one of the lesions grew *Candida albicans*, and biopsy showed budding yeast and pseudohyphae. (*Courtesy of* P.G. Jones, MD.)

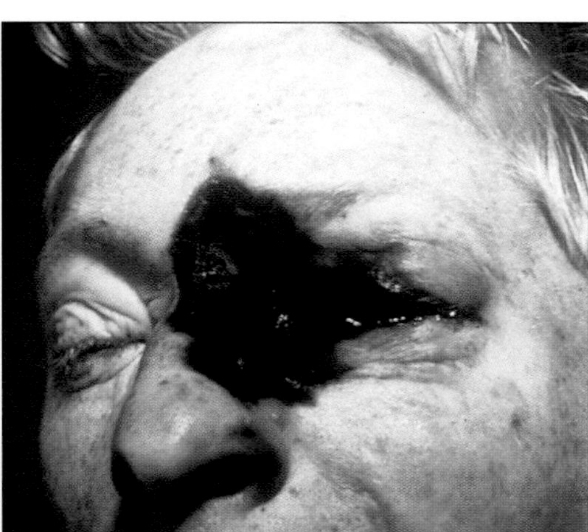

Figure 8-103 Rapidly progressive rhinocerebral mucormycosis. A middle-aged man with insulin-dependent diabetes mellitus and recurrent ketoacidosis presented with rapidly progressive mucormycosis of the sinus, leading to cerebral infarction and death. (*Courtesy of* T. Walsh, MD; *from* Walsh *et al.* [33].)

Manifestations of Protozoal and Helminthic Diseases in Latin America

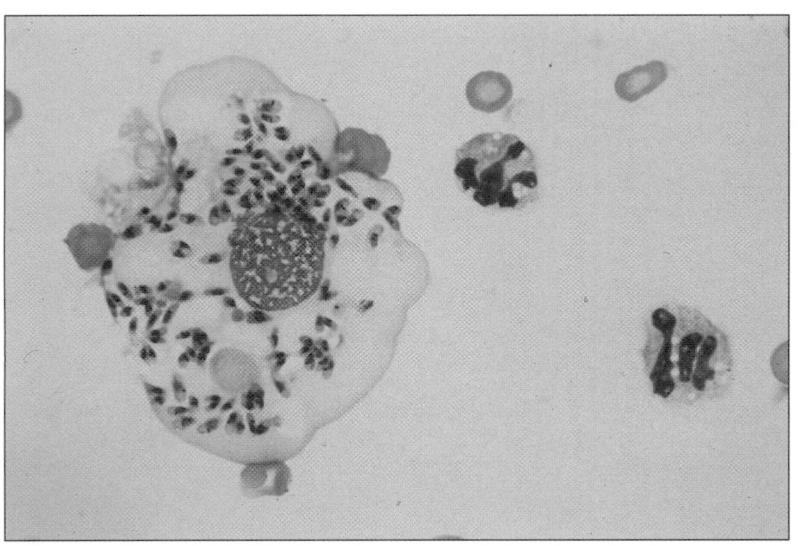

Figure 8-104 *Leishmania* amastigotes in an infected macrophage (Wright-Giemsa stain), seen in a cytocentrifuged preparation of pleural fluid from a patient with visceral leishmaniasis and AIDS. *Leishmania* exist within mononuclear phagocytes as intracellular amastigotes. Although slight ultrastructural differences exist among amastigotes of different *Leishmania* species, they are not sufficient to allow for species-specific identification [34]. (*Courtesy of* D.M. Markovitz, MD, and R.F. Betts, MD.)

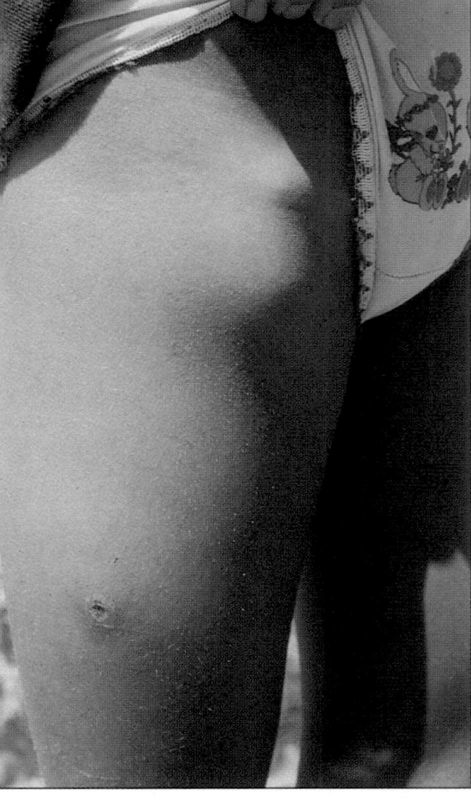

Figure 8-105 Early American cutaneous leishmaniasis with associated regional lymphadenopathy due to *Leishmania (Vianna) braziliensis*. A number of *Leishmania* species can produce cutaneous leishmaniasis. The skin lesion develops weeks to months after promastigotes are inoculated by an infected sandfly. Some persons infected with *L. (V.) braziliensis*, such as this patient, develop regional lymphadenopathy, fever, malaise, and constitutional symptoms prior to the appearance of the skin lesion. The systemic findings resolve as the skin lesion develops.

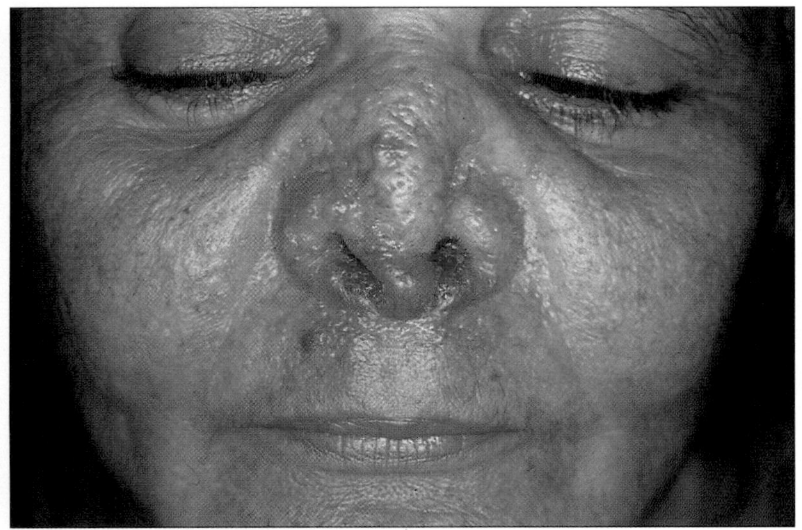

Figure 8-106 American mucosal leishmaniasis due to *Leishmania (Vianna) braziliensis* with involvement of the nasal septum. A small subset of persons with skin lesions due to *L. (V.) braziliensis* manifest mucosal disease months to years after the initial cutaneous lesion(s) resolves. Those affected frequently present with chronic nasal stuffiness.

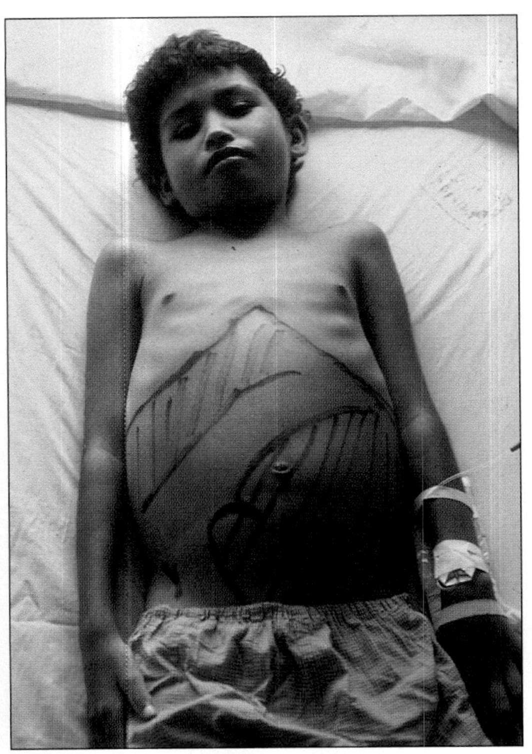

Figure 8-107 American visceral leishmaniasis with hepatosplenomegaly due to *Leishmania (L.) chagasi*. Amastigotes are found in macrophages throughout the reticuloendothelial system in persons with visceral leishmaniasis. The spleen is often massively enlarged.

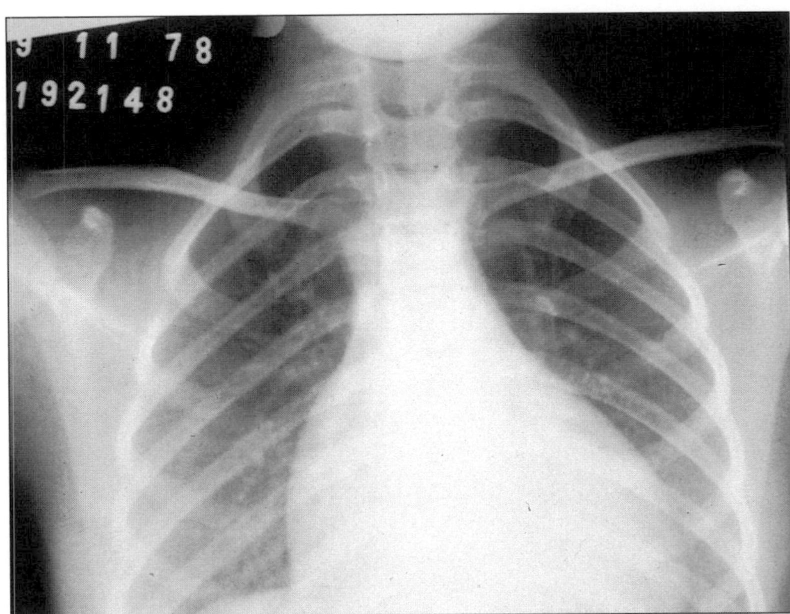

Figure 8-108 Cardiomegaly in a patient with chronic Chagas' disease. Although acute *Trypanosoma cruzi* infections can be fatal, most are asymptomatic or mild and resolve spontaneously. However, parasitemia can persist for decades. A subset of infected persons develop chagasic cardiomyopathy with congestive heart failure, conduction abnormalities, arrhythmias, and thromboemboli.

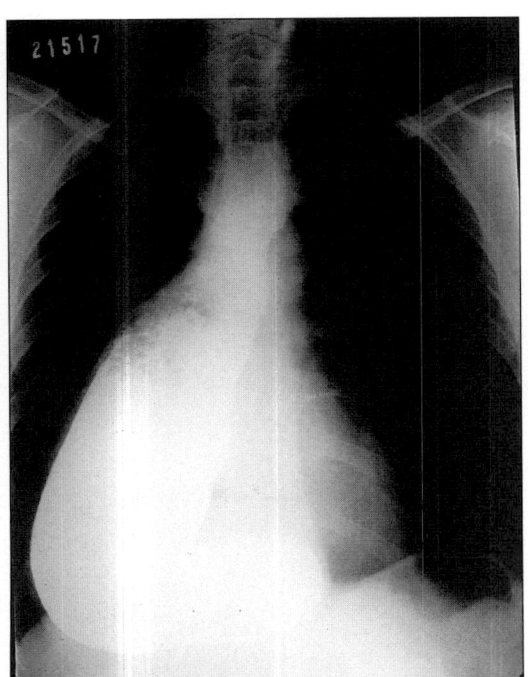

Figure 8-109 Barium swallow demonstrating megaesophagus in chronic Chagas' disease. Progressive esophageal dilatation occurs as a result of autoimmune destruction of the myenteric plexus. Affected persons experience dysphagia, odynophagia, chest pain, and regurgitation. Aspiration pneumonia can complicate advanced disease.

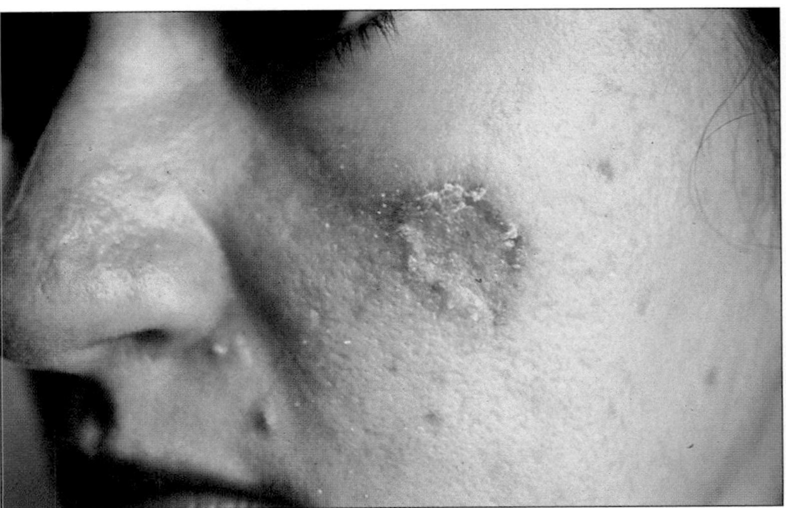

Figure 8-110 American cutaneous leishmaniasis on a patient's cheek. Not all infections result in ulceration. Cutaneous leishmaniasis must be considered in the differential diagnosis of any chronic skin lesion in a person who has been exposed in an endemic area.

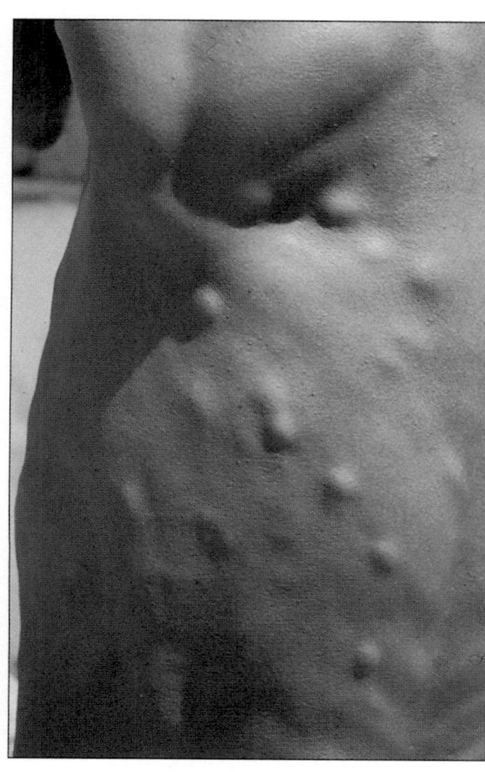

Figure 8-111 Cysticerci in subcutaneous tissue.

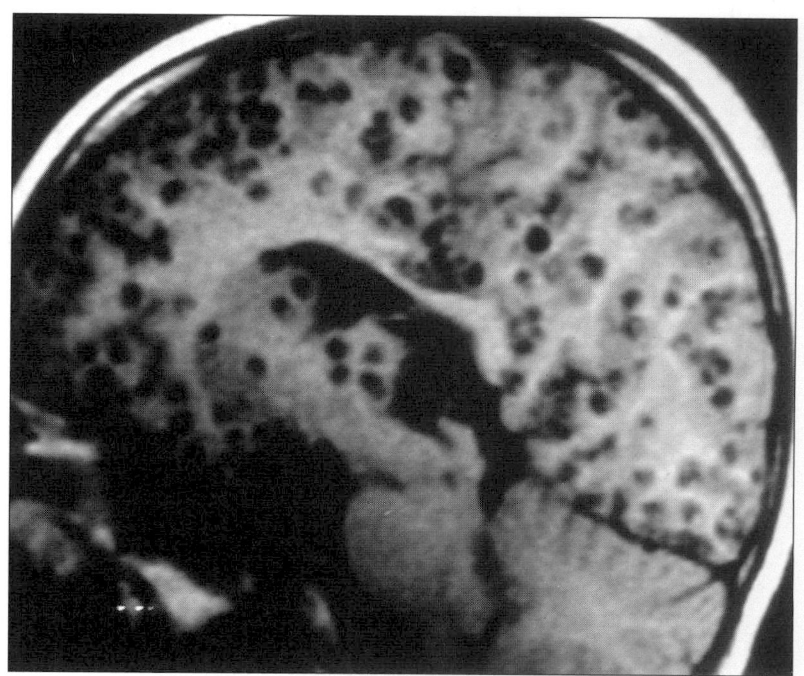

Figure 8-112 Sagittal view of severe neurocysticercosis due to *Taenia solium* seen on a magnetic resonance scan. Neurocysticercosis is a common cause of seizures and focal neurologic abnormalities in Latin America.

Cutaneous Manifestations of Infection in the Immunocompromised Host

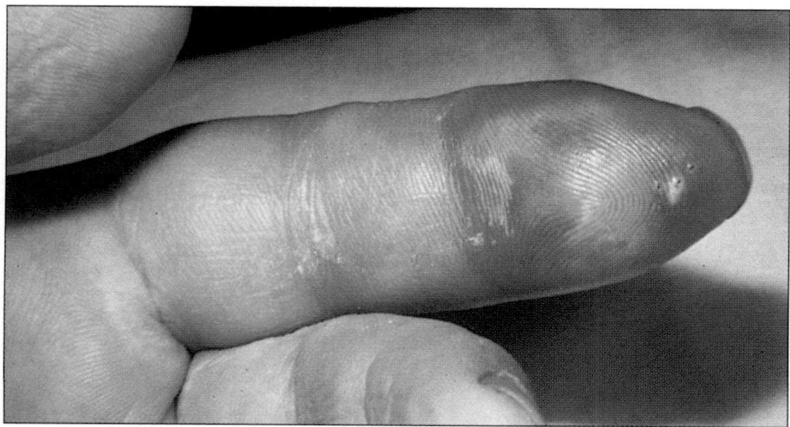

Figure 8-113 Skin lesion on a finger due to *Staphylococcus aureus*. Skin lesions due to *S. aureus* in the immunocompromised host can take many forms, ranging from papules to pustules to ulcers or blebs. Cellulitis also may be seen. The bleb on this patient's finger was at the site of a skin puncture for a complete blood count. On aspiration, the bleb yielded gram-positive cocci on staining and *S. aureus* in culture. Sensitivity studies showed it to be sensitive to methicillin. The patient responded to intravenous therapy with oxacillin. We have isolated mixed cultures of *S. aureus* and *Clostridium perfringens* from such lesions and have added high-dose penicillin to the oxacillin. Mixed infections with *Streptococcus pyogenes* and *S. aureus* also may be seen. Viridans streptococci can cause acute septic syndromes with a maculopapular skin rash and rapid progression to septic shock. The organisms may be resistant to β-lactam antibiotics and require vancomycin. Smears, cultures, and susceptibility studies are all important studies in the patient's evaluation.

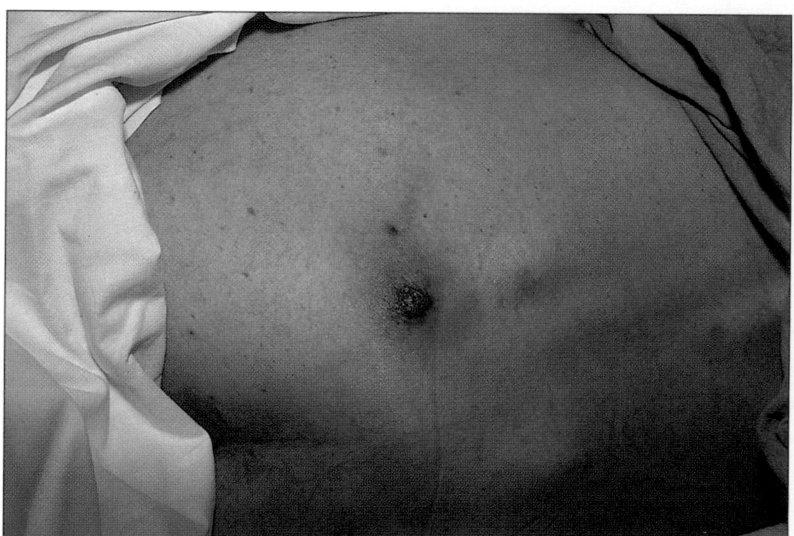

Figure 8-114 Lesion due to mixed infection on a patient's lower back. This lesion, in a neutropenic patient, was due to a mixture of *Staphylococcus aureus* and *Pseudomonas aeruginosa*. Patients may become septic due to more than one organism when they are profoundly neutropenic or when intravenous catheters become contaminated and result in polymicrobial sepsis.

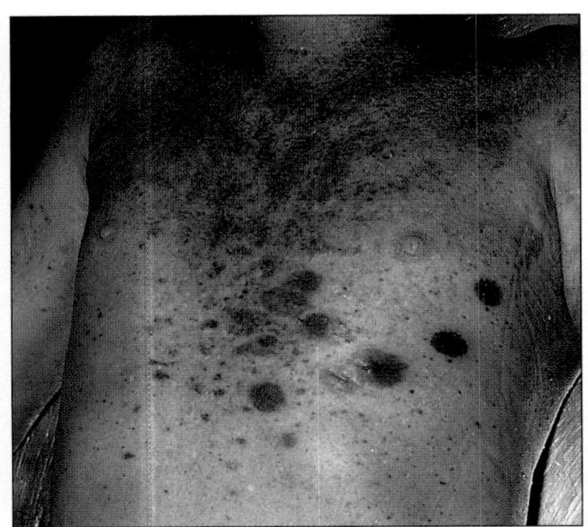

FIGURE 8-115 Classic ecthyma gangrenosum secondary to *Pseudomonas aeruginosa* infection. The black centers set on a red raised papule result from invasion of blood vessels, with clotting and subsequent infarction and necrosis of tissue. *P. aeruginosa* also can produce vesicles, blebs, and cellulitis.

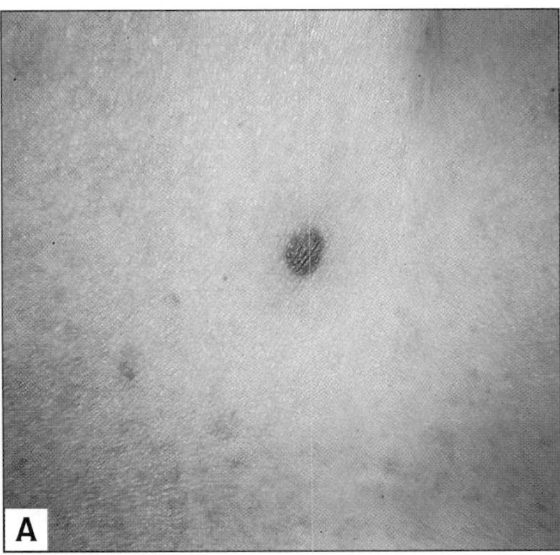

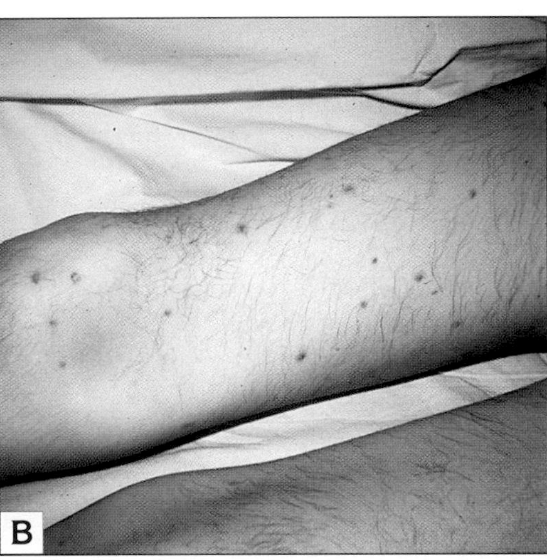

FIGURE 8-116 Skin lesions in disseminated candidiasis. Candidiasis may result in few or many lesions, and the lesions can be expected to contain the organisms. If a Gram stain of an aspirate is negative, a biopsy should be done immediately. **A**, A patient with a few isolated lesions due to *Candida*. **B**, A patient with many scattered lesions over the legs due to *Candida*. These lesions have a purplish hue due to hemorrhage into them.

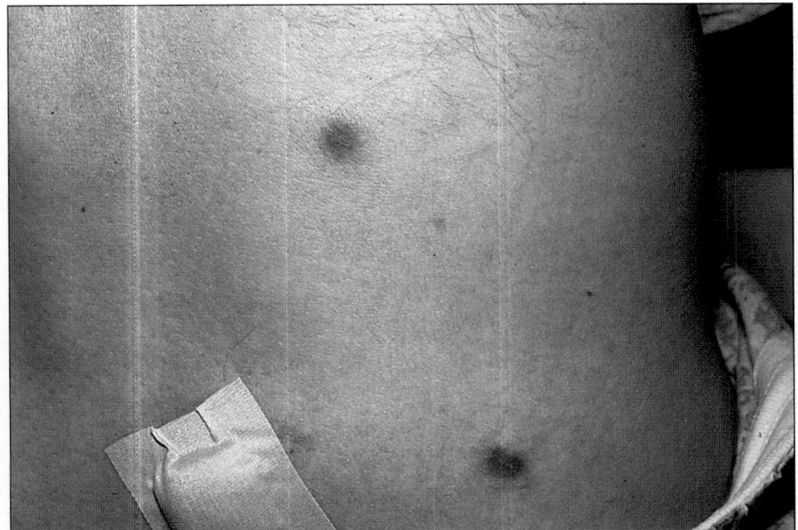

FIGURE 8-117 Skin lesions of trichosporosis. This febrile neutropenic patient developed skin lesions while receiving broad-spectrum antibacterial therapy. He also had a hemorrhagic pharyngitis. Biopsy of a skin lesion and the hemorrhagic material from the throat yielded *Trichosporon beigelii*. It is important to isolate the organism, because *T. beigelii* may be resistant to amphotericin B and most azoles except miconazole.

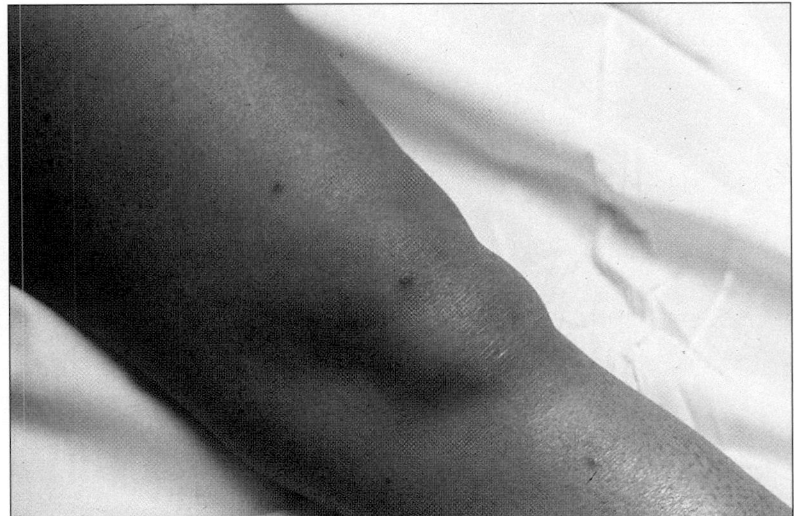

FIGURE 8-118 Vesicular skin lesions and joint disease due to *Mycobacterium haemophilum* in a bone marrow transplant recipient. The patient developed papular, vesicular, and pustular lesions along with an arthritis of the knee. Aspirate of a vesicular skin lesion revealed numerous acid-fast bacilli but no growth on routine mycobacterial cultures. The specimen was, however, grown at room temperature with hemosiderin to encourage the growth of *M. haemophilum*. The laboratory must be alerted to the need for special culture requirements when *M. haemophilum* is suspected. The disease is seen in patients with AIDS, lymphomas, multiple myeloma, and bone marrow or solid organ transplants and should be anticipated in anyone with a T-cell defect and skin and joint disease. In severe cases, pneumonia may result.

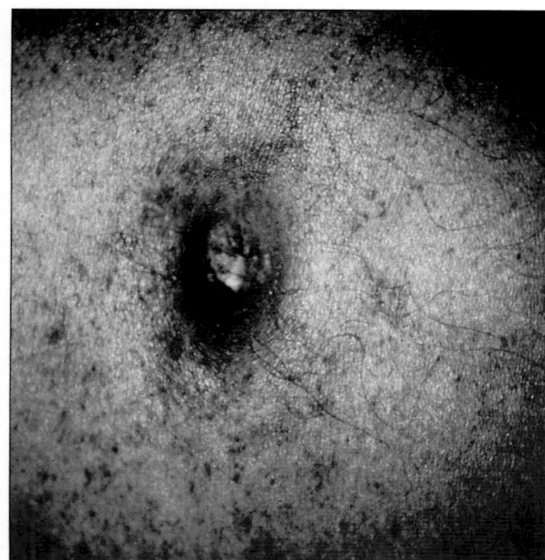

Figure 8-119 Disseminated strongyloidiasis. This bone marrow transplant recipient developed abdominal signs and a pneumonia. A "thumbprint" rash developed around his umbilicus due to distended venules in that area secondary to a disseminated (hyperinfection syndrome) *Strongyloides stercoralis* infection. (*From* Raffalli *et al.* [35]; with permission.)

References

1. Modlin JF: Coxsackieviruses, echoviruses, and newer enteroviruses. *In* Mandell GL, Bennett JE, Dolin (eds.): *Principles and Practice of Infectious Diseases*, 4th ed. New York: Churchill Livingstone; 1995:1620–1636.
2. Scheld WM, Sande MA: Endocarditis and intravascular infections. *In* Mandell GL, Bennett JE, Dolin R (eds.): *Principles and Practice of Infectious Diseases*. 4th ed. New York: Churchill Livingstone; 1995:740–783.
3. Sande MA, Strausbaugh LJ: Infective endocarditis. *In* Hook EW, Mandell GL, Gwaltney JM Jr, *et al.* (eds.): *Current Concepts in Infectious Diseases*. New York: Wiley; 1977.
4. Durack DT, Lukes AS, Braight DK, *et al.*: New criteria for diagnosis of infective endocarditis. *Am J Med* 1995, 96:200–209.
5. Beutler B, Cerami A: Biology of cachectin/TNF—A primary mediator of the host response. *Annu Rev Immunol* 1989, 7:625–655.
6. Rahn D: Lyme disease: Clinical manifestations, diagnosis, and treatment. *Semin Arthritis Rheum* 1991, 20:201–218.
7. Rahn D, Malawista SE: Clinical judgement in Lyme disease. *Hosp Pract* 1990, 25(Mar 30):39–56.
8. Steere AC, *et al.*: The early clinical manifestations of Lyme disease. *Ann Intern Med* 1983, 99:76–82.
9. Klempner MS: Lyme disease [images in clinical medicine]. *N Engl J Med* 1992, 327:1793.
10. Steere AC: Lyme disease: *In* Kelley WN, Harris ED, Ruddy S, Sledge CB (eds.): *Textbook of Rheumatology*, 4th ed. Philadelphia: W.B. Saunders; 1993:1484–1493.
11. Rahn DW, Malawista SE: Treatment of Lyme disease. *In* Rogers DE, Bone R, Clin MJ, *et al.*: *1994 Year Book of Medicine*. St. Louis: Mosby-Year Book; 1995:xxi–xxxvi.
12. Anderson BE, Sims KG, Olson JG, *et al.*: *Amblyomma americanum*: A potential vector of human ehrlichiosis. *Am J Trop Med Hyg* 1993, 49:239–244.
13. Dawson JE, Anderson BE, Fishbein DB, *et al.*: Isolation and characterization of an *Ehrlichia* sp. from a patient diagnosed with human ehrlichiosis. *J Clin Microbiol* 1991, 29:2741–2745.
14. Rikihisa Y: The tribe *Ehrlichiae* and ehrlichial diseases. *Clin Microbiol Rev* 1991, 4:286–308.
15. Chen SM, Dumler JS, Bakken JS, Walker DH: Identification of a granulocytotropic *Ehrlichia* species as the etiologic agent of human disese. *J Clin Microbiol* 1994, 32:589–595.
16. Bakken JS, Dumler JS, Chen SM, *et al.*: Human granulocytic ehrlichiosis in the upper Midwest United States: A new species emerging? *JAMA* 1994, 272:212–218.
17. Fishbein DB, Dawson JE, Robinson LE: Human ehrlichiosis in the United States, 1985 to 1990. *Ann Intern Med* 1994, 120:736–743.
18. Bakken JS, Dumler JS: Human granulocytic ehrlichiosis (HGE): Clinical and laboratory characteristics of 41 patients from Minnesota and Wisconsin. *JAMA* 1996, 275:199–205.
19. Eng TR, Harkness JR, Fishbein DB, *et al.*: Epidemiologic, clinical, and laboratory findings of human ehrlichiosis in the United States, 1988. *JAMA* 1990, 264:2251–2258.
20. Krause PJ, Telford SR III, Persing DH, *et al.*: Increased severity of Lyme disease due to concurrent babesiosis (in press).
21. Pruthi RK, Marshall WF, Wiltsie JC, Persing DH: Human babesiosis. *Mayo Clin Proc* 1995, 70:853–862.
22. Persing DH, Herwaldt BL, Glaser C, *et al.*: Infection with *Babesia*-like organisms in northern California. *N Engl J Med* 1995, 332:298–303.
23. Quick RE, Herwaldt BL, Thomford JW, *et al.*: Babesiosis in Washington State: A new species of *Babesia*? *Ann Intern Med* 1993, 119:284–290.
24. Thomford JW, Conrad PA, Telford SR, *et al.*: Cultivation and phylogenetic characterization of a newly recognized human pathogenic protozoan. *J Infect Dis* 1994, 169:1050–1056.
25. Regnery RL, Perkins BA, Olson JG, Bibb W: Serological response to "Rochalimaea henselae" antigen in suspected cat scratch disease. *Lancet* 1992, 339:1443–1445.
26. Koehler JE, Glaser CA, Tappero JW: *Rochalimaea henselae* infection: A new zoonosis with the domestic cat as reservoir. *JAMA* 1994, 271:531–535.
27. Spach DH, Kanter AS, Dougherty MJ, *et al.*: *Bartonella (Rochalimaea) quintana* bacteremia in inner-city patients with chronic alcoholism. *N Engl J Med* 1995, 332:424–428.
28. LeBoit PE, Berger TM, Egbert BM, *et al.*: Bacillary angiomatosis: The histopathology and differential diagnosis of a pseudoneoplastic infection in patients with human immunodeficiency virus disease. *Am J Surg Pathol* 1989, 13:909–920.
29. Dalton MJ, Robinson LE, Cooper J, *et al.*: Use of *Bartonella* antigens for serologic diagnosis of cat-scratch disease at a national referral center. *Arch Intern Med* 1995, 155:1670–1676.

30. Margileth AM: Antibiotic therapy for cat-scratch disease: Clinical study of the therapeutic outcome in 268 patients and a review of the literature. *Pediatr Infect Dis J* 1992, 11:474–478.

31. Willimas DL, Gillis TP, Fiallo P, *et al.*: Detection of *Mycobacterium leprae* and the potential for monitoring antileprosy drug therapy directly from skin biopsies by PCR. *Mol Cell Probes* 1992, 6:401–410.

32. Kauffman CA: Fungal infections. *Clin Geriatr Med* 1992, 8:777–791.

33. Walsh T, Rinaldi M, Pizzo PA: Zygomycosis of the respiratory tract. *In* Sarosi GA, Davies SF (eds.): *Fungal Diseases of the Lung*. New York: Raven Press; 1993.

34. Chenoweth CE, Singal S, Pearson RD, *et al.*: AIDS-related visceral leishmaniasis presenting in a pleural effusion. *Chest* 1993, 103:648–649.

35. Raffalli J, Friedman C, Reid D, *et al.*: Diagnosis: Disseminated *Strongyloides stercoralis* infection. *Clin Infect Dis* 1995, 21:1459.

CHAPTER 9

Urinary Tract Infections and Infections of the Female Pelvis

Editor
Jack D. Sobel

Contributors
Michel G. Bergeron
Claude Delage
Harry A. Gallis
Dominique Giroux
Elaine T. Kaye
Edward D. Kim
J. Curtis Nickel
Lindsay E. Nicolle
Paul Nyirjesy
Anthony J. Schaeffer
Jack D. Sobel
David E. Soper
Richard L. Sweet
Harold C. Wiesenfeld
Edward S. Wong

Cystitis

Epidemiology of bacterial cystitis

20%–30% of women experience an episode of cystitis during their lifetime
~20% of women experience recurrent infections
Recurrent infections are often clustered: two thirds occur within 6 months
Annually, in the United States, bacterial cystitis accounts for:
- 7 million visits to physicians' offices
- 1% of clinic visits
- $1 billion in outpatient care costs

Figure 9-1 Epidemiology of bacterial cystitis. The incidence of bacterial cystitis varies by age and sex. Women in their reproductive years are particularly prone to symptomatic episodes and account for the majority of visits to physicians in private offices and clinics. Approximately 20% of these women will experience recurrent urinary tract infections. Most recurrences are uncomplicated and can be managed by short courses of antibiotics or, if recurrences are frequent, by chronic suppression or postcoital antibiotics. The annual cost for the management of bacterial cystitis in the ambulatory care setting is estimated to be approximately $1 billion.

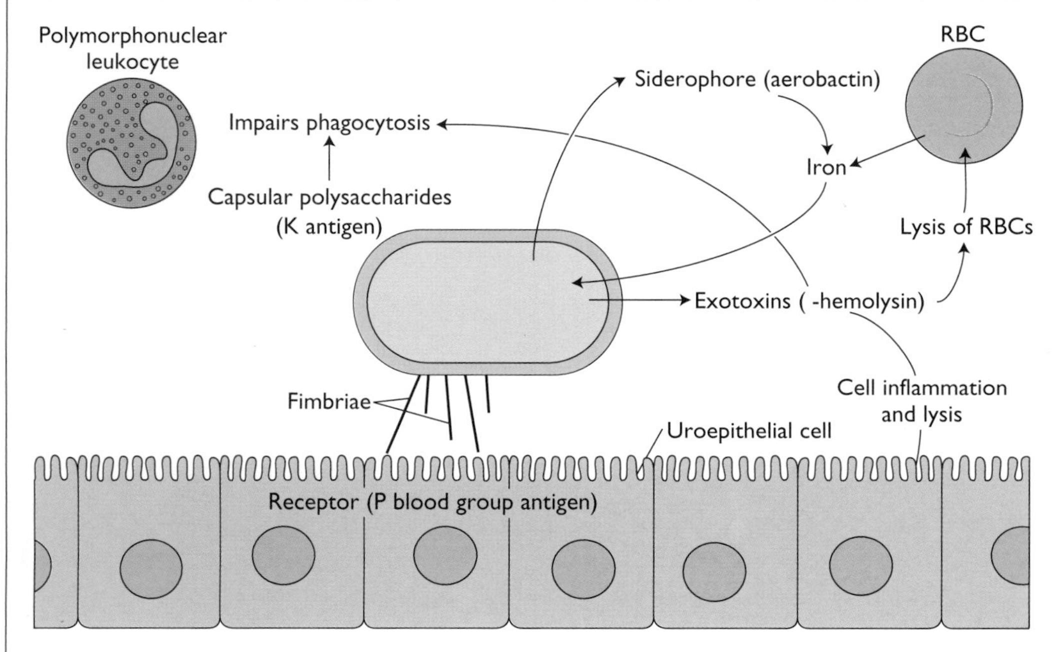

Figure 9-2 Interaction of bacterial virulence factors with host cell. Virulence factors interact in a complex manner. Fimbriae mediate attachment of the bacterium to uroepithelial cells, facilitating colonization and infection. Patients with certain P blood group antigens have receptors on their uroepithelial cells consisting of a Gal (α 1–4)Gal β terminal moiety that provides high-affinity attachment sites for *Escherichia coli* with P-fimbriae. These patients are more prone to recurrent infections, including pyelonephritis. The polysaccharide capsule is both antiphagocytic and anticomplementary. Other virulence factors include the elaboration of exotoxins (α-hemolysin), which mediate inflammation and cell lysis, and siderophores (aerobactin), which scavenge for iron necessary for bacterial growth. (RBC—red blood cell.)

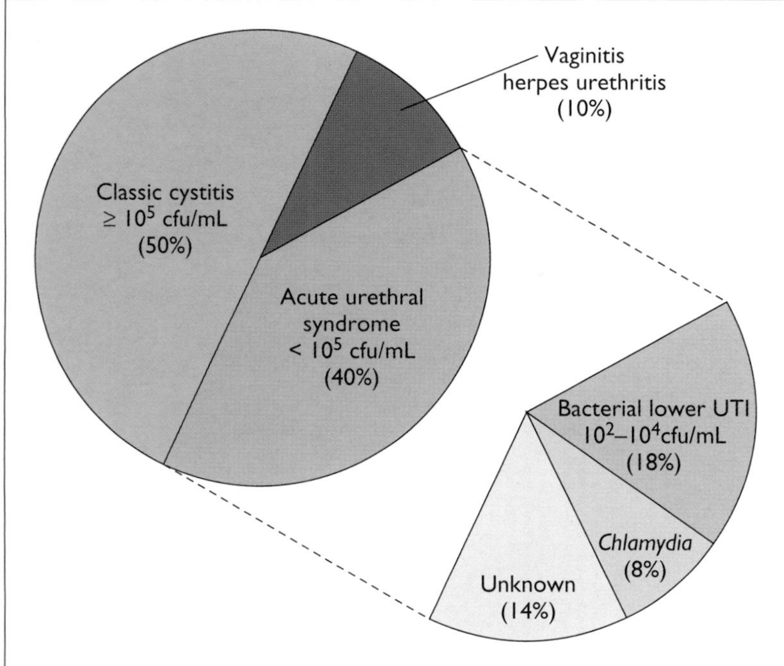

Figure 9-3 Relative frequencies of causes of acute onset of frequency/dysuria in young women. Half of the women who present with acute symptoms of dysuria and frequency have classic cystitis with $\geq 10^5$ colony-forming units (cfu) per mL on urine culture. Forty percent have $< 10^5$ cfu/mL of urine (acute urethral syndrome). Of this latter group, most (18%) have a urinary tract infection (UTI) with low counts of bacteria (10^2 to 10^4 cfu/mL of urine). Some (8%) have a urethral infection due to *Chlamydia*, the remainder (14%) have no identifiable causative agent [1].

Characteristics of complicated versus uncomplicated urinary tract infections

Uncomplicated	Complicated
Female sex	Male sex
Young adults	Older age
Functionally and anatomically intact urinary tract	Functionally or anatomically abnormal urinary tract
Outpatient	Hospitalized
> 80% *Escherichia coli*	Broad range of pathogens
Antimicrobial resistance infrequent	Antibiotic resistance common
Oral therapy	Oral/parenteral therapies
Respond to short courses	Longer courses needed

Figure 9-4 Characteristics of complicated versus uncomplicated urinary tract infections (UTIs). Uncomplicated and complicated UTIs differ significantly in their underlying pathogenesis and their treatment. Uncomplicated infections occur most commonly in young adult women. They are not associated with abnormalities (either functional or anatomic) in the urinary tract and are generally caused by *Escherichia coli*. Complicated infections occur in both sexes. In fact, all UTIs in men should be considered complicated. Complicated infections are often associated with alterations in urinary flow or instrumentation or involve the upper urinary tract (pyelonephritis) and thus are prone to recur. Causative organisms in complicated infections are often antibiotic-resistant. As a result, treatment often requires extended-spectrum antibiotics or parenteral antibiotics, and longer courses are needed.

Treatment of uncomplicated cystitis

Antibiotic regimens	Comments
Single-dose antibiotics with TMP-SMX or quinolones	Less effective than multiple-day regimens
3-day regimens of TMP-SMX, TMP alone, fluoroquinolones, nitrofurantoin, β-lactam agents	Optimal balance between efficacy and side effects Fluoroquinolones are effective but expensive
7-day regimen of TMP-SMX, TMP, oral fluoroquinolones, β-lactam agents	Consider longer course in patients with diabetes, pregnancy, symptoms > 7 days, age > 65 yrs Longer regimens associated with more side effects

TMP-SMX—trimethoprim-sulfamethoxazole.

Figure 9-5 Treatment of uncomplicated cystitis. Uncomplicated cystitis can be managed by one of three strategies. Single-dose antibiotics is the most convenient method but is less effective than multiple-day regimens, in part because it does not reliably eradicate rectal and vaginal carriage. Single-dose β-lactam regimens have been particularly disappointing and should not be used. The 7-day regimen is the most effective but exposes the patient to the greatest amount of antibiotics and thus the most side effects. The 3-day regimen appears to be the optimal balance between efficacy and potential for side effects.

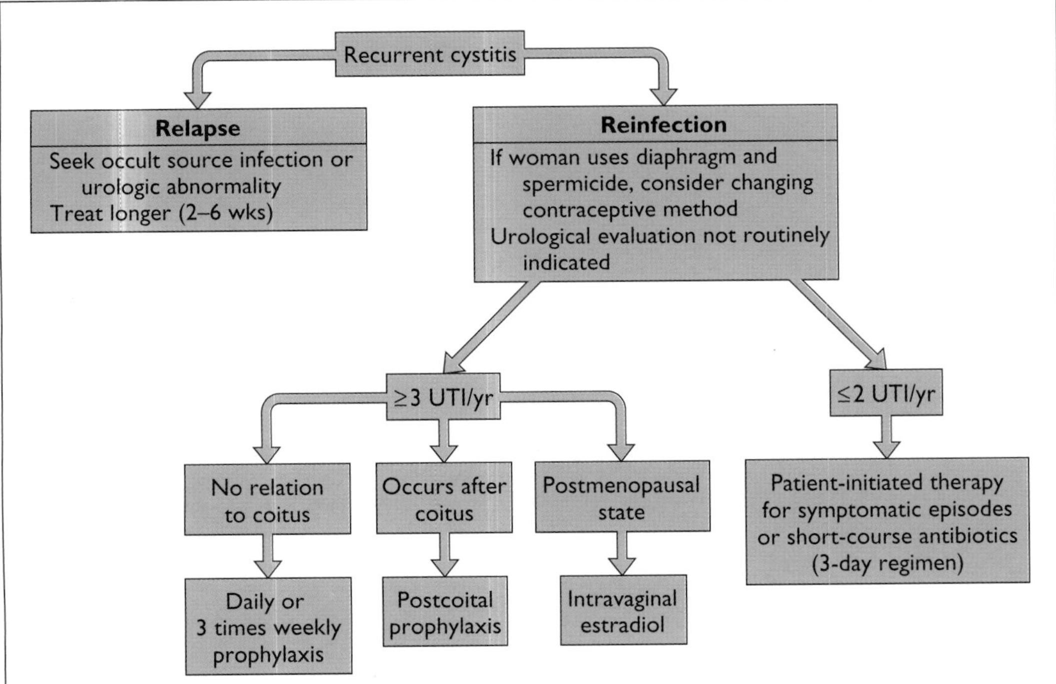

Figure 9-6 Approach to management of recurrent cystitis. The management of recurrent cystitis in women depends on whether the recurrent episode of infection is caused by the same uropathogen (relapse) or one different from that isolated from a prior episode (reinfection). Relapses are complicated infections, requiring longer courses of antibiotics for eradication (≥ 2 weeks of antibiotics). Reinfections occur in patients with normal urinary tracts, and therefore, urologic evaluations are not indicated routinely. The treatment options for recurrent uncomplicated cystitis depend on its frequency and underlying pathogenesis. Women with two or less episodes per year can be managed by patient-initiated single-dose antibiotics when symptoms occur or with short-course antibiotics (*eg*, 3-day regimen) on presentation to the physician. Women who suffer three or more reinfections per year are managed most cost-effectively by continuous or thrice-weekly antibiotic prophylaxis or, if their cystitis occurs after intercourse, by postcoital prophylaxis. Recurrent cystitis in postmenopausal women is related to altered vaginal flora with colonization by Enterobacteriaceae. Recurrent infections can be reduced by intravaginal administration of estriol [2]. (UTI—urinary tract infection.)

Pyelonephritis

Microbiology in pyelonephritis

Uncomplicated	Complicated
Escherichia coli (≥ 80%)	*Escherichia coli* (± 50%)
Proteus mirabilis	*Klebsiella* spp
Klebsiella pneumoniae	*Proteus* spp
Staphylococcus saprophyticus	*Pseudomonas* spp
Staphylococcus epidermidis	*Serratia* spp
	Enterobacter spp
	Enterococcus spp
	Staphylococcus spp
	Yeast

Figure 9-7 Microbiology in pyelonephritis. *Escherichia coli* is the most common cause of uncomplicated and complicated pyelonephritis, but the relative frequency of other pathogens increases in complicated pyelonephritis and varies depending on the underlying pathology or abnormality. Although pyelonephritis is generally caused by one pathogen, multiple bacteria may be isolated when structural abnormalities are present. Microorganisms observed in complicated infections are more a reflection of hospital flora. *Corynebacterium* group D2 and cell-wall deficient bacteria have also been observed rarely in patients with pyelonephritis [3].

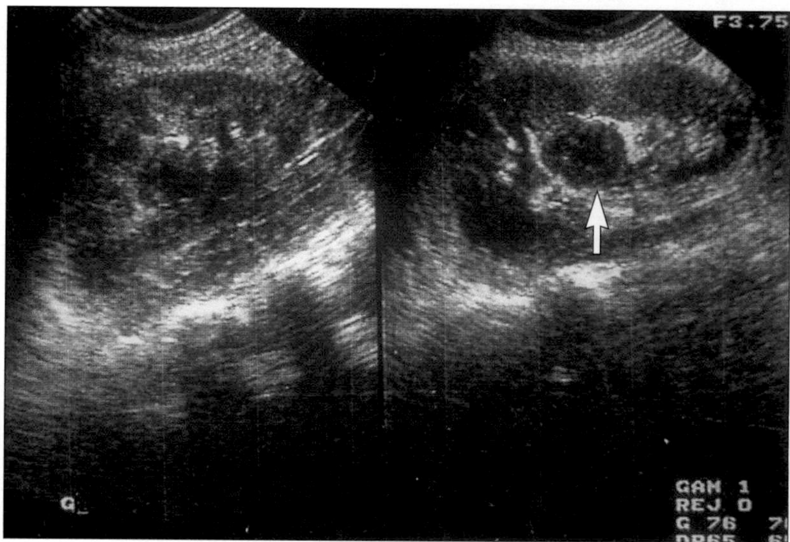

Figure 9-8 Ultrasound imaging in acute pyelonephritis. Ultrasound has the advantages of being rapid, noninvasive, relatively inexpensive, and accessible, and there is no exposure to radiation. It has now replaced intravenous pyelogram as the first means of evaluation of uncomplicated and complicated pyelonephritis. In acute pyelonephritis, the kidney shows renal enlargement, and in complicated pyelonephritis, hypoechoic lesions (*arrow*) may be observed. Ultrasound can detect abscesses of ≥ 2 cm in size and gas. Ultrasound is extremely useful for the confirmation of pyelonephritis during pregnancy and may be used to detect lower urinary tract obstruction and the presence of residual urine.

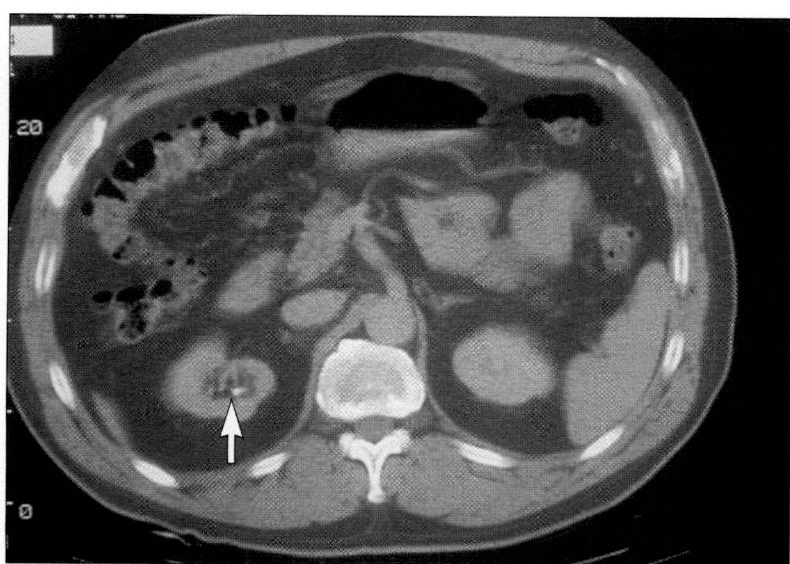

Figure 9-9 Computed tomography (CT) scan showing renal atrophy in acute pyelonephritis. The CT scan shows irregular surface (atrophy) of the right kidney (seen on the left side), as compared with the left kidney, and distended calyces (*arrow*). Although CT is extremely sensitive to define intra- and perirenal suppuration, it is not as effective as intravenous pyelogram to detect abnormalities of the collecting system. Wedged-shaped lesions are seen in > 90% of patients with acute uncomplicated pyelonephritis. Focal and multifocal masslike lesions have also been observed in > 90% of patients with complicated pyelonephritis. Because intravenous pyelogram requires the administration of contrast material, it should thus be reserved for patients in whom ultrasonography is negative. Magnetic resonance imaging offers no advantages over CT scan.

Uropathogens and their susceptibility to antibiotics used in pyelonephritis

	Escherichia coli (492)*, %	*Klebsiella pneumoniae* (105), %	*Proteus mirabilis* (37), %	*Pseudomonas aeruginosa* (78), %	*Serratia marcescens* (40), %
Aminoglycosides					
Gentamicin	98	99	100	96	100
β-Lactams					
Ampicillin	67	4	84	0	2
Ceftriaxone	100	100	100	72	95
Aztreonam	99	100	100	94	95
Ticarcillin/clavulanate	98	100	100	95	97
Imipenem/cilastatin	100	100	100	91	100
Fluoroquinolones					
Ciprofloxacin	100	100	100	100	100
Other antibiotics					
Trimethoprim-sulfamethoxazole	91	96	92	3	98

*Number of isolates. All these bacteria were isolated in the blood of patients.

Figure 9-10 Uropathogens and their susceptibility to antibiotics used in pyelonephritis. The susceptibility of *Escherichia coli* to antibiotics is changing. *E. coli* resistance to ampicillin, amoxicillin, and first-generation cephalosporins is increasing rapidly (25%–35%) so that these drugs cannot be considered anymore as the first choice for empirical treatment of pyelonephritis. In North America, *E. coli* and many other Enterobacteriaceae are still susceptible to trimethoprim-sulfamethoxazole (TMP-SMX), but resistance is rising (10%–15%). In many parts of Europe, *E. coli* is highly resistant to TMP-SMX. Although variable from country to country, aminoglycosides and the quinolones are still, in general, highly effective against many gram-negative bacteria responsible for uncomplicated and complicated pyelonephritis. (*Adapted from* Chamberland *et al.* [4].)

Recommended antibiotics for the treatment of uncomplicated pyelonephritis syndromes

Syndromes (women or men)	Route	Duration, *d*	First choice(s)	Alternative
Subclinical pyelonephritis Acute moderate pyelonephritis (outpatient)	Oral	14	TMP-SMX *or* fluoroquinolones (ciprofloxacin)	Amoxicillin *or* amoxicillin-clavulanate
Severe pyelonephritis (hospitalization)	IV	≈3	Aminoglycoside *or*	Ceftriaxone
	IV	≈3	TMP-SMX *or*	
	IV	≈3	Fluoroquinolones	
	followed by		*followed by*	
	Oral	10	TMP-SMX *or*	Amoxicillin
	Oral	10	Fluoroquinolones (ciprofloxacin)	Amoxicillin-clavulanate
Recurrent pyelonephritis	IV or oral	14–60	Same as severe pyelonephritis	
Pyelonephritis in pregnancy (hospitalization)	IV	≈3	Ceftriaxone *or*	Aztreonam *or* aminoglycosides
	IV	≈3	TMP-SMX	
	followed by		*followed by*	
	Oral	10	Amoxicillin or cephalosporin	TMP-SMX

IV—intravenous; TMP-SMX—trimethoprim-sulfamethoxazole.

Figure 9-11 Recommended antibiotics for the treatment of uncomplicated pyelonephritis syndromes [3].

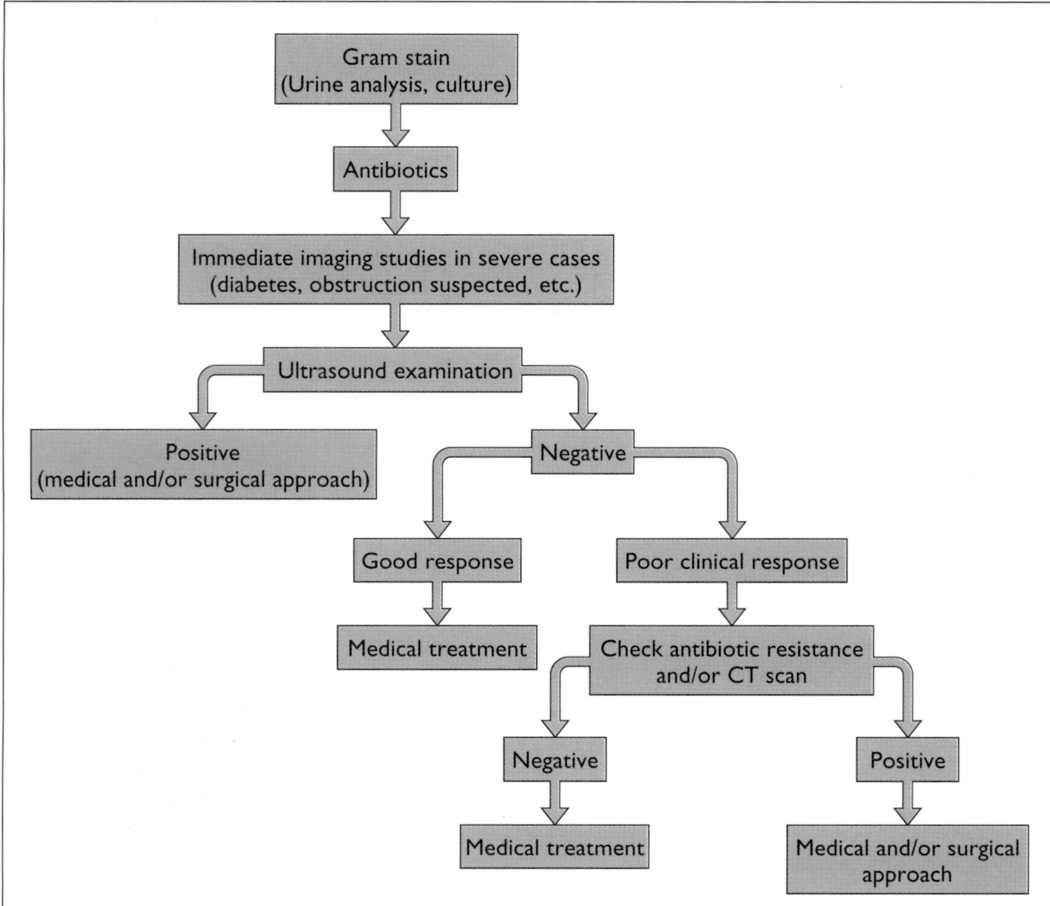

FIGURE 9-12 Clinical management of complicated pyelonephritis. Complicated pyelonephritis usually necessitates hospitalization, thorough investigation of the urinary tract using imaging studies, and, when indicated depending on the underlying anomalies, aggressive medicosurgical procedures. (CT—computed tomography.)

COMPLICATED URINARY TRACT INFECTIONS

Complicated urinary tract infection: Clinical situations
Presence of an indwelling catheter or use of intermittent catheterization
> 100 mL of residual urine retained after voiding
Obstructive uropathy due to bladder outlet obstruction, calculus, or other causes
Vesicle ureteral reflux or other urologic abnormalities, including surgically created ileal loops
Azotemia due to intrinsic renal disease
Renal transplantation

FIGURE 9-13 Specific clinical situations defining a complicated urinary tract infection [5].

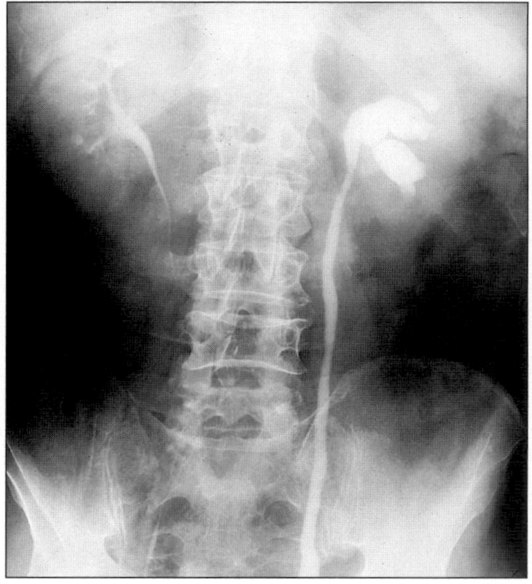

FIGURE 9-14 Intravenous pyelogram showing ureteric stricture due to renal tuberculosis. Ureteric strictures may be associated with proximal dilatation of the urinary system and urinary tract infection because of incomplete emptying. This prone 45-minute intravenous pyelogram film demonstrates amputation of the infundibula to the left upper pole and a stricture of the distal left ureter. In this case, the ureteric stricture is due to tuberculosis of the genitourinary tract.

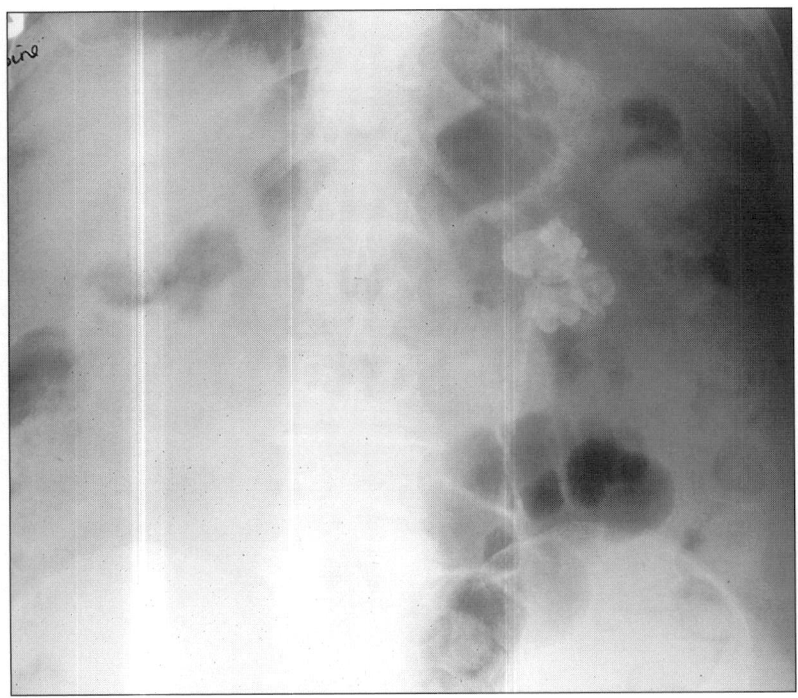

Figure 9-15 Staghorn calculus seen on abdominal radiograph. Staghorn calculi are "infection stones" (struvite and calcium carbonate apatite), produced in association with infection with urease-producing organisms, primarily *Proteus mirabilis*. These are generally large calculi that follow the contours of the renal pelvis and may destroy the kidney. This abdominal film shows a staghorn calculus of the left kidney with associated calcification of the left upper ureter in a woman presenting with recurrent abdominal pain.

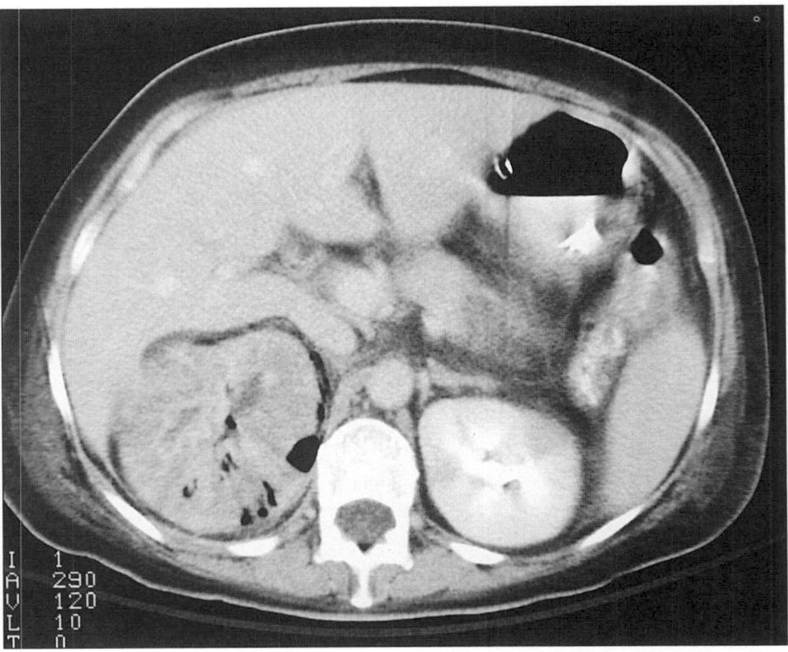

Figure 9-16 Emphysematous pyelonephritis in a patient with diabetes. A rare presentation of urinary tract infection in diabetic patients is that of emphysematous pyelonephritis. This condition occurs in the presence of hyperglycemia with glucose excreted in the urine. Uropathogens may produce gas in the presence of elevated glucose. The computed tomography scan shows an enlarged, inflamed, right kidney with air within the parenchyma and subcapsular space.

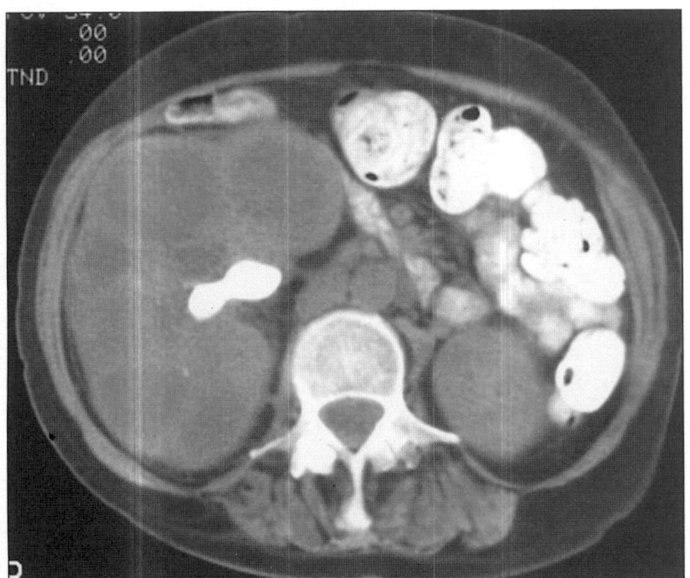

Figure 9-17 Xanthogranulomatous pyelonephritis. Xanthogranulomatous pyelonephritis is a rare disease associated with *Escherichia coli* or *Proteus mirabilis* infection, with replacement of the renal parenchyma by an inflammatory mass. The computed tomography scan shows replacement of the right kidney by a huge multilobulated inflammatory mass. *P. mirabilis* was grown from the urine of this patient.

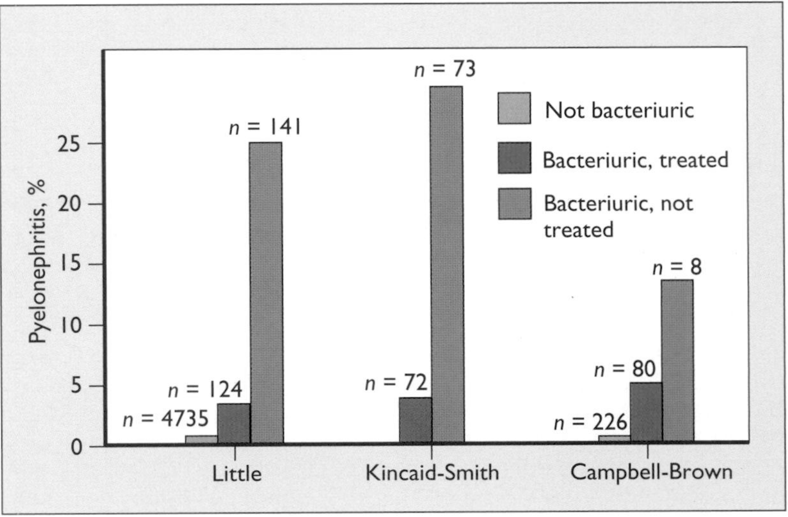

Figure 9-18 Pyelonephritis in pregnancy. Women with asymptomatic bacteriuria early in pregnancy have a high risk of pyelonephritis later in the pregnancy (end of the second trimester or early third trimester) if untreated. This increased occurrence of pyelonephritis is likely secondary to the physiologic hydronephrosis and obstruction associated with pregnancy. Treatment of asymptomatic bacteriuria decreases the risk of subsequent pyelonephritis tenfold. Studies reporting pyelonephritis in women identified with asymptomatic bacteriuria early in pregnancy and subsequently randomized to treatment or nontreatment are summarized in this figure. The risk of pyelonephritis is approximately 30% for women identified with asymptomatic bacteriuria in early pregnancy who are not treated [6–8].

Infections of the Prostate

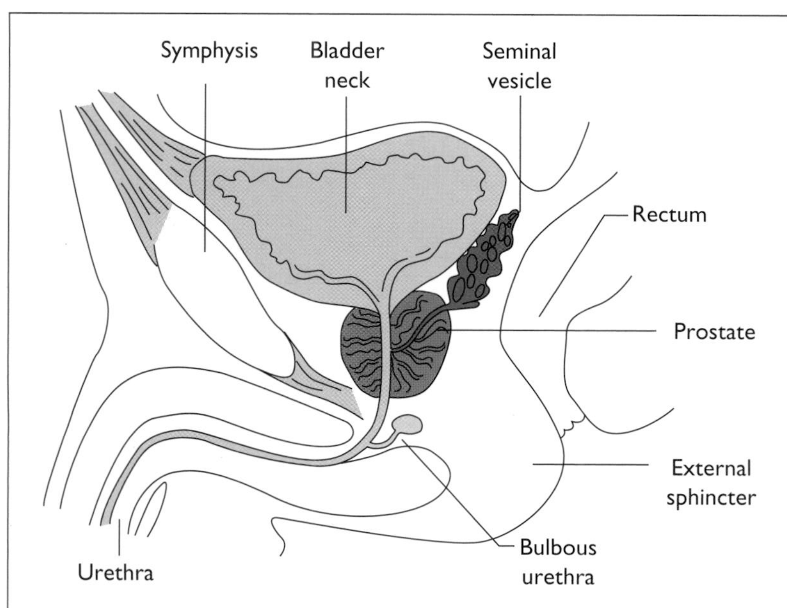

Figure 9-19 Anatomy of the prostate. Coronal view.

Types of prostatitis, by EPS and culture

Classification	EPS	Culture (EPS)	Rectal examination
Acute bacterial prostatitis	↑ PMNs* (++++)	Positive—Enterobacteriaceae	Exquisitely tender
Chronic bacterial prostatitis	↑ PMNs (++)	Positive—Enterobacteriaceae	Normal
Nonbacterial prostatitis	↑ PMNs (++)	Absent bacteria (sterile)	Normal
Prostatodynia	Normal	Sterile	Variable

*EPS contraindicated in acute bacterial prostatitis; urine examination will provide diagnosis (pyuria, bacteriuria).

EPS—expressed prostatic secretions; PMNs—polymorphonuclear cells.

Figure 9-20 Types of prostatitis, by expressed prostatic secretions (EPS) and culture. The various prostatitis syndromes have been classified based on EPS and urine culture findings. This classification system is important for therapy, because the various categories are treated differently. The presence of ≥ 10 leukocytes per high-power field (hpf) in the EPS is considered clinically significant inflammation [9]. In acute bacterial prostatitis (ABP), EPS (as obtained by massage) should not be obtained for risk of precipitating bacteremia. If EPS is obtained inadvertently, sheets of leukocytes (polymorphonuclear cells) are present. Significant bacterial growth is present in the voided urine due to the presence of an accompanying cystitis. In chronic bacterial prostatitis, the EPS is usually associated with ≥ 10 leukocytes/hpf and should be obtained. Unlike patients with ABP, these patients are not acutely ill. Urine culture shows no growth unless the patient develops an acute urinary tract infection, in which case culture would demonstrate the same spectrum of organisms as in ABP. With nonbacterial prostatitis, significant inflammation is present in the prostate as characterized by ≥ 10 leukocytes/hpf. However, routine bacterial culture does not demonstrate growth of organisms. Cultures for fungi, *Chlamydia*, *Ureaplasma*, and *Mycoplasma* rarely demonstrate growth. In prostatodynia, no inflammation in the EPS or bacterial growth in culture is present. "Pelviperineal pain" is an appropriate name to describe the symptoms in this condition.

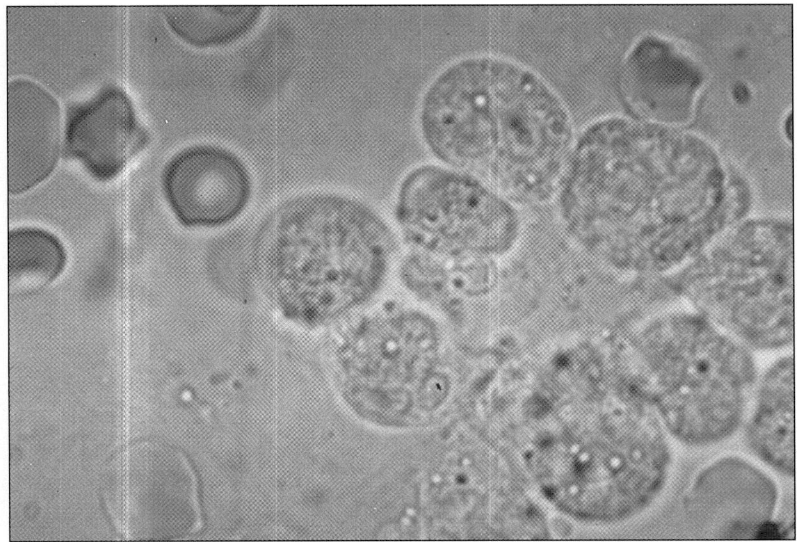

Figure 9-21 Pyuria in acute bacterial prostatitis. Pyuria is the presence of leukocytes in the voided urine. This inflammatory response is caused by the concurrent cystitis present in acute bacterial prostatitis. Pyuria, which is always present in untreated acute bacterial prostatitis, is not specific for this condition. The urinalysis typically demonstrates numerous leukocytes per high-power field.

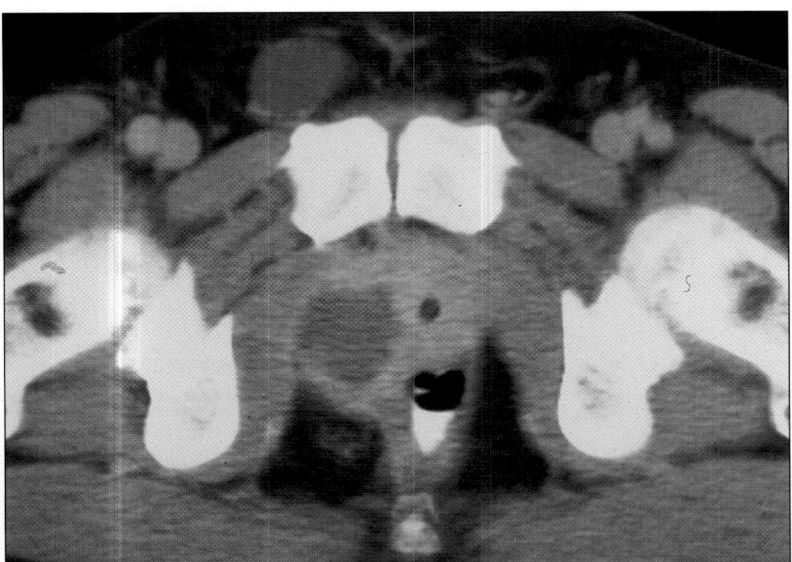

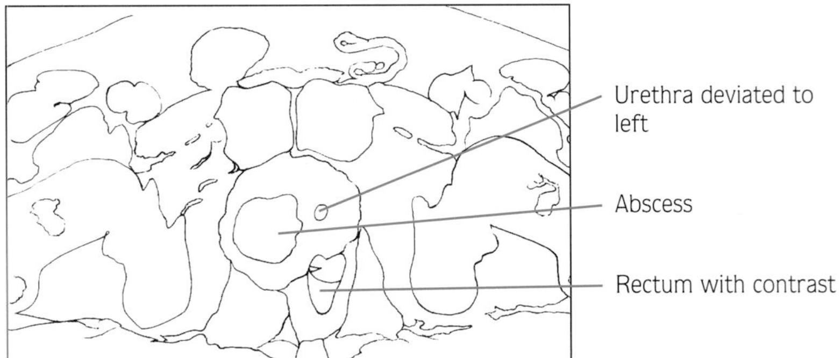

Figure 9-22 Computed tomography scan demonstrating a prostatic abscess. Patients with diabetes, indwelling urinary catheters, immunocompromised status, and urinary tract instrumentation and who are on maintenance hemodialysis are especially prone to the development of prostatic abscess. Clinical symptoms include acute urinary retention, fever, dysuria, urinary frequency, and perineal pain. *Escherichia coli* is the predominant organism identified.

Cardinal clinical manifestations of chronic bacterial prostatitis
Most common cause of relapsing urinary tract infection in men
Asymptomatic periods between episodes of recurrent bacteriuria
Obstruction or irritative voiding symptoms (occasional)
Vague discomfort in pelvis and perineum (infrequent)
Physical findings on palpation normal
Expressed prostatic secretions or postmassage urine culture needed for precise diagnosis

Figure 9-23 Cardinal clinical manifestations of chronic bacterial prostatitis. Relapsing urinary tract infections, with asymptomatic periods between, are common in chronic bacterial prostatitis. Although some men are diagnosed because of asymptomatic bacteriuria, most have varying degrees of irritative voiding symptoms, such as dysuria, frequency, and urgency. In addition, feelings of vague discomfort in the pelvis and perineum may be present. Fevers and chills are uncommon. Rectal palpation of the prostate is not painful and has no specific findings. Prostatic fluid and postmassage urine cultures, which should be obtained for precise diagnosis, demonstrate bacterial growth.

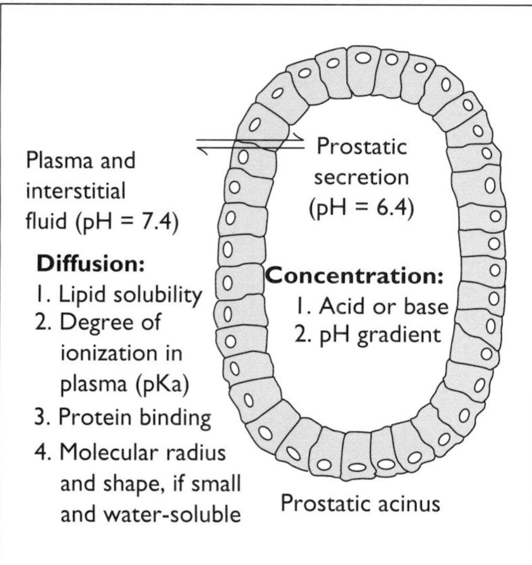

FIGURE 9-24 Factors determining diffusion and concentration of antimicrobial agents in the prostate. The reasons for relapsing urinary tract infections include the poor penetration of most antimicrobial agents into the prostatic fluid and/or bacterial sequestration, which protects them from antimicrobial exposure. Only small molecular size, un-ionized, lipid-soluble drugs not firmly bound to plasma proteins are able to diffuse across the epithelial membrane. (*Adapted from* Stamey *et al.* [10].)

CANDIDURIA

Trends in nosocomial *Candida* UTIs
Candida spp accounted for 7% of nosocomial infections in 1986–1989
Candida UTIs accounted for 9% of nosocomial UTIs, making them the 4th most common etiology
Overall, the frequency of *Candida* infections has increased by 200%–300% in the 1980s
90% of *Candida* UTIs are related to catheters or other instrumentation

UTI—urinary tract infection.

FIGURE 9-25 Trends in nosocomial *Candida* urinary tract infections. *Candida* infections have increased in frequency in all sites over the past 25 years. This increase is primarily due to the increased complexity of illness seen in hospitalized patients, such as immunocompromise and multiple trauma, as well as the increased use of broad-spectrum antibacterial agents [11–13].

Microbiology of candiduria	
Candida albicans	> 50%
Torulopsis glabrata	≈ 25%
Candida tropicalis	5%–15%
Candida parapsilosis	5%–10%
Other *Candida* spp	5%–20%

FIGURE 9-26 Microbiology of candiduria. The percentage of individual species causing candiduria is approximated because many hospitals do not speciate non-*albicans* isolates from the urine. Non-*albicans Candida*, especially *C. glabrata*, is more commonly found in the urinary tract than in the oropharynx, esophagus, and vagina. Mixed infections with two or more *Candida* species are common in complicated urinary tract infections in catheterized patients.

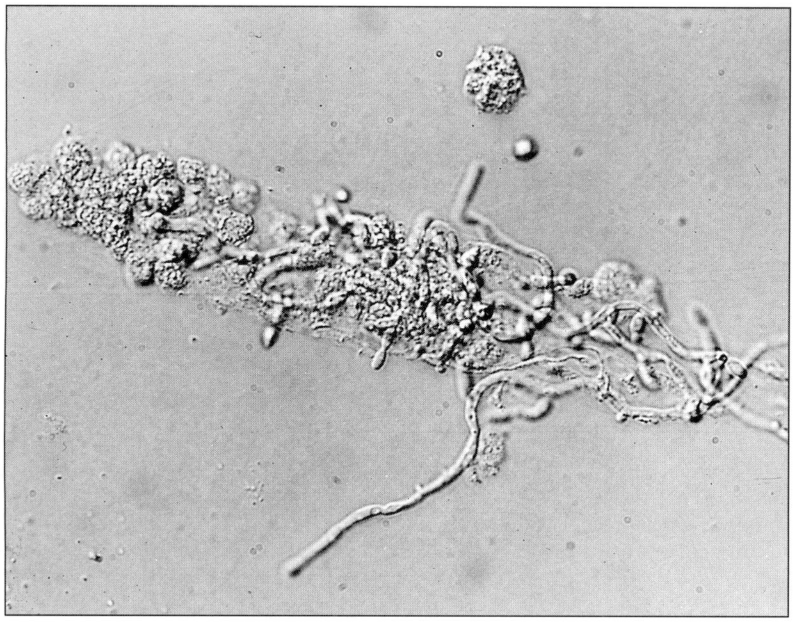

FIGURE 9-27 Light microscopy of renal tubular casts containing *Candida albicans* blastospores and mycelia, indicating renal parenchymal origin. When found on urine examination, this rare finding localizes infection to the kidney. (*Courtesy of* T. Walsh, MD.)

Candiduria as a source of candidemia
A rare occurrence (3%–10% of candidemias) Usually associated with: Urologic procedures Obstruction/stasis Anatomic abnormalities Foreign bodies A large multicenter observational study found positive blood cultures in only 1% of randomly selected patients with candiduria

FIGURE 9-28 Candiduria as a source of candidemia. Despite the common occurrence of candiduria, ascending infection with candidemia rarely occurs. Only 3% to 10% of candidemias result from an ascending infection [14].

Treatment of noncatheter-related symptomatic *Candida* cystourethritis: Systemic therapy
1. Oral fluconazole (200 mg/day × 7 days) 2. Ketoconazole or itraconazole—less effective due to low urinary drug concentrations 3. Oral flucytosine—effective but less experience and more toxicity 4. Intravenous amphotericin B (0.3 mg/kg × single dose) 5. Conventional systemic intravenous amphotericin B (5–7 days of 0.3 mg/kg/day)

FIGURE 9-29 Systemic therapy in the treatment of noncatheter-related *Candida* cystourethritis. Ketoconazole and itraconazole achieve poor urinary drug concentrations and produce unreliable therapeutic results. Oral fluconazole in limited studies appears highly effective, especially given the high concentrations of fluconazole achieved in urine [15].

Antifungal therapy for ascending pyelonephritis	
Amphotericin B	Previous "gold standard" for systemic and renal candidiasis Has never been subjected to rigorous analysis Depending on setting and patient, use 0.3–0.6 mg/kg/day If more prolonged therapy is required, oral fluconazole could be continued after initial therapy with amphotericin B
Fluconazole	Considered equivalent to amphotericin B Well-absorbed with high urinary excretion; low toxicity 400 mg/day intravenous or oral

FIGURE 9-30 Antifungal therapy for ascending pyelonephritis. Treatment of ascending pyelonephritis requires systemic therapy with agents that achieve adequate levels in renal tissue and urine, such as amphotericin B and fluconazole. The other azole drugs, itraconazole and ketoconazole, are not excreted in the urine in sufficient quantity to be predictable. Flucytosine, although having excellent absorption and renal distribution, is limited by its toxicities and relatively narrow spectrum of activity [16–18].

Catheter-Associated Urinary Tract Infections

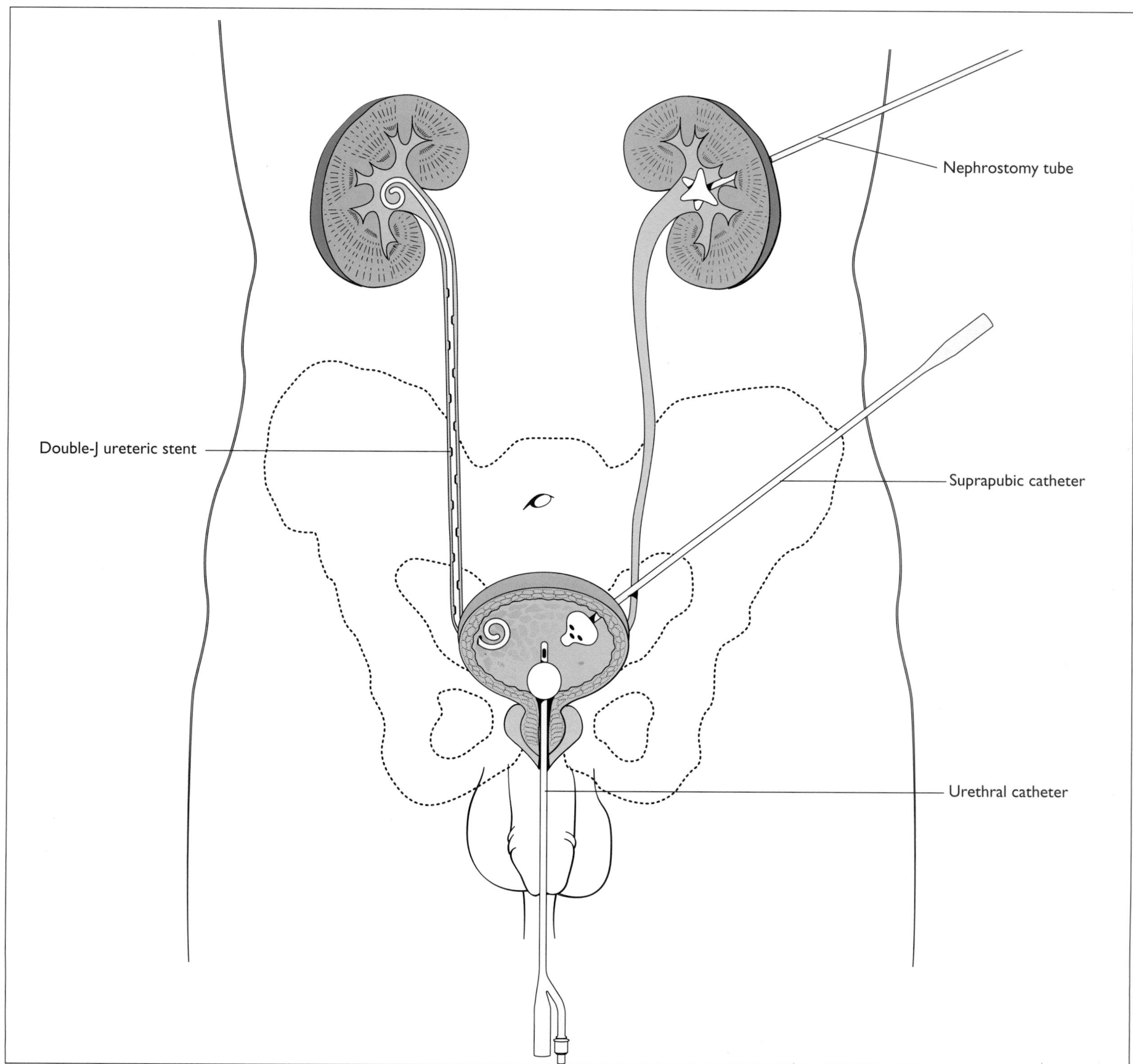

Figure 9-31 Sites and routes of urinary catheters. Catheters and stents are used to drain the bladder and kidneys. Catheters may be inserted into the bladder via the urethra or the percutaneous suprapubic route. The kidney can be drained with a percutaneous nephrostomy catheter or with a ureteric stent into the bladder. Approximately 15% of patients admitted to an acute care hospital will have some form of urinary catheter inserted during their hospital stay.

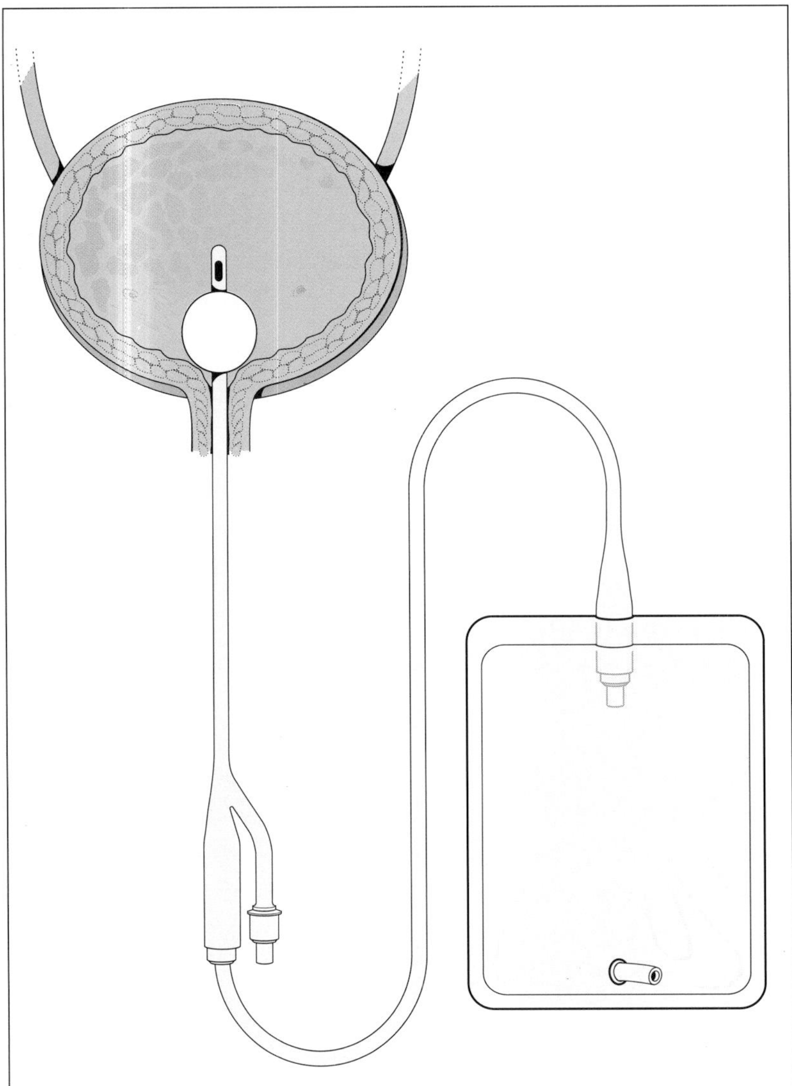

Figure 9-32 Closed urinary catheter system. Introduction of the closed urinary drainage system has been the most important technologic advance in the development of urinary drainage systems. The rate and frequency of acquired catheter-associated bacteriuria decreased significantly when these systems were universally employed. Although these systems have been modified many times over the past two decades, it is not entirely clear whether any of these modifications have subsequently reduced the infection rate from that attained with the original closed system.

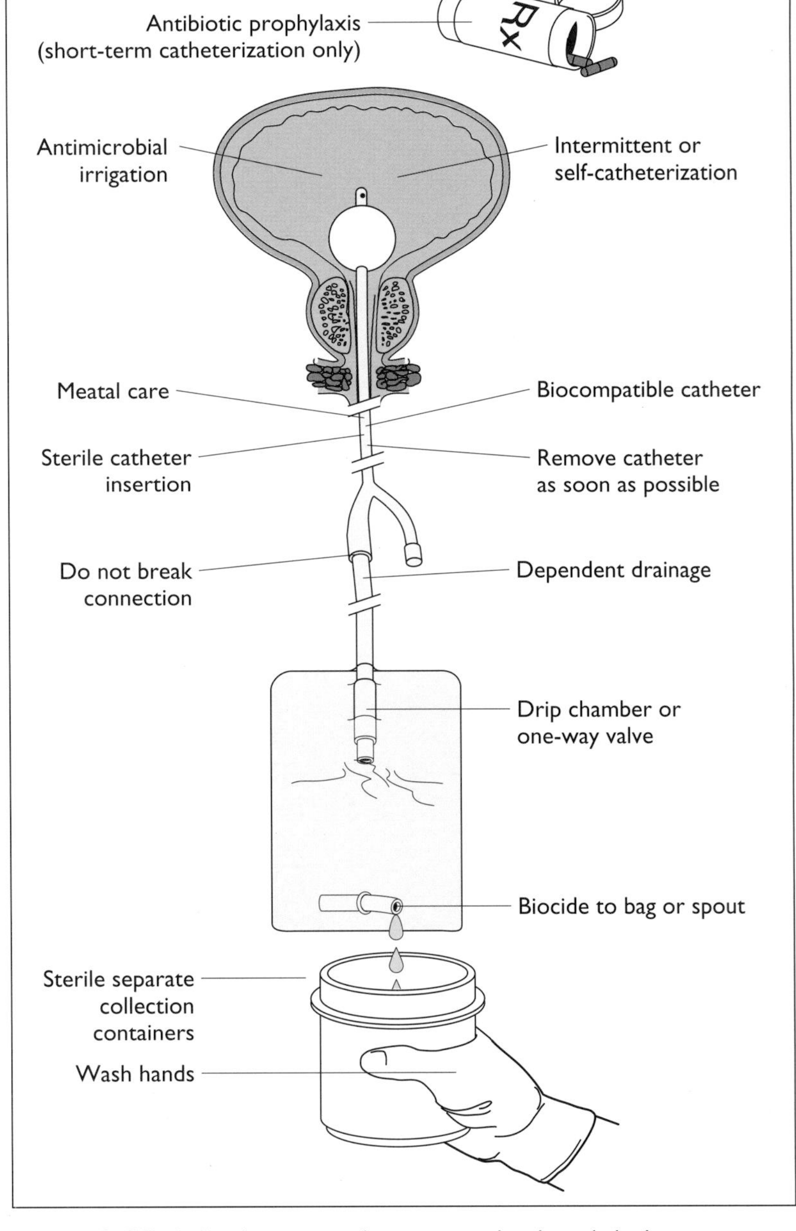

Figure 9-33 Infection control measures in closed drainage systems.

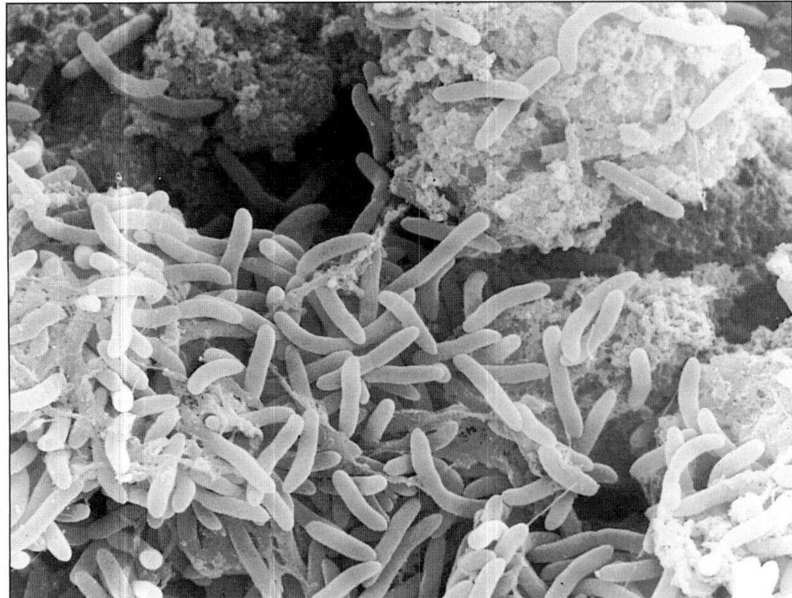

Figure 9-34 Scanning electron micrograph of an experimental bacterial biofilm ascending the luminal surface of a Foley catheter. The bacteria are seen advancing from the lower left, onto the catheter surface in the upper right. (*From* Nickel *et al.* [19]; with permission.)

Selection of antibiotics in catheter-associated urinary tract infections
1. Asymptomatic bacteriuria
Rarely if ever treated
2. Symptomatic cystitis
Trimethoprim-sulfamethoxazole, quinolones, β-lactams
3. Systemic
Ampicillin and gentamicin
Third-generation cephalosporin
Quinolones
Extended-spectrum penicillin

FIGURE 9-35 Selection of antibiotics in catheter-associated urinary tract infections. Asymptomatic bacteriuria should be treated rarely. Symptomatic cystitis is preferably treated with one of the broad-spectrum quinolones combined with catheter removal. Treatment of systemic catheter-associated urinary tract infections should include intravenous antibiotics that cover both gram-positive and gram-negative bacteria.

INFECTIONS OF THE VULVA

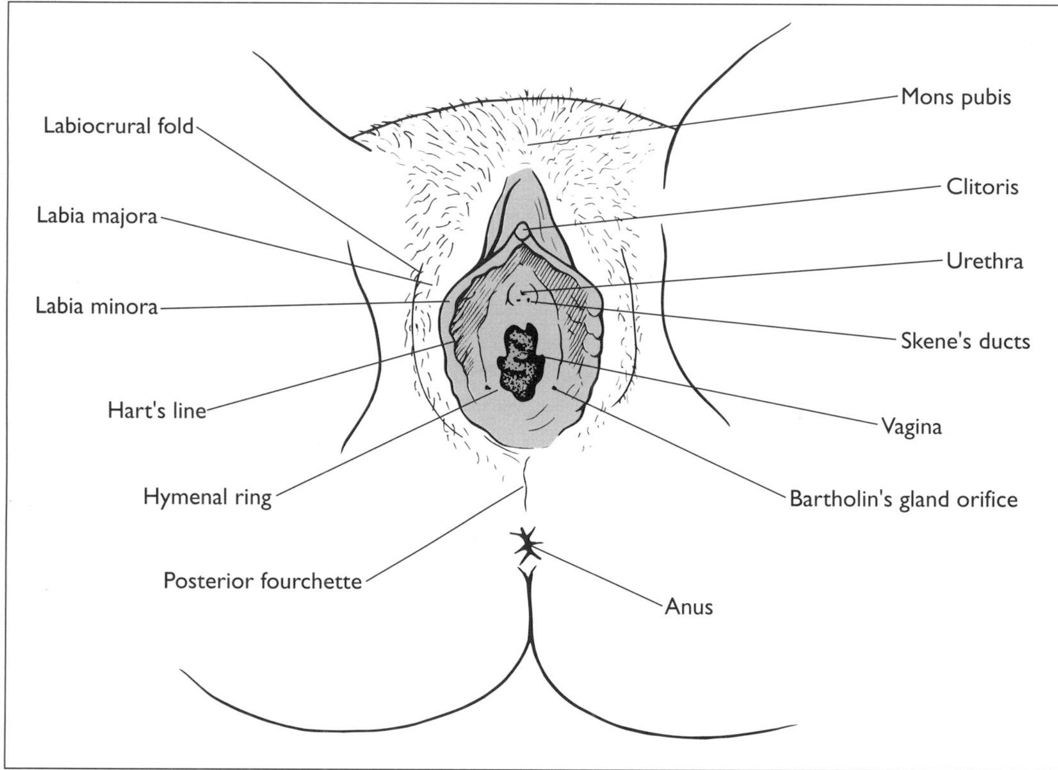

FIGURE 9-36 Schematic depiction of the vulva. The vulva includes the labia majora, labia minora, clitoris, and vulvar vestibule. Its lateral borders are the labiocrural folds, and its central boundary is the hymen. The anterior and posterior boundaries are the mons pubis and anus, respectively.

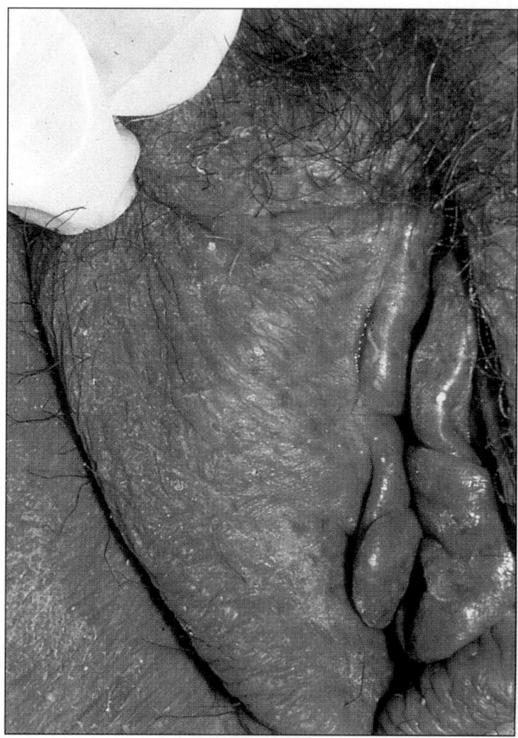

FIGURE 9-37 Lichen simplex chronicus secondary to a candidal infection. Although the *Candida* infection had been treated successfully and cleared, the initial dermatitis led to a "itch-scratch-itch" cycle, which persisted. The pruritus, usually more intense at night, leads to scratching and results in lichenification, fissures, and even distinct papules and nodules called *prurigo nodularis*. Because of similar symptoms of chronic itching and burning, these patients are sometimes misdiagnosed as having recurrent chronic candidiasis. (*Courtesy of* L. Edwards, MD.)

Differential diagnostic features of vaginitis in adult women

Feature	Normal	Candida vaginitis	Bacterial vaginosis	Trichomonal vaginitis
Symptoms	None or physiologic leukorrhea	Vulvar pruritus, soreness, ↑ discharge, dysuria, dyspareunia	Moderate malodorous discharge	Profuse, purulent, offensive discharge; pruritus; dyspareunia
Discharge				
Amount	Scant to moderate	Scant to moderate	Moderate	Profuse
Color	Clear or white	White	White or gray	Yellow
Consistency	Floccular, nonhomogeneous	Clumped but variable	Homogeneous, uniformly coating walls	Homogenous
Bubbles	Absent	Absent	Present	Present
Appearance of vulva and vagina	Normal	Introital and vulvar erythema, edema, occasional pustules, vaginal erythema	No inflammation	Erythema and swelling of vulvar and vaginal epithelium, "strawberry" cervix
pH of vaginal fluid	< 4.5	< 4.5	> 4.7	5–6.0
Amine test (16% KOH)	Negative	Negative	Positive	Occasionally present
Saline microscopy	Normal epithelial cells, lactobacilli predominate	Normal flora, blastospores (yeast) 40%–50%, pseudohyphae	Clue cells, coccobacillary flora predominate, absence of leukocytes, motile curved rods	PMNs +++, motile trichomonads (80%–90%), no clue cells or abnormal flora
10% KOH microscopy	Negative	Positive (60%–90%)	Negative (except in mixed infections)	Negative

KOH—potassium hydroxide; PMNs—polymorphonuclear cells.

FIGURE 9-38 Clinical and laboratory features of candidal, bacterial, and trichomonal vaginitis in adult women. Women who complain of abnormal discharge or vulvar discomfort should be evaluated for vaginitis. Vaginal discharge associated with vaginitis can act as an irritant to the vulva causing erythema and pain. (*Adapted from* Sobel [20].)

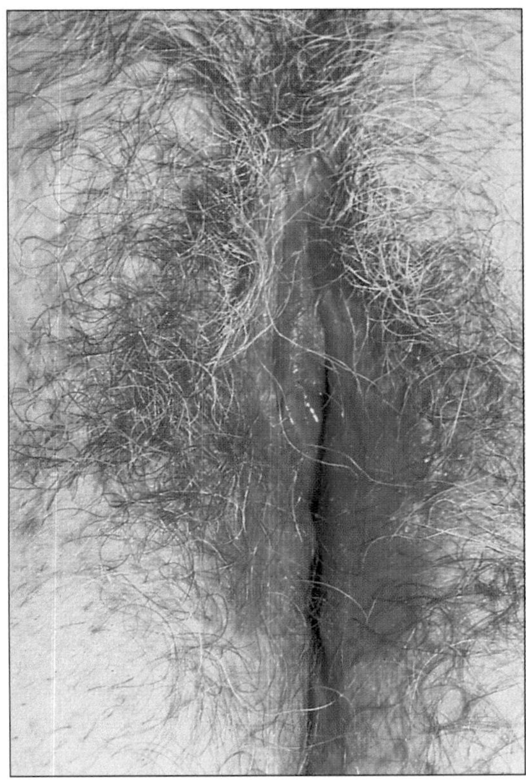

FIGURE 9-39 Candidal infection causing "beefy" red appearance of the vulva. (*Courtesy of* L. Edwards, MD.)

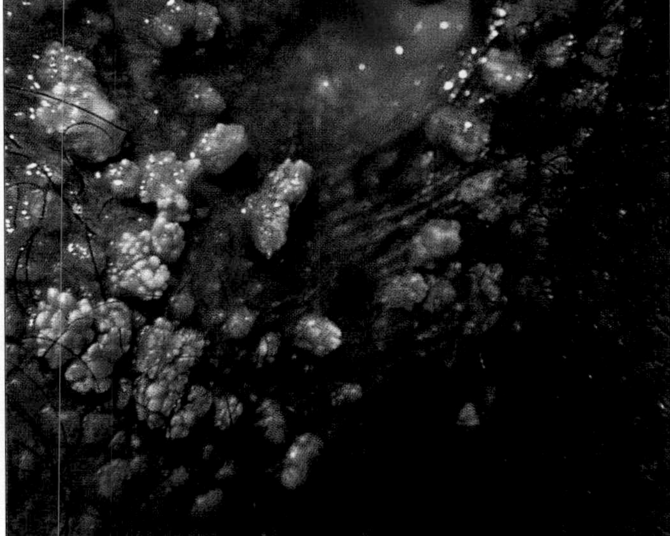

FIGURE 9-40 Close-up view of condyloma acuminata with multiple, pedunculated, and sessile venereal warts. (*From* Tovell and Young [21]; with permission.)

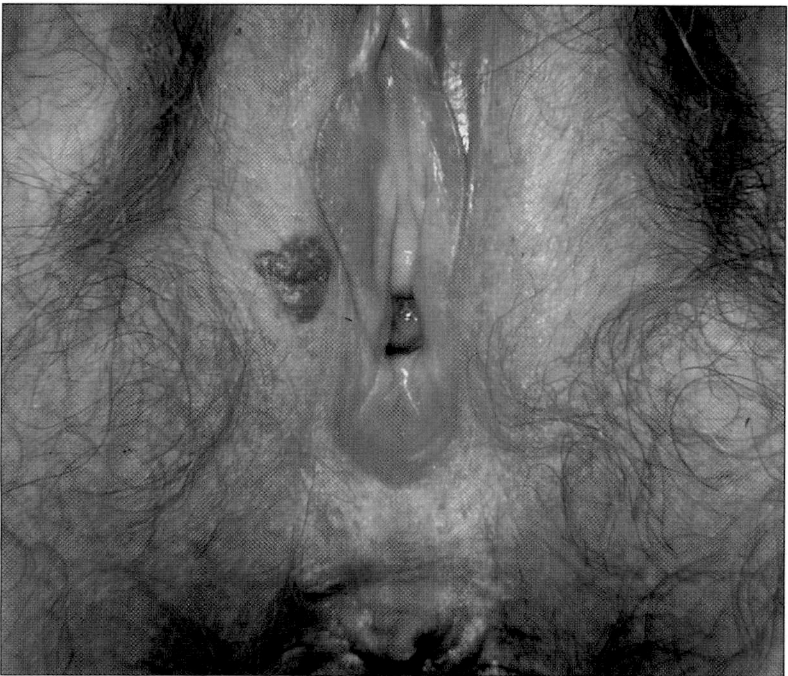

Figure 9-41 Malignant melanoma of the vulva. The lesion is a gray-black plaque with irregular borders on the right labia majora. Approximately 2% to 5% of melanomas occur on the vulva. Vulvar melanomas have a poorer prognosis than melanoma of the torso, reflecting their tendency to be thicker and more advanced at the time of diagnosis. (*Courtesy of* E. Hernandez, MD.)

Cervicitis and Endometritis

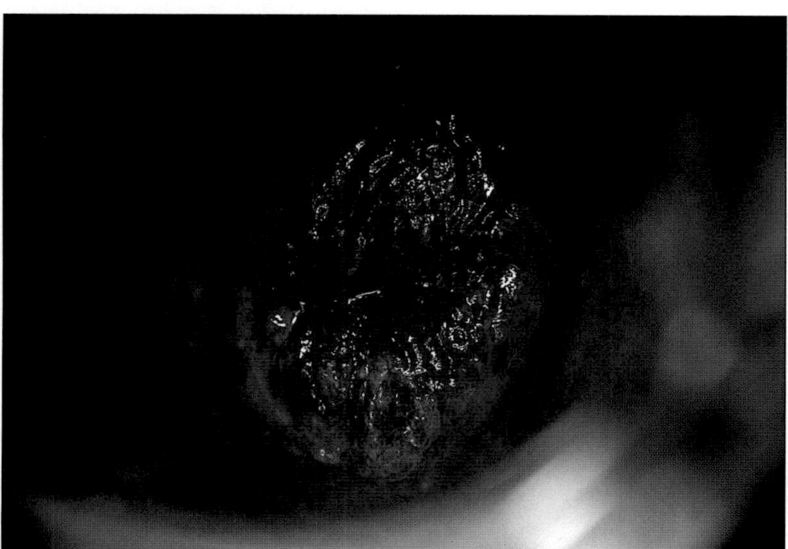

Figure 9-42 Cervical ectopy. The eversion of the endocervical columnar cells causes the normal finding of "ectopy." This commonly occurs in women on oral contraceptives. Cervical ectopy may predispose women to infection with *Chlamydia* [22]. (*Courtesy of* P. Wolner-Hanssen, MD.)

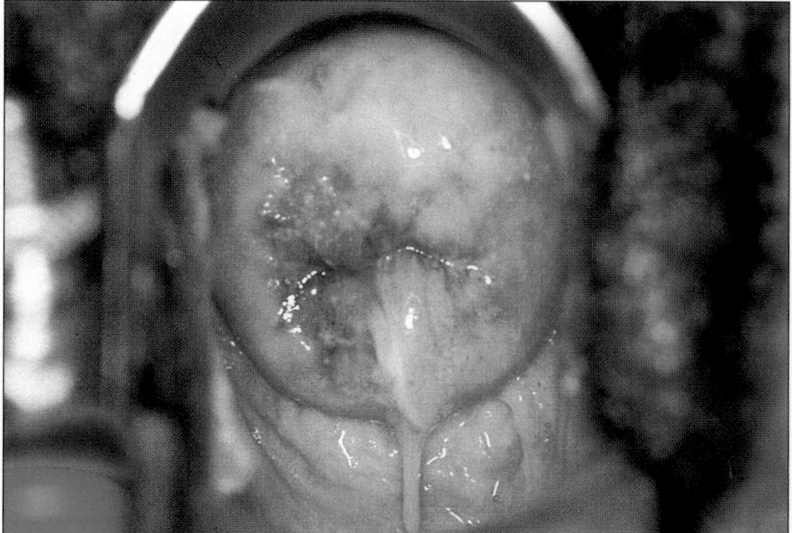

Figure 9-43 Mucopurulent endocervical discharge in gonococcal endocervicitis. Note the thick, yellow exudate escaping from the endocervical canal.

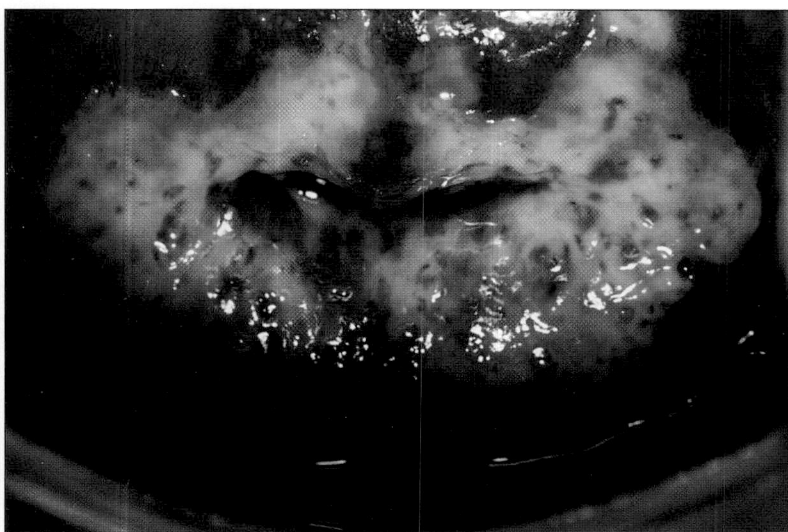

Figure 9-44 Gross appearance of herpes cervicitis. Primary herpes cervicitis may also be characterized by increased surface vascularity and microulcerations without necrotic areas. (*Courtesy of* P. Wolner-Hanssen, MD.)

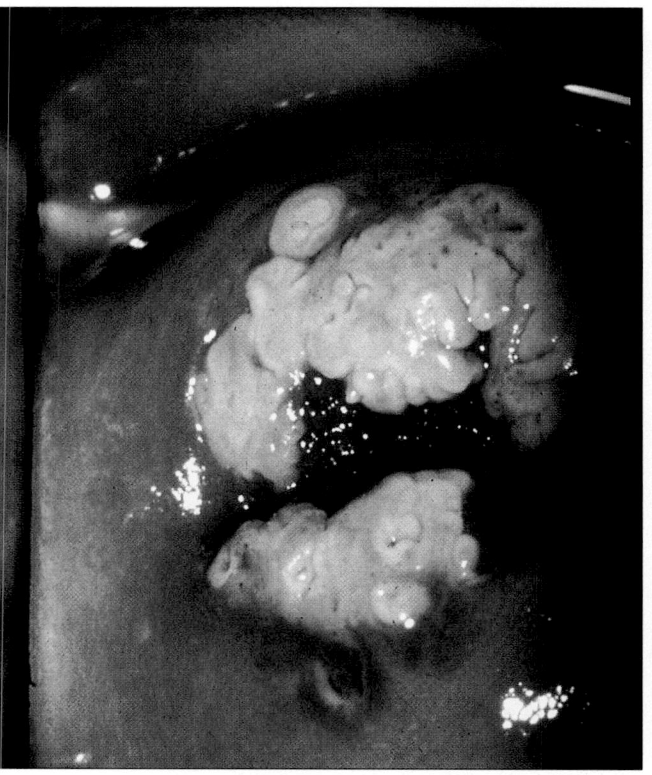

Figure 9-45 Cervical dysplasia manifested by acetowhitening of the squamous epithelium. Advanced degrees of dysplasia are associated with surface vascular changes described as punctation and mosaicism, as shown in the figure. (*Courtesy of* H. Krebs, MD.)

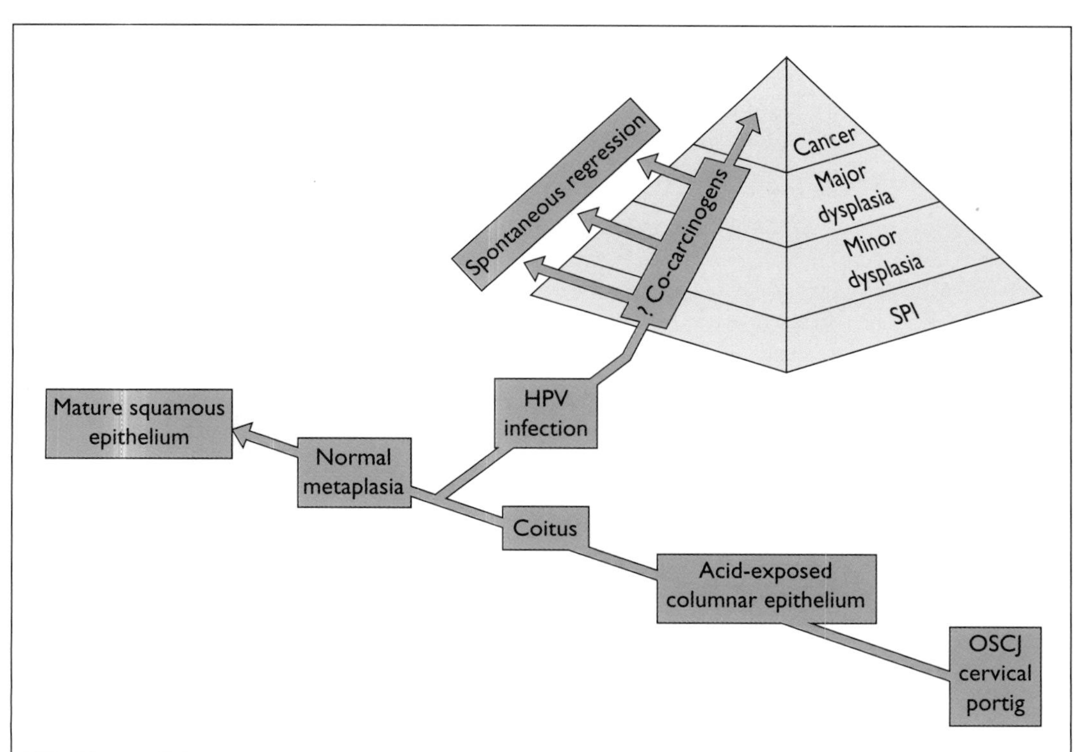

Figure 9-46 Progress of squamous metaplasia in the transformation zone. The process of squamous metaplasia leads to the formation of the transformation zone. Carcinogens, including human papillomavirus (HPV), acting at the squamocolumnar junction result in the dysplastic transformation of the cervical epithelial cells. (OSCJ—original squamocolumnar junction; SPI—subclinical papillomavirus infection.) (*Adapted from* Reid *et al.* [23].)

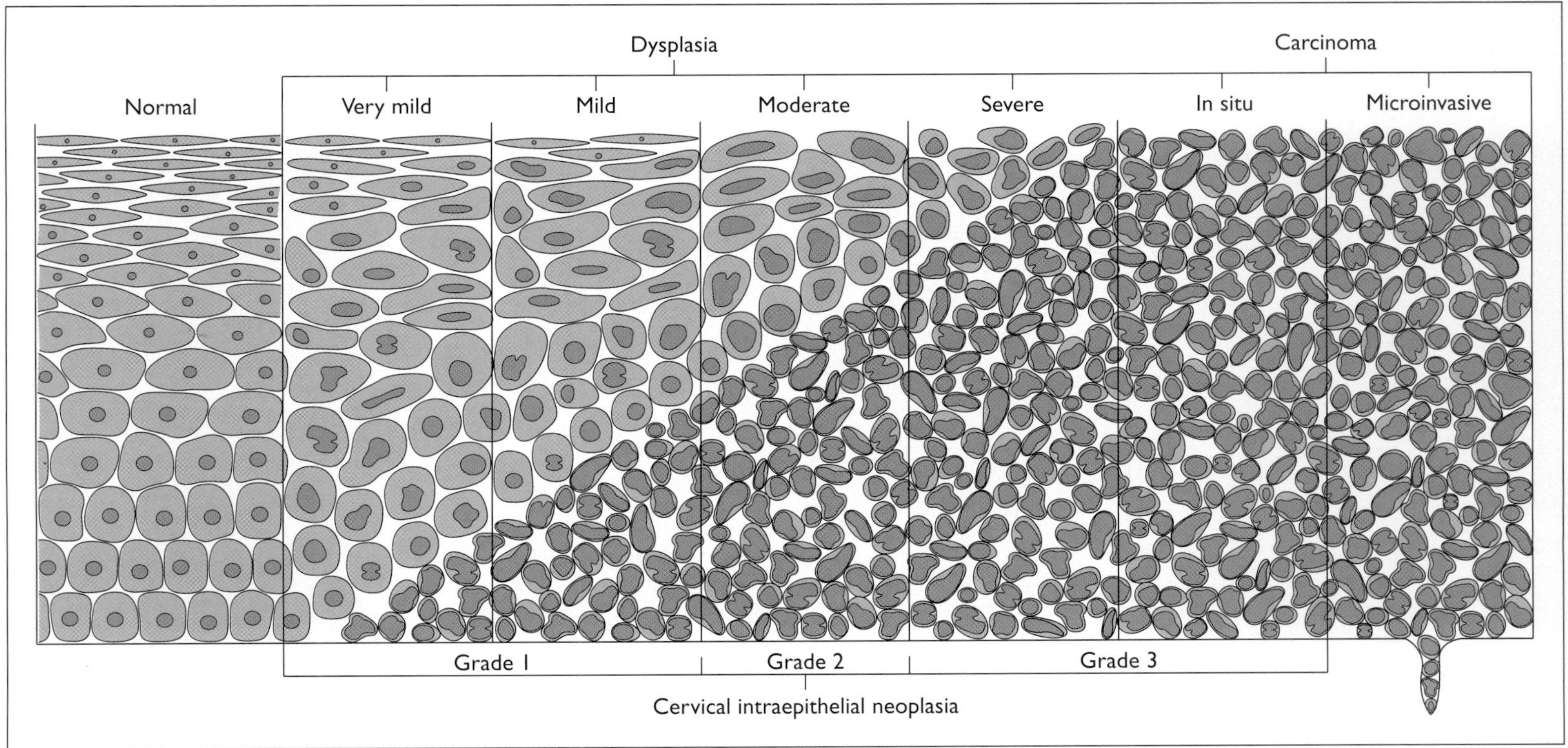

FIGURE 9-47 Depth of dysplastic involvement indicating grade of dysplasia. The depth of involvement of the cervical epithelium with dysplastic cells as reflected in a cervical biopsy determines the grade of dysplasia.

SEPTIC ABORTION

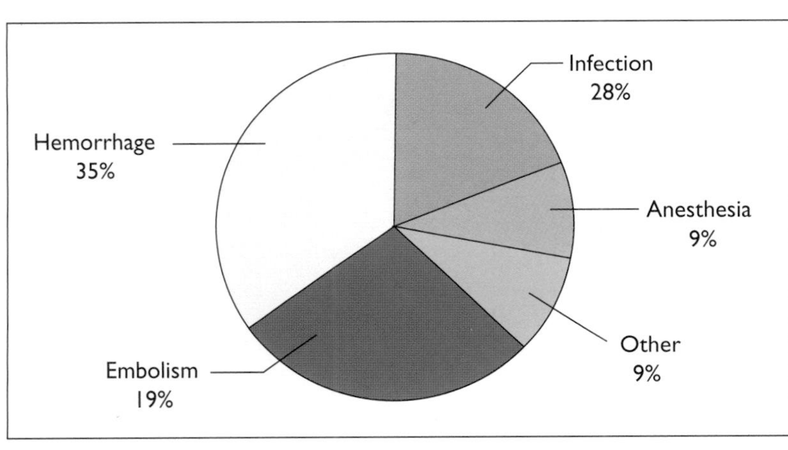

FIGURE 9-48 Causes of deaths due to abortion in the United States between 1979 and 1986. Although infection accounts for only 7.6% of total maternal deaths in the United States, it caused 28% of abortion-related deaths from 1979 to 1986. (*Adapted from* Koonin *et al.* [24].)

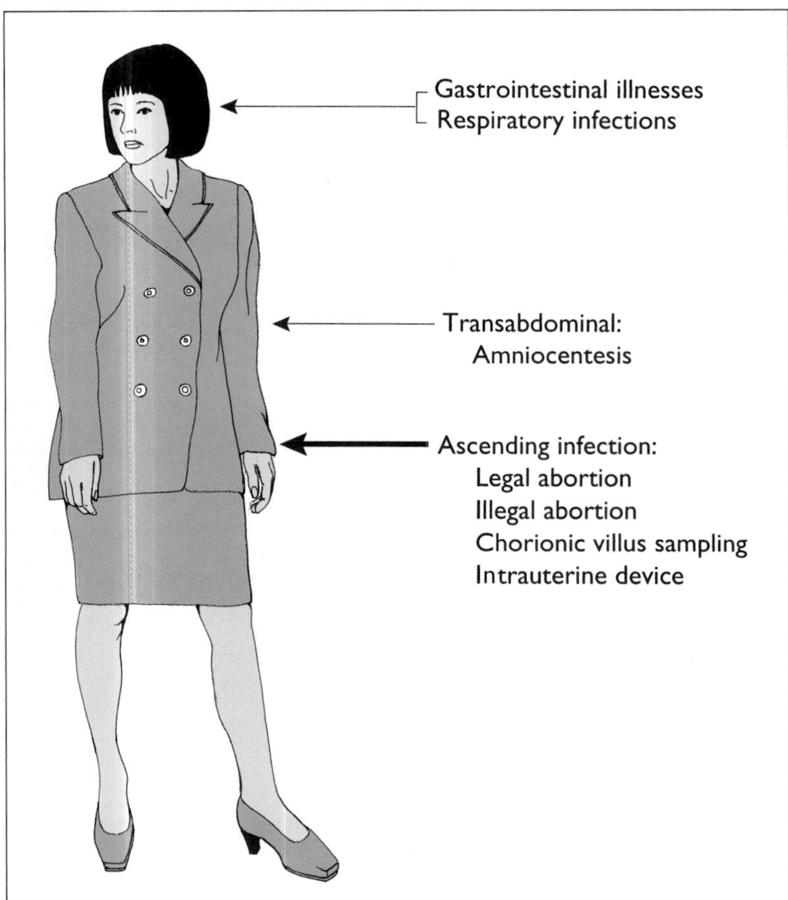

FIGURE 9-49 Pathogenesis of septic abortion. The vast majority of septic abortions occur as a result of ascending infection from the vagina, frequently with some associated traumatic event. However, cases of septic abortion in which the infecting organism was thought to be ingested (*Listeria monocytogenes, Clostridium jejuni*), inhaled (*Haemophilus influenzae*), or introduced transabdominally have been reported.

Signs of septic abortion
Fever, tachycardia, tachypnea, hypotension
Lower abdominal tenderness
Bloody or malodorous vaginal discharge
Cervical os may be open or closed
Uterine tenderness
Adnexal masses
Septic shock and disseminated intravascular coagulation

FIGURE 9-50 Signs of septic abortion. The signs of septic abortion are those arising as a result of bacteremia and its sequelae as well as of the local uterine infection.

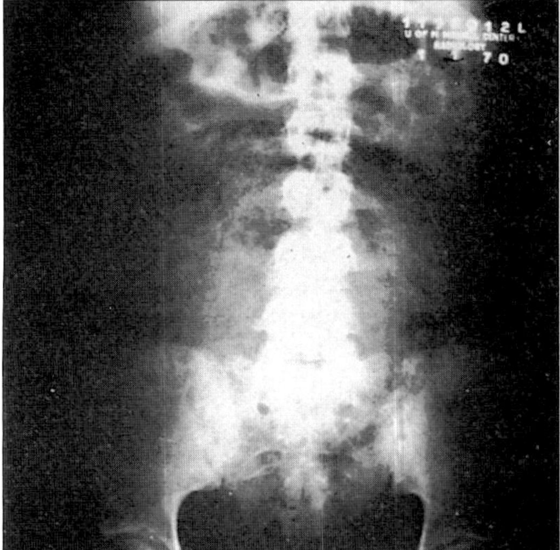

FIGURE 9-51 Abdominal radiograph of patient with a postabortal *Clostridium perfringens* infection. Whereas gas beneath the diaphragm is suggestive of a bowel perforation occurring during the abortion, gas within the myometrium typically results from *C. perfringens* infection. In either situation, operative management of the patient becomes mandatory. (*From* Eaton *et al.* [25]; with permission.)

Antibiotic selection in septic abortion
Ampicillin, gentamicin, and clindamycin
Other aminoglycosides or aztreonam may be substituted for gentamicin
Cefoxitin and doxycycline
Alternatives to cefoxitin include cefotetan, ticarcillin/clavulanate, ampicillin/sulbactam, piperacillin/tazobactam, and imipenem

FIGURE 9-52 Antibiotic selection in septic abortion. Antibiotic selection for the treatment of septic abortion is similar to that for treatment of other pelvic infections. Initial antibiotics should mainly cover the normal vaginal flora and sexually transmitted organisms such as *Neisseria gonorrhoeae* and *Chlamydia trachomatis*. Although penicillin G is generally considered the drug of choice for patients with clostridial infections, alternatives such as clindamycin, metronidazole, tetracycline, and imipenem demonstrate *in vitro* activity against most strains and sidestep concerns about growing penicillin resistance.

Surgical treatment of septic abortion
Curettage of retained products
Laparoscopy if uterine perforation suspected
Laparotomy with possible:
Drainage or removal of abscess
Total abdominal hysterectomy

Figure 9-53 Surgical treatment of septic abortion. Dilation and curettage should be performed routinely to remove any infected debris within the uterus. If uterine perforation is suspected or if the patient fails to respond to therapy, laparoscopy or laparotomy is indicated to look for hemoperitoneum, bowel perforation, or adnexal abscess. Although the exact role of hysterectomy remains controversial, it should be considered in the presence of clostridial infection, unless the patient responds rapidly to medical therapy.

Tuboovarian Abscesses

Clinical findings in tuboovarian abscesses: Physical and laboratory findings
Fever (60%–80% of patients)
Lower abdominal tenderness
"Signs of peritonitis" (*eg,* guarding/rebound)
Excess cervicovaginal secretions
Evidence of cervicitis
Palpation of adnexal mass
Leukocytosis (66%–80% of patients)

Figure 9-54 Clinical findings in tuboovarian abscess. Physical and laboratory findings. The clinical presentation of patients with tuboovarian abscesses is similar to that of women with acute pelvic inflammatory disease. Most women present with abdominal and/or pelvic pain. The presence of other symptoms and findings, such as fever, increased vaginal discharge, and leukocytosis may be variable. Palpation of an adnexal mass may be inadequate due to the pelvic pain and tenderness [26].

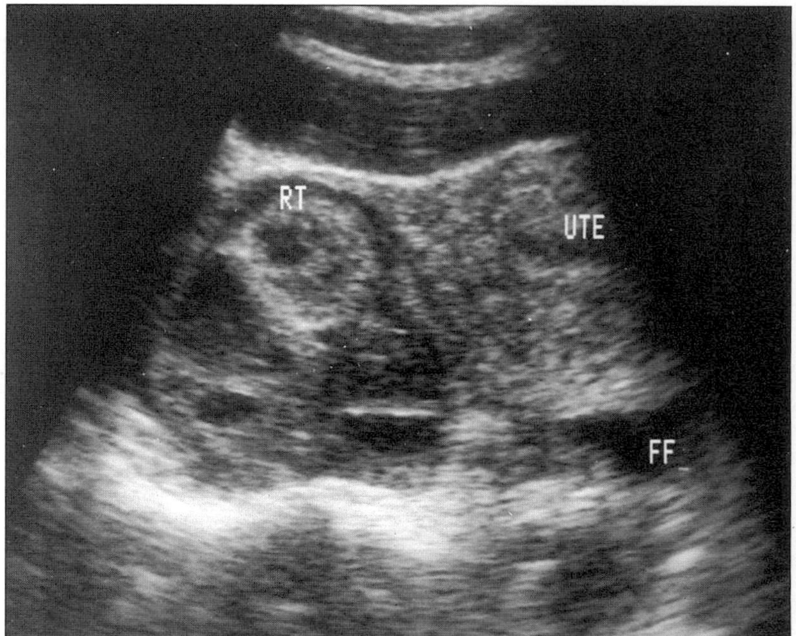

Figure 9-55 Ultrasound image of tuboovarian abscess. The mass in the right adnexa (RT) demonstrates a complex architecture with septations, internal echoes, and thickened walls. Free fluid (FF), which may represent a purulent exudate, is often seen. (UTE—uterus.)

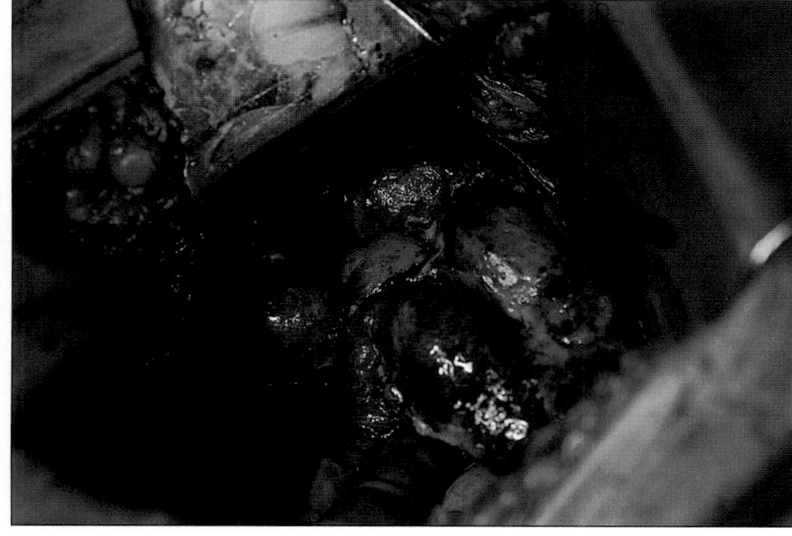

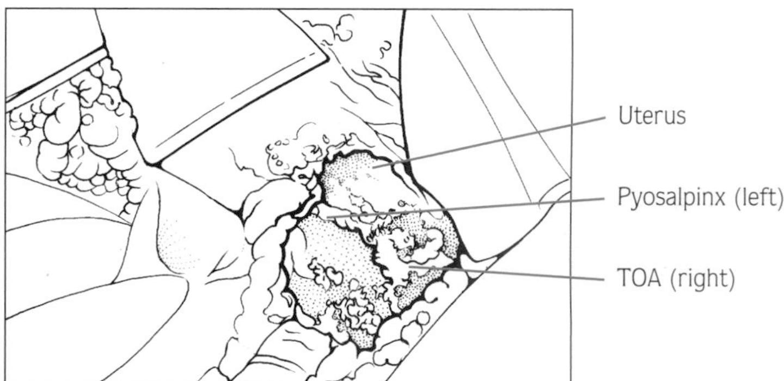

Figure 9-56 Operative view at laparotomy of a patient with a right-sided tuboovarian abscess (TOA) and a left pyosalpinx. Fresh adhesion formation and fibrinous exudate can be easily appreciated.

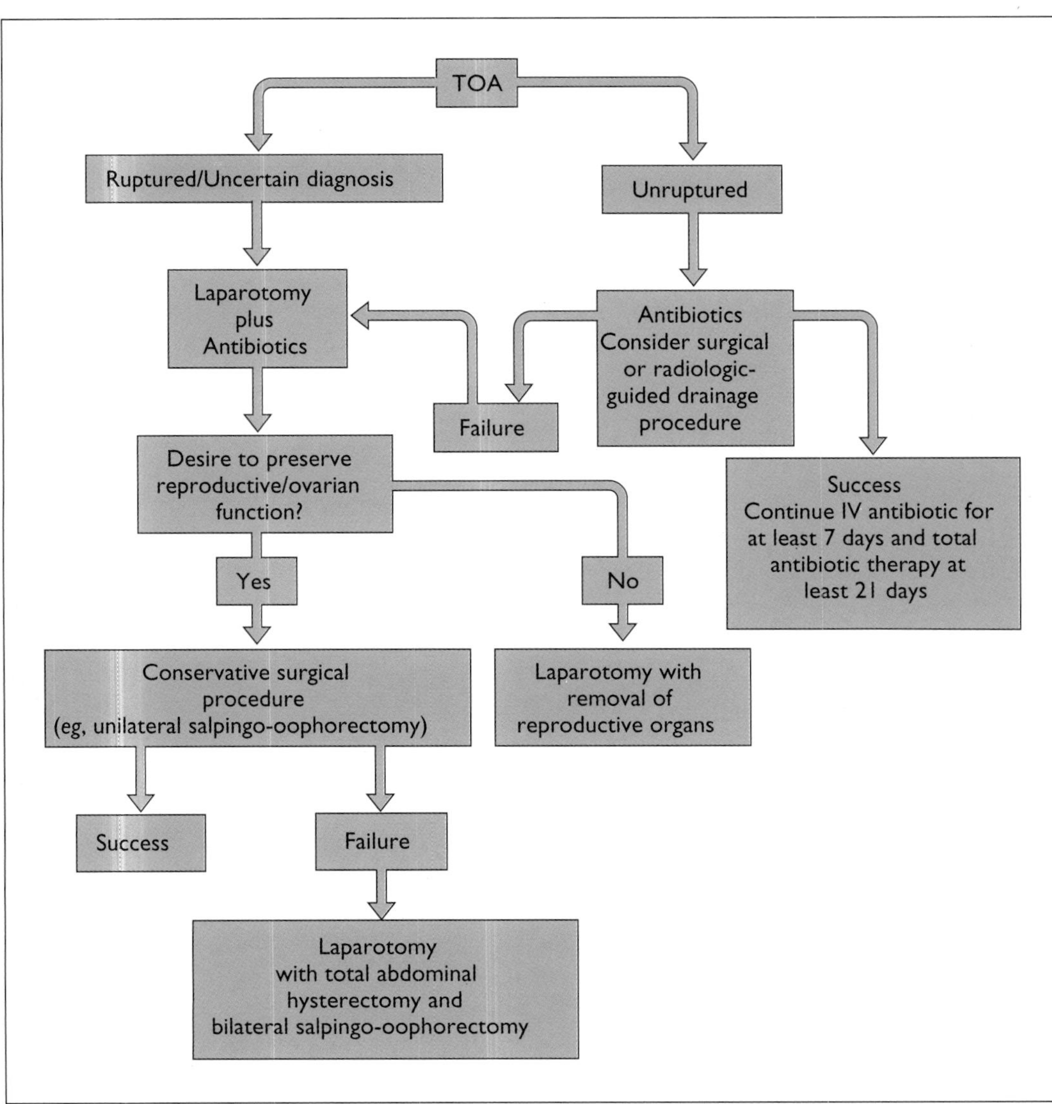

FIGURE 9-57 Approach to the management of tuboovarian abscess(TOA). Medical management utilizing broad-spectrum antimicrobials may be selected when there is certainty of diagnosis, the patient is clinically stable, and the abscess is unruptured. Otherwise, operative intervention with either conservative or definitive procedures is often necessary. Radiologic-guided drainage procedures (ultrasound or computed tomography–guided) may be useful as adjunct measures in addition to antibiotic therapy. (IV—intravenous.)

Medical therapy for tuboovarian abscesses

Clindamycin, 900 mg IV every 8 hrs, *plus*
Gentamicin, 2 mg/kg IV loading dose followed by 1.5 mg/kg every 8 hrs
After discharge continue clindamycin, 450 mg orally five times a day, to complete a 21-day course
or
Cefoxitin 2 g IV every 6 hrs, *or*
Cefotetan, 2 g IV every 12 hrs, *plus*
Doxycycline, 100 mg every 12 hrs orally or IV
After discharge continue doxycycline, 100 mg orally twice a day to complete a 21-day course

*Intravenous therapy should be administered for at least 7 days.
IV—intravenously.

FIGURE 9-58 Medical therapy for tuboovarian abscess. These antibiotic regimens provide adequate coverage against organisms commonly found in tuboovarian abscesses. Specifically, these regimens target anaerobic organisms and both gram-positive and gram-negative aerobic microbes, including *Neisseria gonorrhoeae* and *Chlamydia trachomatis*. The safety of these two regimens is excellent.

Pelvic actinomycosis and IUD use

Tuboovarian abscesses due to *Actinomyces israelii* typically seen with prolonged IUD use
Approximately 10% of IUD users are colonized with *A. israelii*
Removal of IUD usually eradicates *A. israelii* colonization

IUD—intrauterine device.

FIGURE 9-59 Pelvic actinomycosis and intrauterine device (IUD) use. *Actinomyces israelii* is a gram-positive anaerobic bacteria with a filamentous branching appearance. It commonly colonizes the gastrointestinal tract, and it does not cause invasive disease unless mucosal barriers are interrupted, as in IUD use. There are no data on the ideal approach to the management of women with incidental findings of *A. israelii* colonization. Currently, many authorities recommend removal of the IUD followed by repeat testing for *A. israelii* by Papanicolaou smear in 2 to 3 months [27,28].

References

1. Stamm WE, Wagner KF, Amsel R, *et al.*: Causes of the urethral syndrome in women. *N Engl J Med* 1980, 303:409–415.
2. Raz R, Stamm WE: A controlled trial of intravaginal estradiol in post-menopausal women with recurrent urinary tract infections. *N Engl J Med* 1993, 329:753–756.
3. Bergeron MG, Treatment of pyelonephritis. *Med Clin North Am* 1995, 79:619–649.
4. Chamberland S, L'Ècuyer J, Lessard C, *et al.*: Antibiotic susceptibility profiles of 941 gram-negative bacteria isolated from septicemia patients throughout Canada. *Clin Infect Dis* 1992, 15:615–628.
5. Rubin RH, Shapiro ED, Andriole VT, *et al.*: Evaluation of new anti-infective drugs for the treatment of urinary infection. *Clin Infect Dis* 1992, 15:S216–S227.
6. Little PJ: The incidence of urinary infection in 5,000 pregnant women. *Lancet* 1966, 2:925–928.
7. Kincaid-Smith P, Bullen M: Bacteriuria in pregnancy. *Lancet* 1965, i:395–399.
8. Campbell-Brown M, McFadyen R, Seal DJ, Stephenson ML: Is screening for bacteriuria in pregnancy worthwhile? *BMJ* 1987, 294:1579–1582.
9. Schaeffer AJ, Wendel EF, Dunn JK, Grayhack JT: Prevalence and significance of prostatic inflammation. *J Urol* 1981, 125:215–219.
10. Stamey TA, Meares EM Jr, Winningham DG: Chronic bacterial prostatitis and the diffusion of drugs into prostatic fluid. *J Urol* 1970, 103:187–194.
11. Schaberg DR, Culver DH, Gaynes RP: Major trends in the microbial etiology of nosocomial infection. *Am J Med* 1991, 91(suppl 3B):72S–75S.
12. Weber DJ, Rutala W, Samsa WA, *et al.*: Relative frequency of nosocomial pathogens at a university hospital during the decade 1980–1989. *Am J Infect Control* 1992, 20:192–197.
13. Stamm WE: Catheter-associated urinary tract infection: Epidemiology, pathogenesis, and prevention. *Am J Med* 1991, 91(suppl 3B):65S–71S.
14. Ang BSP, Telenti A, King B, *et al.*: Candidemia from a urinary tract source: Microbiological aspects and clinical significance. *Clin Infect Dis* 1993, 17:662–666.
15. Fisher JF, Hicks BC, Dipiro JT, *et al.*: Efficacy of a single intravenous dose of amphotericin B in urinary tract infections caused by *Candida* [letter]. *J Infect Dis* 1987, 156:685–687.
16. Hsu CCS, Ukleja B: Clearance of *Candida* colonizing the urinary bladder by a two-day amphotericin B irrigation. *Infection* 1990, 18:280–282.
17. Wong-Beringer A, Jacobs RA, Guglielmo BJ: Treatment of funguria. *JAMA* 1992, 267:2780–2785.
18. Fisher JF, Newman CL, Sobel JD: Yeast in the urine: Solutions for a budding problem. *Clin Infect Dis* 1995, 20:183–189.
19. Nickel JC, Grant SK, Costerton JW: Catheter associated bacteriuria: An experimental study. *Urology* 1985, 26:369–375.
20. Sobel JD: Vaginal infections in adult women. *Med Clin North Am* 1990, 74:1576.
21. Tovell HMM, Young AW Jr: *Diseases of the Vulva in Clinical Practice*. New York: Elsevier; 1991.
22. Critchlow CW, Wolner-Hanssen P, Eschenbach DA, *et al.*: Determinants of cervical ectopia and of cervicitis: Age, oral contraception, specific cervical infection, smoking, and douching. *Am J Obstet Gynecol* 1995, 173:534–543.
23. Reid R, Fu YS, Herschman BR, *et al.*: Genital warts and cervical cancer: VI. The relationship between aneuploid and polyploid cervical lesions. *Am J Obstet Gynecol* 1984, 150:189.
24. Koonin LM, Atrash HK, Lawson HW, Smith JC: Maternal mortality surveillance, United States, 1979–1986. *MMWR* 1991, 40(SS-2):10.
25. Eaton CJ, Peterson EP: Diagnosis and acute management of patients with advanced clostridial sepsis complicating abortion. *Am J Obstet Gynecol* 1971, 109:1162–1166.
26. Sweet RL, Gibbs RS: Mixed anaerobic-aerobic pelvic infection and pelvic abscess. *In* Sweet SL, Gibbs RS (eds.): *Infectious Diseases of the Female Genital Tract*, 3rd ed. Baltimore: Willams & Wilkins, 1995.
27. Fiorino AS: Intrauterine contraceptive device-associated actinomyces detection on cervical smear. *Obstet Gynecol* 1996, 87:142.
28. Keebler C, Chatwani A, Schwartz R: Actinomycosis infection associated with intrauterine contraceptive devices. *Am J Obstet Gynecol* 1983, 145:596–599.

INDEX

Abdominal infections, 7.2–7.5
Abortion, septic, 9.18–9.20
Abscess
- amebic, of liver, 6.15
- brain, 3.8–3.10
  - papilledema in, 3.20
  - in sinusitis, 3.16, 4.10
- epidural, 3.12–3.13
  - in sinusitis, 3.16, 4.10
- intra-abdominal, 7.5
- kidney, 7.28
- liver, 6.15, 7.26
- lung, 6.11
  - in transplantation, 6.21–6.22
- neck, 4.21–4.22
- orbital, 4.3–4.4
- ovarian, 7.28
- parapharyngeal, 4.21
- periappendiceal, 7.27
- periodontal, 4.10
- prostatic, 9.9
- retropharyngeal, 4.22, 8.14
- spleen, in endocarditis, 8.8
- sublingual space, 4.22
- subperiosteal
  - frontal bone, 4.9
  - orbital, 4.3–4.4
- tuboovarian, 7.28, 9.20–9.21

Acetic acid test, for wart detection, 5.18
Acquired immunodeficiency syndrome *see* Human immunodeficiency virus infection
Acrodermatitis chronica atrophicans, in Lyme disease, 3.3–3.4
Actinomycetoma, 2.12
Actinomycosis
- brain abscess, 3.10
- mycetoma, 2.12
- pelvic, 9.21
- pleural space, 6.18
- pulmonary manifestations of, 6.23

Acyclovir
- in herpes simplex virus infections, 1.45, 5.20–5.21
- in herpes zoster ophthalmicus, 1.19, 3.19
- in varicella-zoster infections, 8.3

Adhesions, in pelvic inflammatory disease, 5.6
Adult respiratory distress syndrome, in toxic shock syndrome, 6.2
African trypanosomiasis (sleeping sickness), 3.10
AIDS *see* Human immunodeficiency virus infection
AIDS dementia complex, 3.7
Alopecia, in syphilis, 5.13
Amantadine, in influenza, 6.13
Ambylomma americanum, ehrlichiosis from, 8.20
Amebiasis
- dysentery in, 7.19
- liver abscess in, 6.15

Amoxicillin, in Lyme disease, 3.4, 8.18–8.19
Amoxicillin-clavulanate, in bite infections, 2.9
Amphotericin B, in candiduria, 9.11
Ampicillin
- in meningitis, 3.2–3.3
- in pyelonephritis, 9.5

Anaerobic infections
- abdominal, 7.2
- appendicitis, 7.3–7.4
- bacterial vaginosis, 5.5
- of bites, 2.8–2.9
- culture specimen collection in, 7.2
- pulmonary, 6.11
- of skin and soft tissue, 2.24

Anemia
- in ehrlichiosis, 8.21
- in HIV infection, 1.32

Aneurysm
- aortic, in syphilis, 5.15
- mycotic, in endocarditis, 8.8

Angina, Ludwig's, 4.22
Angiomatosis
- bacillary, 8.22–8.24
- bacillary epithelioid, in HIV infection, 1.18

Animals
- bites of, infections of, 2.7–2.9
- contact with
  - babesiosis from, 8.19–8.20
  - ehrlichiosis from, 8.19–8.20
  - skin and soft-tissue infections from, 2.9–2.10

Antibiotics
- in bites, 2.9
- in cystitis, 9.3
- in meningitis, 3.2–3.3
- in osteomyelitis, 2.25–2.27
- prophylactic, for traveler's diseases, 7.13
- in pyelonephritis, 9.5
- in septic abortion, 9.19
- in tuboovarian abscess, 9.21
- in urinary tract infections, catheter-associated, 9.13
- *see also specific antibiotic and infection*

Antibodies, Forssman, in syphilis, 5.16
Antibody-dependent cellular cytotoxicity, in HIV infection, 1.11
Anus
- neoplasia of, in HIV infection, 1.44
- warts at, 5.18

Aortic aneurysm, in syphilis, 5.15
Aphthous stomatitis, 4.12
Aphthous ulcers, in HIV infection, 1.23
Apoptosis, HIV-induced, 1.11
Appendicitis, 7.27
- gangrenous or perforated, 7.3–7.4

Appendicolith, 7.27
Arbovirus infections, encephalitis, 3.5
Arthritis
- in HIV infection, 1.14
- in Lyme disease, 8.18–8.19
- reactive, 2.31
- septic, 2.28–2.29, 8.15

Arthrocentesis, in septic arthritis, 2.28
Ascariasis, 7.22

Ascites, in syphilis, 5.16
Aspergillosis
  bronchitis in, 6.24
  external ear, 4.7
  gastrointestinal, 7.25
  pulmonary, 6.10, 8.31
    in cancer, 6.20
    in transplantation, 6.22
Aspiration pneumonia, staphylococcal, 6.3
Azithromycin
  in bite infections, 2.9
  in Lyme disease, 8.18
  in *Mycobacterium avium* complex infections, 1.42
Aztreonam, in pyelonephritis, 9.5

B

Babesiosis, 8.19–8.22
Bacillary angiomatosis, 8.22–8.24
Bacillary epithelioid angiomatosis, in HIV infection, 1.18
Bacillary peliosis, 8.22–8.24
Back pain, in spinal tuberculosis, 2.30
Bacteremia, 8.9–8.11
  Bartonella, 8.22–8.24
  staphylococcal, 6.3, 8.15
  streptococcal, gangrene in, 2.7
Bacterial vaginosis, 5.4–5.5, 9.15
Bacteriuria
  catheter-associated, 9.13
  in pregnancy, 9.7
Bacteroides infections
  appendicitis, 7.4
  brain abscess, 3.10
Balanoposthitis, candidal, 5.9
Ballooned cells, in viral hepatitis, 7.7
Barium studies, of gastrointestinal syphilis, 7.25
Bartholinitis, gonococcal, 5.2
Bartonella infections, 8.22–8.24
  in HIV infection, 1.18
Bell's palsy, in Lyme disease, 8.18
Bismuth preparations, in traveler's diarrhea, 7.13
Bites
  animal, infections of, 2.7–2.9
  mosquito
    encephalitis from, 3.5
    myiasis from, 2.17
  spider, 2.15
  tick
    ehrlichiosis from, 8.19–8.20
    encephalitis from, 3.5
    Lyme disease from, 8.16–8.17
Blastomycosis, 8.29
  pulmonary, 6.9, 6.24
  of skin, 2.12
Blindness, river (onchocerciasis), 2.16
Blisters
  infections with, 2.2
  in syphilis, 5.16
Boils (furuncles), 2.3
Bolivian hemorrhagic fever, 8.27–8.28
Bone
  infections of *see* Osteomyelitis
  lesions of, in syphilis, 5.16
Bone marrow, biopsy of, in HIV infection, 1.33
Borderline lepromatous leprosy, 2.19, 2.22, 8.25–8.26
Borderline leprosy, 2.19
Borderline tuberculoid leprosy, 2.19–2.21, 8.25
Borreliosis (Lyme disease), 8.16–8.19
  vs. babesiosis, 8.21
  erythema migrans in, 2.22
  neurologic disorders in, 3.3–3.4
Bovine spongiform encephalopathy, 3.21
Brain
  abscess of, 3.8–3.10
    papilledema in, 3.20
    in sinusitis, 3.16, 4.10
  edema of, in encephalitis, 3.6
  encephalitis of
    in HIV infection, 1.28
    viral, 3.5–3.8
  hemorrhage of, in sepsis, 3.17
  lymphoma of, 3.7–3.8
    in HIV infection, 1.29, 1.43
  mycotic aneurysm in, in endocarditis, 8.8
  parasitic diseases of, 3.10–3.12
Brain stem disorders, in endocarditis, 3.18
Bronchitis, 6.24–6.25
Brown recluse spider bites, 2.15
Buboes, in chlamydial infections, 5.4
Bullae, infections with, 2.2
Bullous myringitis, 4.8
Bursitis, septic, 2.30

C

Calculi
  kidney, in infection, 9.7
  in Stensen's duct, 4.19
Calicivirus infections, enteritis, 7.17–7.19
Cancer
  in *Helicobacter pylori* infections, 7.15
  in HIV infection, 1.42–1.44
    cervical, 1.48
    see also Kaposi's sarcoma
  pneumonia in, 6.18–6.20
Candidemia, in candiduria, 9.11
Candidiasis
  disseminated, 2.12, 7.23
  esophageal, 1.25, 7.23
  in HIV infection, 1.22–1.23, 1.25
    treatment of, 1.41
  oral, 1.22–1.23, 4.11
  of skin and soft tissue, 2.11–2.12, 8.31
    in immunodeficiency, 8.35
  vulvovaginal, 5.9–5.10, 9.15
    lichen simplex chronica after, 9.14
Candiduria, 9.10–9.11
Capnocytophaga infections, of animal bites, 2.9
Carbuncles, 2.4
Cardiomyopathy, in HIV infection, 1.45
Caries, dental, 4.11

Cat bites, infections of, 2.8
Cat scratch disease, 4.17, 8.22, 8.24
Catheterassociated infections
 intravenous, 6.3
 urinary, 9.12–9.14
Cavernous venous sinus infections, 3.15
Cefotaxime, in meningitis, 3.2
Cefotetan, in tuboovarian abscess, 9.21
Cefoxitin
 in bite infections, 2.9
 in tuboovarian abscess, 9.21
Ceftazidime, in meningitis, 3.2–3.3
Ceftriaxone
 in Lyme disease, 3.4, 8.19
 in meningitis, 3.2
 in pyelonephritis, 9.5
 in septic arthritis, 2.29
Cefuroxime
 in bite infections, 2.9
 in Lyme disease, 8.18
Cellulitis
 in animal bites, 2.7
 orbital, 4.2
  lymphadenopathy in, 4.17
 prepatellar bursitis with, 2.30
 preseptal, 3.19, 4.3
 staphylococcal, 2.4
 streptococcal, 2.6, 8.13
 sublingual space, 4.22
 after tracheoesophageal puncture, 4.22
Central nervous system
 endocarditis effects on, 3.18
 sepsis effects on, 3.17–3.18
Central nervous system infections, 3.2–3.18
 bony sinuses, 3.16
 brain abscess *see* Brain, abscess of
 cryptococcal, 3.9
 encephalitis, 1.28, 3.5–3.8
 epidural abscess, 3.12–3.13
 meningitis
  bacterial, 3.2–3.3
  chronic, 3.3–3.5
 parasitic, 3.10–3.12
 prion diseases, 3.21–3.22
 skull, 3.16
 subdural empyema, 3.12–3.13
 toxoplasmosis, 3.7, 3.9
 venous sinus, 3.14–3.15
Cephalosporins
 in bite infections, 2.9
 in brain abscess, 3.10
 in meningitis, 3.2–3.3
Cerebellum, dysfunction of, in Gerstmann-Strässler syndrome, 3.22
Cerebrospinal fluid analysis, in meningitis, 3.2
 tuberculous, 3.4
Cervicitis, 9.16–9.18
 chlamydial, 5.4
 gonococcal, 5.2
 herpes simplex virus, 5.20
Cervix
 cancer of, in HIV infection, 1.48
 chancre of, 5.12
 dysplasia of, 9.17–9.18
 ectopy of, 9.16
 neoplasia of, in HIV infection, 1.44, 1.49
Chagas' disease, 3.11
 esophageal dilatation in, 8.33
 soft-tissue manifestations of, 2.17
Chancre, in syphilis, 5.11–5.12
Chancroid, 5.21–5.22
Chemical mediators, in sepsis, 8.9
Chemotherapy
 for Hodgkin's disease, 1.44
 for Kaposi's sarcoma, 1.42
 for lymphoma, in HIV infection, 1.43
 pneumonia in, 6.20
Chickenpox, 2.14, 8.3
Chlamydial infections, 5.3–5.4
 psittacosis, 6.6
Chloramphenicol
 in Lyme disease, 8.18–8.19
 in meningitis, 3.3
Cholecystitis, 7.4–7.5
 emphysematous, 7.27
Cholera, 7.10
Cholesteatoma, 4.6
Chorioretinitis, in toxoplasmosis, 3.20
 in HIV infection, 1.21
Chronic wasting syndrome, 3.21
Cidofovir, in cytomegalovirus infections, in HIV infection, 1.41
Cierry-Mader classification, of osteomyelitis, 2.25–2.27
Ciprofloxacin
 in *Bartonella* infections, 8.24
 in *Mycobacterium avium* complex infections, 1.42
 in pyelonephritis, 9.5
Clarithromycin
 in bite infections, 2.9
 in *Mycobacterium avium* complex infections, 1.42
Clindamycin
 in deep neck abscess, 4.21
 in tuboovarian abscess, 9.21
Clofazimine, in *Mycobacterium avium* complex infections, 1.42
Clostridial infections
 brain abscess, 3.10
 sepsis, 8.10
 of skin and soft tissue, 2.23–2.24
  abdominal wall, 7.3
Clostridium difficile infections, 7.26
Clostridium histolyticum infections, gangrene, 2.23
Clostridium perfringens infections
 gangrene, 2.23
 Gram stain in, 2.23
 septic abortion, 9.19
Clostridium septicum infections
 gangrene, 2.23
 necrotizing fasciitis, 2.23
CLOtest, in *Helicobacter pylori* infections, 7.16
Clue cells, in bacterial vaginosis, 5.5
Coagulation disorders
 in HIV infection, 1.34
 in sepsis, 8.11
Coccidioidomycosis, 8.30–8.31
 pulmonary, 6.10

Colitis
cytomegalovirus, 7.26
in HIV infection, 1.26
pseudomembranous, imaging of, 7.26
Colony-stimulating factors, in HIV infection, 1.12
Colpitis macularis, 5.7
Complement deficiency, gonococcal infections in, 2.29
Condyloma acuminatum, 5.17–5.18, 9.15
Condyloma lata, 5.13
in HIV infection, 1.44
Congenital syphilis, 5.15–5.16
Conjunctiva
hemorrhage of, in endocarditis, 8.7, 8.15
suffusion of, in Lassa fever, 8.27
Conjunctivitis, 3.19
in Reiter's syndrome, 2.31
Consciousness alterations, causes of, 3.18
Contact lens, corneal ulcer from, 3.20
Cornea, ulcer of, 3.20
in HIV infection, 1.20
Corticosteroids
in erythema nodosum leprosum, 2.20
in *Pneumocystis carinii* pneumonia, 1.40
Corynebacterium infections, pyelonephritis, 9.4
Cottage cheese discharge, in vulvovaginal candidiasis, 5.9
Coxiella burnetii infections, pneumonia, 6.6
Coxsackievirus infections, 8.5
hand, foot, and mouth disease, 2.14–2.15, 4.13
skin, 2.14–2.15
Crab lice, 2.15, 5.18
Cranial nerve dysfunction, in endocarditis, 3.18
Croup, 4.15
Crusted lesions, 2.2
ecthyma, 2.3
impetigo, 2.3
Cryoglobulinemia, mixed, in hepatitis C, 2.31
Cryptococcoma, of brain, 3.9
Cryptococcosis
in HIV infection, 1.35
meningitis in, 3.4–3.5
pulmonary, 6.10
of skin, 8.31
Cryptosporidiosis, in HIV infection, 1.26, 7.14, 7.20
Culture
of anaerobic bacteria, 7.2
of *Helicobacter pylori*, 7.16
Cyclospora infections
enteritis, 7.20
in HIV infection, 1.26, 1.36
Cyst(s), hydatid
of brain, 3.12
of lung, 6.16, 6.24
Cystic fibrosis, *Pseudomonas aeruginosa* empyema in, 6.17
Cysticercosis, 2.18, 3.11, 8.34
Cystitis, 9.2–9.3
Cytokines
in HIV infection, 1.12
in sepsis, 8.9–8.10
Cytomegalovirus infections
colitis, 7.26
encephalitis, 1.28
in HIV infection, 7.14
encephalitis, 1.28
gastrointestinal, 1.26
retinitis, 1.20, 1.37, 1.41, 3.21
in pediatric patients, 8.4
pneumonia, in cancer, 6.20
retinitis, 1.20, 1.37, 1.41, 3.21

Dacryoadenitis, 4.2
Dacryocystitis, 4.2
Debridement, in osteomyelitis, 2.25–2.27
Deer tick bites, Lyme disease from, 8.16–8.17
Dementia
in Gerstmann-Strässler syndrome, 3.22
in Jakob-Creutzfeldt disease, 3.22
Dental caries, 4.11
Dental infections, brain abscess in, 3.10
Dermacentor, ehrlichiosis from, 8.20
Dermatobia hominis infections, of skin and soft tissue, 2.17
Dermatobia medinensis infections (dracunculiasis), 2.18
Diabetes mellitus
pyelonephritis in, 9.7
retropharyngeal abscess in, 8.14
Dialysis, peritoneal, peritonitis in, 7.3
Diarrhea
bacterial, 7.9–7.14
diagnosis of, 7.12
algorithm for, 7.11
in HIV infection, 1.31, 7.14
Mycobacterium avium complex, in HIV infection, 1.25
traveler's, 7.12–7.13
treatment of, 7.12
algorithm for, 7.11
types of, 7.9
viral, 7.17–7.19
Dicloxacillin, in bite infections, 2.9
Didanosine, in HIV infection, 1.52–1.53, 1.55
hematologic effects of, 1.34
Dilation and curettage, in septic abortion, 9.20
Dirofilariasis, 6.15
Discharge, vaginal
in bacterial vaginosis, 5.5
in candidiasis, 5.9
evaluation of, 9.15
in trichomoniasis, 5.7
Dog bites, infections of, 2.7–2.8
Dog tick, ehrlichiosis from, 8.20
Doxycycline
in *Bartonella* infections, 8.22, 8.24
in Lyme disease, 3.4, 8.18–8.19
in tuboovarian abscess, 9.21
Dracunculiasis, 2.18
Drugs
consciousness alterations from, 3.18
intravenous use of, HIV infection transmission in, 1.4
Duodenal ulcer, in *Helicobacter pylori* infections, 7.15–7.16
Dural venous sinus infections, 3.14
Dysentery, amebic, 7.19
Dysuria
in cystitis, 9.2
in prostatitis, 9.9

E

Ear infections
- external (otitis externa), 4.6–4.8
- middle (otitis media), 4.4–4.6

Eardrum
- disorders of, 4.3–4.4
- normal, 4.3

Ebola virus infections, 8.29
Echinococcosis
- of brain, 3.12
- of lung, 6.16, 6.24

Echovirus infections, 8.5
Ecthyma, staphylococcal, 2.3
Ecthyma gangrenosum
- in bacteremia, 8.11
- in immunodeficiency, 8.35

Ectoparasitic diseases, of skin, 2.15–2.16, 5.18–5.19
Edema
- brain, in encephalitis, 3.6
- facial, in hemorrhagic fever, 8.28
- pulmonary, in hantavirus pulmonary syndrome, 8.29

Effusion, pleural, 6.16–6.18
Eggs, helminth, relative sizes of, 7.21
Ehrlichiosis, 8.19–8.21
Eikenella corrodens infections, of bites, 2.8–2.9
Elephantiasis, 2.16
ELISA (enzyme-linked immunosorbent assay), for HIV, 1.6, 1.8
Embolism
- mesenteric artery, in candidiasis, 7.23
- pulmonary, in sepsis, 8.10

Emphysema, subcutaneous, 6.18
Emphysematous cholecystitis, 7.27
Emphysematous pyelonephritis, 9.7
Empyema
- epidural, in sinusitis, 3.16
- pleural
  - anaerobic, 6.11
  - pneumonia with, 6.2
  - *Pseudomonas aeruginosa*, 6.17
- subdural, 3.12–3.13

Encephalitis
- in HIV infection, 1.28
- viral, 3.5–3.8

Encephalopathy
- mink, 3.21
- in sepsis, 3.17
- spongiform, 3.21
- toxic, 3.18

Endocarditis, infective
- *Bartonella*, 8.22
- brain abscess in, 3.10
- central nervous system manifestations of, 3.18
- external manifestations of, 8.6–8.9
- staphylococcal, 8.15

Endocervicitis, 9.16–9.18
Endotoxin, systemic effects of, 8.9
Entamoeba histolytica infections, liver abscess, 6.15
Enteritis
- bacterial, 7.9–7.14
- fungal, 7.23–7.25
- parasitic, 7.19–7.22
- viral, 7.17–7.19

Enterobacteriaceae infections
- brain abscess, 3.10
- meningitis, 3.3
- prostatitis, 9.8

Enterobius vermicularis (pinworm) infections, 7.22
Enterococcal infections
- appendicitis, 7.3
- endocarditis, 8.7

Enterocytozoon infections, in HIV infection, 7.21
Enterovirus infections
- encephalitis, 3.5
- pneumonia, 6.12

Enthesitis, in Reiter's syndrome, 2.31
Enthesopathy, in Reiter's syndrome, 2.31
Enzyme-linked immunosorbent assay, for HIV, 1.6
Epidural abscess, 3.12–3.13
- in sinusitis, 3.16, 4.10

Epidural empyema, in sinusitis, 3.16
Epiglottitis, 4.14
Epiphysitis, in syphilis, 5.16
Epstein-Barr virus infections, 8.6
- hepatitis in, 7.8

Erysipelas, 2.6, 8.13
- auricular, 4.7

Erythema
- in Bolivian hemorrhagic fever, 8.27
- in pharyngotonsillitis, 4.12
- in sepsis, 8.11

Erythema infectiosum, 8.2
Erythema marginatum, in rheumatic fever, 4.13
Erythema migrans, in Lyme disease, 2.22, 8.18
Erythema multiforme major (Stevens-Johnson syndrome), 4.14
Erythema nodosum leprosum, 2.20, 8.26
Erythromycin
- in *Bartonella* infections, 8.24
- in bite infections, 2.9
- in Lyme disease, 3.4

Eschar, infections with, 2.2
Escherichia coli infections
- appendicitis, 7.3
- cystitis, 9.2–9.3
- enteroaggregative, in HIV infection, 1.27
- enterotoxigenic, 7.13
- pyelonephritis, 9.4–9.5, 9.7
- septic arthritis, 2.29

Esophagitis
- *Candida*, 7.23
  - in HIV infection, 1.25
- herpes simplex virus, 7.25

Esophagography, 7.25
Esophagus, in Chagas' disease, 8.33
Ethambutol, in *Mycobacterium avium* complex infections, in HIV infection, 1.42
Ethmoid sinusitis, 4.9
Eubacterium infections, appendicitis, 7.4
Eumycetoma, 2.12
Exotoxins, in streptococcal infections, 8.12
Eye
- Chagas' disease manifestations in, 2.17, 3.11
- HIV infection manifestations in, 1.19–1.21
- Roth spots in, in endocarditis, 8.8

Eye infections, 3.19–3.21, 4.2
- onchocerciasis, 2.16
- orbital, 3.19–3.21, 4.2–4.4

Eyelid infections, 4.2–4.3
  cellulitis, 3.19
  molluscum contagiosum, in HIV infection, 1.19

F

Facial palsy, in Lyme disease, 8.18
Failure to thrive, in HIV infection, 1.47
Fasciitis, necrotizing, 2.2
  abdominal, 7.27
  abdominal wall, 7.2
  clostridial, 2.24
  streptococcal, 2.6
Fatal familial insomnia, 3.21
Fatty liver, 7.8
Feline spongiform encephalopathy, 3.21
Female, pelvic infections in *see under* Pelvic infections
Femur, osteomyelitis of, 2.26–2.27
Fever
  with consciousness alterations, causes of, 3.18
  viral hemorrhagic, 8.27–8.29
Fifth disease (erythema infectiosum), 8.2
Filariasis, elephantiasis in, 2.16
Finger(s)
  gonococcal infection manifestations in, 5.3
  necrosis of, in bacteremia, 8.11
  paronychia of, 2.3
Fluconazole, in candiduria, 9.11
Flucytosine, in candiduria, 9.11
Folliculitis, 2.2
  eosinophilic pustular, in HIV infection, 1.16
  Pityrosporon, 2.11
Food, safety of, in tropical regions, 7.13
Foot
  hand, food, and mouth disease of, 2.14–2.15, 4.13
  mycetoma of (Madura foot), 2.12
Forma miliar, in *Bartonella* infections, 8.23
Forssman antibodies, in syphilis, 5.16
Foscarnet, in cytomegalovirus infections, 1.41
Fournier's gangrene, 2.24
Francisella tularensis infections, pulmonary manifestations of, 6.23
Frontal bone, abscess of, 4.9
Frontal sinus, infections of, 3.16, 4.9
Fulminant hepatitis, 7.7
Fungal infections
  candiduria in, 9.10–9.11
  endocarditis, 8.7
  enteritis, 7.23–7.25
  nails, in HIV infection, 1.15
  pulmonary, 6.9–6.10
    in transplantation, 6.21
  pyelonephritis, 9.11
  skin and soft-tissue, 2.10–2.12
  systemic, 8.29–8.31
  see also Candidiasis
Furuncles, 2.3
Fusobacterium infections
  appendicitis, 7.4
  brain abscess, 3.10

G

Gallbladder infections, 7.4–7.5, 7.27
Gammopathies, in HIV infection, 1.33
Ganciclovir, in cytomegalovirus infections, 1.41
  retinitis, 1.20
Gangrene
  in appendicitis, 7.3–7.4
  Fournier's, 2.24
  gas, 2.23
    of abdominal wall, 7.3
  streptococcal, 2.7, 7.2
Gardnerella vaginalis infections, 5.5
Gas gangrene, 2.23
  of abdominal wall, 7.3
Gastritis, *Helicobacter pylori*, 7.14–7.17
Gastrointestinal infections
  bacterial, 7.9–7.14
  fungal, 7.23–7.25
  hepatitis, 2.31, 7.5–7.9
  in HIV infection, 1.25–1.27
  host defenses and, 7.10
  imaging of, 7.25–7.28
  infectious doses for, 7.11
  microbial virulence factors in, 7.10
  parasitic, 7.19–7.22
  viral, 7.17–7.19
Genital herpes, 2.13, 5.20–5.21
Genital warts, 5.17–5.18, 9.15
Gentamicin
  in *Bartonella* infections, 8.24
  in brain abscess, 3.10
  in pyelonephritis, 9.5
  in tuboovarian abscess, 9.21
Gerstmann-Strässler syndrome, 3.21–3.22
Giardiasis, 7.19
Gingiva
  hemorrhage of, in hemorrhagic fever, 8.28
  Kaposi's sarcoma of, in HIV infection, 1.22
Gingivitis, acute necrotizing ulcerative, 4.10
Gingivostomatitis, herpetic, 4.11
Globi, of acid-fast bacilli, in leprosy, 2.20
Gonococcal infections, 5.2–5.3
  endocervicitis, 9.16
  septic arthritis, 2.29
  skin and soft tissue, 2.29
Gram-negative infections
  peritonitis, 7.3
  pulmonary, 6.3–6.5
Gram-positive infections
  peritonitis, 7.3
  pulmonary, 6.2–6.3
Granulocyte-macrophage colony-stimulating factor
  in HIV infection, 1.12
  in lymphoma, 1.43
Granuloma
  in leprosy, 2.20
  of liver, in Q fever, 7.9
  in tuberculosis, 6.7
Growth failure, in HIV infection, 1.47
Guinea worm infections (dracunculiasis), 2.18
Gummas, in syphilis, 5.14

Haemophilus ducreyi infections (chancroid), 5.21–5.22
Haemophilus infections
  of bites, 2.9
  brain abscess, 3.10
Haemophilus influenzae infections
  epiglottitis, 4.14
  meningitis, 3.3
  orbital cellulitis, 4.2
  pneumonia, 6.5
Hair loss, in syphilis, 5.13
Hairy leukoplakia, in HIV infection, 1.16, 1.22–1.23
Hand
  hand, food, and mouth disease of, 2.14–2.15, 4.13
  osteomyelitis of, from human bites, 2.8
  scabies of, 5.19
Hansen's disease (leprosy), 2.19–2.22, 8.25–8.27
Hantavirus pulmonary syndrome, 6.14, 8.28–8.29
Head, infections of *see specific region*
Headache, in endocarditis, 3.18
Heart
  congenital disease of, brain abscess in, 3.10
  infections of *see* Endocarditis
Heartworm infections, 6.15
Helicobacter pylori infections, 7.14–7.17
Helminth eggs, relative sizes of, 7.21
Hemolysis
  in sepsis, 8.10
  of streptococcal culture, 2.5
  in syphilis, 5.16
Hemorrhage
  cerebral, in sepsis, 3.17
  conjunctival, in endocarditis, 8.7, 8.15
  gingival, in hemorrhagic fever, 8.28
  subarachnoid, in endocarditis, 3.18
  subconjunctival, in conjunctivitis, 3.19
Hepatitis, 7.5–7.9
  diagnostic algorithm for, 7.6
  fulminant, 7.7
  histology of, 7.7–7.9
Hepatitis A, 7.5–7.6
Hepatitis B, 7.5–7.8
Hepatitis C, 7.6, 7.8
  skin lesions in, 2.31
Hepatitis D, 7.6
Hepatitis E, 7.6
Herpes simplex virus infections
  cervicitis, 9.17
  encephalitis, 1.28, 3.5–3.7
  esophagitis, 7.25
  genital, 2.13, 5.20–5.21
  gingivostomatitis, 4.11
  in HIV infection
    chronic mucocutaneous, 1.37
    encephalitis, 1.28
    keratitis, 1.20
    proctitis, 1.26
    retinitis, 1.21
    stomatitis, 1.45
  keratitis, 1.20
  in pediatric patients, 8.4
  proctitis, 1.26
  retinitis, 1.21
  of skin and soft tissue, 2.13
  stomatitis, 1.45
  tracheobronchitis, 6.25
Herpes zoster, 2.14
Herpes zoster ophthalmicus, 3.19
  in HIV infection, 1.19
Heusner classification, of spinal epidural abscess, 3.13
Hip
  osteomyelitis of, 2.25
  septic arthritis of, 2.29
Histoplasmosis
  disseminated, 7.24
  in HIV infection, 1.35, 1.38
  of oral cavity, 2.12, 8.30
  pulmonary, 6.9
  tracheobronchitis in, 6.25
HIV infection *see* Human immunodeficiency virus infection
Hodgkin's disease, in HIV infection, treatment of, 1.44
Hospital (streptococcal) gangrene, 7.2
Human bites, infections of, 2.8–2.9
Human granulocytic ehrlichiosis, 8.19–8.21
Human immunodeficiency virus
  antibodies to, 1.10
  antiretroviral drugs effects on, 1.50
  evolution of, 1.5
  levels of, vs. disease course, 1.8
  life cycle of, 1.4
  replication of, 1.5
Human immunodeficiency virus infection, 1.2–1.58
  anogenital neoplasia in, 1.44
  aphthous ulcers in, 1.23
  apoptosis induced by, 1.11
  asymptomatic, 1.3, 1.9–1.10
  bacillary epithelioid angiomatosis in, 1.18
  bronchitis in, 6.24–6.25
  candidiasis in
    esophageal, 7.23
    oral, 1.22–1.23
    treatment of, 1.41
  cardiomyopathy in, 1.45
  central nervous system complications in, 3.7–3.9, 3.11
  cervical neoplasia in, 1.44
  classification of, 1.3, 1.12
  clinical features of, 1.13–1.14
    cutaneous, 1.15–1.19
    gastrointestinal, 1.25–1.27
    hematologic, 1.32–1.34
    metabolic, 1.30–1.32
    neurologic, 1.27–1.29
    ophthalmic, 1.19–1.21
    in opportunistic infections, 1.37–1.38
    oral cavity, 1.22–1.23
    pulmonary, 1.24–1.25
  coccidioidomycosis in, 6.10
  condyloma lata in, 1.44
  containment of, 1.10
  cryptococcosis in, 1.35, 3.4, 6.10
  cryptosporidiosis in, 1.26, 7.20
  Cyclospora infections in, 1.26, 1.36
  cytokine action in, 1.12

Human immunodeficiency virus infection (*continued*)
  cytomegalovirus infections in
    encephalitis, 1.28
    gastrointestinal, 1.26
    retinitis, 1.20, 1.37, 1.41
  diagnosis of, 1.6–1.8
  diarrhea in, 1.31, 7.14
  encephalitis in, 1.28
  Enterocytozoon infections in, 7.21
  epidemiology of, 1.2–1.3
    in women, 1.48–1.49
  Escherichia coli infections in, enteroaggregative, 1.27
  genotypic variation in, 1.5
  growth failure in, 1.47
  hairy leukoplakia in, 1.22
  hematologic manifestations of, 1.32–1.34
  herpes simplex virus infections in
    chronic mucocutaneous, 1.37
    keratitis, 1.20
    proctitis, 1.26
    skin, 2.13
    stomatitis, 1.45
  histoplasmosis in, 1.35, 1.38
    disseminated, 7.24
  Hodgkin's disease in, 1.44
  immune response in, 1.9–1.12
  Isospora infections in, 7.20
  Kaposi's sarcoma in, 1.18–1.19, 1.22
  latent period in, 1.3, 1.9–1.10
  leishmaniasis in, 1.36
  lymphoid interstitial pneumonitis in, 1.46
  lymphoma in
    brain, 1.29
    treatment of, 1.43
  malignancies in, 1.42–1.44
  microsporidiosis in, 1.26
  molluscum contagiosum in, 1.17, 1.19
  Mycobacterium avium complex infections in, 1.35, 1.42
  Mycobacterium kansasii infections in, 1.38
  natural history of, 1.3
    immune response in, 1.9–1.10
    variations in, 1.10
    vs. viral burden, 1.8
  neurologic disorders in, 1.46–1.47
  neurosyphilis in, 1.29
  nonprogressing, 1.10
  opportunistic infections in
    clinical features of, 1.37–1.38
    epidemiology of, 1.39
    microbiology of, 1.35–1.36
    prevention of, 1.39–1.42
    treatment of, 1.39–1.42
  oral cavity infections in, 1.45
  parotid gland enlargement in, 1.44
  in pediatric patients, 1.44–1.47
  perinatal transmission of, 1.47
    prevention of, 1.3
  periodontitis in, 1.23
  Pneumocystis carinii infections in
    disseminated, 1.38
    pneumonia, 1.24, 1.36, 1.39
  pneumonia in
    pneumococcal, 6.2
    Pneumocystis carinii, 1.24, 1.36, 1.39
  prevention of, 1.3–1.4
  primary, differential diagnosis of, 1.13
  Pseudomonas aeruginosa infections in, 1.20
  Reiter's syndrome in, 2.31
  retinitis in, cytomegalovirus, 1.37, 1.41
  salmonellosis in, 1.35
  scabies in, 1.17
  spectrum of, 1.12–1.14
  survival trends in, in women, 1.49
  syphilis in, 1.29, 5.12
    testing for, 5.10
  T lymphocyte count in, vs. clinical category, 1.3
  toxoplasmosis in, 1.36
    cerebral, 1.29
    chorioretinitis, 1.21
  transmission of, prevention of, 1.3–1.4
  treatment of
    drugs for, 1.51–1.55
    hematologic effects of, 1.34
    opportunistic infection manifestations, 1.39–1.42
    rationale for, 1.12, 1.50–1.52
    virologic response in, 1.9
  tuberculosis in, 1.25
  varicella-zoster virus infections in
    acute retinal necrosis syndrome in, 1.37
    disseminated, 1.38
    of ophthalmic nerve, 1.19
  viral dynamics in, 1.50–1.52
  virus characteristics in, 1.4–1.5
  wasting in, 1.30–1.32
  in women, 1.47–1.49
Human monocytic ehrlichiosis, 8.19–8.21
Human papillomavirus infections, 5.17–5.18, 9.15
  of respiratory system, 4.16
Hutchinson's sign, in herpes zoster ophthalmicus, 3.19
Hutchinson's teeth, in syphilis, 5.16
Hyaluronidase, in streptococcal infections, 8.12
Hydatid cysts
  of brain, 3.12
  of lung, 6.16, 6.24

Imaging, of gastrointestinal infections, 7.25–7.28
Imipenem-cilastin, in pyelonephritis, 9.5
Immune globulin, in varicella-zoster infections, 8.3
Immune response, in HIV infection, 1.9–1.12
Immunization, for varicella-zoster infections, 8.3
Immunodeficiency
  babesiosis in, 8.21
  candidiasis in, 7.23, 8.35
  diarrhea in, 7.12
  mucormycosis in, 7.24
  Mycobacterium haemophilum infections in, 8.35
  necrotizing otitis in, 4.8
  pneumonia in, in cancer, 6.18–6.20
  Pseudomonas aeruginosa infections in, 8.11, 8.35
  respiratory infections in, in transplantation, 6.21–6.22
  staphylococcal infections in, 8.34

strongyloidiasis in, 6.15, 8.36
trichosporosis in, 8.35
see also Human immunodeficiency virus infection
Immunoglobulins, patterns of, in HIV infection, 1.33
Impetigo
staphylococcal, 2.3, 8.13
streptococcal, 8.12
Indinavir, in HIV infection, 1.54–1.55
hematologic effects of, 1.34
"Infection stones," in kidney, 9.7
Infectious mononucleosis, 8.6
hepatitis in, 7.8
Inflammatory response, in sepsis, 8.9
Influenza, pneumonia in, 6.12–6.13
Insomnia, fatal familial, 3.21
Interferon-α, for Kaposi's sarcoma, in HIV infection, 1.43
Interferon(s), in HIV infection, 1.12
Interleukins
in HIV infection, 1.12
in sepsis, 8.9–8.10
Intra-abdominal infections, 7.2–7.5
Intrauterine device, infection in, 9.21
Isospora infections, in HIV infection, 7.20
Itching
in lichen simplex chronica, 9.14
in swimmer's itch, 2.10
Itchy red bump disease, in HIV infection, 1.16
Itraconazole, in candiduria, 9.11
Ixodes bites, Lyme disease from, 8.16–8.17

Jakob-Creutzfeldt disease, 3.21–3.22
Janeway lesions, in endocarditis, 8.7, 8.16
Job's syndrome, furuncles in, 2.3
Jock itch (tinea cruris), 2.11
Joint(s), infections of, 2.28–2.31

Kaposi's sarcoma, in HIV infection, 1.18–1.19
of oral cavity, 1.22
treatment of, 1.42–1.43
Kawasaki disease, 4.13, 8.13
Keratitis, in HIV infection
herpes simplex virus, 1.20
Pseudomonas aeruginosa, 1.20
Ketoconazole, in candiduria, 9.11
Kidney
abscess of, 7.28
infections of, 9.4–9.6
catheter-associated, 9.12
complicated, 9.6–9.7
stones of, in infection, 9.7
Klebsiella pneumoniae infections
pneumonia, 6.5
pyelonephritis, 9.5
Knee
septic arthritis of, 2.29
septic bursitis of, 2.30
Kuru, 3.21

Lacrimal system, infections of, 4.2
Lamivudine, in HIV infection, 1.53–1.55
hematologic effects of, 1.34
Langhans' giant cells
in leprosy, 2.19–2.20
in tuberculosis, 6.7
Laparoscopy, in pelvic inflammatory disease, 5.6
Larva migrans, cutaneous, 2.17
Laryngitis, 4.15
Larynx, papillomatosis of, 4.16
Lassa fever, 8.27–8.28
Legionella pneumophila pneumonia, 6.6, 6.12
in transplantation, 6.22
Leishmaniasis, 8.32–8.33
in HIV infection, 1.36
mucocutaneous, 2.17
Leonine facies, in leprosy, 2.22
Leopard skin, in onchocerciasis, 2.16
Lepra type-1 reaction, 2.20
Lepromatous leprosy, 2.19–2.21, 8.26–8.27
Lepromin skin test, 2.19
Leprosy (Hansen's disease), 2.19–2.22, 8.25–8.27
Leukocytes, fecal, in diarrhea evaluation, 7.12
Leukopenia, in ehrlichiosis, 8.21
Leukoplakia, hairy, in HIV infection, 1.16, 1.22–1.23
Lice, 2.15
Bartonella infections from, 8.22
pubic, 2.15, 5.18
Lichen simplex chronica, of vulva, 9.14
Lipopolysaccharides, systemic effects of, 8.9
Listeria monocytogenes infections, meningitis, 3.3
Lithiasis
kidney, in infection, 9.7
in Stensen's duct, 4.12
Liver
abscess of, 7.26
amebic, 6.15
candidiasis of, 7.23
viral hepatitis of, 7.5–7.9
Lone star tick, ehrlichiosis from, 8.20
Loxosceles reclusa (recluse spider) bites, 2.15
Ludwig's angina, 4.22
Lung infections
abscess, 6.11
in transplantation, 6.21–6.22
in HIV infection, 1.24–1.25
see also Pneumonia; Tuberculosis
Lyme disease, 8.16–8.19
vs. babesiosis, 8.21
erythema migrans in, 2.22
neurologic disorders in, 3.3–3.4
Lymphadenopathy
in *Bartonella* infections, 8.24
cervical, 4.17–4.18
in chlamydial infections, 5.4
Lymphocytes
in leprosy, 2.19–2.20
see also T lymphocytes
Lymphoid interstitial pneumonitis, in HIV infection, 1.46
Lymphoma
brain, in HIV infection, 1.29
central nervous system, 3.7–3.8
gastric, in *Helicobacter pylori* infections, 7.15, 7.17

Lymphoma (*continued*)
in HIV infection, 1.14, 1.19
treatment of, 1.43
of skin, in HIV infection, 1.19

M protein, as toxin, 8.12
Macrophage(s), differentiation of, in leprosy, 2.19
Macrophage colony-stimulating factor, in HIV infection, 1.12
Madura foot, 2.12
Malignant melanoma, of vulva, 9.16
Malignant (necrotizing) otitis, 4.8
Mastoiditis
brain abscess in, 3.10
sigmoid sinus thrombosis in, 3.15
Maxillary sinusitis, 4.8–4.9
Mechanical ventilation, necrotizing pneumonia in, 6.12
Medullary osteomyelitis, 2.25–2.27
Melanoma, of vulva, 9.16
Meningitis
bacterial, 3.2–3.3
chronic, 3.3–3.5
in endocarditis, 3.18
in sinusitis, 3.16
viral, 3.2
Meningococcal infections
sepsis, 8.11
septic arthritis, 2.29
skin and soft tissue, 2.29
Mesenteric artery embolism, in candidiasis, 7.23
Metabolic disorders, in HIV infection, 1.30–1.32
Metronidazole, in brain abscess, 3.10
Microsporidiosis, in HIV infection, 1.26, 7.14
Mink encephalopathy, 3.21
Mites, scab, 2.15
Molluscum contagiosum, 2.13, 5.19
in HIV infection, 1.17, 1.19
Mononucleosis, infectious, 8.6
hepatitis in, 7.8
Mosquito bites
encephalitis from, 3.5
myiasis from, 2.17
Mouth *see* Oral cavity
Mucopyocele, 3.16
Mucormycosis
disseminated, 7.24
pulmonary, 6.10
in cancer, 6.20
in transplantation, 6.21
rhinocerebral, 8.31
Mumps
encephalitis in, 3.5
parotitis in, 4.19
Murmurs, in endocarditis, 8.7
Mycetoma, 2.12
Mycobacterium avium complex infections
in HIV infection, 1.35
small intestinal, 1.25
treatment of, 1.42
lymphadenopathy in, 4.18
pulmonary, 6.8
Mycobacterium haemophilum infections, in immunodeficiency, 8.35
Mycobacterium kansasii infections, 6.8
in HIV infection, 1.38
Mycobacterium leprae infections (leprosy, Hansen's disease), 2.19–2.22, 8.25–8.27
Mycobacterium tuberculosis infections *see* Tuberculosis
Mycoplasma pneumoniae pneumonia, 6.6
Mycotic aneurysm, in endocarditis, 8.8
Myiasis, cutaneous, 2.17
Myoclonus, in Jakob-Creutzfeldt disease, 3.22
Myonecrosis, clostridial, 7.3
Myositis, 2.2
streptococcal, 2.6
Myringitis, bullous, 4.8

Nafcillin, in meningitis, 3.3
Nails
fungal infections of, in HIV infection, 1.15
paronychia of, 2.3
Natural killer cells, action of, in HIV infection, 1.11
Neck
deep infections of, 4.20–4.22
fascial layers of, 4.20–4.21
lymphadenopathy of, 4.17–4.18
Necrosis, of digits, in bacteremia, 8.11
Necrotizing fasciitis, 2.2
abdominal, 7.27
abdominal wall, 7.2
clostridial, 2.24
nonclostridial, 2.24
streptococcal, 2.6
Necrotizing otitis (malignant), 4.8
Necrotizing ulcerative gingivitis, acute, 4.10
Neisseria meningitidis infections
meningitis, 3.3
sepsis, 8.11
Nephrostomy tube, infections from, 9.12
Neurocysticercosis, 2.18, 3.11, 8.34
Neurologic disorders
in HIV infection, 1.27–1.29, 1.46–1.47
in leprosy, 2.19, 2.21, 8.25–8.27
in Lyme disease, 8.18–8.19
Neuroretinitis, in cat scratch disease, 4.17
Neurosyphilis, in HIV infection, 1.29
Neutropenia
candidiasis in, 7.23
pneumonia in, in cancer, 6.18–6.20
Nevirapine, in HIV infection, 1.52, 1.55
hematologic effects of, 1.34
Nits, 5.18
Nocardiosis
brain abscess in, 3.10
lymphadenopathy in, 4.18
mycetoma in, 2.12
pneumonia in, 6.7
Norwalk virus infections, enteritis, 7.17
Nosocomial infections
candiduria, 9.10–9.11
pneumonia, 6.3, 6.12
Nutrition, in HIV infection, 1.47

Onchocerciasis, 2.16
Onychomycosis, in HIV infection, 1.15
Opportunistic infections, in HIV infection
  clinical features of, 1.37–1.38
  epidemiology of, 1.39
  microbiology of, 1.35–1.36
  prevention of, 1.39–1.42
  treatment of, 1.39–1.42
Optic nerve, pressure on, in brain abscess, 3.20
Oral cavity
  Kaposi's sarcoma of, in HIV infection, 1.19
  ulceration of, in histoplasmosis, 7.24
Oral cavity infections, 4.10–4.12
  hand, food, and mouth disease, 2.14–2.15, 4.13
  histoplasmosis, 2.12, 8.30
  in HIV infection, 1.16, 1.22–1.23, 1.45
  Ludwig's angina, 4.22
  syphilis, 5.11, 5.14
Oral contraceptives, cervical ectopy in, 9.16
Oral rehydration solution, in diarrhea, 7.12
Orbital infections, 3.19–3.21, 4.2–4.4
  cellulitis, lymphadenopathy in, 4.17
Oroya fever, 8.22, 8.24
Osler's nodes, in endocarditis, 8.8, 8.16
Osteomyelitis
  classification of, 2.25–2.27
  of hand, from human bites, 2.8
  host factors in, 2.25
  in septic arthritis, 2.29
  of skull, 3.16
  treatment of, 2.27
Otitis, necrotizing (malignant), 4.8
Otitis externa, 4.6–4.8
Otitis media, 4.4–4.6
  brain abscess in, 3.10
Otomycosis, 4.7
Ova, helminth, relative sizes of, 7.21
Ovary, abscess of, 7.28, 9.20–9.21
Oxacillin
  in meningitis, 3.3
  in septic arthritis, 8.15

P24 antigen, in HIV infection, 1.8–1.9
Pain
  back, in spinal tuberculosis, 2.30
  pelviperineal, in prostadynia, 9.8
  in tuboovarian abscess, 9.20
Palate, Kaposi's sarcoma of, in HIV infection, 1.22
Papanicolaou smear, in trichomoniasis, 5.8
Papilledema, in brain abscess, 3.20
Papillomatosis, laryngeal, 4.16
Parainfluenza virus infections, pneumonia, 6.12
Paranasal sinusitis, 3.16, 4.8–4.10
  brain abscess in, 3.10
  venous sinus infections in, 3.15
Parapharyngeal abscess, 4.21
Parasitic diseases
  of central nervous system, 3.10–3.12
  ectoparasitic, of skin, 2.15–2.16, 5.18–5.19
  gastroenteritis, 7.19–7.22
  of Latin America, 8.32–8.34
  of respiratory system, 6.15–6.16
  of skin and soft tissue, 2.17–2.18
Paronychia, 2.3
Parotid gland enlargement, in HIV infection, 1.44
Parotitis, 4.19–4.20
  staphylococcal, 4.19, 8.14
Parrot fever (psittacosis), 6.6
Parvovirus B19 infections, rash in, 8.2
Pasteurella multocida infections, of animal bites, 2.8–2.9
Pastia's lines, in scarlet fever, 4.13
Pediatric patients
  congenital syphilis in, 5.15–5.16
  HIV infection in, 1.44–1.47
    transmission to, 1.3–1.4, 1.47
  Lyme disease in, treatment of, 3.4
  rotavirus infections in, 7.17–7.18
  viral exanthems in, 8.2–8.6
Peliosis, bacillary, 8.22–8.24
Pelvic infections, in female, 9.14–9.21
  cervicitis *see* Cervicitis
  pelvic inflammatory disease, 5.6, 7.28
  septic abortion, 9.18–9.20
  tuboovarian abscess, 9.20–9.21
  vulvar, 9.14–9.16
Pelvic inflammatory disease, 5.6, 7.28
Pelviperineal pain, in prostadynia, 9.8
Penicillin(s)
  in *Bartonella* infections, 8.22
  in bite infections, 2.9
  in brain abscess, 3.10
Penicillin G
  in deep neck abscess, 4.21
  in Lyme disease, 3.4, 8.19
  in meningitis, 3.2–3.3
Penis
  candidiasis of, 5.9
  chancres on, 5.11
  chancroid of, 5.21
  herpes simplex virus infections of, 5.20–5.21
  molluscum contagiosum of, 5.19
  scabies of, 5.19
  warts of, 5.17
Pentamidine, in *Pneumocystis carinii* pneumonia, 1.39
  prophylactic, 1.24
Peptic ulcer disease, *Helicobacter pylori* in, 7.14–7.17
Peptostreptococcus infections, appendicitis, 7.4
Periadenitis mucosa necrotica recurrens (Sutton's disease), 4.12
Periappendiceal abscess, 7.27
Periodontal abscess, 4.10
Periodontitis, in HIV infection, 1.23
Peripheral neuropathy, in HIV infection, 1.28
Peritoneal dialysis, peritonitis in, 7.3
Peritonitis, in peritoneal dialysis, 7.3
Petechiae
  in hepatitis C, 2.31
  in toxic shock syndrome, 8.13
Petriellidium infections, mycetoma, 2.12
Phagocytosis defects, pneumonia in, in cancer, 6.19–6.20
Pharyngitis, viral, 8.14
Pharyngotonsillitis, 4.12–4.14
Pinworms, 7.22
Piroplasma infections, newly identified, 8.22

Pityrosporon folliculitis, 2.11
Pleural effusion, 6.16–6.18
Pneumococcal infections, pneumonia, 6.2
Pneumocystis carinii infections
  in HIV infection
    disseminated, 1.38
    pneumonia, 1.24
    prophylaxis of, 1.40
    treatment of, 1.39
  in transplantation, 6.21–6.22
Pneumonia
  atypical, 6.6–6.7
  in cancer, 6.18–6.20
  Chlamydia psittaci, 6.6
  gram-negative, 6.3–6.5
  gram-positive, 6.2–6.3
  Haemophilus influenzae, 6.5
  Klebsiella pneumoniae, 6.5
  Legionella pneumophila, 6.6
  Mycoplasma pneumoniae, 6.6
  necrotizing, 6.12
  Nocardia, 6.7
  nosocomial, 6.3, 6.12
  pleural effusion in, 6.16–6.18
  pneumococcal, 6.2
  Pneumocystis carinii, in HIV infection, 1.24, 1.36, 1.39
  Pseudomonas aeruginosa, 6.5
  staphylococcal, 6.3
  streptococcal, 6.2
  in transplantation, 6.21–6.22
  viral, 6.12–6.14
Pneumonitis, lymphoid interstitial, in HIV infection, 1.46
Pneumothorax, 6.18
Polyarthritis, in HIV infection, 1.14
Polymerase chain reaction
  in HIV infection, 1.8
  in leprosy diagnosis, 8.27
Polymicrobial infections
  of animal bites, 2.7
  of skin and soft tissue, 2.24
Polyneuropathy, in HIV infection, 1.28
Potassium hydroxide test, in fungal infections, 2.10
Pott's disease, 4.18
Pott's puffy tumor, 4.9
Prednisone, in *Pneumocystis carinii* pneumonia, 1.40
Pregnancy
  HIV transmission in, 1.47
  pyelonephritis in, 9.7
  septic abortion in, 9.18–9.20
Prepatellar bursitis, cellulitis with, 2.30
Preseptal cellulitis, 3.19, 4.3
Prion diseases, 3.21–3.22
Probenecid, in Lyme disease, 3.4
Proctitis, in HIV infection, 1.26
Progressive multifocal leukoencephalopathy, in HIV infection, 3.7
Prostadynia, 9.8
Prostatitis, 9.8–9.10
Proteases, in streptococcal infections, 8.12
Proteus mirabilis infections, pyelonephritis, 9.5
Prurigo nodularis, of vulva, 9.14
Pruritic papular dermatoses of HIV disease, 1.16
Pseudomembranous colitis, imaging of, 7.26
Pseudomonas aeruginosa infections
  appendicitis, 7.3
  bacteremia, 8.11
  meningitis, 3.3
  osteomyelitis, 2.27
  pneumonia, 6.5, 6.19
  pyelonephritis, 9.5, 9.7
  sclerokeratitis, in HIV infection, 1.20
  skin and soft tissue, in immunodeficiency, 8.35
Pseudoparalysis, in syphilis, 5.16
Psittacosis, 6.6
Psoriasis, in HIV infection, 1.15
Psychiatric disorders, in endocarditis, 3.18
Pubic lice, 2.15, 5.18
Pulmonary edema, in hantavirus pulmonary syndrome, 8.29
Pulmonary embolism, in sepsis, 8.10
Pulmonary infections *see* Lung infections; Pneumonia; Tuberculosis
Pyelonephritis, 9.4–9.6
  complicated, 9.6–9.7
  fungal, 9.11
Pyosalpinx, 9.20–9.21
Pyuria, in prostatitis, 9.9

Q fever, 6.6
  liver pathology in, 7.9
Quinolones
  in bite infections, 2.9
  in cystitis, 9.3
  in traveler's diarrhea, 7.13

Rabbit fever, pulmonary manifestations of, 6.23
Rapid urease tests, in *Helicobacter pylori* infections, 7.16
Rash
  in erythema infectiosum, 8.2
  in gonococcal infections, 5.3
  in hand, food, and mouth disease, 4.13
  in hepatitis C, 2.31
  in infectious mononucleosis, 8.6
  in scarlet fever, 4.13
  in staphylococcal infections, 8.15
  in strongyloidiasis, in immunodeficiency, 8.36
  swimmer's itch, 2.10
  in syphilis, 5.12—5.14
  in toxic shock syndrome, 8.13
Reactive arthritis, 2.31
Recluse spider bites, 2.15
Rehydration, oral solutions for, 7.12
Reiter's syndrome, 2.31
Respiratory infections, 4.14—4.16
  brain abscess in, 3.10
  bronchiolitis, 6.25
  bronchitis, 6.24—6.25
  dacryoadenitis in, 4.2
  fungal, 6.9—6.10
  in HIV infection, 1.24—1.25
  orbital infections in, 4.2—4.4
  parasitic, 6.15—6.16
  in transplantation, 6.21—6.22
  see also Lung infections; Pneumonia; Tuberculosis

Respiratory syncytial virus infections, pneumonia, 6.12, 6.14
Respiratory system, extrapulmonary infection manifestations in, 6.23—6.24
Retinitis
- in cat scratch disease, 4.17
- cytomegalovirus, 3.21
  - in HIV infection, 1.20, 1.37, 1.41
- herpetic, 1.21
- in HIV infection
  - cytomegalovirus, 1.20, 1.37, 1.41
  - herpetic, 1.21
  - *Pneumocystis carinii*, 1.38
  - toxoplasmic, 1.21
  - varicella-zoster virus, 1.37
- *Pneumocystis carinii*, 1.38
- toxoplasmic, 1.21
- varicella-zoster virus, 1.37

Retinochoroiditis, in toxoplasmosis, 3.20
Retinopathy, in hemorrhagic fever, 8.28
Retonavir, in HIV infection, hematologic effects of, 1.34
Retropharyngeal abscess, 4.22, 8.14
Reye's syndrome, liver pathology in, 7.8
Rheumatic fever, 4.13
Rhinocerebral mucormycosis, 8.31
Rhinovirus infections, pneumonia, 6.12
Rhizopus infections, gastrointestinal, 7.24
Ridley-Jopling classification, of leprosy, 2.19
Rifabutin, in *Mycobacterium avium* complex infections, in HIV infection, 1.42
Rift Valley fever, 8.28
Rimantadine, in influenza, 6.13
Ringworm, of body (tinea corporis), 2.11
Ritonavir, in HIV infection, 1.52, 1.54–1.55
River blindness (onchocerciasis), 2.16
Rocky Mountain spotted fever, pulmonary manifestations of, 6.23
Romaña's sign, in Chagas' disease, 2.17, 3.11
Rotavirus enteritis, 7.17–7.18
Roth spots, in endocarditis, 8.8

Salmonellosis, in HIV infection, 1.35
Sandfly, *Bartonella* infections from, 8.22
Saquinavir, in HIV infection, 1.55
- hematologic effects of, 1.34

Sarcoma, Kaposi's, in HIV infection, 1.18–1.19, 1.42–1.43
- of oral cavity, 1.22

Scabies, 2.15, 5.19
- in HIV infection, 1.17

Scalded skin syndrome, staphylococcal, 2.4
Scarlet fever, 4.12–4.13, 4.17, 8.13, 8.15
Schistosomiasis
- hepatosplenic, 2.18
- pulmonary, 6.16

Sclerokeratitis, *Pseudomonas aeruginosa*, in HIV infection, 1.20
Scrapie, 3.21
Scrofula, 4.18
Scrotum, Fournier's gangrene of, 2.24
Seizures, in endocarditis, 3.18
Sepsis, 8.9–8.11
- central nervous system manifestations of, 3.17–3.18
- in streptococcal infections, 8.12

Septic abortion, 9.18–9.20
Septic arthritis, 2.28–2.29
- staphylococcal, 8.15

Septic bursitis, 2.30
Septic thrombosis, of venous sinuses, 3.14–3.15
Serratia marcescens infections, pyelonephritis, 9.5
Sexually transmitted diseases, 5.2–5.22
- bacterial vaginosis, 5.4–5.5
- candidiasis, 5.9–5.10, 9.15
- chancroid, 5.21–5.22
- chlamydial infections, 5.3—5.4
- ectoparasitic, 2.15, 5.18–5.19
- gonococcal *see* Gonococcal infections
- herpes simplex virus infections, 2.13, 5.20–5.21
- human immunodeficiency virus infection *see* Human immunodeficiency virus infection
- human papillomavirus infections, 5.17–5.18, 9.15
- molluscum contagiosum, 2.13, 5.19
- pelvic inflammatory disease, 5.5
- syphilis *see* Syphilis
- trichomoniasis, 5.7–5.8, 9.15

Shigellosis, 7.12
Shingles (herpes zoster), 2.14
- in HIV infection, 1.19, 1.38
- ophthalmic nerve involvement in, 3.19
  - in HIV infection, 1.19

Shock
- septic, 8.9
- in streptococcal infections, 8.12

Sickle cell disease, septic arthritis in, 2.29
Sigmoid venous sinus infections, 3.14–3.15
Sinusitis, 3.16, 4.8–4.10
- brain abscess in, 3.10
- venous sinus infections in, 3.15–3.16

Skin, systemic infection manifestations in
- babesiosis, 8.19–8.22
- bacteremia, 8.9–8.11
- *Bartonella* infections, 8.22–8.24
- ehrlichiosis, 8.19–8.21
- fungal infections, 8.29–8.31
- HIV infection, 1.14–1.19
- in immunodeficiency, 8.34–8.36
- infective endocarditis, 8.6–8.9
- leprosy, 8.25–8.27
- Lyme disease, 8.16–8.19
- parasitic diseases, 8.32–8.34
- sepsis, 8.9–8.11
- *Staphylococcus aureus* infections, 8.14–8.16
- streptococcal infections, 8.12–8.14
- viral exanthems, 8.2–8.6
- viral hemorrhagic fevers, 8.27–8.29

Skin and soft-tissue infections
- anatomic considerations in, 2.2
- in animal bites, 2.7–2.9
- from animal contact, 2.9–2.10
- bullous, 2.2
- chancroid, 5.21–5.22
- clostridial, 2.23–2.24
- crusted lesions in, 2.2
- ectoparasitic, 2.15–2.16, 5.18–5.19
- external ear, 4.6–4.8
- folliculitis, 2.2
- fungal, 2.10–2.12, 8.29–8.31
- gonococcal, 5.3
- in immunodeficiency, 8.34–8.36
- leprosy, 2.19–2.22, 8.25–8.27

Skin and soft-tissue infections (*continued*)
  molluscum contagiosum, 2.13, 5.19
  myositis, 2.2
  parasitic, 2.17–2.18, 8.32–8.33
  spirochetal, 2.22
  staphylococcal, 2.3–2.5
  streptococcal, 2.5–2.7
  syphilis, 5.11–5.14
  ulcerated, 2.2
  vesicular, 2.2
  viral, 2.12–2.15, 8.2–8.6
  vulvar, 5.9–5.10, 9.14–9.16
Skin test, lepromin, 2.19
Skull, osteomyelitis of, 3.16
"Slapped cheek" appearance, in erythema infectiosum, 8.2
Sleeping sickness, 3.10
Small intestine, *Mycobacterium avium* complex infections of, 1.25
Soft-tissue infections *see* Skin and soft-tissue infections
South American trypanosomiasis (Chagas' disease)
  esophageal dilatation in, 8.33
  soft-tissue manifestations of, 2.17
Spider bites, 2.15
Spinal cord dysfunction, in endocarditis, 3.18
Spine
  epidural abscess of, 3.13
  tuberculosis of, 2.30, 4.18
Spirochetal infections, of skin and soft tissue, 2.22
Spleen
  abscess of, in endocarditis, 8.8
  candidiasis of, 7.23
Spongiform encephalopathy, 3.21
Sporotrichosis, 2.9, 8.30
Staphylococcal infections
  appendicitis, 7.3
  catheter-associated, 6.3
  impetigo, 8.13
  meningitis, 3.3
  peritonitis, 7.3
  of skin and soft tissue, 2.3–2.5, 4.17
Staphylococcus aureus infections
  abdominal, 7.2
  of bites, 2.7, 2.9
  brain abscess, 3.10
  cellulitis, 2.4, 3.19
  ecthyma, 2.3
  endocarditis, 8.6–8.8
  external manifestations of, 8.14–8.16
  furuncles, 2.3
  impetigo, 2.3
  meningitis, 3.3
  osteomyelitis, 2.26
  paronychia, 2.3
  parotitis, 4.19
  pneumonia, 6.3
    in transplantation, 6.21
  preseptal cellulitis, 3.19
  sepsis, 8.10
  septic arthritis, 2.28–2.29
  of skin and soft tissue, 8.14–8.15
    in immunodeficiency, 8.34
  in skin and soft-tissue trauma, 2.4
Staphylococcus epidermidis endocarditis, 8.7
Staphylococcus intermedius infections, of animal bites, 2.7, 2.9
Stavudine, in HIV infection, 1.55
  hematologic effects of, 1.34
Stevens-Johnson syndrome, 4.14
Stomatitis
  aphthous, 4.12
  herpes simplex virus, in HIV infection, 1.45
Stones
  kidney, in infection, 9.7
  in Stensen's duct, 4.19
Strawberry tongue
  in scarlet fever, 4.12
  in streptococcal infections, 8.13
Streptococcal infections
  abdominal wall, 7.2
  appendicitis, 7.3
  brain abscess, 3.10
  endocarditis, 8.7
  external manifestations of, 8.12–8.14
  group A, 8.12–8.13
  orbital cellulitis, 4.2
  peritonitis, 7.3
  pharyngotonsillitis, 4.12
  Reiter's syndrome in, 2.31
  scarlet fever, 4.12–4.13
  of skin and soft tissue, 2.5–2.7, 8.12–8.14
  toxic shock syndrome, 6.2
Streptococcus agalactiae meningitis, 3.3
Streptococcus pneumoniae infections
  meningitis, 3.3
  pneumonia, 6.2
Streptococcus pyogenes infections, 2.5
  abdominal, 7.2
  cellulitis, 2.4
  ecthyma, 2.3
  Gram stain in, 2.5
  of human bites, 2.8
  impetigo, 2.3
Streptococcus sanguis infections, of oral cavity, 4.12
Streptolysins, in streptococcal infections, 8.12
Stroke
  in endocarditis, 3.18
  in sepsis, 3.17
Strongyloidiasis, 7.22
  disseminated, 6.15
    in cancer, 6.20
    in transplantation, 6.22
  in immunodeficiency, 8.36
Subarachnoid hemorrhage, in endocarditis, 3.18
Subconjunctival hemorrhage, in conjunctivitis, 3.19
Subdural empyema, 3.12–3.13
Sublingual space, abscess of, 4.22
Subperiosteal abscess
  frontal bone, 4.9
  orbital, 4.3–4.4
Sutton's disease, 4.12
Swimmer's ear, 4.6
Swimmer's itch, 2.10
Synovial fluid analysis, in septic arthritis, 2.29
Syphilis, 5.10–5.16
  congenital, 5.15–5.16
  epidemiology of, 5.10
  gastrointestinal, 7.25
  in HIV infection, 1.29

laboratory tests for, 5.10
late, 5.14–5.15
primary, 5.10–5.11
secondary, 5.12–5.14
Systemic infections, external manifestations of
babesiosis, 8.19–8.22
bacteremia, 8.9–8.11
Bartonella infections, 8.22–8.24
ehrlichiosis, 8.19–8.21
fungal infections, 8.29–8.31
in immunodeficiency, 8.34–8.36
infective endocarditis, 8.6–8.9
leprosy, 8.25–8.27
Lyme disease, 8.16–8.19
parasitic diseases, 8.32–8.34
sepsis, 8.9–8.11
Staphylococcus aureus infections, 8.14–8.16
streptococcal infections, 8.12–8.14
viral exanthems, 8.2–8.6
viral hemorrhagic fevers, 8.27–8.29

T lymphocytes
CD4+, HIV infection of, 1.4–1.5
depletion of, 1.3, 1.8–1.12, 1.50
defects of, pneumonia in, in cancer, 6.19–6.20
Taenia saginata infections, 7.22
Taenia solium infections
of brain, 2.18, 3.11, 8.34
of skin and soft tissue, 2.18
Tapeworms, 7.22
Teeth, Hutchinson's, in syphilis, 5.16
Tenosynovitis
in gonococcal infections, 2.29, 5.2
in meningococcal infections, 2.29
Tetracycline
in *Bartonella* infections, 8.22, 8.24
in bite infections, 2.9
Thalidomide, in erythema nodosum leprosum, 2.20
Thrombocytopenia
in ehrlichiosis, 8.21
in HIV infection, 1.32
Thrombosis, septic, of venous sinuses, 3.14–3.15
Thrush, 4.11
Thyroiditis, 4.20
Tibia, osteomyelitis of, 2.26–2.27
Ticarcillin-clavulanate, in pyelonephritis, 9.5
Tick bites
ehrlichiosis from, 8.19–8.20
encephalitis from, 3.5
Lyme disease from, 8.16–8.17
Tinea corporis, 2.11
Tinea cruris, 2.11
Tinea versicolor, 2.10
Toes, necrosis of, in bacteremia, 8.11
Tongue
hairy leukoplakia of, in HIV infection, 1.22
histoplasmosis of, 2.12
strawberry
in scarlet fever, 4.12
in streptococcal infections, 8.13
syphilis manifestations in, 5.14
Tonsillitis, 4.12–4.14
Toxic encephalopathy, 3.18
Toxic epidermal necrolysis, 2.4
Toxic shock syndrome
staphylococcal, 2.5, 8.15
streptococcal, 2.7, 6.2, 8.13
Toxins, in streptococcal infections, 8.12
Toxoplasmosis
cerebral, 1.29, 3.7, 3.9, 3.11
chorioretinal, 1.21, 3.20
in HIV infection, 1.21, 1.29, 1.36
Trachea, papillomatosis of, 4.16
Tracheitis, 4.16
Tracheobronchitis, 6.24
Tracheoesophageal puncture, cellulitis in, 4.22
Transforming growth factors, in HIV infection, 1.12
Transplantation, respiratory infections in, 6.21–6.22
Trauma
brain abscess in, 3.10
skin and soft-tissue infections in, 2.4
clostridial, 2.23
streptococcal, 4.2
Traveler's diarrhea, 7.12–7.13
Trench fever, 8.22, 8.24
Trench mouth, 4.10
Treponema pallidum infections *see* Syphilis
Trichomoniasis, 5.7–5.8, 9.15
Trichosporosis, in immunodeficiency, 8.35
Trimethoprim-sulfamethoxazole
in brain abscess, 3.10
in cystitis, 9.3
in *Pneumocystis carinii* pneumonia, 1.39
in pyelonephritis, 9.5
in traveler's diarrhea, 7.13
Tropical regions, food safety in, 7.13
Trypanosoma cruzi infections (Chagas' disease), 3.11
esophageal dilatation in, 8.33
soft-tissue manifestations of, 2.17
Trypanosomiasis
African (sleeping sickness), 3.10
South American (Chagas' disease), 3.11
esophageal dilatation in, 8.33
soft-tissue manifestations of, 2.17
Tuberculoid leprosy, 2.19, 8.25
Tuberculosis
meningitis in, 3.4
miliary, in HIV infection, 1.25
pulmonary, 6.7–6.8
in cancer, 6.19
empyema in, 6.17
scrofula in, 4.18
of spine, 2.30
of urinary tract, 9.6
Tuboovarian abscess, 9.20–9.21
imaging of, 7.28
Tularemia, pulmonary manifestations of, 6.23
Tumor(s), Pott's puffy, 4.9
Tumor necrosis factors
in HIV infection, 1.12
in sepsis, 8.9–8.10
Tympanic membrane
disorders of, 4.3–4.4, 4.8
normal, 4.3

Tympanosclerosis, 4.6
Tzanck stain, in herpes simplex virus infection, 2.14

Ulceration
- aphthous, in HIV infection, 1.23
- corneal, 3.20
  - in HIV infection, 1.20
- ecthyma, 2.3
- gastric, *Helicobacter pylori* in, 7.14–7.17
- in herpes simplex virus infections, 2.13, 4.11, 5.20–5.21
- in HIV infection, 1.12
- in leprosy, 2.20
- oral cavity
  - in aphthous stomatitis, 4.12
  - in herpes simplex virus infections, 4.11
  - in histoplasmosis, 2.12, 7.24
- skin, 2.2
- in syphilis, 5.11–5.12
- in trench mouth, 4.10

Urease tests, in *Helicobacter pylori* infections, 7.16
Ureter, stent in, infections from, 9.12
Urethritis
- chlamydial, 5.4
- gonococcal, 5.2–5.3
- in Reiter's syndrome, 2.31

Urinary frequency, in cystitis, 9.2
Urinary tract infections, 9.2–9.14
- candiduria, 9.10–9.11
- catheter-associated, 9.12–9.14
- complicated, 9.3, 9.6–9.7
  - pyelonephritis, 9.4, 9.6
- cystitis, 9.2–9.3
- prostate, 9.8–9.10
- pyelonephritis, 9.4–9.6
- recurrent, cystitis, 9.3
- uncomplicated
  - cystitis, 9.3
  - pyelonephritis, 9.4–9.5

Urination, disorders of, in cystitis, 9.2
Urine
- bacteria in
  - catheter-associated, 9.13
  - in pregnancy, 9.7
- *Candida* in, 9.10–9.11
- pus in, in prostatitis, 9.9

UTIs *see* Urinary tract infections
Uvulitis, 4.12

Vagina, chancre of, in syphilis, 5.12
Vaginitis, 9.15
- candidal, 5.9–5.10

Vaginosis, bacterial, 5.4–5.5, 9.15
Vancomycin
- in brain abscess, 3.10
- in meningitis, 3.3

Varicella-zoster virus infections, 2.14, 8.3
- in HIV infection
  - acute retinal necrosis syndrome in, 1.37
  - disseminated, 1.38
- pneumonia, 6.14

Vasculitis
- in hepatitis C, 2.31
- in HIV infection, 1.14

Venereal warts, 9.15
Venous sinus infections, 3.14–3.16
Verruga peruana, 8.22, 8.24
Vesicles, infections with, 2.2
Vibrio cholerae infections, 7.10
Vincent's infection, of oral cavity, 4.10
Violin-string adhesions, in pelvic inflammatory disease, 5.6
Viral infections
- of central nervous system, 3.5–3.8
- enteritis, 7.17–7.19
- exanthems in, 8.2–8.6
- hemorrhagic fever, 8.27–8.29
- hepatitis, 7.5–7.9
  - diagnostic algorithm for, 7.6
  - histology of, 7.7–7.9
- pharyngitis, 8.14
- pneumonia, 6.12–6.14
  - in transplantation, 6.21
- of skin and soft tissue, 2.13–2.15
- *see also specific infections*

Viridans streptococcal infections, endocarditis, 8.7
Vulva
- chancroid of, 5.22
- herpes simplex virus infections of, 5.20
- infections of, 5.9–5.10, 9.14–9.16

Warts, genital, 5.17–5.18, 9.15
Wasting, in HIV infection, 1.30–1.32
Weight loss, in HIV infection, 1.30–1.32
Western blot test, for HIV infection, 1.7–1.8
Wrist, septic arthritis of, 2.28
Wuchereria bancrofti infections, 2.16

Xanthogranulomatous pyelonephritis, 9.7

Zalcitibine, in HIV infection, 1.53, 1.55
- hematologic effects of, 1.34

Zidovudine
- in HIV infection, 1.51–1.55
  - hematologic effects of, 1.34
- prophylactic, in pregnancy, 1.47

Zoster, 2.14
- in HIV infection, 1.19, 1.38
- ophthalmic nerve involvement in, 3.19